Noninvasive Electrocardiology

Clinical Aspects of Holter Monitoring

Frontiers in Cardiology

Series Advisors:

MICHEL BERTRAND
JOHN CAMM
DESMOND JULIAN
NORMAN KAPLAN
ULRICH SIGWART

Published

Management of Acute Myocardial Infarction
Edited by Desmond Julian and Eugene Braunwald

Molecular Interventions and Local Drug Delivery
Edited by Elazer R. Edelman

Forthcoming

Endoluminal Stenting
Edited by Ulrich Sigwart

Noninvasive Electrocardiology

Clinical Aspects of Holter Monitoring

Edited by

Arthur J. Moss

Professor of Medicine and Director of the Heart Research
Follow-up Program, University of Rochester Medical Center,
Rochester, NY, USA

and

Shlomo Stern

Professor of Medicine, Hebrew University,
and Director of the Department of Cardiology,
Bikur Cholim Hospital, Jerusalem, Israel

W. B. Saunders Company Ltd
London • Philadelphia • Toronto • Sydney • Tokyo

W. B. Saunders Company Ltd 24–28 Oval Road
London NW1 7DX, UK

The Curtis Center
Independence Square West
Philadelphia, PA 19106-3399, USA

Harcourt Brace & Company
55 Horner Avenue
Toronto, Ontario M8Z 4X6, Canada

Harcourt Brace & Company, Australia
30–52 Smidmore Street
Marrickville, NSW 2204, Australia

Harcourt Brace & Company, Japan
Ichibancho Central Building, 22-1 Ichibancho
Chiyoda-ku, Tokyo 102, Japan

A catalogue record for this book is available from the British Library

ISBN 0-7020-1925-9

Typeset by Paston Press Ltd, Loddon, Norfolk
Printed in Great Britain by The University Press, Cambridge

Contents

Contributors

Fabio Badilini
Hôpital Lariboisiere, Paris, France

S. Serge Barold
Department of Cardiology, Genessee Hospital, Rochester, New York, USA

Antonio Bayés de Luna
Department of Cardiology and Cardiac Surgery, Hospital de la Santa Creu i Sant Pau, Universitat Autònoma de Barcelona, Barcelona, Spain

Antoni Bayés Genís
Department of Cardiology and Cardiac Surgery, Hospital de la Santa Creu i Sant Pau, Universitat Autònoma de Barcelona, Barcelona, Spain

Jesaia Benhorin
Heiden Department of Cardiology, Bikur Cholim Hospital, Jerusalem, Israel

Anna M. Bianchi
Department of Biomedical Engineering, Polytechnic University, Milan, Italy

Lee A. Biblo
Department of Medicine, Division of Cardiology, Case Western Reserve University/University Hospitals of Cleveland, Cleveland, Ohio, USA

J. Thomas Bigger Jr
Division of Cardiology, Department of Medicine, Columbia University, New York, USA

Martin Borggrefe
Westfälische Wilhelms-Universität, Medizinische Klinik und Poliklinik, Münster, Germany

Matthew S. Bosner
Department of Medicine, The Jewish Hospital of St Louis, Washington University School of Medicine, St Louis, Missouri, USA

Günter Breithardt
Westfälische Wilhelms-Universität, Medizinische Klinik und Poliklinik, Münster, Germany

A. John Camm
Department of Cardiological Sciences, St George's Hospital Medical School, London, England

Didier Catuli
Hôpital Lariboisiere, Paris, France

Sergio Cerutti
Department of Biomedical Engineering, Polytechnic University, Milan, Italy

Richard J. Cohen
Harvard–MIT Center for Biomedical Engineering, Massachusetts Institute of Technology, Cambridge, Massachusetts, USA

Peter F. Cohn
Department of Medicine, Division of Cardiology, State University of NY Health Sciences Center, Stony Brook, New York, USA

J. Ph. Couderc
Hôpital Cardiologique, Lyon, France

Philippe Coumel
Hôpital Lariboisiere, Paris, France

Prakash C. Deedwania
Cardiology Division, Department of Medicine, VAMC/UCSF Medical Education Program, Fresno, California, USA

Lucia Dumaresq
Department of Cardiology and Cardiac Surgery, Hospital de la Santa Creu i Sant Pau, Universitat Autònoma de Barcelona, Barcelona, Spain

Frederick A. Ehlert
Division of Cardiology, Department of Medicine, St Luke's–Roosevelt Hospital Center, New York, NY, USA

Nabil El-Sherif
Cardiology Division, State University of NY Health Sciences Center, Brooklyn, New York, USA

Jocelyne Fayn
Hôpital Cardiologique, Lyon, France

Lü Fei
Department of Cardiological Sciences, St George's Hospital Medical School, London, England

Thomas Fetsch
Westfälische Wilhelms-Universität, Medizinische Klinik und Poliklinik, Münster, Germany

Jeffrey J. Goldberger
Division of Cardiology, Department of Medicine, Northwestern University, Chicago, Illinois, USA

Josep Guindo
Department of Cardiology and Cardiac Surgery, Hospital de la Santa Creu i Sant Pau, Universitat Autònoma de Barcelona, Barcelona, Spain

W. Jackson Hall
Department of Biostatistics, University of Rochester, New York, USA

Martin Höher
University Hospital of Ulm, Ulm, Germany

Vinzenz Hombach
University Hospital of Ulm, Ulm, Germany

Eduard Homs
Department of Cardiology and Cardiac Surgery, Hospital de la Santa Creu i Sant Pau, Universitat Autònoma de Barcelona, Barcelona, Spain

Alan H. Kadish
Division of Cardiology, Department of Medicine, Northwestern University, Chicago, Illinois, USA

Harold L. Kennedy
Rush–Presbyterian–St Luke's Medical Center, Chicago, Illinois, USA

Robert E. Kleiger
Cardiology Division, The Jewish Hospital of St Louis, Missouri, USA

Mathias Kochs
University Hospital of Ulm, Ulm, Germany

Emanuela H. Locati
Instituto di Clinica Medica Generale e Terapia Medica, University of Milan, Milan, Italy

Federico Lombardi
Ospedale L. Sacco, University of Milan, Milan, Italy

Luca T. Mainardi
Department of Biomedical Engineering, Polytechnic University, Milan, Italy

Pierre Maison Blanche
Hôpital Lariboisiere, Paris, France

Markku Mäkijärvi
Westfälische Wilhelms-Universität, Medizinische Klinik und Poliklinik, Münster, Germany

Marek Malik
Department of Cardiological Sciences, St George's Hospital Medical School, London, England

Frank I. Marcus
Cardiology Section, University of Arizona Health Sciences Center, Tucson, Arizona, USA

Vicenç Martí
Department of Cardiology and Cardiac Surgery, Hospital de la Santa Creu i Sant Pau, Universitat Autònoma de Barcelona, Barcelona, Spain

Antoni Martinez-Rubio
Westfälische Wilhelms-Universität, Medizinische Klinik und Poliklinik, Münster, Germany

Mario Merri
Formerly with the Department of Electrical Engineering, University of Rochester, Rochester, New York, USA

D. Morlet
Hôpital Cardiologique, Lyon, France

Arthur J. Moss
Department of Medicine, University of Rochester School of Medicine and Dentistry, Rochester, New York, USA

David Mulcahy
Cardiology Branch, National Institutes of Health, Bethesda, Maryland, USA

Thomas J. Mullen
Medical Engineering and Medical Physics Program, Harvard–MIT Division of Health Sciences and Technology, MIT, Cambridge, Massachusetts, USA

James E. Muller
Deaconess Hospital, Boston, Massachusetts, USA

Bruce D. Nearing
Institute for the Prevention of Cardiovascular Disease, New England Deaconess Hospital, Harvard Medical School, Boston, Massachusetts, USA

Hans-Heinrich Osterhues
University Hospital of Ulm, Ulm, Germany

F. Peyrin
LTSU/CREATIS, CNRS URA 1216, Villeurbanne, France

Silvia G. Priori
Istituto di Clinica Medica Generale e Terapia Medica, University of Milan, Milan, Italy

Arshed A. Quyyumi
Cardiology Branch, National Institutes of Health, Bethesda, Maryland, USA

Lutz Reinhardt
Westfälische Wilhelms-Universität, Medizinische Klinik und Poliklinik, Münster, Germany

Marc Roelke
Cardiac Unit, Massachusetts General Hospital, Boston, Massachusetts, USA

Paul Rubel
Hôpital Cardiologique, Lyon, France

Jeremy N. Ruskin
Cardiac Unit, Massachusetts General Hospital, Boston, Massachusetts, USA

Peter J. Schwartz
Institute of Cardiology, University of Pavia, Pavia, Italy

J. Sobral
Department of Cardiology and Cardiac Surgery, Hospital de la Santa Creu i Sant Pau, Universitat Autònoma de Barcelona, Barcelona, Spain

Jonathan S. Steinberg
Division of Cardiology, Department of Medicine, St Luke's–Roosevelt Hospital Center, New York, NY, USA

Shlomo Stern
Department of Cardiology, Bikur Cholim Hospital, Jerusalem, Israel

Edward L. Titlebaum
Department of Electrical Engineering, University of Rochester, Rochester, New York, USA

Geoffrey H. Tofler
Institute for the Prevention of Cardiovascular Disease, Deaconess Hospital, Boston, Massachusetts, USA

P. Touboul
Hôpital Cardiologique, Lyon, France

Richard L. Verrier
Institute for the Prevention of Cardiovascular Disease, Deaconess Hospital, Harvard Medical School, Boston, Massachusetts, USA

Xavier Viñolas
Department of Cardiology and Cardiovascular Surgery, Hospital de la Santa Creu i Sant Pau, Universitat Autònoma de Barcelona, Barcelona, Spain

Albert L. Waldo
Department of Medicine, Division of Cardiology, Case Western Reserve University/University Hospitals of Cleveland, Cleveland, Ohio, USA

Takashi Yanaga
Department of Bioclimatology and Medicine, Medical Institute of Bioregulation, Kyushu University, Oita, Japan

Wojciech Zareba
Department of Medicine, University of Rochester Medical Center, New York, USA

Prologue

Shlomo Stern

The science of noninvasive electrocardiology has its roots with Einthoven and other pioneers of electrocardiology in the late 19th and early 20th centuries. Subsequently, this new science matured through numerous theoretical, laboratory and clinical contributions made by physiologists, electrophysiologists, clinicians and other investigators during the first five to six decades of this century. The contribution of Norman J. Holter to the science of electrocardiology in the late 1950s opened a totally new channel in this development, as it permitted recording of the ECG signal under dynamic conditions and for extended periods. This advance heralded a new era in our understanding of what we can learn by studying the dynamic aspects of P-QRS-T waves.

Holter's words in 1962, based on the experience he accumulated by using his system in Montana, seem to have been prophetic. In his publication in *Science*, he envisioned the use of long and continuous ECG records for the study of 'the outside influences [which] disturb the steadiness seen in the isolated heart', to conduct 'new pharmacological research', to explore the 'pulse microstructure', to better comprehend the nature of 'changes [which] might occur during the normal active day of a clinically normal individual', and to achieve a better understanding of 'the correlation of heart activity with eating, exercise, sexual and other emotional activities, fatigue, sleep and so on'.

The detection of evanescent arrhythmias, establishing the frequency of disturbances of heart rate and rhythm in normal individuals, the study of spontaneous variability of rhythm and rate in diseased states, the prognostic significance of postinfarction ventricular arrhythmias, as well as the proarrhythmic effects of certain antiarrhythmic drugs – all these occupied the interest of investigators during the 1960s and early 1970s. Subsequently, ST segment variation during daily activities was studied and our current understanding of 'silent ischemia' has emerged. Concurrently, exercise electrocardiology, also scrutinizing mainly the ST segment of the surface ECG, developed further and provided important new clinical information.

In the late 1980s and early 1990s, a quantum leap took place in the noninvasive study of the electrocardiographic signal. Careful assessment of the continuous 24-hour recording opened new channels of information centering on circadian variations; not only were ischemic episodes, silent or painful, shown to have a definite circadian rhythm, but also the 'ischemic threshold', the QT interval and other ECG parameters were documented to vary rhythmically during a 24-hour period. The circadian variations in the appearance of acute ischemic events helped elucidate much about the mechanism of sudden cardiac death. During the 1980s, Holter-like devices became part also of implanted defibrillators.

New techniques involving digitization of the analog Holter data and later direct digital acquisition from the patient have permitted more sophisticated investigations of the electrocardiologic signal: high-resolution electrophysiological recordings from Holter tapes, not only of the QRS complex but also of the P wave, opened the door for the signal-averaging technique and the study of late potentials. The impact of the knowledge derived from these data on risk stratification of postinfarction patients, or those suffering from other ischemic conditions with or without overt ventricular arrhythmias, is considerable. Another emerging new area of study, heart rate variability, was also facilitated and extended by long-term recordings of the electrocardiogram. It is now clear not only that variations in heart rate occur secondarily to physical and mental stress and to many other external influences, but also that these variations are under parasympathetic and sympathetic influences throughout the day and the night. Bioengineering analysis of heart rate variability in both the time and frequency domains have enhanced our knowledge of the autonomic control of the cardiovascular system in health and disease.

QT dispersion, nonvisible T-wave alternans, new quantification of the ST segment, spectrocardiagrams, and various other investigations during the 1990s opened a treasure chest full of new, intriguing and relevant information about the electrical activity of the heart. The electrocardiogram has stood the test of time, and the surface electrocardiographic signal, after nearly a century of use, continues to sprout new information.

The editors of this book and its publisher are fortunate to have many pioneers and innovators of these exciting new developments as authors of the various chapters in this book. This is the first collection in print of the newest information derived from the surface electrocardiogram, some based on recently published articles and others printed for the first time. The reader is offered not only the electrophysiological background of the data but also the technology involved, the methodologic developments, and the applications in day-to-day clinical practice. The rich quality of electrocardiologic information derived noninvasively should enhance the clinical and research use of the methods described to improve patient care and to expand our scientific understanding of the electrical activity of the heart.

SECTION I

Technical Considerations

Introduction by Federico Lombardi

In 1957, Norman J. Holter introduced a radiotelemetry system for recording the ECG signal during ambulatory activity. His cumbersome equipment was soon replaced by an analog, tape-based recorder and a complicated analysis system. Subsequent technical advances have miniaturized the recorder and vastly improved the analytic system so that it is now, for the most part, semiautomatic with minimal requirement for technician interaction. High-frequency (200–1000 Hz) digital recorders with large hard-disk capacity (above 100 Mbyte) are becoming available. Such recording systems permit three-channel, 24-hour ECG data acquisition with minimal or no data compression. This new generation of recorders permits downloading of the acquired data into personal computers with software that permits automatic evaluation of an enormous amount of information contained within the ECG signal.

The technical requirements for the recorder, the signal processing, and the analysis need to be viewed in terms of the clinical applications for which the system is intended. Holter monitoring was initially used to detect rhythm disturbances, principally the frequency and complexity of ventricular ectopic activity. The ventricular ectopics are generally of large amplitude with high-frequency content, and various templates have been used to identify such beats reliably. More recently, there has developed an increased interest in the detection and classification of atrial ectopic beats and rhythms. This will be a challenge because the atrial signal is of low amplitude and frequency, and the signal-to-noise ratio is such that sophisticated signal processing will be required to properly identify various atrial arrhythmias.

Non-arrhythmic features of ambulatory ECG monitoring that appear particularly suitable for automatic computer analysis include QRS width, amplitude, and frequency content, RR intervals, and ST and T waves changes. With the availability of three-channel digital recorders with frequency capability in the 1000 Hz range, it should be possible to obtain high-resolution analysis of the QRS complex to identify the presence or absence of late potentials; i.e. a signal-averaged ECG by Holter. QRS detection and RR interval histograms are available on all current Holter recorders. Software for time and frequency analysis of the RR time series is commercially available, but the power spectral analysis processing techniques for quantification of heart rate variability in the frequency domain have not yet been standardized. Sophisticated signal processing is required since artifact and ectopic beats can introduce serious errors. Automatic analysis of ST segment displacement is a difficult problem because the very-low-frequency components of the

ST signal may be difficult to separate from low-frequency baseline drift. The baseline fluctuations need to be removed from the digitized tracing without compromising the important components of the baseline position and the ST segment itself. Quantification of the various components of the T wave can now be done reliably with sampling frequencies of 250 Hz, but higher frequencies may be required when investigating such phenomena as T-wave alternans.

The two chapters of this section provide detailed descriptions of the currently available recorder and analytic systems and of the fundamental bioengineering principles underlying the science of signal processing. Although the latter is highly technical, it provides a succinct and useful summary of the critical features required for the proper extraction of a clean ECG signal – an essential first step in the analysis of electrocardiologic data from Holter monitoring.

1

Holter Recorders and Analytic Systems

Harold L. Kennedy

Introduction

Ambulatory (Holter) electrocardiography is a widely used noninvasive test to evaluate electrocardiographic abnormalities of patients in a variety of cardiac disease states. The clinical utility of the ambulatory ECG recording lies in its ability to examine a patient over an extended period of time, permitting patient ambulatory activity and facilitating the diurnal electrocardiographic examination of a patient in a changing environment (both physical and psychological). In contrast to the standard ECG, which provides a wide-scoped fixed picture of 12 leads portraying cardiac electrical events over a brief (<30 seconds) duration, the 24-hour ambulatory ECG (in general) provides a more narrow view of two or three leads of electrocardiographic data, but has the strength of recording changing dynamic cardiac electrical phenomena that often are transient and of brief duration. The recording is a record of past events that permits detailed analysis of dynamic and transient electrocardiographic changes, although technology exists that permits online continuous monitoring.[1]

In the past it has been readily apparent that 12-lead ECG instruments were neither small enough nor durable enough to permit ambulatory measurements, but that viewpoint must now be questioned in view of the technological advances of the 1990s. There are now available ambulatory recording instruments which either derive[2] or directly record[3] 12-lead electrocardiograms continuously. However, such instruments have not gained widespread clinical popularity in the workplace, possibly for the following reasons:

1. It is not readily apparent what great advantage they offer over a state-of-the-art 3-channel ambulatory ECG.
2. Intuitively it would seem that 12-lead data are likely to be more difficult to obtain in a truly ambulatory state (if not simply recording resting prolonged ambulatory ECG data), because of the need for continuous placement of multiple electrode leads subject to muscle and motion artifacts.
3. Most importantly, the variety of data provided by present-day 3-channel recorders (ST segment changes, signal-averaged ECG, QT or QRS interval measurements, and heart rate variability) has not been fully explored or completely understood for its clinical value, and such investigations are ongoing.

Early ambulatory ECGs using single-channel data in the 1960s focused attention entirely on cardiac arrhythmias. Later, 2-channel ambulatory ECGs refined this interest

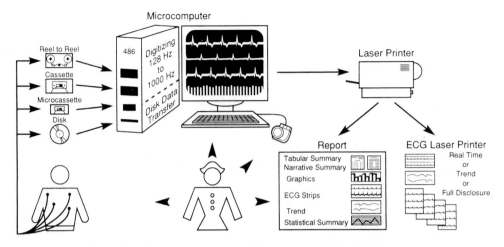

Figure 1.1   Schematic of conventional ambulatory (Holter) ECG system.

in cardiac arrhythmias and added ST segment observations in the 1970s and 80s. Subsequently, the emergence of 3-channel ambulatory ECGs in the late 1980s, coupled with other technological advancements (microcomputers, software analysis algorithms, and digital storage), spawned electrocardiographic analysis advancement to examine RR interval changes (for heart rate variability), QRS complex measurements (for specific intervals, such as QT, QTc, QTm), and the high-resolution signal-averaged ECG (for electrophysiological myocardial substrate abnormality, such as late potentials).[4–7]

These diverse scientific parameters available from the current 3-channel ambulatory ECG offer enormous insights into the genesis, mechanism of action, or sustained presence of specific cardiac arrhythmias and other electrophysiologic abnormalities, and may require another decade or more of scientific investigation to explore. Thus it is not surprising that 3-channel Holter recorders are currently preferred for ambulatory ECG.

Complicating this complex picture is the emergence of cellular facsimile, and digital or optical fiber transmission of data by computer information systems that are readily adaptable to currently available ambulatory ECG systems. It would appear that, for the time being at least, both clinically and in the laboratory, 3-channel ambulatory ECG will constitute the mainstay of ambulatory (Holter) ECG technology.

Ambulatory ECG Technology

Ambulatory ECG recorders may be divided into those that use magnetic-tape recording systems and those that use electronic storage systems. Both types utilize the same analytic systems (Figure 1.1).

Recorders

The conventional 3-channel Holter recorder is a small, lightweight (11 oz or 312 g), battery-operated electromagnetic tape-recorder that records, from bipolar leads, three channels of electrocardiographic data on cassette or microcassette magnetic tape (Figure 1.2). The recorder contains a patient-activated event button, a quartz digital clock, a built-in calibrator (1 mV, 60 bpm, 100 ms rectangular pulse, automatically activated for 6 minutes when energized), and is powered by a 9-volt disposable alkaline battery.

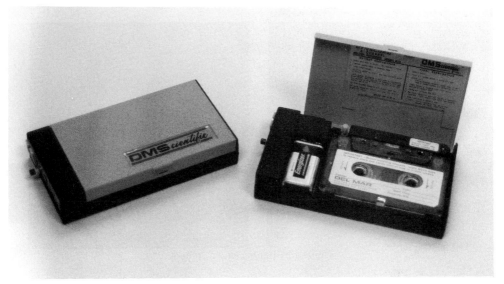

Figure 1.2 Ambulatory (Holter) ECG recorder.

Reel-to-reel recorders were quite reliable and were often used, but the necessity for accurate timing and the avoidance of phase shifts for accurate ST segment changes led to the popularity of cassette recorders with quartz timing.[8] It was questionable, still, whether a tape-recorded signal could accurately reproduce the frequencies needed for reliable signal-averaged ECG data.[9] Nevertheless, comparison studies showed that tape-based ambulatory ECG systems did reliably reproduce the high-resolution ECG, with some limitations.[7,9]

More recently, 3-channel 24-hour cassette-tape recorders have been improved to contain a timing track channel (32 Hz) with phase-locked motor accuracy for extremely precise timing (1 mm/s). This permits reliable recording of RR intervals for accurate heart rate variability data.[10] In the author's experience, this requirement is absolutely necessary to ensure the accuracy of heart rate variability measurements, and it has been recommended by an authoritative Task Force on Heart Rate Variability.[12]

These evolutionary developments have kept cassette-tape Holter recorders in the mainstream of the marketplace as the most cost-effective method for recording the ambulatory ECG, with an average price per unit of $1000–1500.

Nevertheless, the 1980s and 90s have seen the evolution of solid-state electronic storage technology that has been applied to Holter recorders. These solid-state recorders started out as real-time analysis devices,[1] and evolved to solid-state storage recorders capable of 11–15 Mbyte storage. They could produce ambulatory ECG data as a full-disclosure printout or download the data to an analytic system.[12]

More recent developments of digital technology have led to the ambulatory ECG disk recorder (Figure 1.3). The disk allows 80–200 Mbytes of storage, a vast increase. As a result, manufacturers have improved standard ECG measurements of the ST segment by digital recording, and have also given more precision and enhanced dimensions (in terms of signal-sampling capability) to measurements of heart rate variability and signal-averaging. Thus, employing disk technology, ECG measurements can be made at 1000 Hz (therefore recording 500 Hz) for brief periods, to examine the signal-averaged ECG; whereas at other times the ambulatory ECG examination can be programmed to record at 200 Hz for standard arrhythmia and ST segment measurements. This digital

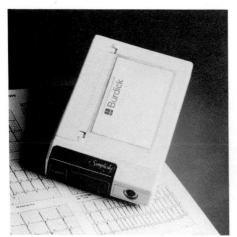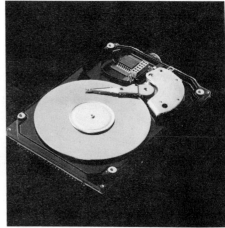

Figure 1.3 Burdick disk recorder.

accuracy and recording assures the user of more precise interval measurements, providing reliable time and frequency domain data.

Obviously, such technology comes at an increased price, which currently is at two to three times the cost of a conventional 3-channel ambulatory ECG tape-recorder.

Analytic Systems

Perhaps the greatest change in ambulatory electrocardiography during the past decade has resulted from the emergence of the personal computer. In the mid-1980s there was a necessity for specialized computers utilizing operator interaction and specifically designed components for arrhythmia detection, ST segment change detection, RR interval measurements and signal-averaging. Now these functions are all performed by software operating on a personal computer, so the need for specially designed computers has, in the author's opinion, been obviated.

A standard PC (usually with an AT486 microprocessor, 33, 50 or 66 MHz), a super-VGA high-resolution graphics video monitor, and a high-quality laser printer, are now state-of-the-art (Figure 1.4). Such a system is practical and cost-effective, and maintenance and repair services are readily available. This worldwide availability of the personal computer, and the ease of updating software (often by telephone modem), has facilitated the expansion of ambulatory electrocardiography to many countries and locations in which it could not previously be maintained.

Such systems provide the time-tested ambulatory ECG modalities of audio-visual superimposition, the RR arrhythmiagraph, full-disclosure paging, template matching, and operator interaction to provide accurate analysis of Holter recorded data. Features of color-coded ECG abnormalities, zoom capability, electronic calipers, multiple ECG size and time presentations, and various 'window' screens, are all enhancements now added by current commercial personal computers to the process of ambulatory ECG analysis. Audio systems, an ever-increasing option on personal computers, can be used to prompt or identify specific ECG phenomena during operator interaction.

In addition, local area networks (LANs), batch processing, and megabyte or gigabyte storage, have all been adapted to ambulatory ECG analysis systems. Faster and more

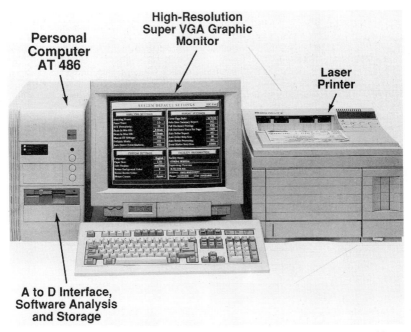

Figure 1.4   Commercially available personal computer, super-VGA graphics screen, and laser printer.

powerful microprocessor chips have, however, resulted in more costly Holter models, and the majority of ambulatory ECG users may recognize no major technical advantages to justify the additional cost. The author suspects that cost-effective technology enhancements of the commercial PC will be the driving force of new ambulatory ECG analysis systems.

Conclusions

As we enter the last half of the 1990s, ambulatory ECG Holter recorders and analysis systems are keeping pace with the electronic developments of the technology marketplace. We can anticipate in the future that multimedia CD–ROM disks will provide educational and storage features to analytic systems. Distant satellite locations could easily transmit their digital data over the Internet for either interpretation or reporting; but this would not seem practicable for the day-to-day examinations of patient care. Thus, the rapid pace of technological development currently in progress may not supersede the cost-effective Holter recorders and analytic systems presently being used. For workers in the field, this is a welcome economic respite.

References

1. Kennedy HL, Wiens RD. Ambulatory (Holter) electrocardiography using real-time analysis. *Am J Cardiol* 1987; **59**: 1190–5.
2. Drew BJ, Koops RR, Adams MG, Dower GE. Derived 12-lead ECG. Comparison with the standard ECG during myocardial ischemia and its potential application for continuous ST segment monitoring. *J Electrocardiol* 1994; **27**(Suppl): 249–55.
3. Mortara instrument. H-12 Recorder Milwaukee, WI.

4. Yanaga T, Maruyama T, Kumanomido A, Adachi M, Noguchi S, Taguch J. Usefulness of automatic measurement of GT interval using Holter tape in patients with hyperthyroidism. *J Amb Monitor* 1993; **6**: 27–34.

5. Laguna P, Caminal P, Jane R, Thakor NV, Bayesdeluna A, Marti V. Automatic QT interval analysis in post-myocardial infarction patients. *J Amb Monit* 1991; **4**: 93–111.

6. Coumel P, Fayn J, Maison-Blanche P, Rubel P. Clinical relevance of assessing QT dynamicity in Holter recordings. *J Electrocardiol* 1994; **27**(Suppl): 62–6.

7. Kennedy HL, Bavishi NS, Buckingham TA. Ambulatory (Holter) electrocardiography signal-averaging: a current perspective. *Am Heart J* 1992; **124**: 1339–46.

8. Taylor DI, Vincent R. Artefactual ST segment abnormalities due to electrocardiograph design. *Br Heart J* 1985; **54**: 121–8.

9. Berbari EJ, Rajagopalan CV, Lander P, Lazzara R. Changes in late potential measurements as a function of decreasing bandwidth. *J Cardiovasc Electrophysiol* 1991; **2**: 503–8.

10. DM Scientific. Model 423 Dynacord Holter recorder. Del Mar Avionics, Irvine, CA.

11. Task Force of the European Society of Cardiology and The North American Society of Pacing and Electrophysiology. Heart rate variability: standards of measurement, physiological interpretation, and clinical use. *Europ Heart J* (in press).

12. Kennedy HL. Role of Holter monitoring for arrhythmia (bradyarrhythmia and tachycarrhythmia) assessment and management. In: Podrid PJ, Kowery PR (eds), *Cardiac Arrhythmia*. Baltimore: Williams & Wilkins, 1995: 219.

2

Signal Processing

Anna M. Bianchi, Luca T. Mainardi and Sergio Cerutti

Digital signal processing techniques have had a tremendous impact on the interpretation of cardiovascular signals, with particular emphasis on the ECG. Relevant physiological data and clinical information are enhanced through the proper application of algorithms, more or less sophisticated. In this chapter, the main approaches in the area of digital signal processing are reviewed, including the traditional analog to digital (A/D) and pre-processing procedures, digital filtering of signals, synchronized averaging, baseline shift recognition and correction, and filtering and time-variant parameter estimation. A few applications are discussed regarding wave recognition and classification, data compression, frequency-domain analysis and the time–frequency approach. All these methods constitute an important background for the processing of cardiovascular signals, thus improving the phase of parameter extraction for advanced procedures in cardiological diagnosis, patient monitoring and control of therapy.

Signal Acquisition

Analog signals are usually converted into digital form for processing by computerized techniques. However, discrete representations of continuous data present problems because digital signals are discretized both in time (sampling) and amplitude (quantization) after A/D conversion.

Figure 2.1 shows the effect of sampling and quantization on an original analog signal. The signal is first represented by a discrete time series and this series of numbers is converted to a numerical form by forcing the values of each sample to one of a predefined set of values. Obviously, the numerical conversion, by affecting the characteristics of the input analog signal, can modify or distort the information contained in it. In order to obtain a reliable digital representation of analog measurements, a few simple principles need to be followed. In the following section we discuss basic concepts of sampling theory and describe errors involved with digital conversion.

Sampling

Biological magnitudes that change continuously in nature are usually observed at discrete time instants. For example, the body temperature is typically measured two or three times a day. It is plain that when measurements are more frequent, the sample series better reproduces the original. A correct choice of the observation rate is crucial in order to be sure that all the relevant information about the dynamics of the signal is still

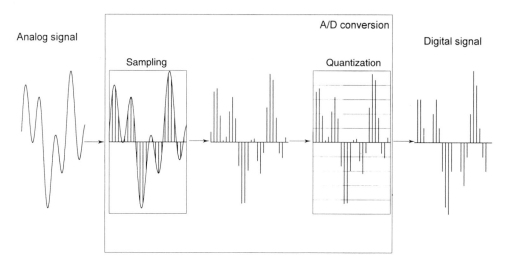

Figure 2.1 Block diagram of the A/D conversion procedure. The analog input signal is sampled and quantized in order to produce the output digital signal.

contained in these observations: a low sampling rate may fail to capture faster changes in the signal, while too high a rate may provide redundancy, with problems during data processing and storage.

From a theoretical point of view, Shannon's theorem[1] defines the minimum value of sampling rate (f_s) for band-limited signals (i.e. signals with frequency content up to a maximum frequency f_b). The theorem ensures that sampling with at least twice the original signal bandwidth ($f_s \geq 2 f_b$) safeguards the frequency content of the analog signal and allows perfect reconstruction of the original signal from its sampled values by proper interpolation techniques.

In fact, the sampled signal $x_s(t)$ can be obtained by multiplying the original continuous signal $x(t)$ with an impulse train $i(t)$:

$$x_s(t) = x(t) \cdot i(t) = x(t) \sum_{k=-\infty,+\infty} \delta(t - kT_s) = \sum_{k=-\infty,+\infty} x(t)\delta(t - kT_s) \qquad (2.1)$$

where $\delta(t)$ is the delta (Dirac) function, k is an integer and T_s is the sampling interval. Taking into account that multiplication in the time-domain implies convolution in the frequency-domain, we obtain:

$$X_s(f) = X(f)^*I(f) = \frac{1}{T_s} \sum_{f=-\infty,+\infty} X(f - kf_s) \qquad (2.2)$$

where $X(f)$ and $I(f)$ are the Fourier transforms of $x(t)$ and $i(t)$ respectively, and $f_s = 1/T_s$ is the sampling frequency.

The Fourier transform of the sampled signal, $X_s(f)$ in Figure 2.2(b), consists of identical repeats of $X(f)$ centered around multiples of the sampling frequency. Such repeats partially overlap each other when $f_s < 2f_b$; frequencies placed above $f_s/2$ are folded back, summing up to the lower frequencies. This phenomenon is known as *frequency aliasing* and when it occurs the original information cannot be recovered. Otherwise, when $f_s > 2f_b$, the original signal waveform can be retrieved by lowpass filtering of the sampled signal as presented in Figure 2.2(c).[2] Such observations are the basis of the sampling theorem previously noted.

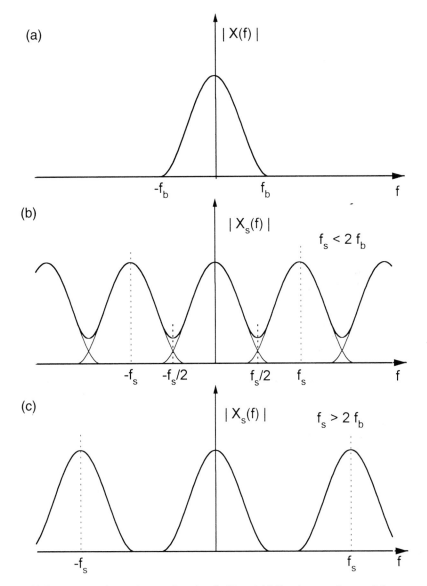

Figure 2.2 (a) Fourier transform of an analog signal. (b) and (c) Fourier transforms of the same signal after sampling (see text for an explanation).

Quantization

The second block in Figure 2.1 represents the quantization process: continuous signal amplitudes are converted into a set of predefined values. Binary representation of real numbers provides a finite set of values: N bits of code give 2^N different numbers. Each digital sample differs from the original one by a quantity, named *quantization error*, which depends on the selected coding procedure.

Errors due to quantization can be treated as noise $e(n)$ added to the signal $y(n)$ and its effect on the measured quantities can be described statistically. If we assume that quantization error follows a uniform distribution between two quantization levels (Δ is the interval between the two levels, i.e. the value of the least significant bit (LSB)), then the probability distribution $p(e)$ of $e(t)$ will be:

$$p(e) = \begin{cases} 1/\Delta & -\Delta/2 < e < \Delta/2 \\ 0 & \text{otherwise} \end{cases} \tag{2.3}$$

if we decide to round the $x(t)$ values to the nearest quantization level (rounding), or

$$p(e) = \begin{cases} 1/\Delta & -\Delta < e < 0 \\ 0 & \text{otherwise} \end{cases} \tag{2.4}$$

if the values of $x(t)$ are truncated to the lower quantization level (truncation).

First and second momentum properties of $e(n)$ can be computed. In particular, the mean value of $e(n)$, m_e, is zero and $-\Delta/2$ in the two cases, respectively. The variance is the same for the two distributions; that is:

$$\sigma_e^2 = \int_{-\infty}^{\infty} (e - m_e)^2 p(e) de = \frac{1}{\Delta} \int_{-\Delta/2}^{\Delta/2} e^2 de = \frac{\Delta^2}{12} \tag{2.5}$$

depending only on the value of the quantization interval.

Finally, it is possible to evaluate the signal-to-noise ratio (SNR) for the quantization process:

$$\text{SNR} = 10 \log_{10} \left(\frac{\sigma_x^2}{\sigma_e^2} \right) = 10 \log_{10} \left(\frac{\sigma_x^2}{2^{-2N}/12} \right) = 6.02N + 10.79 + 10 \log_{10}(\sigma_x^2), \tag{2.6}$$

having set $\Delta = 2^{-2N}$ and where σ_x^2 is the variance of the signal and N is the number of bits used for coding. It should be noted that the SNR increases by almost 6 dB for each added bit of coding. Several forms of quantization are usually employed: uniform, non-uniform (preceding the uniform sampler with a nonlinear block) or roughly (small number of quantization levels and high quantization step). Details can be found in references 3–5.

From a practical point of view, the choice of the proper sampling rate and the value of Δ may be adapted to the characteristics of the signal and to the particular measurements that should be extracted from it. As an example, in electrocardiography, different bandwidths are usually considered for different applications. For diagnostic applications, minimum sampling rate is suggested at 500 Hz,[6] implying a bandwidth up to 200 Hz (the lower frequency cutoff has to be maintained at 0.05 Hz). In 24-hour Holter tapes a bandwidth of 0.05–100 Hz is generally accepted[7] in order to properly detect ST displacements, arrhythmias and morphology changes in the main waves. The upper band limit is extended up to 500 Hz in order to detect ventricular late potentials[8] or fetal ECG, and reduced bandwidth (up to 50/70 Hz) may be accepted for monitoring patients in intensive care units. Similar considerations apply in defining standards for the choice of quantization levels. Generally, a 12-bit quantization is used. In order to correctly describe low-amplitude signals, like cardiac late potentials, the value of Δ (in μV) should be specified, and Δ is usually set lower than $1 \mu V$; it can be higher for more traditional clinical ECG acquisition.

Digital Filtering

A digital filter is a system which transforms a digital input $x(n)$ into a digital output series $y(n)$ in an attempt to enhance or depress some desirable or undesirable characteristics of $x(n)$. Schematically, a digital filter is usually represented by the block diagram shown in Figure 2.3, where $T[\ ]$ is the transformation that defines the input/output relationship of the filter.

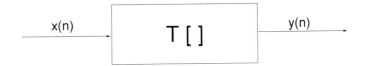

Figure 2.3 Block diagram of a digital filter.

For linear time-invariant filters, $T[\ ]$ can be expressed by the following differential equation:

$$y(n) = \sum_{m=0}^{M} b_m x(n-m) - \sum_{k=1}^{N} a_k y(n-k) \tag{2.7}$$

where the current output $y(n)$ depends on linear combination of both input $\{x(n),$ $x(n-1), \ldots, x(n-M)\}$ and output $\{y(n-1), y(n-2), \ldots, y(n-N)\}$ values. If all the a_k values are zero, the filter is said to be implemented in a *non-recursive form*; otherwise the filter is said to be implemented in *recursive form*.

A common way of investigating the characteristics of a filter is by observing its response (output) to different input testing signals. Among the various inputs, the impulse function $\delta(n)$ and sinusoidal signals at different frequencies are most useful in defining the properties of linear time-invariant filters.

The filter's *impulse response* to $\delta(n)$ can be used to determine the filter output to any input sequence. In fact, a generic input $x(n)$ can be seen as a sum of weighted and delayed impulses:

$$x(n) = \sum_{k=-\infty}^{+\infty} x(k)\delta(n-k). \tag{2.8}$$

Let us assume that $h(n)$ is the impulse response of a generic filter. By the time-invariant properties of the filter, each impulse $\delta(n-k)$ will produce the same response $h(n-k)$ but shifted in time. By linearity, all these responses will sum at the output, thus producing:

$$y(n) = \sum_{k=-\infty}^{+\infty} x(k)h(n-k) = \sum_{k=-\infty}^{+\infty} h(k)x(n-k). \tag{2.9}$$

Therefore, the response $y(n)$ to any input $x(n)$ is obtained by convolution of $x(n)$ and the impulse response of the filter. The impulse response describes the input/output relationship of the filter and it characterizes the filter behavior. According to the structure of $h(n)$, filters are classified as Finite Impulse Response (FIR) or Infinite Impulse Response (IIR). For FIR filters $h(n)$ is composed of a finite number of non-zero values, while for IIR filters $h(n)$ oscillates up to infinity with nonzero values. It is clearly evident that, in order to obtain an infinite response to an impulse in input, the IIR filter must contain a feedback which sustains the output as the input vanishes.

Another way to characterize a filter is to look at its response to sinusoidal inputs at different frequencies. Let us consider the complex sinusoid $x(n) = \exp(j\omega n T_s)$ and let us compute the filter response to this input. We have:

$$y(n) = \sum_{k=0,\infty} h(k)\exp(j\omega T_s(n-k)) = \exp(j\omega n T_s) \sum_{k=0,\infty} h(k)\exp(j\omega k T_s) = x(n) \cdot H(\omega). \tag{2.10}$$

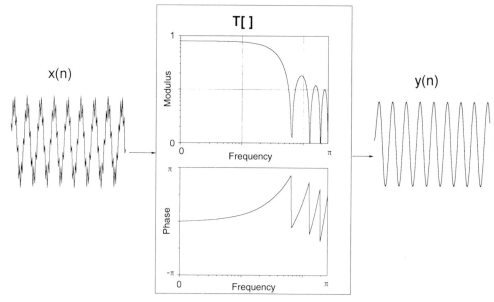

Figure 2.4   The transfer function of a digital filter can be described in terms of modulus and phase diagrams.

Thus the input sinusoid appears at the filter output as the same sinusoid but multiplied by a quantity $H(\omega)$, called the *frequency response* of the filter. $H(\omega)$ is a complex function which defines the response of the filter for each sinusoid of ω pulse frequency in the input. As a complex function, $H(\omega)$ will be defined by its modulus $|H(\omega)|$ and its phase $\angle H(\omega)$ as shown in Figure 2.4 for a moving-average filter of order 5. Figure 2.4 shows the effects of such a filter on an input signal: the higher frequencies in the signal are suppressed by this filter. Filters are usually classified as lowpass, highpass, bandpass and bandstop, according to their frequency response.

Characterization of a digital filter through its impulse or frequency responses allows one to completely describe the filter properties. Nevertheless, analysis and design of digital filters are greatly simplified by the use of the z-transform.[9] Applying the z-transform to equation (2.7) we obtain:

$$H(z) = \frac{\sum_{m=0,M} b_m z^{-m}}{1 + \sum_{k=1,N} a_k z^{-k}} \tag{2.11}$$

where $H(z)$ is the transfer function of the filter. $H(z)$ is expressed as the ratio of two polynominal expressions. It is possible to express it in a more useful form by evidencing the roots of the two polynomials:

$$H(z) = \frac{b_0 z^{N-M} \Pi_{m=1,M}(z - z_m)}{\Pi_{k=1,N}(z - p_k)} \tag{2.12}$$

where p_k are the poles and z_m are the zeros of $H(z)$.

Considerable insight into the behavior of the digital filter can be gained by plotting the positions of poles and zeros in the complex z-plane. In fact, a stable filter has all the poles inside the unit circle ($|p_k| < 1$), while the frequency response can be roughly estimated by visual inspection. In fact it can be shown that:

$$H(\omega) = H(z)|_{z=\exp(j\omega T_s)}. \tag{2.13}$$

$H(\omega)$ is evaluated in the complex z-plane on the point locus which describes the unit circle ($|\exp(j\omega T_s)| = 1$). At a given frequency $\omega = \omega_0$, the value of $H(\omega)$ is obtained by the product of the distance from that point to each of the zeros, divided by the product of the distances to the poles. Therefore, zeros close to the unit circle make $|H(\omega)|$ approach zero. Poles close to the unit circle mean high values of $|H(\omega)|$: the closer the pole, the higher the modulus. A phase diagram $\angle H(\omega)$ can also be estimated from the poles/zeros diagram: nonlinearity in $\angle H(\omega)$ is the result of zeros (positive phase shift) or a pole (negative phase change) close to the unit circle. Compare the modulus and phase diagrams of Figure 2.5(a) and (b) with the relative geometry of poles and zeros of Figure 2.5(c). Hence a filter with a desired frequency response can be designed by placing poles and zeros in appropriate points in the z-plane.

Design Criteria

It is known that ideal filters are not physically possible (they would require an infinite number of coefficients in the impulse response), so we can design FIR or IIR filters which can only mimic, with an acceptable error, the ideal response. In many cases the filter is designed in order to satisfy some requirements, usually on the frequency response, which depend on the characteristic of the particular application for which the filter is projected. Such requirements may be limitations on ripples in the passband and in the stopband and constraints on the width of the transition between passband and stopband. Figure 2.6 shows the comparison between real and ideal responses.

When the filter is intended to process biological signals there is a requirement for a zero (or at least linear) phase response in order to preserve the original signal shape. Nonlinear phase response can introduce distortions that are not acceptable, especially if the signal is to be used for diagnostic purposes.

An example is shown in Figure 2.7. A noisy ECG in (a) is filtered by three bandpass filters with different phase-response characteristics. The zero (b) and linear (c) phase filters produce undistorted waves, which can be time-delayed as is the case in (f). On the other hand, the nonlinear phase filter in (g) drastically modifies the signal waveform, the monophasic T waves in particular becoming biphasic after filtering.

FIR filters can be designed to fulfil the requirement for a linear phase response by constraining the coefficients of the impulse response to have symmetry around their midpoint. Several design techniques are available, some of them requiring heavy computational tasks, which are capable of developing filters with specific requirements. For FIR filters, they include the window technique, the frequency sampling method or equiripple design filters. For IIR filters, Butterworth, Chebychef and elliptic designs are employed using impulse-invariant or bilinear transformations. For detailed analysis of digital filter techniques, see references 2 and 10.

Other Digital Signal Processing Procedures

Traditional filtering is based on the hypothesis that signals and noise have different frequency contents. Then the noise can be easily removed or decreased by means of a linear digital filter.

However, in many cases noise and signal bandwidths overlap, and sometimes the amplitude of the noise is much higher than that of the signal. A traditional filter, designed

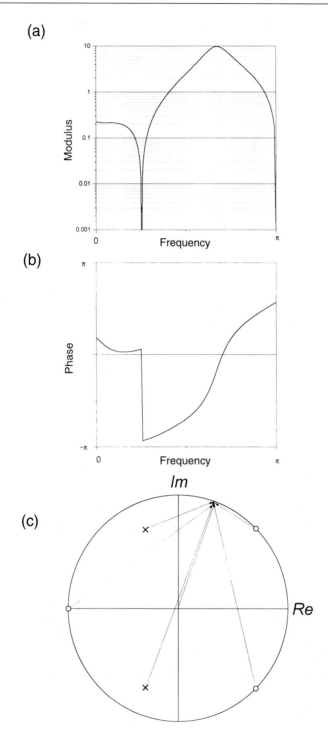

Figure 2.5 (a) Modulus and (b) phase diagrams of a filter, with (c) the corresponding poles and zeros in the z-transform domain.

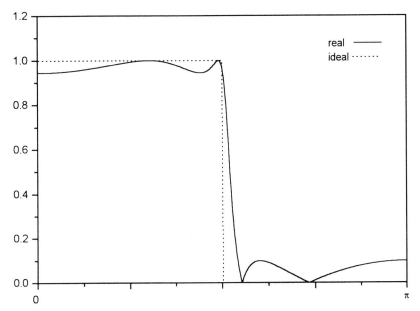

Figure 2.6 Comparison of the responses of an ideal and a real lowpass filter.

for attenuating a frequency band, will then introduce signal cancellations, or at least distortion. Examples of situations where noise overlaps the signal are:

ECG + 50/60 Hz interference
ECG + EMG
ECG + respiration.

Since correct diagnostic evaluation of biomedical signals, and in particular of an ECG, requires that both low and high frequency contents be preserved, some alternative filtering methods should be adopted. In such cases the filter is based on the different statistical properties of signal and noise, and on *a priori* knowledge of some signal and/or noise characteristics, or on their interaction modalities, etc.

In the following, various types of digital signal processing procedures employed in electrocardiography are illustrated, with some examples of applications.

Averaging

When the signal repeats identically with a certain synchronization (for example, the PQRST activity in correspondence with each sinusal cardiac beat), and furthermore signal and noise are related by well-defined statistical interactions, the averaging technique (synchronous with a defined trigger) can satisfactorily increase the signal-to-noise ratio (SNR).[11,8]

The three hypotheses on which the averaging is based are the following:

1. All the signal realizations contain a deterministic signal component $x(n)$, which does not vary for all the epochs considered.
2. The superimposed noise $w(n)$ is a broadband stochastic process with zero mean and variance σ^2:

$$E[w(n)] = 0 \quad E[w(n)^2] = \sigma^2. \tag{2.14}$$

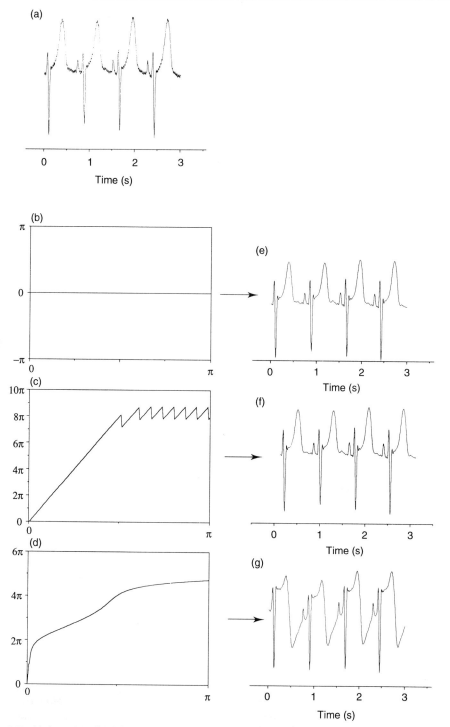

Figure 2.7 (a) An original ECG signal. (b) A zero-phase digital filter. (c) A linear-phase digital filter. (d) A nonlinear-phase filter. The outputs of the filters are (e) in phase, (f) delayed by a constant number of samples, (g) presented with phase distortion more significant in the T and P waves.

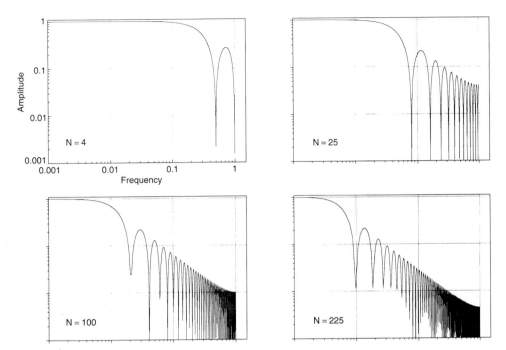

Figure 2.8 Amplitude spectral characteristics of an averaging procedure as the number N of averaged cycles is increased.

3. The signal $x(n)$ and the noise $w(n)$ are *uncorrelated*, so that the recorded signal $y(n)$ at the ith realization can be expressed as:

$$y_i(n) = x(n) + w_i(n). \tag{2.15}$$

If the time epochs are properly aligned, with the trigger as a reference point, the signal waveform directly sums up, and the averaging process yields:

$$y_t(n) = \frac{1}{N}\sum_{i=1}^{N} y_i(n) = \frac{1}{N}\left(\sum_{i=1}^{N} x(n) + \sum_{i=1}^{N} w_i(n)\right). \tag{2.16}$$

The noise term is an estimate of the mean by taking the average on N realizations. The variance of such an average (σ_a) is related to the noise variance according to:

$$\sigma_a^2 = \sigma^2/N. \tag{2.17}$$

Thus the amplitude of the signal is maintained, while the variance of the noise is reduced by a factor of N. Evaluating the improvement of SNR in terms of RMS values, it is possible to calculate:

$$\text{SNR} = \text{SNR}_i \cdot \sqrt{N}. \tag{2.18}$$

The signal averaging improves the SNR on the single tracings by a factor of $\sqrt{N}$.

The averaging procedure is equivalent to a moving-average lowpass filter where the output is a function of the preceding values with a lag of h samples, where h is the distance, measured in samples, between corresponding samples in consecutive epochs: in practice, the filter operates not on a time sequence, but in the sweep sequence, on corresponding samples. Figure 2.8 shows the frequency response of the filter in

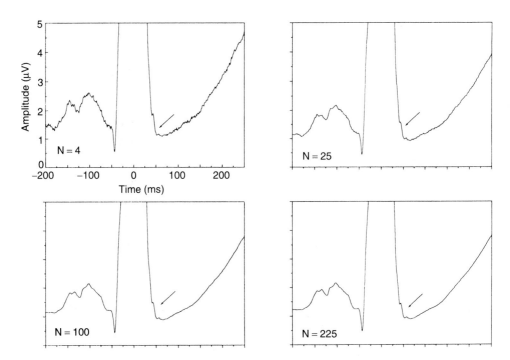

Figure 2.9 SNR improvement in a high-amplification ECG signal with progressive number N of cardiac cycles averaged. The arrows mark low-amplitude activity at the end of the QRS, which is better recognizable when the SNR is improved.

correspondence to different values of N, while Figure 2.9 shows the results of the corresponding averages on the ECG signal.

Misleading results may occur if the assumptions (i.e. wide band of noise, or non-correlation between signal and noise) are not valid. Further, particular attention must be paid to time alignment of the sweeps in order to avoid the jitter that may cause loss of higher-frequency components in the signal.

Adaptive Filters

When no *a priori* information is available on the interaction between signal and noise, or when the signal, the noise or their relationship is nonstationary, an adaptive optimal filter can be successively employed.

According to the input signal configuration, an adaptive filter can be used as a *noise canceller* or as a *signal enhancer*. In the present section a noise canceller implementation is considered.

Figure 2.10 shows a general block diagram of an adaptive filter. The recorded signal $d(t)$ is the sum of a contribution $s(t)$, not related to the noise, and a second one, $n(t)$, related to the noise. A second sequence $u(t)$ is related, in some unknown way, to the noise.

In practice, the filter extracts from the input signal the components that are cross-correlated to the noise and can automatically adjust its parameters, based on the incoming signals and the prediction error.

The output of the adaptive filter, $y(t)$, is an estimation of the signal portion correlated to the noise $\hat{n}(t)$. Thus the error

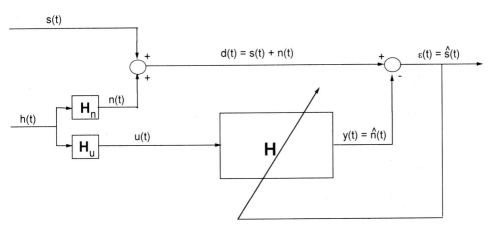

Figure 2.10 Block diagram of an adaptive filtering procedure (see text).

$$\varepsilon(t) = d(t) - y(t) \qquad (2.19)$$

is an estimation of the signal portion uncorrelated to the noise: $\varepsilon(t) = \hat{s}(t)$; hence:

$$\varepsilon = \hat{s} = s + n - \hat{n}. \qquad (2.20)$$

By squaring and calculating the expectation value, under the hypothesis of noncorrelation between s and n, we obtain:

$$E[\hat{s}^2] = E[s^2] + E[(n - \hat{n})^2]. \qquad (2.21)$$

On minimizing $E[(n - \hat{n})^2]$, an optimal estimation, in the least-squares sense, is provided for $s(t)$.

The minimization algorithm is performed recursively and a 'forgetting factor' is employed in order to track the varying characteristics of the noise or of the signal.

Adaptive filters may be described and classified from the following features:

1. the performance index which is to be optimized;
2. the algorithm that updates the parameters of the filter;
3. the structure of the filter that actually performs the required operation on the signal.

Figure 2.11 shows what happens when the adaptive filter is used to cancel 50 Hz interference from an ECG signal. At the beginning of the filtering procedure the adaptation interval is well visible.

Other applications are in separating the maternal and fetal ECGs recorded by abdominal leads, or recipient and donor heart activity in transplanted patients, etc. A detailed theoretical description and examples of applications in the biomedical field can be found in reference 12.

Baseline Correction

The first step in all ECG processing is baseline noise reduction that is required for a more correct evaluation of fiducial points and parameters of the signal.

Simple highpass filtering is frequently unacceptable because the baseline can oscillate with high frequency. A filter, to be sufficiently robust to remove noise and to be implemented with a reasonable low number of coefficients, should have the lower -3 dB

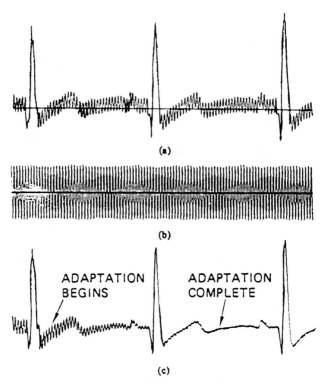

Figure 2.11   50 Hz noise reduction by means of an adaptive filter. (a) Original signal. (b) Noise interference. (c) Filtered signal. (Reproduced with permission from reference 12; © IEEE)

frequency point above 0.05 Hz. Such characteristics will influence the low-frequency components of the ECG, such as the ST segment, that have diagnostic relevance.[13,14] Thus, it is generally advisable to use alternative methods that employ more sophisticated digital filter criteria and are strictly related to the signal under analysis.

As, in the ECG, pre-P-wave and post-T-wave periods of each cardiac cycle are isoelectric intervals, the baseline is supposed to pass through these points. The baseline is thus detected as the fitting of the isoelectric segments by means of different-order polynomials or other non-polynomial functions (sinusoids, cubic splines, Lagrange functions, etc.).

A critical step in the procedure is the correct choice of the isoelectric interval. The regressions are carried out on a set of contiguous points selected between the T wave of a cycle and the P wave of the successive one which are by definition considered isoelectric. Other authors choose the isoelectric segment between the P wave and the QRS complex. The former solution may present disadvantages in cases of tachycardia, while the latter has available only a limited number of points.

If the baseline is estimated as the sequence of straight lines connecting two isoelectric points per cardiac cycle, low-frequency heart activity will be preserved and the baseline will be accurately tracked with regard to the very low frequencies. Increasing the order of the estimator and selecting one point (node or knot) per cardiac cycle (for example, between the P wave and the QRS complex) through which the estimated line must pass, higher-frequency baseline wandering will be removed and low-frequency signal information is preserved.

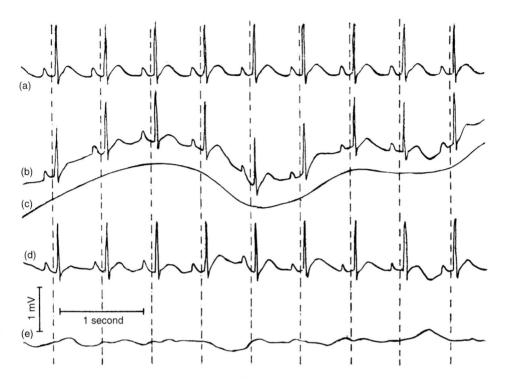

Figure 2.12 Example of baseline noise reduction. (a) Original signal. (b) Corrupted ECG (ECG + base-line noise). (c) Baseline estimate. (d) Improved ECG. (e) Error (original ECG − improved ECG).

A parameter for evaluation of the goodness of the fit is the residual variance z of the isoelectric points, $P(k)$, referred to the interpolating function $y(k)$:

$$z(\mathbf{a}) = \frac{1}{N} \sum_{k=1}^{N} [y(k) - P(k)]^2 \tag{2.22}$$

where $\mathbf{a}$ is the parameter vector defining the interpolating function, and N is the number of points in the isoelectric line.

An example of baseline wandering removal is shown in Figure 2.12.

Wave Recognition and Classification

A common problem in biomedical signal processing, especially when dealing with diagnostic devices, is the detection, measurement and classification of waveforms.

Sometimes it is necessary only to detect the occurrence of an event, in other instances the exact shape of the signal is required. Usually, the general shape of the wave is known, so the recognition methods are based on *a priori* assumptions. Different approaches are used to solve the problem of wave detection and modified versions of the same approaches are sometimes employed for classification. In the following, the methods most commonly used in ECG analysis will be presented.

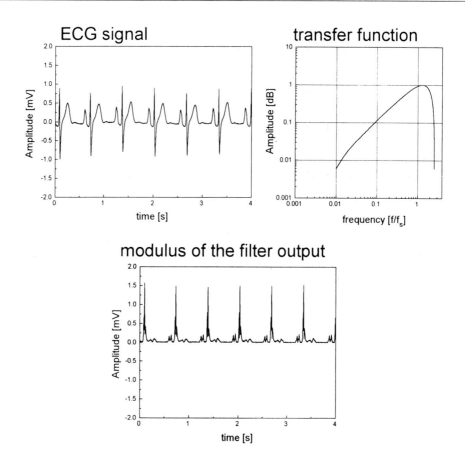

Figure 2.13   The original ECG signal is filtered via a derivative lowpass filter in order to obtain the output signal.

The *structural feature* methods are generally heuristic and are specific to a given wave. An approximate and general knowledge of the wave shape is needed for selection of typical structural characteristics of the signal.

The waves to be detected, even if consecutive, are not generally identical, as the system generating the signal may change, or different kinds of noise may be superimposed. Otherwise, they are characterized by a common structure. For example, in the ECG, the QRS complex is the most easily identified part of the signal for amplitude and frequency content and can be easily recognized even in noisy recordings. Various problems may prevent detection of the R wave by the simple threshold technique. For example, other waves in the signal (e.g. the T wave), under particular recording conditions, may have a comparable amplitude (Figure 2.13). Alternatively, baseline shift due to movements of electrodes, or to movements of the patient, may make such a technique unreliable and an adaptive threshold may be required. Another possibility is that there may be line-frequency noise.

To overcome these problems, preprocessing of the signal is required that can enhance peculiar features of the QRS complex and attenuate other waves. As the QRS complex is characterized by higher-frequency content, a highpass filter can perform well. Similar results may be obtained by a derivative filter (Figure 2.13 shows the ECG after differentiation). Since the differential operator has removed the baseline trend and the slower components, a threshold technique can now be applied.

The algorithm may be made more specific by considering duration and slope of the wave, in the neighborhood of the threshold overcoming.

The *contour limiting* method is more flexible than the previous one, and can easily be adapted to various waves. It consists of an extention of the thresholding method.

This method uses a template which may be obtained by averaging typical waves detected and aligned manually. The variance of each sample of the template is evaluated and is used to generate the upper and the lower limits of the wave with a given probability (i.e. confidence interval of the template). An observation vector $x(k)$ is obtained from the signal by taking into account a number of samples equal to the samples in the template. At each time instant k, the observation vector is compared with the limits. A waveform is assumed to be present in the observation window if the signal vector is contained inside the contours for each time k. A critical point is the construction of the limit functions. Large limits will lead to false-positive detection, while small limits may lead to rejection of some true waves. In addition, in order to avoid missing beats, and for a classification of the waves, different templates should be calculated for each possible type of waveform.

A common procedure for wave detection is the *matched filter*. The output of a moving-average filter is given by:

$$y(k) = \sum_{j=0}^{N-1} b_j x(k-j) \tag{2.23}$$

as previously described. The filter coefficients are chosen in order to maximize the output SNR

$$\text{SNR}_o = \frac{(E[s_i + n_i] - E[n_i])^2}{E[n_i^2]} \tag{2.24}$$

where $y_i = s_i + n_i$ when the input signal contains the wave of interest, and $y_i = n_i$ when the input signal does not contain the wave. The noise output is supposed to have zero mean and variance σ^2 and is not correlated with the signal. Under these hypotheses, equation 2.24 becomes:

$$\text{SNR}_o = \frac{\left(\sum_{j=0}^{N} b_j E[x_i(j)]^2\right)}{\sigma^2 \sum_{i=0}^{N-1} b_i^2}. \tag{2.25}$$

The expression is maximized for $b_i = E[s(i)]$, so the impulse response of the filter is a template of the wave of interest, and the filter output is a cross-correlation between the template and the input signal.

In summary, the matched filtering procedure consists of the choice of a template, and a cross-correlation between incoming signal and template. A wave is detected when the filter output overcomes a given threshold. The method can be adapted for signal classification if different templates are chosen, one for each possible class of morphology. The detected beat will be assigned to the class corresponding to the template that causes the output to overcome the threshold. The matched filter only determines the presence of a wave, not its exact shape.[15]

Finally, in *syntactic methods* (also known as *linguistic, structural* or *grammatical*), the signal is decomposed in a sequence of subpatterns (primitives) and rules (grammar) are given describing the subpattern compositions resulting in the given wave. If a classification of the signal is required, each class will be defined by its own grammar. A deterministic finite-state automata is generally used for the recognition and classification operation. For further details, see references 16 and 17.

In practice, in ECG processing, detection and classification of waves is performed by means of a combination of the methods outlined above. Derivative filters are employed for feature enhancement of the QRS; when the derivative overcomes the threshold, a syntactic method is used in order to recognize the correctness of the derivative configuration; and finally, once the presence of the wave has been detected, a template procedure allows its classification.

Other approaches are currently being studied for the solution of critical points in wave recognition and classification. For example, neural networks are providing satisfactory results in the recognition and classification of ST segment changes.

Data Compression

Compressing ECG traces is a practical task employed for efficient signal transmission and data storage. Compression is necessary for real-time transmission over telephone lines, or when requirements on memory size and cost are critical – such as in archiving a large database or during 24-hour solid-state Holter recordings.

In general, compression is obtained by encoding only those parts of the signal that contain useful new information, discharging the redundancy (i.e. samples which correlate with the neighboring ones, predictable parts of each sample, etc.). With regard to the ECG signal, sampling at high frequency (500 Hz) is necessary for a correct description of the high-frequency diagnostic attributes of the QRS complexes,[6] but it is not necessary for slowly varying parts of the signal (mainly the baseline). Along these parts several samples can be neglected with no appreciable loss of information. Sometimes compression is obtained by taking the derivative of the ECG signal and encoding the series of the differences. In such a way we convert the original ECG into a new signal with a lower dynamic excursion that can be encoded by a lower number of bits.

Even if the ECG has several features which may help the compression task (it is periodic; a stable baseline occupies a significant portion of the beat), it is difficult to obtain the desired amount of compression without introducing some (hopefully small) errors on the decompressed signals. The amount of compression and the consequent reconstruction errors are the two parameters that should be taken into account in comparing different compression methods. They are usually in conflict: greater data reductions are obtained at the expense of greater errors in the reconstructed signal.[18]

The compression ratio (CR) – i.e. the ratio between the number of bits required to represent the original signal and the number of bits in the compacted data – determines the number of bits of memory needed before and after compression.

Evaluation of the reconstruction errors is more difficult. The best way to evaluate these errors is to measure their effects on the clinical usefulness of the signal, because of course the reconstructed signal should not lose diagnostic accuracy. The only way to measure the diagnostic relevance of a reconstructed signal is by the qualitative evaluation of original and reconstructed ECGs by one or more cardiologists. Usually, a quantification of reconstruction error is given in terms of the percentage root–mean–square difference (PRD):

$$PRD = \sqrt{\frac{\sum_{k=1}^{N} (y(k) - \hat{y}(k))^2}{\sum_{k=1}^{N} y(k)^2}} \times 100 \qquad (2.26)$$

where $y(k)$ and $\hat{y}(k)$ are the original and the reconstructed sequences. Such an index is easy to compute and therefore it is frequently employed. Nevertheless, it is too general: errors are weighted equally wherever they are on the baseline or on the ST–T segment, but the clinical implications of equal errors is not the same in different points of ECG tracing.

Several compression techniques have been presented in the literature. Some of them handle the ECG samples directly (direct methods), others operate a linear transformation on the signal before compression (transformational methods). Examples of direct methods are the TP (turning-point) algorithm and the ATZEC (Amplitude Zone Time Epoch Code) method. They retain the samples which contain information and dispense with the others. The ATZEC method decomposes a raw ECG into a sequence of plateaux and slopes, providing a piece-linear approximation of the original ECG. In the transform-ation methods, a Fourier transform, a Karunen–Loewe transform or a discrete cosine transform (DCT) are usually employed.

Sometimes preprocessing techniques are applied to the raw data. They are used to extract some typical features which are coded and then used to reconstruct the original waveform (parameter extraction methods). Linear predictions, neural nets or syntactic methods are employed to extract the signal features.

Further details on compression techniques can be found in references 19 and 20.

Frequency Domain Analysis

Frequency domain analysis becomes a fundamental tool when interest focuses on evaluation of the rhythms present in a signal. The signal is then represented in terms of a power spectral density (PSD), and the contributions of the various frequencies present in the overall signal are determined. Methods to estimate the PSD are classified as *nonparametric* and *parametric*.

Nonparametric Methods

Nonparametric methods are the traditional tools for frequency analysis of a signal. They are based on the Fourier transform (FT) and can be easily and efficiently evaluated by means of the fast Fourier transform (FFT) algorithm.[21] Expression of the PSD can be obtained directly from the time series by means of the periodogram expression:

$$\text{PSD}(f) = \frac{1}{N\Delta t} \left| \Delta t \sum_{k=0}^{N-1} y(k) \exp(-j2\pi k f \Delta t) \right|^2 = \frac{1}{N\Delta t} |Y(f)|^2 \tag{2.27}$$

where Δt is the sampling period, N is the number of samples, and $Y(f)$ is the discrete Fourier transform of $y(k)$. Alternatively, on the basis of the Wiener–Khintchine theorem, the PSD can be evaluated indirectly from the FT of the autocorrelation function R_{yy} of the signal, where R_{yy} is estimated as:

$$R_{yy}(\tau) = \frac{1}{N} \sum_{k=0}^{N} y(k)y(k+\tau). \tag{2.28}$$

However, both the autocorrelation function and this Fourier transform are theoreti-cally defined on infinite data sequences. Thus errors are introduced by the need to operate on finite data sets, which means an implicit rectangular windowing of the data (i.e. multiplication of a hypothetical infinite sequence of data with a rectangular function) that results in a convolution, in the frequency domain, between signal and window transforms. This leads to leakage in the PSD. Different windows, which smoothly connect the sides to zero, are often used to solve this problem; however, they introduce reduction in the frequency resolution. Further, the frequency resolution Δf is a function of the number N of samples in the window; thus, a large data set is needed for a sufficient spectral resolution.

Various methods of spectral averaging and smoothing have been proposed in the literature. These are needed to improve the statistical consistency of the estimated spectra.[21]

Parametric Methods

Parametric approaches assume the time series under analysis to be the output of a mathematical model. The PSD is calculated as a function of the model parameters according to appropriate expressions. The first step in this approach is to make a choice of the model structure that can well represent the signal generating mechanism.

It is worth noting that the model is completely independent from the physiological, anatomical and physical characteristics of the biological system, but simply provides an input–output relationship of the process under analysis in the so-called black–box approach.

Among the numerous modeling possibilities, autoregressive (AR) models are used to describe a wide number of different processes. They are a particular case of the more general autoregressive moving-average (ARMA) model, but have higher efficiency in terms of identification procedure and parameter calculation.

The autoregressive PSD is obtained as a function of the model parameters:

$$\text{PSD}(f) = \frac{\lambda^2 \Delta t}{\left| 1 + \sum_{i=1}^{p} a_i z^{-i} \right|^2_{z = \exp(j2\pi f \Delta t)}} \tag{2.29}$$

where λ^2 is the input noise variance, a_i are the model parameters, and p is the model order (i.e. the number of parameters) which has to be chosen high enough to make the model fit the data. As a help in the correct choice of p, various criteria have been proposed in the literature.[23,23] In addition, tests have been suggested on the residual of the identification in order to verify *a posteriori* the correctness of the identification.[24]

Comparison of Parametric and Nonparametric Methods

Parametric methods suffer less leakage than nonparametric methods owing to the time-limited period of analysis. In fact, parametric approaches give a stochastic description of the signal and no assumptions are made about the samples outside the analysis window. In addition, parametric approaches have a better spectral resolution that does not depend on the number of samples. Finally, when using parametric identification an automatic spectral decomposition may be achieved, through residual integration, for the post-processing of the spectra and for the evaluation of the spectral parameters (see the example reported in Figure 2.14).

On the other hand, nonparametric methods are methodologically and computationally less complex because the PSD is evaluated from the data without the need for *a priori* choice of the structure and complexity of the model, and without *a posteriori* verification of the model's suitability.

Figure 2.14(a) shows the interval tachogram (i.e. the series of consecutive RR intervals expressed in seconds as a function of the beat number) obtained from the ECG recording

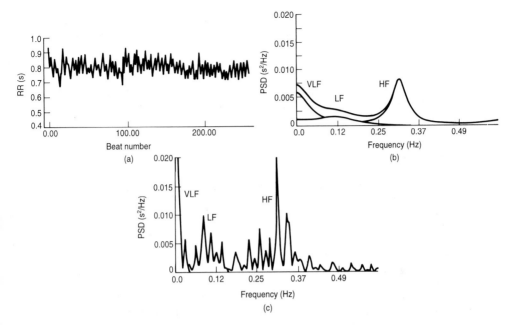

Figure 2.14 (a) An RR interval tachogram of a normal subject in control conditions. (b) PSD of the signal obtained by a parametric method. (c) PSD of the signal obtained by a nonparametric method.

of a normal subject during resting conditions. Figure 2.14(b) shows the corresponding PSD obtained by means of an AR model of order 8. An automatic spectral decomposition has been applied and the central frequency and total power of each spectral component have been calculated. In particular, some of them represent a well-defined physiological meaning: the component centered around 0.1 Hz, marked LF (low frequency), has been found to be associated with the sympathetic activity on the heart, while the component synchronous with respiration, marked as HF (high frequency), can be considered a marker of the vagal activity controlling heart rate.[25] Thus, the frequency and power of these components are quantitative indices relating to the autonomic control of the heart.

Figure 2.14(c) shows the PSD obtained by a nonparametric method.

Time–Frequency Analysis

One of the basic assumptions, when applying frequency analysis, is signal stationarity; i.e. the signal is assumed to have its statistical characteristics unchanged during the analysis period. However, many biological signals and phenomena are time-dependent, and sometimes the interest is mainly in tracking and quantifying these changes.

Different approaches have been proposed for this purpose. The simplest one is the short-time Fourier transform (STFT): a running window is obtained on the data record and the FT is evaluated for different time positions of the window. The procedure can be summarized as in the following expression:

$$\text{STFT}(\tau, f) = \int x(t) g^*(t - \tau) \exp(-2i\pi f t)\, dt. \tag{2.30}$$

The signal $x(t)$ is assumed to be stationary when seen through the window $g(t - \tau)$ centered on the time instant t. A sequence of PSDs is obtained which is able to reflect the

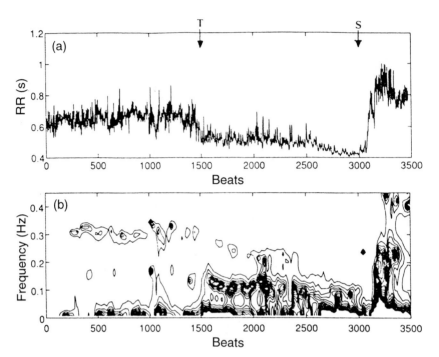

Figure 2.15   (a) Interval tachogram of a subject during a vasovagal syncope episode (marked by S). (b) Contour plot in the time–frequency plane where the time is measured by beat number.

temporal changes in the frequency content of the signal. A tradeoff does exist between an acceptable frequency resolution, that requires a longer time interval, and a time resolution, that requires shorter time intervals. On the other hand, the indetermination principle states that one of the two parameters can be maximized, at the expense of the second one. The following expression summarizes the concept:

$$\Delta t \Delta f \geq 1/4\pi. \tag{2.31}$$

Once a window has been chosen for the STFT, then the time–frequency resolution is fixed over the entire time–frequency plane, since the same window is used at all frequencies.

In order to overcome this problem, the resolutions Δt and Δf may be made variable in the time–frequency plane and a multiresolution analysis is obtained. Δt and Δf still satisfy expression (2.31), but the time resolution becomes arbitrarily good at high frequencies, while the frequency resolution becomes arbitrarily good at low frequencies. On this concept is based the wavelet transform, an innovative and powerful tool for time frequency analysis. A detailed description of the method can be found in reference 26 while examples of applications on biomedical signals are in reference 27.

Alternatively, the Wigner distribution (WD) is able to describe a signal in the time–frequency plane. It is a nonparametric approach that allows one to map nonstationary signals as a function of both time and frequency, and variations in signal dynamics can be easily identified.

The WD is a nonlinear transformation and cross-terms may appear when analyzing multicomponent signals. Modified versions of the WD distribution has been proposed in the literature with the aim of reducing the cross-terms. Applications in the biomedical

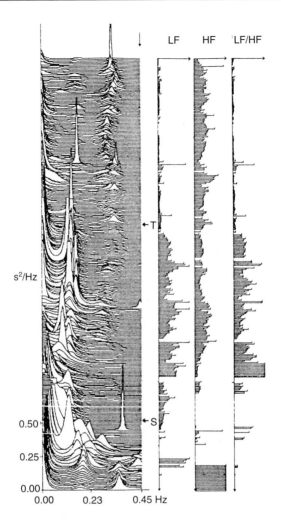

Figure 2.16 Compressed spectral array of the episode in Figure 2.15(a), with the spectral parameters LF, HF, LF/HF indicated on a beat-to-beat basis.

field are, for example, in the study of heart rate variability and in the recognition of ventricular late potentials.[28,29]

A different approach to the time-variant evaluation of the PSD of a signal consists of recursive implementation of AR models. The vector **a** of the model coefficients is corrected on a sample-by-sample basis:

$$\mathbf{a}(n) = \mathbf{a}(n-1) + \mathbf{K}(n)e(n) \tag{2.32}$$

where n is the discrete time index, $\mathbf{K}$ is the gain of the algorithm and $e(n)$ is the prediction error of the model, implemented in prediction form at time $n-1$.

The structure of the gain can be obtained by means of different procedures, which minimize the figure of merit step-by-step:

$$J = \sum_{n=1}^{N} \omega^{N-n} \cdot e(n)^2 \tag{2.33}$$

where ω is a parameter ($0 < \omega \le 1$) that exponentially weights the error terms, allowing the algorithm to track signal modification.[30]

Figure 2.15 shows an example of time-variant AR identification performed on an RR series obtained during a syncope event in Figure 2.15(a). Figure 2.15(b) shows the PSD represented in countour-graph form, and Figure 2.16 shows the compressed spectral array (CSA). Both representations permit a visual identification of the LF power decreasing in correspondence with syncope, denoting a withdrawal in sympathetic activity. Quantification of the phenomenon can be obtained through a beat-to-beat calculation of the spectral parameters (LF, HF, LF/HF) that quantify the sympathovagal balance (represented on the side of the CSA plot).

References

1. Shannon CE. Communication in presence of noise. *Proc IRE 1949;* **37**: 10–21.
2. Oppenheim AV, Schafer RW. *Digital Signal Processing.* Englewood Cliffs, NJ: Prentice-Hall, 1975.
3. Widrow B. A study of rough amplitude quantization by means of Nyquist sampling theory. *IRE Trans Circ Theory 1956;* **3**: 266–88.
4. Jaeger RC. Tutorial: Analog data acquisition technology: part II, analog to digital conversion. *IEEE Micro 1982;* **8**: 46–56.
5. Carassa F. *Communicazioni Elettriche.* Turin: Boringhieri Ed., 1983.
6. Pipberger HV, Arzbaecher RC, Berson AS, Briller SA, Brody DA, Flowers NC, Geselowitz DB, Lepeschkin E, Oliver GC, Schmitt OH, Spach M. Recommendations for standardization of leads and of specification for instruments in electrocardiography and vectorcardiography. Report of the Committee of Electrocardiography, American Heart Association. *Circulation* 1975; **31**(52): 11.
7. Bailey JJ, Berson AS, Garson A, Horan LG, Macfarland PW, Mortara DW, Zywietz C. Recommendations for standardization and specification in automated electrocardiography: bandwidth and digital signal processing. A report for health professionals by *ad hoc* writing group of the committee on electrocardiography and cardiac electrophysiology of the council on clinical cardiology, American Heart Association. *Circulation* (special report) 1990; **81**: 2.
8. Breithardt G, Cain ME, El-Sherif N, Flowers N, Hombach V, Janse M, Simson B, Steinback G. Standards for analysis of ventricular late potentials using high-resolution or signal-averaged electrocardiography: statement by a Task Force Committee between the European Society of Cardiology, the American Heart Association and the American College of Cardiology. *Europ Heart J* 1991; **12**: 473–80.
9. Rainer LR, Cooley JW, Helms HD, Jackson LB, Kaiser JF, Rader CM, Shafer RFW Steigglitz K, Weinstein CJ. Terminology in digital signal processing. *IEEE Trans Audio Electroac 1972;* **AU-20**: 322–37.
10. Antoniou A. *Digital Filters: Analysis and Design.* New York: McGraw Hill, 1979.
11. Simson MB. Use of signals in the terminal QRS complex to identify patients with ventricular tachycardia after myocardial infarction. *Circulation 1981;* **64**: 235–42.
12. Widrow B, Glover JRJ, Kaunitrz J, Charles SJ, Hearn RH, Zeidler JR, Dong E, Goodlin RC. Adaptive noise cancelling: principles and applications. *Proc IEEE 1975;* **63**(12): 1692–716.
13. Bartoli F, Cerutti S, Gatti E. Digital filtering and regression algorithms for an accurate detection of the baseline in ECG signals. *Med Inform 1983;* **8**(2): 71–82.
14. Meyer CR, Keiser HN, Electrocardiogram baseline noise estimation and removal using cubic splines and state-space computation techniques. *Comput Biomed Res 1977;* **10**: 459–70.
15. Cohen A. *Biomedical Signal Processing: Time and Frequency Domains Analysis.* Boca Raton, FL: CRC Press, 1983.
16. Gonzales RC, Thomson MG. *Syntactic Pattern Recognition: An Introduction.* London: Addison-Wesley, 1978.
17. Papakonstantinou G, Gritzali F. Syntactic filtering of ECG waveforms. *Comput Biomed Res 1981;* **14**: 158.
18. Nave G, Cohen A. ECG compression using long-term prediction. *IEEE Trans Biomed Eng 1993;* **40**(9): 877–85.
19. Jalaleddine SMS, Hutchens CG, Strattan RD, Coberly WA. ECG data compression techniques – a unified approach. *IEEE Trans Biomed Eng 1990;* **37**: 329–43.
20. Tompkins WJ (eds). *Biomedical Digital Signal Processing.* Englewood Cliffs, NJ: Prentice Hall, 1993.
21. Marple SL. *Digital Spectral Analysis with Applications.* Englewood Cliffs, NJ: Prentice Hall, 1987.
22. Akaike H. Statistical predictor identification. *Ann Inst Statist Math 1970;* **22**: 203–17.
23. Akaike H. A new look at the statistical model identification. *IEEE Trans Autom Contr 1974;* **AC-19**: 716–23.
24. Box GEP, Jenkins GM. *Time Series Analysis: Forcasting and Control.* San Francisco: Holden Day, 1976.
25. Malliani A, Pagani M, Lombardi F, Cerutti S. Cardiovascular neural regulation explored in the frequency domain. *Circulation Research Advanced Series* 1991; **84**: 482–92.
26. Rioul O, Vetterli M. Wavelets and signal processing. *IEEE SP Magazine.* Oct 1991: 14–38.
27. Bartnik EA, Blinowka KJ, Durka PJ. Single evoked potential reconstruction by means of wavelet transform. *Biol Cybern 1992;* **67**: 175–81.

28. Venturi M, Conforti F, Macerata A, Varanini M, Emdin M, Marchesi C. Power spectrum estimation for the analysis of variability of non-stationary cardiovascular signals. In: *Spectral Analysis of Heart Rate Variability Signal*, workshop held in Veruno (NO), 19 October 1990: 69–86.
29. Novak P, Novak V. Time/frequency mapping of the heart rate, blood pressure and respiratory signals. *Med Biol Eng Comp* 1993, March: 103–10.
30. Bianchi AM, Mainardi LT, Petrucci E, Signorini MG, Mainardi M, Cerutti S. Time-variant power spectrum analysis for the detection of transient episodes in HRV signal. *IEEE Trans Biomed Eng 1993;* **40**(2): 136–43.

SECTION II

Arrhythmia Monitoring

Introduction by Takashi Yanaga

Current indications for the use of Holter monitoring to detect clinically meaningful cardiac arrhythmias include:

1. Evaluation of patients with syncope, palpitations, or other symptoms that may be due to arrhythmias.
2. Evaluation of patients with known arrhythmias in order to improve the quantification of the frequency and/or the rate of the rhythm disorder.
3. Assessment of the potential for malignant cardiac arrhythmias and sudden death in high-risk patients with known cardiac disease.
4. Evaluation of antiarrhythmic drug efficacy.
5. Surveillance of the function of implanted pacemakers. During the past decade, there has been a dramatic increase in catheter ablation procedures and in the implantation of cardiac defibrillators, and Holter monitoring has assumed an important role in evaluating the safety and efficacy of these interventions.

The chapters in this section expand on these indications. Holter monitoring provides a unique insight into some of the electrophysiological phenomena associated with the triggering of various arrhythmias, and one chapter has a particularly enlightening description and interpretation of the electrical events immediately preceding the onset of torsade de pointes. Although implantation of the cardioverter–defibrillator requires an invasive procedure, the recorded premalignant and malignant arrhythmias uncovered by this device in this especially high-risk group of patients have important relevance to noninvasive electrocardiology.

The chapter on pacemaker-related arrhythmias emphasizes the deductive reasoning that needs to be applied to understand pacemaker malfunction. The figures and the accompanying legends provided in the pacemaker chapter are enormously instructive.

When Norman J. Holter first commented on the potential uses of his new ambulatory ECG monitoring technique in 1957, he believed his system had particular applicability in the detection and analysis of various cardiac arrhythmias. How right he was!

3

Supraventricular Arrhythmias

Lee A. Biblo and Albert L. Waldo

Introduction

Ambulatory electrocardiographic monitoring is an important diagnostic tool in patients with supraventricular arrhythmias. The ambulatory ECG can also be used to assess therapeutic procedures. Most sustained supraventricular arrhythmias are diagnosed upon presentation of the patient at a medical facility by recording of a standard 12-lead ECG, either alone or with an appropriate rhythm strip. However, transient arrhythmias may cause symptoms that may not last long enough for patients to travel to a medical facility to obtain an ECG. For those patients, the ambulatory ECG is critical for diagnosis. If the arrhythmic events are sufficiently frequent in a 24-hour period, or if the expectation is that the arrhythmia will occur in a 24-hour period, then the continuous 24-hour ambulatory ECG is most useful.

If the events are episodic and cannot be expected to occur on a daily basis, a transtelephonic monitor (a device which patients can carry with them and which permits rapid placement of electrodes, such as a wrist bracelet or chest electrodes) is better suited for recording the rhythm. Some symptoms are so fleeting that they do not permit patients to apply electrodes in sufficient time to capture the arrhythmia. In those instances, the continuous-loop transtelephonic monitor is indicated.

In patients whose symptoms include syncope or near syncope, the use of event monitors is difficult. For these patients, the continuous ambulatory ECG is critical for diagnosis. It is also critical to diagnose events that may occur during sleep, or events that may be suspected but which are associated with either no symptoms or such minimal symptoms that they do not elicit a response from the patient that would urge the use of an event monitor.

The continuous 24-hour ambulatory ECG is essential for the diagnosis of the sick sinus syndrome. Invasive electrophysiologic tests, such as sinus node overdrive suppression and sinoatrial conduction time assessment, may be completely normal in patients with marked sinus node dysfunction. Thus, the best diagnostic tool for this disorder is continuous ECG monitoring. Abnormalities of AV conduction can also be recognized using 24-hour ambulatory ECG monitoring. In addition, continuous ambulatory ECG monitoring is useful in the assessment of autonomic dysfunction. For instance, in many patients atrial fibrillation may be vagally mediated.

Assessment of therapy for supraventricular arrhythmias is often facilitated by 24-hour ECG monitoring. In fact, both drug therapy and nonpharmacologic therapy are often best assessed using the ambulatory ECG. An example of the former is assessing the efficacy of drug therapy to control the ventricular response rate in patients with chronic atrial fibrillation. An example of the latter is the assessment of the adequacy of radiofrequency modulation of AV conduction in patients with chronic atrial fibrillation.

The major current applications of ambulatory ECG monitoring of supraventricular arrhythmias include:

1. Assessment of symptoms (frequent, preferably daily) possibly associated with a transient arrhythmia.
2. Characterization of known or suspected supraventricular arrhythmias.
3. Assessment of sinus node dysfunction.
4. Correlation of the effects of the activities of daily living with supraventricular arrhythmias.
5. Assessment of AV conduction.
6. Determination of the effectiveness of antiarrhythmic therapy (drug therapy, pacemaker therapy, ablative therapy, or surgical therapy).

Ambulatory ECG monitoring supplements the role of invasive electrophysiologic testing in characterizing some tachyarrhythmias, such as AV re-entrant tachycardia (associated with an overt or concealed accessory AV connection) and AV nodal re-entrant tachycardia, and in characterizing some AV conduction abnormalities, such as aberrant ventricular conduction during a supraventricular arrhythmia.

Sinus Node Dysfunction

Continuous 24-hour ambulatory ECG remains the most reliable tool for diagnosing sinus node dysfunction.[1] Recordings have to be quite long, as abnormalities which are diagnostic may be episodic. Sinus pauses or sinus bradycardia when associated with appropriate symptoms are usually diagnostic of sinus node dysfunction (Figure 3.1). The correlations with symptoms is invaluable though not always a requisite. Furthermore, it is important to emphasize that markers of apparent sinus node dysfunction may be normal under certain circumstances. For instance, in the well-trained athlete, sinus bradycardia and even sinus pauses greater than 3 seconds may reflect normal sinus node function.[2] Many of the markers of sinus node dysfunction which occur when awake are not abnormal when asleep. Standards for abnormal sinus node function during sleep are not well established. Thus, abnormal findings which occur during the day almost always have more significance, especially when associated with symptoms.

The following ECG data on Holter monitoring are the primary diagnostic criteria for establishing sinus node dysfunction:

1. Sustained sinus bradycardia present throughout the 24-hour period at rates of 50 bpm or less.
2. Sinus pauses up to 6 seconds, although sinus pauses between 3 and 6 seconds may be indicative of sinus node dysfunction.
3. Permanent or intermittent periods of symptomatic AV junctional rhythm.
4. Documentation of bradycardia–tachycardia syndrome, particularly as classically described with failure of the prompt return of sinus rhythm following spontaneous termination of supraventricular tachyarrhythmia (presumably due to exaggerated overdrive suppression) (Figure 3.1).

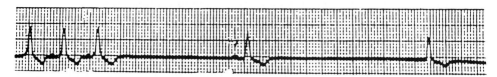

Figure 3.1 An ECG event recording from a 76-year-old man who complained of frequent near-syncopal spells. Tachycardia–bradycardia syndrome with sinus node dysfunction is documented on the recording.

The latter syndrome is frequently associated with abnormalities of AV conduction and of the AV junctional escape pacemaker. In fact, the abnormal AV junctional escape pacemaker is ultimately responsible for the clinical symptoms of lightheadedness or syncope leading to a period of ventricular asystole.

Suspected Supraventricular Arrhythmia Associated with Palpitation

Of course, palpitation has many potential etiologies, and will not always prove to be secondary to a cardiac rhythm disorder. When associated with arrhythmia, the ambulatory ECG is useful for accurate correlation of the symptoms with the cardiac rhythm.

If palpitation is infrequent but daily, obtaining a 24-hour ambulatory ECG is quite appropriate. If palpitation is more episodic, an event monitor is indicated. When the events are fleeting though episodic, a continuous-loop ECG recorder should be used (Figure 3.2). If the episodes are sufficiently long to allow wrist bracelet application, use of a transtelephonic monitor is usually more convenient for the patient. Occasionally, one has to be quite persistent in the application of any of these techniques to obtain a diagnosis, or to find a lack of correlation of the rhythm with the symptoms. Emphasis must be placed on keeping an accurate log, particularly when using a 24-hour ambulatory ECG.

Atrial Fibrillation/Flutter

Atrial fibrillation can be documented by many different methods. When the rhythm is sustained, patients can present to a medical facility, permitting the rhythm to be documented by a 12-lead ECG. However, in some instances, it is preferable to make the diagnosis using a 24-hour ambulatory ECG or an ECG event monitor. Clearly, the ambulatory ECG is useful when symptoms are episodic. In addition, asymptomatic episodes of atrial fibrillation are not uncommon.[3] Furthermore, there are unique applications of the 24-hour ambulatory ECG in atrial fibrillation, particularly in understanding the relationship to autonomically mediated atrial fibrillation. The patterns of vagally mediated or adrenergically mediated paroxysmal atrial fibrillation should be identifiable on 24-hour ambulatory ECG.[4] These patterns should fit the clinical history. Close attention to heart rate changes which occur in proximity to the onset of the arrhythmia is necessary. A mixed picture of vagal and adrenergic atrial fibrillation may be difficult to identify.

Atrial fibrillation of vagal origin is associated with a predominance of men over women at a ratio of about 4:1. The age when the first symptoms appear is usually between 40 and

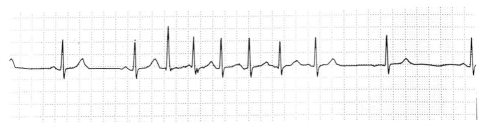

Figure 3.2 An ECG strip from a continuous-loop recorder, demonstrating a short paroxysm of a supraventricular arrhythmia in a patient with fleeting palpitations.

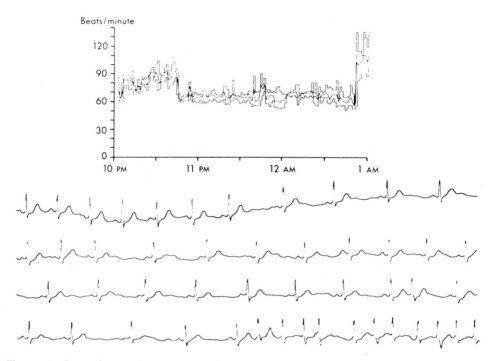

Figure 3.3 Onset of an episode of vagally mediated nocturnal paroxysmal atrial fibrillation. The patient probably went to sleep a few minutes before 11 pm, as suggested by the fall in the heart rate at that time in the rate–time plot. The atrial fibrillation started two hours later, as shown by the trend of heart rates in the diagram (mean, maximal, and minimal frequencies), and the bottom ECG traces. Note in the two top ECG tracings the important beat-to-beat cycle length variations, and the presence of an atrial premature beat in the third tracing. (Reproduced with permission from reference 4)

50 years, with extremes ranging from 25 to 60 years. The clinical history may be as short as weeks and as long as 15 or 20 years. An important part of the syndrome is the striking absence of the development of chronic atrial fibrillation in these patients. Furthermore, the arrhythmia should be classified as so-called 'lone atrial fibrillation', as it is not associated with any underlying structural heart disease or obvious cause. The number of attacks of atrial fibrillation is variable from patient to patient. Commonly, there are weekly episodes lasting from a few minutes to several hours. An essential feature is the occurrence of episodes at night, not infrequently ending by morning. Rest, relationship to eating, particularly after dinner, and alcohol ingestion also are factors associated with this form of atrial fibrillation. In terms of the Holter monitor, the arrhythmia is heralded by a progressive bradycardia (55–60 bpm) that reflects increased vagal tone (Figure 3.3). The onset of atrial fibrillation is usually immediately preceded by a further prolongation of the sinus cycle length. Due to increased vagal tone, characteristic of this etiology of atrial fibrillation is a ventricular response less than 100 bpm. Sinus node dysfunction is not a part of this syndrome, so it should be readily distinguished from the so-called tachycardia–bradycardia syndrome.

Adrenergically mediated atrial fibrillation is quite different, and is rather uncommon. It is principally found in patients with hyperthyroidism, pheochromocytoma, or cardio-myopathy with heart failure. Palpitation occurs predominantly or exclusively during the daytime hours, particularly in the morning, during exercise, or during emotional stress. The electrocardiographic features may be those of atrial fibrillation, but frequently,

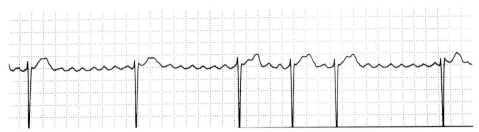

Figure 3.4 A Holter monitor ECG strip recorded during atrial fibrillation while the patient was at rest. It demonstrates a slow ventricular response. The first, second and fifth cycle lengths are constant, indicating high-degree AV block with AV junctional escape beats. This suggests either an intrinsic AV conduction abnormality or, more likely, excessive block at the AV node due to therapy in this patient receiving both digoxin and diltiazem.

particularly in the early stages of the episodes, they consist of runs of atrial tachycardia alternating with sinus rhythm. Typically, the onset of the arrhythmia occurs with an increase in sinus rate, usually to at least 90 bpm.

After the diagnosis of atrial fibrillation has been made, the principal use of the Holter monitor is to assess the efficacy of antiarrhythmic drugs in suppression of atrial fibrillation, or the adequacy of the control of the ventricular response during atrial fibrillation both during rest (Figure 3.4) and in association with activity. Furthermore, the Holter monitor can be used to assess therapy in other regards. Virtually all antiarrhythmic agents have the potential for proarrhythmic adverse effects.[5] These can include:

1. Recurrence of the arrhythmia, not as atrial fibrillation, but as 'slow' atrial flutter such that 1:1 AV conduction may occur (class IA or IC antiarrhythmic agents, usually class IC agents).
2. Torsade de pointes (class IA or class III antiarrhythmic agents).
3. Development of, or worsening of, sinus node dysfunction (virtually all the antiarrhythmic agents, calcium-channel blockers, and beta-blockers).
4. Development of, or worsening of, various forms of AV conduction abnormalities (virtually all the antiarrhythmic classes of agents, but in particular, beta-blockers, calcium-channel blockers, and amiodarone).
5. Development of other conduction abnormalities such as bundle branch block.

Holter monitoring may assess the efficacy of nonpharmacologic therapy of atrial fibrillation. The Holter monitor can examine the adequacy of radiofrequency ablation performed either to cause complete heart block or to modify AV nodal conduction. In patients who have undergone His bundle ablation due to paroxysmal atrial fibrillation, some form of dual chamber pacemaker system is placed. The idea is that during sinus rhythm, the pacemaker will sense the atrial activity and initiate ventricular pacing at an appropriate interval, providing the patient with a sinus-node mediated rhythm. When paroxysmal atrial fibrillation occurs, depending on the pacemaker system used, a programmed response to maintain a clinically acceptable paced ventricular rate should be expected. The Holter monitor is invaluable in assessing whether or not the pacemaker system is working as designed, or whether programming changes must be made. In addition, for those patients who have had radiofrequency ablation to modify AV nodal conduction as a method to control the ventricular response rate during atrial fibrillation, the Holter monitor is critical for assessing adequacy of the ventricular rate in the presence of atrial fibrillation (paroxysmal or chronic). Close attention to the ventricular response during exercise is necessary.

For patients who undergo a Maze operation or a catheter ablation procedure to prevent atrial fibrillation, a Holter monitor becomes critical to assess the efficacy of the procedure. It is particularly important to evaluate symptoms that may possibly be associated with an arrhythmia in the period following such therapy. And finally, in anticipation of newer therapies such as the implantable automatic atrial defibrillator, once again, the Holter monitor will be invaluable for characterizing the efficacy of therapy.

The application of ambulatory ECG monitoring in the diagnosis and treatment of *atrial flutter* is much the same as for atrial fibrillation. There are, however, a few aspects which apply more particularly to atrial flutter. Class IC agents show the atrial flutter rate, perhaps to rates as low as 180–200 bpm, permitting 1:1 AV conduction, and on occasion, class IA agents may do the same thing. Since atrial flutter, like atrial fibrillation, tends to recur, ambulatory ECG monitoring is essential in evaluating this possibility. In addition, recent advances in radiofrequency catheter ablation have enabled physicians to cure atrial flutter by creating a lesion at an apparent isthmus in the atrial flutter re-entrant circuit. However, late recurrences have been reported, and subsequent presentation with atrial fibrillation in such treated patients has also been recognized. Ambulatory ECG monitoring, therefore, is indicated for the evaluation of such therapies.

Atrial Tachycardia

At present, the rhythms which fall in this category probably have more than one mechanism. A significant number of patients have atrial tachycardia on the basis of some form of re-entry. These patients usually have underlying structural heart disease. A tachycardia mediated cardiomyopathy must be excluded in all such patients with concomitant global left ventricular dysfunction. Effective therapy directed at the rhythm disturbances will often reverse the cardiomyopathy. For patients with atrial tachycardias, the same diagnostic and therapeutic indications for Holter monitoring or ECG event monitoring as for atrial fibrillation or atrial flutter largely pertain.

Patients with lung disease may exhibit so-called 'multifocal atrial tachycardia'. This arrhythmia usually responds to correction of underlying pulmonary abnormalities or drug toxicity. Ambulatory ECG monitoring should help assess the clinical effectiveness of treatment.

A new syndrome, 'inappropriate sinus tachycardia', has been reported.[6] Patients exhibit a sinus rate which is 'set' at a more rapid level. Although the 24-hour Holter monitor shows heart rate variability, average heart rates are greater than 100 bpm. This must be distinguished from sinus node re-entry tachycardia. Sinus node re-entry tachycardia has an abrupt onset as opposed to the warm-up of sinus tachycardia (Figure 3.5). Like all atrial tachycardias, when incessant, a tachycardia mediated cardiomyopathy may result. Thus, slowing of the sinus rate, usually with beta-blockers, is essential. An early experience with sinus node modification by radiofrequency energy has been

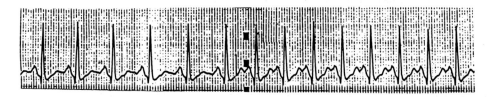

Figure 3.5 An ECG loop recording from a 19-year-old man who used cocaine for many years. He complained of palpitations. A tachycardia with an abrupt onset and a sinus-like P wave morphology is noted. This is consistent with sinus node re-entry tachycardia.

reported.[7] Once again, ambulatory ECG monitoring of some sort is critical both for diagnosis and for evaluation of therapy.

Atrioventricular Re-entrant Tachycardia

These rhythms are associated with the presence of one or more accessory AV connection(s). When antegrade conduction is possible over the accessory AV connection, a delta wave is present in the ECG during sinus rhythm as a result of ventricular pre-excitation. The most common form of ventricular pre-excitation is associated with the Wolff–Parkinson–White syndrome. The presence of one or more accessory AV connections may be associated with a constellation of arrhythmias, the most common of which is atrioventricular re-entrant tachycardia (AVRT). In some patients, the accessory AV connection only conducts in one direction because of the presence of unidirectional block. Unidirectional block may be either antegrade or retrograde. Most commonly, the block is antegrade, and the presence of an accessory AV connection is not apparent from the ECG. Such a pathway may be associated with orthodromic AVRT (O-AVRT), and is referred to as 'concealed' because, without the presence of ventricular pre-excitation, it is usually not possible to know without invasive electrophysiologic studies that such a pathway is present. When the accessory AV connection conducts only in an antegrade direction, it may be associated with antidromic AVRT (A-AVRT), but the accessory pathway is virtually always manifest because of a delta wave present in the 12-lead ECG.

The ambulatory ECG is invaluable in diagnosing and directing therapy of arrhythmias present in patients with the Wolff–Parkinson–White syndrome. There are several reasons why arrhythmias associated with WPW and related syndromes are important to diagnose. First, AVRT can now be cured by radiofrequency ablation of the accessory AV connection during electrophysiologic study. Therefore, identification of the presence of the arrhythmia serves to direct therapy. Additionally, patients with the WPW syndrome are at significant risk to develop atrial fibrillation or atrial flutter, and, critically, the accessory AV connection in some patients will be capable of conducting most or all the atrial impulses to the ventricles, resulting in very rapid, often life-threatening, ventricular rates and rhythms, including ventricular fibrillation.[8] For this reason, even patients with the WPW syndrome who are asymptomatic should at the very least undergo a Holter monitor exam. If any subclinical arrhythmia is detected, electrophysiologic study to characterize the accessory pathway is indicated, possibly with subsequent radiofrequency ablation of the accessory pathway.

The ambulatory ECG can be invaluable in several other ways. In patients with O-AVRT, the change in cycle length observed with spontaneous bundle branch block aberration can help guide accessory pathway location. The cycle length of AVRT which utilizes a free wall pathway on the same side (ipsilateral) as the bundle branch block generally prolongs by greater than 35 ms. In addition, should atrial fibrillation develop, the RR interval during atrial fibrillation can guide the urgency of treatment. Patients with short RR intervals (≤250 ms) are at risk for sudden cardiac death and should be appropriately triaged for therapy. Also, multiple QRS complex morphologies during atrial fibrillation usually indicate the presence of multiple accessory AV connections.[10]

For patients following apparent successful radiofrequency ablation therapy, it is often important to document the efficacy of the procedure. Holter monitoring can demonstrate the absence of a delta wave over a 24-hour period, and may identify the cause of continued symptoms (e.g. palpitation), if present. The latter are frequently due to premature atrial beats which may initiate short runs of intra-atrial re-entrant rhythms, giving the patient symptoms. Once identified, this arrhythmia following successful radiofrequency therapy may be treated, if need be. Also, it is well recognized that the initial radiofrequency ablation therapy may not be successful. Recurrence rates have ranged from 2% to 10%.[11] In such instances, it becomes important to document the presence again of AVRT. In the latter instance, patients are usually well advised to have another radiofrequency ablation procedure performed, as the data clearly show that a second procedure has a high likelihood of success (usually at least 95%).

For those patients in whom, for any number of reasons, antiarrhythmic drug therapy is deemed the appropriate therapy of AVRT, the Holter monitor or ECG event monitor becomes a useful tool to explain symptoms that may persist despite this therapy.

Atrioventricular Nodal Re-entrant Tachycardia (AVNRT)

The relationship of Holter monitoring/ECG event monitoring to the diagnosis and treatment of this arrhythmia is virtually identical to that for the pre-excitation syndromes and AV re-entrant tachycardia. Perhaps the only qualitative difference is that there are many patients whose AVNRT is very easily controlled with simple medication, such as a daily dose of digoxin. Care must be taken to exclude an anterograde conducting accessory AV connection before initiating therapy with AV nodal blocking agents. The absence of a delta wave even during periods of high vagal tone is reassuring, but does not exclude the presence of an anterograde conducting pathway, especially a far left-sided pathway. And once again, if pharmacologic therapy is initiated, the ambulatory ECG is an effective tool to assess efficacy.

Assessment of AV Conduction Abnormalities

The ambulatory ECG is invaluable in assessing abnormalities of AV conduction, particularly when either minimally symptomatic, or episodic. The correlation with symptoms remains essential to the appropriate consideration of permanent pacing (Figure 3.6). On occasion, this evaluation is often in concert with invasive electrophysiologic studies, which include His bundle recording and programmed stimulation studies designed to stress the AV conduction system and elicit underlying abnormalities. Occasionally, these abnormalities may be secondary to a treatable or reversible cause, most often, drug therapy.

Screening for AV block is generally not indicated unless a patient has symptoms. However, in the presence of known cardiac infiltrative disorders like sarcoidosis, or calcified aortic stenosis, a screening Holter monitor to exclude paroxysmal AV block is reasonable.

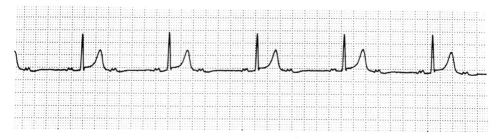

Figure 3.6 An ECG loop recording from a 70-year-old women who had transient episodes of dizziness for 3 months. Holter monitor ECG recordings were normal. An invasive electrophysiologic study documented normal AV node function. This recording documents transient 2:1 AV block.

Inappropriate Use of Outpatient Ambulatory ECG Monitoring

In patients in whom symptoms are severe and thought potentially life-threatening, inhospital telemetered ECG monitoring is a more appropriate strategy. This would include patients with syncope or near syncope in the setting of Wolff–Parkinson–White syndrome or structural heart disease. Structural heart disease can usually be ascertained after a careful history, physical exam, and 12-lead ECG. An echocardiogram to evaluate myocardial and valvular structure is usually reasonable. In this situation, appropriate invasive studies may supplement inhouse ECG monitoring to elicit and characterize any electrical abnormality.

Acknowledgement

The authors acknowledge support in part by grant RO1 HL38408 from the National Institutes of Health, National Heart, Lung and Blood Institute, Bethesda, Maryland, and a grant from the Wuliger Foundation, Cleveland, Ohio.

References

1. Vera Z, Mason DT. Detection of sinus node dysfunction: consideration of clinical application of testing methods. *Am Heart J* 1981; **102**: 308–12.
2. Swiryn S, McDonough T, Hueter DC. Sinus node function and dysfunction. *Med Clin N Am* 1984; **68**: 935–54.
3. Page RL, Wilkinson WE, Clair WK, McCarthy EA, Pritchett ELC. Asymptomatic arrhythmias in patients with symptomatic paroxysmal atrial fibrillation and paroxysmal supraventricular tachycardia. *Circulation* 1994; **89**: 224–7.
4. Coumel P. Role of the autonomic nervous system in paroxysmal atrial fibrillation. Touboul P, Waldo AL (eds), *Atrial Arrhythmias: Current Concepts and Management*. St Louis, MO: C. V. Mosby, 1990, 248–61.
5. Prystowsky EN. Inpatient versus outpatient initiation of antiarrhythmic drug therapy for patients with supraventricular tachycardia. *Clin Cardiol* 1994; **17**: II.7–10.
6. Morillo CA, Klein GJ, Thakur RK, Li H, Zardini M, Yee R. Mechanism of 'inappropriate' sinus tachycardia: role of sympathovagal balance. *Circulation* 1994; **90**: 873–7.
7. Waspe LE, Chien WW, Merillat JC, Stark SI. Sinus node modification using radiofrequency current in a patient with persistent inappropriate sinus tachycardia. *PACE* 1994; **17**: 1569–76.
8. Zardini M, Yee R, Thakur RK, Klein GJ. Risk of sudden arrhythmic death in the Wolff–Parkinson–White syndrome: current perspectives, *PACE* 1994; **17**: 966–75.
9. Kerr CR, Gallagher JJ, German LD. Changes in ventriculoatrial intervals with bundle branch block aberration during reciprocating tachycardia in patients with accessory atrioventricular pathways. *Circulation* 1982; **66**: 196–201.
10. Fananapazir L, German LD, Gallagher JJ, Lowe JE, Prystowsky EN. Importance of pre-excited QRS morphology during induced atrial fibrillation to the diagnosis and localization of multiple accessory pathways. *Circulation* 1990; **81**: 578–85.
11. Kay GN, Epstein AE, Dailey SM, Plumb VJ. Role of radiofrequency ablation in the management of supraventricular arrhythmias: experience in 760 consecutive patients. *J Cardiovasc Electrophysiol* 1993; **4**: 371–89.

4

Ventricular Arrhythmias

Frank I. Marcus

Introduction

Ventricular premature beats (VPBs) are ubiquitous and even short runs of ventricular tachycardia (VT) may by seen in asymptomatic people. In normal, healthy subjects aged 10–30 years, the incidence of VT – defined as three or more consecutive VPBs – is in the range 1–3%.[1] The prevalence of frequent VPBs increases with age, as does the prevalence of ventricular couplets and VT. In a group of healthy elderly people aged 60–85 years, ventricular couplets were observed during 24-hour ambulatory ECG monitoring in 11% and ventricular tachycardia of 3–13 beats in 4%.[2] The prevalence of episodes of transient VT in an elderly population, including those with cardiac disease, was observed in 4.3% of women and 10.3% of men.[3] Multivariant analysis showed that there was a higher prevalence of ventricular arrhythmias including a combination of VT and at least 15 VPBs per hour in subjects with an abnormal left ventricular ejection fraction.

These data indicate that there is an appreciable prevalence of ventricular arrhythmias among an asymptomatic population, as well as in patients who have cardiac disease with impaired left ventricular function. When ambulatory ECG monitoring is used for diagnostic purposes to evaluate the cause of syncope or pre-syncope, there needs to be a correlation between the symptoms and the ventricular arrhythmias. Conversely, the lack of ventricular arrhythmias when pre-syncope or syncope occurs is particularly useful to exclude ventricular arrhythmias as an etiology of the symptoms.[4]

Ambulatory ECG Monitoring after Myocardial Infarction

As an aid in risk assessment

The development and commercial availability of the ambulatory ECG recorder in the 1960s made it possible to study the relationship between the frequency and complexity of ventricular arrhythmias after myocardial infarction and subsequent mortality. The yield of recording VPBs during 6 hours of ambulatory ECG monitoring was increased twelve-fold compared with that of a 36-second ECG.[5] About ten days after a myocardial infarction, only 15–25% of patients have 10 or more VPBs per hour.[6] Mortality rates are 2.5–4 times as great for patients with at least 10 VPBs per hour in a 24-hour ECG recording in comparison with lower VPB frequencies. In addition, pairs or runs of VPBs are associated with death independent of VPB frequency. Transient VT (defined as at least three consecutive ventricular beats at a rate of >100 bpm) occurring on a predischarge 24-hour ECG recording has a strong relationship with subsequent mortality (odds ratio = 4.2) but occurs in only about 12% of patients. Since it is well known that ventricular arrhythmias are more frequent in patients with impaired left ventricular function, the question was raised as to whether the presence of ventricular arrhythmias was simply another marker of decreased left ventricular function. It was found that ventricular arrhythmias are a risk indicator for subsequent mortality independent of the associated left ventricular dysfunction.[6]

Assessment of antiarrhythmic drug efficacy in clinical trials

With the information that ventricular arrhythmias after a myocardial infarction are an independent risk factor, it was reasonable to assume that ventricular premature beats singly or in runs could trigger VT or ventricular fibrillation, and that suppression of the ventricular ectopy would decrease the mortality in the first few years after hospital discharge. Randomized trials evaluating the influence of antiarrhythmic drugs on mortality after infarction did *not* show a significant decrease in mortality, but they did not use serial ECG monitoring to guide therapy.[4] Treatment with beta-blockers was found to blunt the rise in VPB frequency seen in control patients after myocardial infarction. However, there was a similar reduction in both arrhythmic and nonarrhythmic death rates in patients with or without arrhythmias at baseline. It was important to determine whether suppressing ventricular premature beats and repetitive forms would decrease mortality in those patients who had these arrhythmias and who survived a myocardial infarction.

The Cardiac Arrhythmia Pilot Study (CAPS) was undertaken in 1987 as a first step to answer this question. This study was designed to determine whether frequent or repetitive ventricular arrhythmias after myocardial infarction could be suppressed with a drug strategy that incorporated dose ranging and changing drugs. This was answered in the affirmative, and the second phase of these investigations was launched entitled Cardiac Arrhythmia Suppression Trial (CAST). This randomized, placebo-controlled, double-blind, multicentered clinical trial was designed to determine whether suppression of ventricular arrhythmias after myocardial infarction with antiarrhythmic drug treatment would reduce arrhythmic death.[7]

The target group consisted of survivors of myocardial infarction less than 80 years of age who had at least six VPBs per hour on a 24-hour ECG obtained between 6 days and two years after myocardial infarction. The primary end-point was arrhythmic death or cardiac arrest. In April 1989, encainide and flecainide were removed from CAST because of strong evidence that these drugs increased the death rate in comparison with placebo (Table 4.1).

The study design was altered to enroll patients with an increased risk of arrhythmic death by limiting enrollment to patients with a left ventricular ejection fraction ≤40% who had their infarction 6–90 days before enrollment. In addition, the inclusion criteria were broadened for the length of symptomatic ventricular runs >15 beats at a rate of ≥120 bpm up to 30 seconds of this asymptomatic arrhythmia. Subsequently the trial was discontinued since there was no apparent difference in mortality between the placebo-

Table 4.1 Treatment results from the CAST trial

	Placebo	Encainide/flecainide	Odds ratio
Patient numbers	725	730	
Follow-up	10 mo	10 mo	
Sudden cardiac death	9 (1.2%)	33 (4.5%)	3.2 (1.7–5.9)
Other cardiac death	6 (0.8%)	14 (1.9%)	2.2 (0.9–5.4)
Non-cardiac/unclassified	7 (0.9%)	9 (1.2%)	
Total number of deaths or cardiac arrest	22 (3%)	56 (7.6%)	2.5 (1.6–3.9)

and moricizine-treated patients. The findings from the CAST study indicated that suppression of ventricular arrhythmias after myocardial infarction with drugs with class 1C antiarrhythmic action does not predict improved survival and in fact was associated with an increased risk of arrhythmic death. Although moricizine is difficult to categorize according to the Vaughan Williams classification, it has many characteristics of a class 1C drug.

The CAST study also brought into question the role of ambulatory ECG monitoring as a means of assessing drug efficacy, since the antiarrhythmic drugs used effectively suppressed ventricular ectopy but this effect did not predict better outcome. However, the results of CAST should not be generalized to other situations such as assessing antiarrhythmic drug efficacy in patients with sustained VT or patients resuscitated from cardiac arrest. Observations from the CAPS trial provided some insight as to which patients were likely to have VPBs suppressed on the ambulatory ECG by antiarrhythmic drugs used in this trial. In patients treated with encainide or flecainide, the greatest response was observed in the absence of a prior myocardial infarction in patients with a higher ejection fraction and in the younger age population.[8] Ancillary evidence that patients with greater cardiac damage were less likely to respond to antiarrhythmic drugs was the fact that patients who were entered into the CAST study but who were not randomized to double-blind therapy, primarily because of lack of suppression of VPBs or adverse effects during titration, were older, and had a lower left ventricular ejection fraction. Also, these nonrandomized patients had a greater use of digitalis, diuretics and antihypertensive drugs.[9]

Whether antiarrhythmic drugs that have electrophysiological effects different from class 1C, such as amiodarone, may have a favorable effect on mortality and cardiac arrest in patients after myocardial infarction with frequent or complex ventricular ectopy, is being investigated in the Canadian Amiodarone Myocardial Infarction Trial (CAMIAT).[10] Preliminary results are encouraging. The Basel Antiarrhythmic Study of Infarct Survival (BASIS) trial studied patients, one to three days before hospital discharge after myocardial infarction, who had frequent multiform or repetitive ventricular arrhythmias (Lown class 3 or 4 B) in at least two of 24 hours of ECG recording. In this small ($n = 198$) study, the probability of survival was significantly greater than that of control patients, and arrhythmic events (sudden death and sustained VT and VF) were significantly reduced by amiodarone. The European Infarct Amiodarone Trial (EMIAT) is also evaluating the role of amiodarone after myocardial infarction but this study is not testing the VPB suppression hypothesis. Patients are being enrolled with a left ventricular ejection fraction <40% and a 24-hour ECG recording is being performed, but the results do not constitute part of the inclusion criteria and follow-up ambulatory ECG recordings are not being done routinely. The above data suggest that the VPB suppression hypothesis is still viable, although results obtained with amiodarone may not be generalized to other antiarrhythmic drugs since amiodarone is a unique compound with many and varied metabolic effects.

The widespread use of thrombolytic therapy appears to result in fewer post-MI patients with nonsustained VT, but there is probably no decrease in the prevalence of frequent VPBs (>10 per hour). Nevertheless the association of frequent VPBs remains a significant predictor of total as well as sudden death mortality even after the use of thrombolytic agents.[11]

Ambulatory ECG Monitoring in Heart Failure

As an aid in risk assessment

Numerous studies have clearly demonstrated that patients with heart failure not only have frequent VPBs but a significant proportion of these patients have episodes of transient VT.[12] Between 28 and 80% of patients with heart failure evaluated by ambulatory ECG recordings have transient VT. Although the prognostic importance of VPBs alone in these patients is still debatable, it is clear that transient VT in patients with heart failure carries a significantly increased risk for overall cardiac mortality and sudden cardiac death. For example, in the Veterans Administration Cooperative trial, V/HeFT II, that compared the outcome of 804 patients with left ventricular ejection fraction <45%, randomized to enalapril or hydralazine/isosorbide dinitrate, couplets were noted in 56–60% and VT ($\geqslant$3 consecutive beats) in 7–29%. The presence of VT at 3 months, one year and two years, predicted significantly higher mortality during the subsequent year.[13] Patients with more than 10 VPBs per hour also had a higher mortality in the first 18 months than those with either no VPBs or fewer than 10 VPBs per hour. Correlates of VPB frequency appear to be severe left ventricular dysfunction, such as left ventricular ejection fraction <20%, as well as increasing age. In the Captopril–Digoxin Multicenter Study, analysis of various factors as continuous variables showed that VPB frequency coupled with VT frequency were univariate predictors of total mortality. In addition, couplets and ventricular tachycardia frequency were also significant univariate predictors of sudden cardiac death.

The significance of a reduction in ventricular ectopy

Since VT and couplets, and possibly VPB frequency, predict increased mortality in heart failure, it would be expected that a decrease in ventricular ectopy would be associated with a decrease in mortality rate, particularly in sudden cardiac death.

This hypothesis appears to be true in patients treated with ACE inhibitors but not necessarily in patients treated with antiarrhythmic drugs. In the V/HeFT II trial there was a 49% reduction in sudden cardiac death at two years in the enalapril group as compared with the hydralazine–isosorbide dinitrate treated patients.[13] This decrease coincided with the decrease in ventricular tachycardia prevalence and the decrease in new VT emergence. This effect could not be ascribed to a preferential improvement in left ventricular function since left ventricular ejection fraction improved more in patients in the hydralazine–isosorbide dinitrate arm than in the enalapril arm. On the other hand, the suppression of VPBs with class 1 antiarrhythmic drugs does not appear to decrease the risk of sudden death in patients with heart failure. Several small trials of amiodarone in heart failure have shown that this unique drug does in fact effectively reduce ventricular ectopy and most trials have reported a trend towards decreasing mortality.

However, two recently reported large trials have had dissimilar results. In the multicenter trial conducted in Argentina, 516 patients with advanced heart failure (mean left ventricular ejection fraction 19–20%) were randomized to amiodarone 300 mg a day or standard treatment. A 24-hour ambulatory ECG was performed prior to amiodarone.[14] After two years, amiodarone treatment was associated with a 27% reduction in total mortality, and there was a trend towards decreased sudden death mortality and death due to progressive heart failure. The decrease in mortality was independent of the presence of transient VT that was present in 33% of the patients.

The Veterans Cooperative Study recently reported their preliminary results[15] with amiodarone 400 mg/day, compared with placebo in a randomized double-blind trial in 674 patients with congestive heart failure (NYHA class III/IV, left ventricular dilatation, ejection fraction $\leqslant$40% and $\geqslant$10 PVBs/hour). In comparison with placebo, amiodarone significantly suppressed arrhythmia frequency; however, there was no significant difference in all-cause mortality between treatment groups.

From these two recent investigations one can conclude that amiodarone does not increase mortality in patients with congestive heart failure, and it is possible that in selected groups, yet to be defined, this drug may decrease mortality. It can be stated that the VPB suppression theory has not been substantiated in patients with heart failure even with the potent suppression of ventricular ectopy with amiodarone.

Ambulatory ECG Monitoring for Ventricular Ectopy in Hypertrophic Cardiomyopathy

As an aid in risk assessment

It has been particulary difficult to obtain reliable markers to predict the clinical course in patients with hypertrophic cardiomyopathy (HCM). Cardiac death, presumably arrhythmic, in patients with HCM occurs at an annual rate of 2–4% in referral centers.[16] Sudden death is most common in children and young adults at ages between 10 and 35 years. Of note, HCM is the most common cause of unexpected death in young competitive athletes.

The mechanism of sudden death in HCM encompasses the spectrum of paroxysmal atrial fibrillation initiating ventricular fibrillation, ventricular arrhythmias and ischemia. Although in children and adolescents with this condition sudden death is higher than in adults, the occurrence of transient VT on ambulatory monitoring is uncommon, even in patients in this age group who have been resuscitated from cardiac arrest. Thus ambulatory ECG monitoring is not a useful prognostic indicator in patients in this age group.

In the adult with HCM, transient VT, often at a slow rate, can be found in about 25% of these patients. The presence of transient VT on ambulatory ECG monitoring is the single best marker of high risk but its positive predictive value is only about 22%. The absence of this finding has a 97% negative predictive value.

Because the finding of transient VT carries a seven-fold increase in the incidence of sudden death but the positive predictive value of this finding is low, other means are needed to identify which of these patients with transient VT are prone to sudden cardiac death. For example, it has been reported that patients with HCM who are at risk of sudden death have increased dispersion and inhomogeneity of intraventricular conduction determined at electrophysiological study, which may create conditions for arrhythmogenesis.[17] Treatment of asymptomatic patients who have transient VT with amiodarone is controversial.[18]

In summary, findings on the ambulatory ECG are not by themselves sufficient to accurately stratify patients with HCM into a high-risk subgroup to determine further treatment strategies for preventing sudden cardiac death.

Transient ventricular tachycardias in patients with valvular heart disease

Compared with controls, patients with mitral valve prolapse do not have an appreciable excess of complex ventricular arrhythmias.[19] Significant mitral regurgitation is associated with frequent VPBs and transient ventricular tachycardia. Mortality in MVP patients is determined by the degree of left ventricular dysfunction rather than the presence of transient VT *per se*.

Complex ventricular ectopy is common in patients with mitral regurgitation, aortic stenosis or aortic regurgitation. In these conditions the presence and severity of the arrhythmias relates to the degree of left ventricular dysfunction. However, there are insufficient data to indicate that transient VT is an independent adverse prognostic factor for sudden cardiac death.[19]

Ambulatory ECG Monitoring to Predict Antiarrhythmic Drug Efficacy

In 1982, Graboys and associates published the first study with a large number of patients using ambulatory ECG as a guide to evaluate antiarrhythmic drug efficacy.[20] Their data indicated that protection against sudden cardiac death could be achieved in patients with VT or those who were resuscitated from sudden cardiac arrest by suppressing ventricular arrhythmias using ambulatory ECG monitoring.

This approach encompassed a short control monitoring period, followed by ECG monitoring for 3–5 hours after oral administration of a single large dose of an antiarrhythmic drug. If the drug suppressed runs of ventricular tachycardia and was tolerated, a 24-hour ECG recording was obtained while the patient was receiving maintenance doses of the drug. Efficacy prediction required total elimination of transient VT and R-on-T beats, reduction of over 90% of pairs and over 50% of VPBs. Two antiarrhythmic drugs were generally employed to provide 'a so-called fail-safe program of drug protection'. Over an average follow-up of 29.6 months, there were six sudden deaths among 98 patients in whom an antiarrhythmic drug was found that was predicted to be effective with an annual mortality of 2.3%. In contrast, of the 25 patients in whom the drug did not abolish ventricular ectopy to the required extent, 17 died suddenly. There was less possibility of suppressing ventricular tachycardia by antiarrhythmic drugs, the lower the left ventricular ejection fraction or the higher the density of ventricular tachycardia on baseline ambulatory ECG monitoring. Importantly, in a later publication[21] they concluded that ventricular function was the most powerful predictor of survival and, when left ventricular ejection fraction was less than 30%, the control of ventricular arrhythmias did not significantly improve survival.

The initial encouraging results with the use of ambulatory ECG monitoring to guide antiarrhythmic drug efficacy was a major impetus to compare this method with that of electrophysiological testing (EPS) to determine which of the two assessment methods yields the most accurate prediction of drug efficacy. This was the aim of a National Institutes of Health supported multicenter trial with the acronym ESVEM (Electrophysiologic Study Versus Electrocardiographic Monitoring for selection of antiarrhythmic therapy of ventricular arrhythmias). Between 1 October 1985 and 15 February 1991, 2103 patients with sustained VT, aborted sudden cardiac death or unmonitored syncope with inducible VT were screened for enrollment. To qualify for enrollment, patients had to have ventricular tachycardia or ventricular fibrillation induced twice at electrophysiological study *and* have an average of more than 10 PVBs per hour over 48 hours of ambulatory ECG monitoring. A total of 486 patients were randomized, 242 to the EPS limb and 244 to the ambulatory ECG limb (Figure 4.1). The patients received up to six drugs in random order until one was predicted to be effective, as evaluated by suppressing inducible arrhythmias in the EPS group or suppressing ventricular premature beats in the ambulatory ECG group. The patients were then followed over a 6-year period for recurrence of arrhythmia or death.[22]

It was found that there was no significant difference in predicting long-term success in either group, once a drug was determined to be effective. However, ambulatory ECG monitoring had the advantage that it identified an antiarrhythmic drug predicted to be effective more often than EPS in these patients. In addition, the actuarial probability of a recurrence of arrhythmia after a prediction of drug efficacy by either strategy was significantly lower for patients treated with sotalol than for patients treated with other antiarrhythmic drugs.[23]

It was emphasized that the results of this study applied to patients who met the enrollment criteria; i.e. those who had inducible sustained ventricular arrhythmias and at least 10 PVBs per hour. It is not known, therefore, if the results apply to patients who have this density of VPBs who are not inducible, or to patients who are inducible but do not have the required degree of VPBs.

The ESVEM landmark study has evoked considerable controversy relating to the criteria for assessment by EPS and by ambulatory ECG monitoring. Both were criticized as not being sufficiently rigorous, as evidenced by the high recurrence rate of ventricular arrhythmias in both groups which was 37 ± 3% at one year. This rate was lower (21

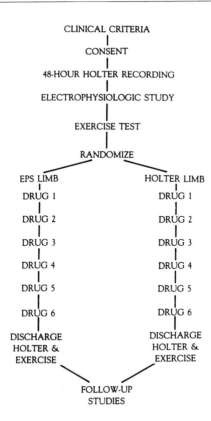

CLINICAL CRITERIA
|
CONSENT
|
48-HOUR HOLTER RECORDING
|
ELECTROPHYSIOLOGIC STUDY
|
EXERCISE TEST
|
RANDOMIZE

EPS LIMB   HOLTER LIMB
| |
DRUG 1   DRUG 1
| |
DRUG 2   DRUG 2
| |
DRUG 3   DRUG 3
| |
DRUG 4   DRUG 4
| |
DRUG 5   DRUG 5
| |
DRUG 6   DRUG 6
| |
DISCHARGE   DISCHARGE
HOLTER &   HOLTER &
EXERCISE   EXERCISE

FOLLOW-UP
STUDIES

Figure 4.1 Schematic of the design of the Electrophysiologic Study Versus Electrocardiographic Monitoring (ESVEM) trial. Patients fulfilling entry criteria must give consent and then meet specific eligibility criteria by Holter monitoring and subsequently by electrophysiologic study. They are then evenly, randomly allocated to undergo assessment of up to six antiarrhythmic drugs by either electrophysiologic study (EPS limb) or electrocardiographic monitoring and exercise testing (Holter limb). An exercise test is performed before drug assessment and before follow-up in patients receiving a drug that is predicted effective. An additional Holter monitor study is obtained at the time of discharge in both limbs but is not used to assess efficacy. (Reproduced with permission from reference 27: © American Heart Association)

± 4%) in patients treated with sotalol. The arrhythmic death rate was relatively low (10 ± 2%), and still lower for patients treated with sotalol (6 ± 3%). These differences were still present at the end of four years. Subsequently a retrospective analysis of the ESVEM database has shown that the major outcome criteria of the study would not be altered by selection of a more rigorous criteria by EPS (3 versus 2 extra stimuli) to routinely determine an efficacy prediction[24] or by demanding a higher degree of suppression of ventricular ectopy[25] or even that suppression of both spontaneous and inducible ventricular arrhythmias identifies a group with a better outcome.[26]

The results of the ESVEM study raise numerous important questions. Since there was no placebo group, and the arrhythmia recurrence rate was high, would the results have been similar if patients had been treated empirically with an antiarrhythmic drug that was well tolerated and did not cause obvious proarrhythmia? Since sotalol has beta-blocking effects, would a beta-blocking drug that does not have class 3 antiarrhythmic properties be as effective? Of the 296 patients who had predictions of drug efficacy, it was found that there was a lower recurrence rate in patients who had not failed an antiarrhythmic drug before enrollment, and that decreased left ventricular ejection fraction as a continuous variable was an independent predictor of arrhythmia recurrence when all 486 randomized patients were studied. This then raises the question of whether arrhythmia recurrence and arrhythmia death are more importantly related to variables other than suppression of ventricular beats by ambulatory ECG or by EPS.

With the advent of the automatic implantable cardioverter–defibrillator as a backup to prevent arrhythmic death, it should now be possible to conduct clinical trials to answer some of the above questions. Until this information becomes available, the results of the ESVEM trial are the best available data to guide antiarrhythmic drug therapy using ambulatory ECG monitoring in selected patients. The results of Lampert et al.[21] suggest that control of ventricular arrhythmias does not significantly improve outcome in patients with left ventricular ejection fraction below 30%. Implantation of an AICD may prove to be superior strategy in this group of patients.

Conclusions

Ambulatory ECG monitoring is now a well-accepted method to identify patients who are at higher risk of subsequent mortality among those who have recovered from an acute myocardial infarction. This information, combined with other data such as heart rate variability, signal-averaged late potentials, or other means of assessing autonomic tone such as carotid sinus sensitivity, may identify a sufficiently high-risk subgroup upon which to base the strategy to prevent sudden cardiac death. Post-MI patients, the best studied group to date, may provide clues to prevention of arrhythmic or sudden cardiac death in other groups of patients, such as hypertrophic cardiomyopathy or patients with valvular heart disease. It may be possible to identify subgroups of patients with cardiac failure who may benefit from empirical therapy with amiodarone, similar to the approach used to treat patients after myocardial infarction with beta-blockers.

The use of ambulatory ECG monitoring to guide selection of antiarrhythmic drugs to prevent recurrent ventricular tachycardia or cardiac arrest remains controversial. In the future, antiarrhythmic drugs may be selected for treatment of serious ventricular arrhythmias on the basis of ambulatory ECG monitoring to determine proarrhythmic effects rather than being used to assess suppression of ventricular arrhythmias. Finally, patients who have severe left ventricular dysfunction, such as an ejection fraction below 30%, may not be suitable for antiarrhythmic drug therapy even when guided by ambulatory ECG monitoring. These many unanswered questions will provide fruitful avenues for further investigation.

References

1. Bjerregaard P. Continuous ambulatory electrocardiography in healthy adult subjects over a 24-hour period. *Danish Med Bull* 1984; **31**: 282–97.
2. Fleg JL, Kennedy HL. Long-term prognostic significance of ambulatory electrocardiographic findings in apparently healthy subjects ≥60 years of age. *Am J Cardiol* 1992; **70**: 748–51.
3. Manolio TP, Furberg CD, Rau Taharju PM, *et al*. Cardiac arrhythmias on 24-hour ambulatory electrocardiography in older women and men: the cardiovascular health study. *J Am Coll Cardiol* 1984; **23**: 916–25.
4. DiMarco JP, Philbrick JT. Use of ambulatory electrocardiographic (Holter) monitoring. *Ann Int Med* 1990; **113**: 53–68.
5. Moss AJ, Schnitzler R, Green R, DeCamilla J. Ventricular arrhythmias 3 weeks after acute myocardial infarction. *Ann Int Med* 1971; **75**: 837–41.
6. Moss AJ, Bigger JT, Odoroff CL. Postinfarction risk stratification. *Prog Cardiovasc Dis* 1987; **29**: 389–412.
7. Bigger JT. Clinical aspects of trial design: what can we expect from the cardiac arrhythmia suppression trial? *Cardiovasc Drugs Ther* 1990; **4**: 657–64.
8. Anderson JL, Hallstrom AP, Griffith LS, *et al*. Relation of baseline characteristics to suppression of ventricular arrhythmias during placebo and active antiarrhythmic therapy in patients after myocardial infarction. *Circulation* 1989; **79**: 610–19.

9. Wyse DG, Hallstrom A, McBride R, *et al*. Events in the cardiac arrhythmia suppression trial (CAST): mortality in patients surviving open label titration but not randomized to double-blind therapy. *J Am Coll Cardiol* 1991; **18**: 20–8.

10. Nademanee K, Singh BN, Stevenson WG, Weiss JN. Amiodarone and post-MI patients. *Circulation* 1993; **88**: 764–74.

11. Maggioni AP, Zuanetti G, Franzosi MG, *et al*. Prevalence and prognostic significance of ventricular arrhythmias after acute myocardial infarction in the fibrinolytic era: GISSI-2 results. *Circulation* 1993; **87**: 312–22.

12. Deedwania PC. Ventricular arrhythmias in heart failure: to treat or not to treat? *Cardiol Clin* 1994; **12**: 137–54.

13. Fletcher RD, Cintron GB, Johnson G, *et al*. Enalapril decreases prevalence of ventricular tachycardia in patients with chronic congestive heart failure. *Circulation* 1993; **87** (Suppl VI): 49–55.

14. Doval NC, Nul DR, Grancelli HO, *et al*. Randomised trial of low-dose amiodarone in severe congestive heart failure. *Lancet* 1994; **344**: 493–8.

15. Singh JN, Fletcher RO, Fisher SG, *et al*. Results of the congestive heart failure survival trial of antiarrhythmic therapy. *Circulation* 1994; **90**: 546(A).

16. Stewart JT, McKenna WJ. Hypertrophic cardiomyopathy: treatment of arrhythmias. *Cardiovasc Drugs Ther* 1994; **8**: 95–9.

17. Saumarez RC, Camm AJ, Panagos A, *et al*. Ventricular fibrillation in hypertrophic cardiomyopathy is associated with increased fractionation of paced right ventricular electrograms. *Circulation* 1992; **86**: 467–74.

18. Maron BJ, Bonow RO, Cannon RO, *et al*. Hypertrophic cardiomyopathy: interrelation of clinical manifestation, pathophysiology and therapy. *New Engl J Med* 1987; **316**: 780–9, 844–52.

19. Kinder C, Tamburro P, Kopp D, *et al*. The clinical significance of nonsustained ventricular tachycardia: current perspectives. *PACE* 1994; **17**: 637–64.

20. Graboys TB, Lown B, Podrid P, *et al*. Long-term survival of patients with malignant ventricular arrhythmias treated with antiarrhythmic drugs. *Am J Cardiol* 1982; **50**: 437–43.

21. Lampert S, Lown B, Graboys TB, *et al*. Determinants of survival in patients with malignant ventricular arrhythmias associated with coronary artery disease. *Am J Cardiol* 1988; **61**: 791–7.

22. Mason JW, for the Electrophysiologic Study Versus Electrocardiographic Monitoring investigators. A comparison of electrophysiological testing with Holter monitoring to predict antiarrhythmic-drug efficacy for ventricular tachycardias. *New Engl J Med* 1993; **329**: 445–51.

23. Mason JW, for the Electrophysiologic Study Versus Electrocardiographic Monitoring investigators. A comparison of seven antiarrhythmic drugs in patients with ventricular tachycardias. *New Engl J Med* 1993; **329**: 452–8.

24. Reiffel JA, Reiter M, Freedman R, *et al*. Did the number of premature stimuli used or the length of unsustained tachycardia induced affect the predictive accuracy of the electrophysiologic study used to guide therapy in the ESVEM trial (abstract). *PACE* 1994; **17**: 826.

25. Reiffel J, Mann D, Reiter M, *et al*. A comparison of Holter suppression criteria for declaring drug efficacy in patients with sustained ventricular tachyarrhythmias in the ESVEM trial (abstract). *J Am Coll Cardiol* 1994; **23**: 279A.

26. Reiter M, Mann D, Reiffel J. Predictive value of combined Holter monitoring and electrophysiological testing in the ESVEM study (abstract). *J Am Coll Cardiol* 1994; **23**: 279A.

27. The ESVEM Investigations. The ESVEM trial: electrophysiologic study versus electrocardiographic monitoring for selection of antiarrhythmic therapy of ventricular tachyarrhythmias. *Circulation* 1989; **79**: 1354–60.

5

Torsades de Pointes

Emanuela H. Locati

Introduction

Torsades de pointes is a French term generally used to identify a rapid polymorphic ventricular tachycardia with a distinctive twisting morphology, and typically occurring in the setting of prolonged repolarization, either congenital or acquired.[1–5]

Torsades de pointes may have variable duration and often stops spontaneously, although longer runs may degenerate into ventricular fibrillation, thus provoking sudden cardiac death. Recently there has been a growing interest in torsades de pointes, as it has been reported with increasing frequency as a potentially lethal complication of several cardiac and noncardiac pharmacologic therapies.[3–7] Also, the diagnosis of torsades de pointes has considerable clinical importance since the treatment is different from other forms of sustained ventricular tachycardia.[6,7]

The electrophysiological mechanisms involved in the genesis of torsades de pointes have not been conclusively established, and either re-entry due to dispersion of repolarization or triggered activity associated with delayed repolarization have been advocated.[3,4,8–10] Both hypotheses could explain some of the features clinically observed in torsades de pointes, such as the long coupling interval of the initial extrasystole,[6] the facilitation by slow heart rate,[7] and the presence of a prodromal pause determining the typical initiating pattern often referred as 'long–short' sequence.[6]

Torsades de pointes are infrequent and paroxysmal arrhythmias that are not easily inducible by programmed electrical stimulation. So far, most clinical studies have been based on brief electrocardiographic tracings, including generally only one or two beats before the onset of the arrhythmias.[6,7,11] Therefore, very little direct information has been available on the sequence of events triggering the onset in real-life clinical conditions.

Although recordings of torsades de pointes during Holter monitoring are rare, the computerized Holter analysis of the heart rate and repolarization changes prior to the onset of torsades de pointes may contribute to our understanding of the mechanisms of arrhythmogenesis acting in individual patients. Some interesting data are already available from recent studies analyzing Holter recordings of patients with torsades de pointes associated with acquired or congenital long QT syndromes.[12–15]

Until recently, Holter analysis of ventricular arrhythmias was generally limited to the simple count of events, without considering the heart rate variations associated with the onset of the arrhythmias. Furthermore, computer algorithms for heart rate variability consider arrhythmias as undesirable accidents, to be eliminated from the analysis.

Nonetheless, study of the heart rate changes preceding the onset of arrhythmias by computerized Holter analysis may provide valuable information on the rate dependence and the adrenergic dependence of arrhythmias.[16] The analysis of heart rate determinants of arrhythmias by computerized Holter techniques was initially applied to repetitive and benign ventricular arrhythmias.[17,18] A recent study analyzed the spontaneous cycle length sequences preceding the onset of torsades de pointes recorded by Holter monitoring in 12 patients with acquired prolonged ventricular repolarization.[13] This showed that a significant heart rate increase, and escalating oscillatory 'short–long–short' sequences, preceded the onset of all ventricular arrhythmias, with greater oscillations preceding torsades de pointes than salvos and premature ventricular beats. These findings suggest that an increased adrenergic activity and pause-dependent mechanisms may interact in the genesis of torsades de pointes.

Thus, computerized quantitative Holter analysis may be viewed as a new *'non-invasive electrophysiologic test'*, exploring at the same time the electrophysiological substrate and the factors triggering the spontaneous onset of arrhythmias in the individual patient in real clinical conditions.

Typical Electrocardiographic Features: Implications for Pathogenesis and Diagnosis

The minimal criteria required for the clinical diagnosis of torsades de pointes are the presence of the typical twisting morphology, and the association with congenital or acquired prolonged ventricular repolarization. Other characteristic features, such as the presence of a prodromal pause, the long coupling of the first ventricular beat, and the rate-dependence are less homogeneous in acquired than congenital long QT syndromes, and thus may not be a requisite for the clinical diagnosis of torsades de pointes.[2–5]

The 'Twisting' Morphology

Torsades de pointes differ from other polymorphic ventricular tachycardias for the typical morphology, with a complete shift in polarity of the ventricular complexes, ordinarily occurring every five to fifteen beats – hence the eponym 'torsades de pointes' (Figure 5.1). Of note, the twisting pattern is not necessarily equally evident in all leads, so in some cases it may be difficult to detect by 2-channel Holter recordings.

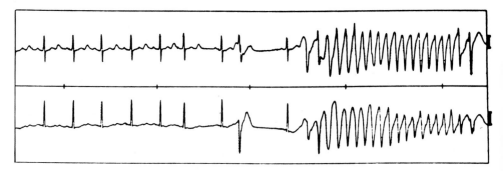

Figure 5.1 Example of torsades de pointes recorded by 2-channel Holter monitoring in a patient with prolonged ventricular repolarization due to therapy with amiodarone (female, age 62 years). Note the typical twisting morphology and abnormalities of the ventricular repolarization, with a prominent late component (T–U complex). Also note the presence of the 'cascade phenomenon', as the entire sequence of events was started by a premature atrial beat, which initiated a 'short–long' pattern leading to an enhancement of the late component of the T–U complex from where the first ventricular beat emerged. Therefore the ventricular beat was followed by a longer compensatory pause, followed by a T–U complex of greater amplitude finally triggering the onset of torsades de pointes. Paper speed = 25 mm/s.

So far, no hypothesis has conclusively explained the origin of the twisting morphology. In the original description, Dessertenne attributed this phenomenon to two automatic foci firing from opposing sides of the heart and competing for excitation of the ventricles.[1] This interpretation has still a potential interest since triggered activity originating from pause-dependent early after-depolarization (EAD) might be indeed a form of focal activity.[3,4,19]

On the other hand, within the framework of re-entrant mechanisms related to dispersion of refractoriness, the undulating pattern could be attributed to the formation of one or more large migrating macro re-entry pathways.[3,4,8,9,19] Of note, triggered activity following after-depolarization and re-entry may not be antithetic mechanisms. Since EADs may arise in specific areas of the myocardium, they may create dispersion of refractoriness and favor the onset of re-entrant arrhythmias.[19] Torsades de pointes generally have a high ventricular rate, usually above 180 beats per minute, and longer runs tend to show a chaotic rhythm that may mimic ventricular fibrillation. Nonetheless, even long and chaotic runs may either degenerate into ventricular fibrillation or spontaneously reconvert to sinus rhythm. Until now no study has identified the mechanisms that favor the spontaneous resolution to sinus rhythm, or conversely, the factors that provoke the degeneration into ventricular fibrillation. It is noteworthy that runs of longer duration or of rhythms that degenerate into ventricular fibrillation may have a higher firing rate after the onset than runs of shorter duration in the same patient. We have recently observed this finding in a study including 105 episodes of torsades de pointes from patients with acquired prolonged ventricular repolarization.[13]

Thus, the detection of a high ventricular rate even in the very initial phase of the arrhythmias may contribute to the early identification of those runs of torsades de pointes more likely to degenerate into ventricular fibrillation.

QT Interval Prolongation

The presence of prolonged ventricular repolarization is generally considered necessary for the diagnosis of torsades de pointes. Prolongation of the QT interval may be either congenital or acquired, and a variety of cardiac and noncardiac medications and metabolic disturbances may prolong the ventricular repolarization process (Table 5.1). Multiple provoking factors may coexist (e.g. a patient taking quinidine and/or terfenadine, and being moderately hypokalemic due to diuretic therapy), and their interaction may contribute to precipitate the onset of torsades de pointes in susceptible individuals.[4,5,11]

Both in acquired and in congenital long QT syndromes, women appear to be more prone than men to the development of torsades de pointes.[3,4,20–22] The pathophysiological basis for this gender disparity is still unknown, but several data seem to indicate a female predisposition to prolonged cardiac repolarization, since even in the normal population women have longer corrected QT interval than men.[22,23]

In acquired forms, rather independently of the provoking agent or condition, torsades de pointes seem to be more likely when the QT interval duration exceeds 600 ms.[7] Also, in congenital long QT syndrome, patients with a longer QT interval have an increased risk for cardiac events.[20] Nonetheless, malignant arrhythmias may occur even in patients with borderline QT interval.[3,20,21] In some borderline cases, the occurrence of torsades de pointes may be associated with a transient prolongation of the QT interval; for example following a sudden adrenergic activation.[3,21]

Thus, the detection of a transient prolongation of QT interval by Holter monitoring in patients with borderline QT interval may help identify patients at higher risk of developing torsades de pointes.

Table 5.1 Causes and conditions leading to torsades de pointes

---

Congenital long QT syndrome
Jervell and Lange–Nielsen syndrome
Romano–Ward syndrome
Sporadic nonfamilial syndrome

Drugs
Antiarrhythmic agents that prolong repolarization
    Class IA (quinidine, dysopiramide, procainamide)
    Class III (d,l sotalol, d-sotalol, amiodarone, *N*-acetilprocainamide, bretylium, dofetilide, sematilide)
    Others (encainide*, ajmaline, aprindine, propafenone)
Tricyclic and tetracyclic antidepressants
    amitryptiline, imipramine, doxepin, maprotiline
Phenothiazine
    thioridazine, chlorpromazine
Neuroleptics
    haloperidol, chloral hydrate
Antihystaminics
    astemizole, terfanadine
Antibiotics and chemotherapeutics
    erytromycine, spyramycine, pentamidine, trimethoprine-sulphametoxazole
    anthramicyne*
Serotonin antagonists
    ketanserin, zimeldine
Miscellaneous
    prenylamine, bepridil, lidoflazyne, terodiline, probucol, cocaine, papaverine, adenosine
Poisoning with arsenic, organophosphorous insecticides
Ionic contrast media

Electrolyte abnormalities
Hypokalemia
Hypomagnesemia
Hypocalcemia*

Bradyarrhythmias
Sinus bradycardia
Atrioventricular block

Altered nutritional states
Anorexia nervosa
Diets, starvation

Cerebrovascular disease
Intracranial and subaracnoidal hemorrhage, stroke, intracranial trauma

Hypothyroidism

---

*Association not well established.
Modified with permission from reference 5.

Stereotyped Patterns of Onset: 'Short–Long' Sequences

As consistently reported by several clinical studies, drug-induced torsades de pointes are typically preceded by a prodromal pause.[3–7,11–13] As the long cycle is generally a post-extrasystolic pause, the entire sequence is more completely defined as a 'short–long–short' phenomenon.[6,8] This pattern has been observed in all acquired forms, regardless of the disparate conditions provoking a prolonged ventricular repolarization.[2–7,11–13,24–27] Nonetheless, 'short–long–short' sequences could be observed even in torsades de pointes associated with congenital long QT syndrome.[2,3,15,21] Finally, it should be underlined that 'short–long' initiating sequences are not uniquely restricted to torsades de pointes, since they have been observed in different benign and malignant ventricular arrhythmias.[10,12,18]

The oscillating pattern may be originated either by a bigeminal rhythm, or by atrioventricular block, or by sudden cycle length variation induced by premature atrial beats or by atrial fibrillation.[2–5,13,24] Different modalities of onset have been observed even within the same patient, in cases with multiple episodes of torsades de pointes recorded on the same Holter monitoring system (Figure 5.2).[13]

Independent of the mechanisms determining the oscillating patterns, the amplitude of the 'short–long' sequences appears to be correlated with the complexity of the following arrhythmias. Specifically, in a recent quantitative analysis of Holter recordings of patients with acquired prolonged ventricular repolarization, we observed that all ventricular arrhythmias were preceded by escalating oscillatory 'short–long–short' patterns, with greater oscillations preceding torsades de pointes than salvos and isolated ventricular beats.[13] Furthermore, the onset of ventricular arrhythmias was preceded in most cases by a distinctive escalating pattern that we defined as 'cascade phenomenon', with two characteristic features:

1. The primary event was a premature atrial beat starting a 'short–long' sequence entraining a first ventricular beat.
2. As the amplitude of the 'short–long–short' oscillatory pattern increased, with shorter 'short' and longer 'long' intervals, the complexity of the subsequent arrhythmias progressively increased, in some cases until the onset of torsades de pointes (Figure 5.3).

Thus, this finding may suggest that in susceptible patients with prolonged ventricular repolarization, sudden variations of heart rate, originated by otherwise benign supraventricular arrhythmias or atrioventricular block, may act as a trigger, initiating an escalating oscillatory 'short–long–short' pattern, ultimately leading to the onset of malignant ventricular arrhythmias.[3,8,10,13]

It is noteworthy that recent studies by Holter monitoring showed that oscillatory 'short–long' sequences were not restricted to drug-induced torsades de pointes, but they could also play a role in arrhythmogenesis associated with the congenital long QT syndrome.[15,21] This may in part explain the beneficial effect of permanent pacing in congenital long QT syndrome[21,25] that is often used in association with antiadrenergic treatment such as beta-blocking agents and left cardiac sympathetic denervation.[20,21,26]

Thus, the detection by Holter monitoring of rhythm disturbances giving rise to 'short–long' oscillating sequences in conditions of prolonged ventricular repolarization may identify patients more likely to develop potentially fatal ventricular arrhythmias.

Pause-Dependent T–U Wave Abnormalities

The onset of torsades de pointes is often preceded by further prolongation of the QT interval and by typical changes of the configuration of the T wave, with the appearance of an enhanced late component corresponding in timing with the U wave, thus defined as T–U complex.[3,4,13,24] The amplitude of the T–U complex is generally greater in the beat following a pause, and often the first ventricular complex of torsades de pointes seems to arise from the peak of the late component.

Several different hypotheses have been proposed for the origin of the U wave in basal conditions. In summary, the U wave may be due either to the late repolarization of certain regions of the myocardium, or to the longer repolarization of the Purkinje network, or to the heterogeneity in the electrical behavior of cells within the ventricular wall, the M cells.[3,24] In any case, the presence of a U wave seems to indicate a certain degree of heterogeneity in the ventricular repolarization process.[3,24]

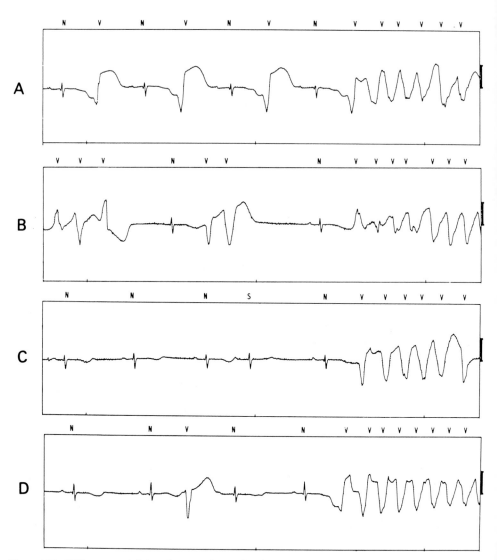

Figure 5.2 Different modalities of onset of torsades de pointes recorded by Holter monitoring in the same patient with prolonged ventricular repolarization due to therapy with quinidine (female, age 80 years). All 34 TdeP episodes observed in this patient in the same Holter recording were preceded by 'short–long–short' sequences, although constituted by different arrhythmias. *Panel A*: The 'first short' interval was due to a ventricular beat belonging to a bigeminal sequence. *Panel B*: The 'first short' interval was the last beat of a salvo (in this case, a couplet). *Panel C*: The 'first short' interval was determined by a PAB. *Panel D*: The 'first short' interval due to an interpolated ventricular ectopic beat. Paper speed = 25 mm/s. N = normal beat; S = supraventricular beat; V = ventricular beat.

Independent of the mechanisms involved in the genesis of the U wave in basal conditions, the pause-dependent T–U wave complex observed in prolonged ventricular repolarization might be the electrocardiographic counterpart of after-depolarizations.[3,8,10,19,24] More specifically, after-depolarizations that may be involved in the genesis of drug-induced torsades de pointes seem to be pause-dependent early after-

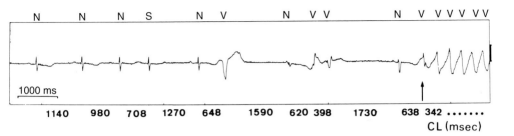

Figure 5.3 Example of 'cascade' phenomenon preceding the onset of torsades de pointes in prolonged ventricular repolarization induced by quinidine (female, age 80 years). This sequence was initiated by a premature atrial beat followed by a pause (1270 ms), leading to a ventricular beat with a longer compensatory pause (1590 ms), then a couplet followed by an even longer pause (1730 ms), finally inducing torsades de pointes. The beat indicated by the arrow was corrected manually, on the basis of ECG aspects seen on the second channel, not shown. Paper speed = 25 mm/s. N = normal beat; S = supraventricular beat; V = ventricular beat.

depolarizations (EADs).[3,8,10,19,24,27–30] Indeed, EAD amplitude is reported to be augmented at longer cycle lengths, particularly following a pause.[8,10,27–29] Ventricular arrhythmias may occur when pause-dependent after-depolarizations reach a critical threshold.[3,8,10,27–29]

An EAD may be a localized phenomenon, possibly arising from specific tissues of the myocardium such as the M cells or the Purkinje fibers,[24] and this may further accentuate the dishomogeneity of the substrate, thus favoring the development of sustained ventricular arrhythmias by re-entrant pathways.[19,30] In this view, after-depolarization and dispersion of ventricular repolarization may both be involved in the genesis of torsades de pointes.[19,30] Typically, 'short–long' sequences and further aberrations of the T–U complex have been observed in all acquired forms, regardless of the disparate conditions provoking the prolongation of ventricular repolarization – thus supporting the definition of drug-induced torsades de pointes as a typical example of pause-dependent arrhythmia.[3–7,11–13] Nonetheless, pause-dependent aberration of the T wave has often been observed also in cases of congenital long QT syndrome[3,15,21] (Figure 5.4), thus suggesting that pause-dependent mechanisms, possibly related to early after-depolarization and triggered activity, may play a role in arrhythmogenesis in both conditions.[3,4,10,15,21,24]

Thus, the detection by Holter techniques of typical aberrations of the T wave, with an enhanced late component or T–U complex in the beats following a pause, may identify patients at higher risk of developing torsades de pointes both in acquired and in congenital long QT syndrome.

Rate Dependency: Bradycardia Dependency Versus Adrenergic Dependency

Until recently, very little quantitative information was available on the heart rate changes occurring in the minutes preceding the onset of torsades de pointes. Some information has been provided by a few studies on sudden arrhythmic deaths recorded during Holter monitoring, where torsades de pointes were occasionally recognized among the arrhythmias degenerating into ventricular fibrillation.[12,31,32] Torsades de pointes appeared to be preceded by a typical pause and by lower basal heart rate when compared with other types of malignant ventricular tachyarrhythmias degenerating into ventricular fibrillation.[12] Marked bradycardia seems to be a constant characteristic finding also in patients with classical congenital long QT syndrome;[21] nonetheless, the onset of torsades de pointes is often preceded by a major increase in heart rate in these patients[15,21] (Figures 5.4 and 5.5). Furthermore, a prodromal pause is often absent, while further prolongation

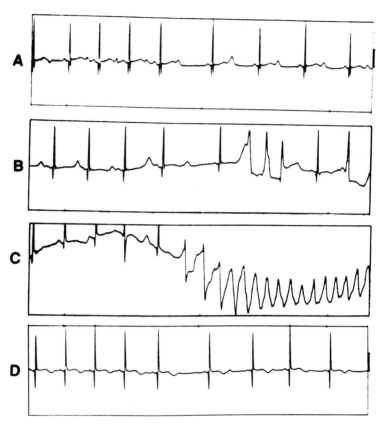

Figure 5.4 Strips of Holter recordings taken at different conditions in a patient with congenital long QT syndrome (female, age 11 years). *Panel A*: Strip recorded in the absence of therapy. Note the evident increase in the amplitude of the late component of the T wave in the beat following a spontaneous sinus pause. *Panel B*: In association with a modest T-wave alternans, pause-dependent aberrations of the T–U complex persist, with the appearance of ventricular premature beats. *Panel C*: A longer episode of torsades de pointes is preceded by a clear increase of the heart rate without any evident prodromal pause. *Panel D*: After left cardiac sympathetic denervations and during verapamil administration, sinus pauses persist, although the amplitude of the T wave is reduced, without the appearance of a clear late component after the pause. (Modified with permission from reference 15)

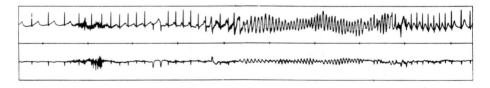

Figure 5.5 Episode of torsades de pointes recorded by 2-channel Holter monitoring in a patient with congenital long QT syndrome (female, age 25 years). This episode happened at night during sleep, while the patient experienced a nightmare. Note the long QT interval at baseline (there was a lack of shortening of the QT interval with increasing heart rate just prior to the onset of torsades de pointes). Note that, although sinus tachycardia appears to be the prominent feature of the initiating sequence, oscillatory short–long sequences due to premature ventricular beats were also detected.

of the QT interval and even overt T-wave alternans are sometimes observed. This profile is likely to be induced by an increased adrenergic stimulation, hence the definition of 'adrenergic-dependent' long QT syndrome,[3] in contrast with the acquired forms where 'pause-dependent' mechanisms seem to be prevalent.[3–7,22–24]

Therefore, delayed after-depolarizations (DADs), typically associated with adrenergic activation, may play a specific role in the genesis of torsades de pointes in the adrenergic-dependent long QT syndromes,[3] and typically in the idiopathic long QT syndrome where arrhythmias are likely to be precipitated by a sudden adrenergic activation.[3,19,21]

It is noteworthy that, at least in experimental conditions, EADs and DADs may appear simultaneously in the presence of catecholamines.[33] Thus it is possible that in clinical conditions, too, EADs and DADs may interact to determine the genesis of arrhythmias associated with prolonged ventricular repolarization.[19] Of note, in a recent analysis of multiple Holter recordings of one patient with idiopathic long QT syndrome, both pause-dependent and adrenergic-dependent arrhythmias could be observed (Figure 5.4), although longer runs of torsades de pointes were generally preceded by sinus tachycardia, thus suggesting that adrenergic activation was required for the genesis of sustained ventricular arrhythmias in this patient.[15] Indeed, in this case as in most patients with idiopathic long QT syndrome, antiadrenergic interventions were able to prevent the occurrence of further malignant ventricular arrhythmias.[15,20,21,26] On the other hand, also in patients with acquired prolonged repolarization the spontaneous onset of torsades de pointes was shown to be preceded by a significant increase of the heart rate, in association with escalating oscillatory 'short–long–short' cycle length patterns.[13] These findings suggest that, even in drug-induced delayed ventricular repolarization, both adrenergic-dependent and pause-dependent mechanisms (possibly inducing after-depolarizations and triggered activity) may have a synergistic role in the genesis of complex ventricular arrhythmias.

Thus, analysis of the heart rate changes in the minutes preceding the onset of arrhythmias by quantitative Holter techniques may help to quantify the relative contributions of pause-dependent and adrenergic-dependent mechanisms to the onset of torsades de pointes, and may provide a rational basis for the therapeutic management in individual patients.

T-Wave Alternans

The onset of torsades de pointes in congenital long QT syndrome may be preceded by typical beat-to-beat changes in shape and polarity of the T wave, defined as 'T-wave alternans'.[3,21,34] T-wave alternans has been described, typically although not exclusively, in patients with congenital long QT syndrome, where the presence of this phenomenon, even in a minor form, is associated with an increased risk of cardiac events.[21,34,35] In congenital long QT syndrome, T-wave alternans events are specifically observed in conditions of adrenergic activation, generally precluding the onset of torsades de pointes.[21,34] In both experimental and clinical conditions, T-wave alternans could typically be induced by activation of the cardiac sympathetic nerves, primarily the left cardiac sympathetic nerves.[21,34]

In general, the presence of T-wave alternans is indicative of heterogeneity of ventricular repolarization,[36] and it is most often observed in cases of major prolongation of the QT interval, such as is frequently observed in congenital long QT syndrome.[34–37] Nonetheless, T-wave alternans is not restricted to the congenital long QT syndrome, but this phenomenon appears to be prevalent in conditions likely to develop malignant ventricular arrhythmias.[36] Therefore, quantitation of T-wave alternans by complex demodulation techniques applied to long-term ECG recordings may have prognostic value in estimating the risk of ventricular fibrillation.[36]

Multiple mechanisms may be responsible for the genesis of T-wave alternans in different clinical conditions. In long QT syndrome, one of the proposed mechanisms suggests that T-wave alternans may reflect rate-dependent differences in duration between subendocardial and subepicardial layers of the ventricular wall.[37] Of note, the cycle length is a powerful determinant of functional refractory period and action potential duration, and a given cycle length might act differentially on different myocardial tissues,[30,37,38] thus setting a substrate of potential dishomogeneity of repolarization duration likely to be arrhythmogenic.[8,10,30,38] The acceleration of heart rate *per se* might also entrain a 2:1 entry block, provoking a localized bradycardia which could potentially induce EADs and trigger the initial beat and facilitate the continuation of a self-maintaining feedback loop and re-entrant arrhythmias in a substrate of prolonged ventricular repolarization.[8,28,29,38] In experimental conditions it has been shown that 2:1 conduction of early after-depolarization may be associated with the appearance of T-wave alternans on the surface tracing.[19] Therefore, an acceleration of the heart rate due to increased adrenergic activity in conditions of prolonged ventricular repolarization may entrain further perturbations of the electrophysiologic substrate, increasing the dispersion of recovery and favoring the onset of triggered activity.

Thus, the detection of T-wave alternans by Holter monitoring may be a marker of electrical instability that might help identify the patients at higher risk of developing torsades de pointes associated with prolonged ventricular repolarization.

Long Versus Short Coupling of Torsades de Pointes

In typical torsades de pointes, one of the characteristic features is the long coupling of the first ventricular beat, generally above 600 ms.[3,4,9] As highlighted previously, the first ventricular complex of torsades de pointes associated with prolonged ventricular repolarization generally appears to emerge from the peak of the late component of the T–U complex,[3,4,21] thus accounting for the typical long coupling of these arrhythmias. Nonetheless, a new variant of polymorphic ventricular tachycardias has recently been described showing several electrocardiographic features of torsades de pointes, such as the typical twisting morphology[5,39] and in some cases even a typical short–long initiating sequence,[5] but without any prolongation of the ventricular repolarization. These arrhythmias show a short coupling of the first ventricular beat, generally less than 300 ms,[5,39] as they appear to originate from the apex of a normal T wave, without overt aberrations of the T wave morphology (Figure 5.6).

Torsades de pointes associated with normal ventricular repolarization may be familial in approximately 30% of cases, could have a higher risk of degenerating into ventricular fibrillation, and does not show a female prevalence.[39]

As to the management, it does not respond to beta-blockers and/or amiodarone, and although some cases may respond to verapamil, the treatment of choice is the implantable cardiac defibrillator.[39] The mechanisms of arrhythmogenesis that may determine this variant of torsades de pointes are not known, as neither triggered activity following after-depolarization nor re-entry can wholly account for the electrocardiographic profile of these malignant arrhythmias.[39]

Thus, analysis of the modalities of onset of torsades de pointes, with particular reference to the initiating sequence and the coupling of the first beat of torsades de pointes, may allow the detection of torsades de pointes with atypical pathogenetic factors, and may guide the therapeutic management of arrhythmias in individual patients.

The Role of Holter Monitoring in Clinical Management

Holter monitoring is a valuable technique to study the spontaneous behavior of cardiac arrhythmias, such as torsades de pointes, which are typically paroxysmal and not easily

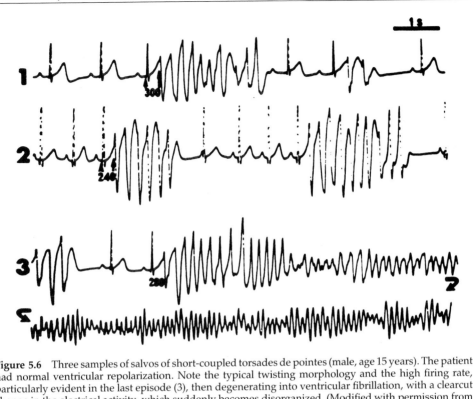

Figure 5.6 Three samples of salvos of short-coupled torsades de pointes (male, age 15 years). The patient had normal ventricular repolarization. Note the typical twisting morphology and the high firing rate, particularly evident in the last episode (3), then degenerating into ventricular fibrillation, with a clearcut change in the electrical activity, which suddenly becomes disorganized. (Modified with permission from reference 15)

induced by programmed electrical stimulation.[10,12,13] The recent wider use of Holter monitoring has allowed identification of the sequence of events leading to the onset of torsades de pointes in an increasing number of patients with acquired or congenital long QT syndromes.[12,13,15] This new information may modify our understanding of the mechanisms of arrhythmogenesis in long QT syndromes, until now generally based on clinical observations performed on brief ECG tracings, including only one or few beats before the onset,[3–7,11] and may have clinical implications in the therapeutic management of affected patients.

Patients with acquired prolonged ventricular repolarization

In these patients, Holter monitoring has shown that the spontaneous onset of ventricular arrhythmias is preceded by an increasing heart rate in the last minute, and escalating oscillatory 'short–long–short' cycle-length patterns, with greater oscillations preceding torsades de pointes than salvos and isolated ventricular beats.[12,13] These findings suggest that adrenergic-dependent and pause-dependent mechanisms (possibly inducing after-depolarizations and triggered activity), may have a synergistic role in the genesis of complex ventricular arrhythmias associated with acquired delayed ventricular repolarization.

These observations may have clinical implications in the treatment of acquired torsades de pointes. Up to now, clinical management has been aimed at the prevention of bradycardia and pauses by cardiac pacing, together with drug or electrolyte therapy, including atropine, isoproterenol, lidocaine, magnesium sulphate, or more recently potassium channel openers or activators such as pinacidil or nicorandil.[5] Nonetheless, in view of the signs of adrenergic activation detected by computerized Holter techniques, beta-blockers may not be contraindicated, but in same cases even indicated, and the choice of such therapy may be guided by analysis of several Holter recordings.

Patients with congenital long QT syndrome

At the other extreme of the spectrum, in patients with congenital long QT syndrome, the onset of malignant arrhythmias is generally preceded by signs of adrenergic activation, such as sinus tachycardia or even overt T-wave alternans. Nonetheless, recent clinical observations have highlighted the role of escalating oscillatory 'short–long' sequences and pause-dependent aberrations of the T–U complex in the genesis of arrhythmias, thus likely to be dependent on pause-dependent after-depolarization and triggered activity.[19,21] Therefore, both adrenergic and pause-dependent mechanisms of arrhythmogenesis may be active also in the congenital long QT syndrome, although the adrenergic activation may play a determinant role in the genesis of malignant ventricular arrhythmias.

These Holter-monitored observations have meaningful clinical implications, as they explain the efficacy of permanent pacing in preventing the onset of ventricular arrhythmias,[25] by inhibiting sudden heart rate variations possibly entraining escalating oscillatory sequences leading to arrhythmogenesis. Nonetheless, pacing alone cannot prevent the genesis of arrhythmias induced by adrenergic hyperactivity. Therefore, antiadrenergic interventions – both beta-blockers and left cardiac sympathetic denervation – remain the therapy of choice against fatal ventricular arrhythmias;[20,21,25,26] while 'triple therapy' – including beta-blockers, left cardiac sympathetic denervation and permanent pacing – may confer the highest degree of protection in patients at higher risk.

Patients with intermediate forms

The presence of intermediate forms, with borderline QT prolongation, with late onset of symptoms in life, and without familial involvement, further support the hypothesis of a common pathway of pause-dependent and adrenergic-dependent mechanisms in the genesis of torsades de pointes.[21] In these forms, even more than in congenital or acquired conditions, the serial analysis of Holter monitoring may explore the electrophysiologic substrate, by quantifying specific features such as rate-dependence, the presence of transient further prolongation of the QT interval, the occurrence of oscillatory short–long patterns, and the appearance of pause-dependent aberrations of the T–U complex. This approach may help evaluate the relative prevalence of pause-dependent and adrenergic-dependent mechanisms of arrhythmogenesis, and may provide a rational basis for therapeutic management of torsades de pointes in the individual patient.

Quantitative Analysis of Holter Monitoring to Identify Vulnerable Substrates

So far no study has systematically explored in torsades de pointes some of the electrocardiographic features known to precede the spontaneous onset of ventricular arrhythmias in different clinical conditions, and specifically the morphologic changes of the depolarization or repolarization process such as the QRS duration, the amplitude of the late potentials, the ST deviation, the QT duration, or the T wave amplitude or T-wave alternans. The inclusion of the dynamic behavior of these parameters might improve our ability to predict the likelihood of onset of torsades de pointes following specific cycle length patterns.

In particular, study of the QT dynamics may have special implications in patients with prolonged ventricular repolarization, either acquired or congenital. Abrupt heart rate changes and pauses may create further prolongation of the QT interval and aberrations in the T wave configuration that may be the electrocardiographic counterpart of after-depolarizations, and may therefore be useful in identifying those patients at higher risk of arrhythmogenesis.

Quantitative Holter analysis may be utilized to identify individual-specific sequences associated with the onset of malignant arrhythmias, such as 'short–long' sequences in patients with prolonged ventricular repolarization. In a preliminary study we have already implemented simple cycle length parameters by a new computer algorithm scanning the 24-hour Holter ECG data in order to obtain the probability of a specific template to be followed by ventricular arrhythmias. Our initial data suggest that in some patients with acquired prolonged ventricular repolarization, individual-specific 'short–long' templates have indeed a higher probability of being followed by ventricular arrhythmias than by sinus rhythm.[40] This approach may have clinical implications in the identification of individual-specific cycle length sequences more likely to be followed by malignant arrhythmias, thus providing a new parameter to be implemented in the algorithms for the detection of arrhythmias by implantable antitachycardia devices.

On these grounds, computerized Holter analyses might become a new 'noninvasive electrophysiologic test', exploring at the same time the individual electrical substrate and the factors triggering the onset of arrhythmias in real-life clinical conditions. Among the other advantages, the use of computerized Holter techniques may allow serial compari-sons of Holter recordings obtained in different clinical conditions, at a low cost and with minimal discomfort for the patient.

References

1. Dessertenne F. La tachycardie ventriculaire à deux foyers opposes variables. *Arch Mal Coeur* 1966; **59**: 263–72.
2. Coumel P, Leclercq JF, Dessertenne F. Torsades de pointes. In: Josephson M, Wellens HJJ (eds), *Tachycardias: Mechanisms, Diagnosis, Treatment*. Philadelphia: Lea & Febiger, 1984: 325–51.
3. Jackman WM, Friday KJ, Anderson JL, Aliot EM, Clark M, Lazzara R. The long QT syndromes: a critical review, new clinical observation and a unifying hypothesis. *Prog Cardiovasc Dis* 1988; **31**: 115–72.
4. Roden D. The long QT syndrome and torsades de pointes: basic and clinical aspects. In: El-Sherif N, Samet P (eds), *Cardiac Pacing and Electrophysiology*. Philadelphia: W.B. Saunders, 1991: 265–83.
5. Haverkamp W, Shenasa M, Bogreffe M, Breithard G. Tosades de pointes. In: Zipes DP, Jalife J (eds), *Cardiac Electrophysiology: From Cell to Bedside* (2nd edn). Philadelphia: W.B. Saunders, 1994: 885–99.
6. Roden DM, Woosley RL, Primm RK. Incidence and clinical features of the quinidine-associated long QT syndrome: implications for patient care. *Am Heart J* 1986; **111**: 1088–93.
7. Keren A, Tzivoni D, Gavish D, Levi J, Gottlieb S, Benhorin J, Stern S. Etiology, warning signs and therapy of torsades de pointes. *Circulation* 1981; **64**: 1167–74.
8. Cranefield PF, Aronson RS. Cardiac arrhythmias: the role of triggered activity and other mechanisms. Mount Kisko, NY: Futura, 1988: 553–79.
9. Surawicz B. Electrophysiologic substrate of torsades de pointes: dispersion of repolarization or early afterdepolariza-tion? *J Am Coll Cardiol* 1989; **14**: 172–84.
10. Coumel P. Early after-depolarization and triggered activity in clinical arrhythmias. In: Rosen MJ, Janse MJ, Wit AL (eds), *Cardiac Electrophysiology: A Textbook*. Mount Kisko, NY: Futura, 1990: 387–411.
11. Kay GN, Plumb VJ, Arciniegas JG, Henthorn WR, Waldo AL. Torsade de pointes: the long–short initiating sequence and other clinical features. Observation in 32 patients. *J Am Coll Cardiol* 1983; **2**: 806–17.
12. Leclercq JF, Maisonblanche P, Cauchemez B, Coumel P. Respective role of sympathetic tone and of cardiac pauses in the genesis of 62 cases of ventricular fibrillation recorded during Holter monitoring. *Eur Heart J* 1988; **9**: 1276–83.
13. Locati EH, Maisonblanche P, Cauchemez B, Coumel P. Determinants of ventricular arrhythmias associated with prolonged repolarization: a computerized quantitative analysis of dynamic Holter recording. In: *Computers in Cardiology*. Los Alamitos, CA: IEEE Comp. Soc. Press, 1991: 605–8.
14. Merri M, Moss AJ, Benhorin J, Locati EH, Alberti M, Badilini F. Relationship between ventricular repolarization and cardiac length during 24-hour electrocardiographic Holter recordings: finding in normals and in patients with long QT syndrome. *Circulation* 1992; **8**: 1916–21.

15. Malfatto G, Rosen MR, Foresti A, Schwartz PJ. Idiopathic long QT syndrome exacerbated by beta-adrenergic blockade and responsive to left cardiac sympathetic denervation: implications regarding electrophysiologic substrate and adrenergic modulation. *J Cardiovasc Electrophysiol* 1992; **3**: 295–305.

16. Coumel P. Noninvasive exploration of cardiac arrhythmias. *Ann New York Acad Sci* 1990; **601**: 312–28.

17. Albrecht P, Cohen RJ, Mark RG. A stochastic characterization of chronic ventricular ectopic activity. *IEEE Trans* 1988; **35**: 539–50.

18. Zimmermann M, Maisonblanche P, Cauchemez B, Leclercq JF, Coumel P. Determinants of the spontaneous ectopic activity in repetitive monomorphic idiopathic ventricular tachycardia. *J Am Coll Cardiol* 1986; **7**: 1219–27.

19. Priori GS, Napolitano C, Schwartz PJ. Electrophysiologic mechanisms involved in the development of torsades de pointes. *Cardiovasc Drugs Ther* 1991; **5**: 203–12.

20. Moss AJ, Schwartz PJ, Crampton RS, Tzivoni D, Locati EH, MacCluer J, Hall JW, Weitkamp L, Vincent GM, Garson A, Robinson JL, Benhorin J, Choi S. The long QT syndrome: prospective longitudinal study of 328 families. *Circulation* 1991; **84**: 1136–44.

21. Schwartz PJ, Locati EH, Napolitano C, Priori SG. The long QT syndrome. In: Zipes DP, Jalife J (eds), *Cardiac Electrophysiology: From Cell to Bedside* (2nd edn). Philadelphia: W.B. Saunders, 1994; 788–811.

22. Makkar RR, Fromm BS, Steinman RT, Meissner MD, Lehmann MH. Female gender as a risk factor for torsades de pointes associated with cardiovascular drugs. *JAMA* 1993; **270**: 2590–7.

23. Merri M, Benhorin J, Alberti M, Locati E, Moss AJ. Electrocardiographic quantitation of ventricular repolarization. *Circulation* 1989; **80**: 1301–8.

24. Antzelevitch C, Sicouri S. Clinical relevance of cardiac arrhythmias generated by afterdepolarization: role of the M cells in the generation of U waves, triggered activity and torsades de pointes. *JACC* 1994; **23**: 259–77.

25. Moss AJ, Liu JE, Gottlieb S, Locati EH, Robinson JL, Schwartz PJ. Efficacy of permanent pacing in the management of long QT syndrome. *Circulation* 1991; **84**: 1524–9.

26. Schwartz PJ, Locati EH, Moss AJ, Crampton RS, Trazzi R, Ruberti U. Left cardiac sympathetic denervation in the therapy of the congenital long QT syndrome: a worldwide report. *Circulation* 1991; **84**: 503–11.

27. El-Sherif N, Bekheit S, Henkin R. Quinidine-induced long QTU interval and torsades de pointes: role of bradycardia-dependent early afterdepolarization. *JACC* 1989; **14**: 252–7.

28. Cranefield PF, Aronson RS. Torsade de pointes and other pause-induced ventricular arrhythmias: the short–long–short sequence and early afterdepolarization. *PACE* 1988; **11**: 670–8.

29. Brachman J, Sherlag BJ, Rosenstraukh LV, Lazzara R. Bradycardia-dependent triggered activity: relevance to drug-induced multiform ventricular tachycardia. *Circulation* 1983; **68**: 846–56.

30. Brugada P. Torsade de pointes. *PACE* 1988; **11**: 2246–9.

31. Pratt CM, Francis MJ, Luck JC, Wyndham CR, Miller RR, Quinones MA. Analysis of ambulatory electrocardiograms in 15 patients during spontaneous ventricular fibrillation with special reference to preceding arrhythmic events. *J Am Coll Cardiol* 1983; **2**: 789–97.

32. Olshausen KV, Witt T, Pop T, Treese N, Bethge KP, Meyer J. Sudden cardiac death while wearing a Holter monitor. *Am J Cardiol* 1991; **67**: 381–6.

33. Priori SG, Corr PB. Mechanisms underlying early and delayed afterdepolarization induced by catecholamines in isolated adult ventricular myocytes. *Am J Physiol* 1990; **258**: 1796–805.

34. Schwartz PJ, Malliani A. Electrical alternation of the T wave: clinical and experimental evidence of its relationship with the sympathetic nervous system and with the long QT syndrome. *Am Heart J* 1975; **89**: 45–50.

35. Zareba W, Moss AJ, LeCessie S, Hall JW. T wave alternans in congenital long QT syndrome. *JACC* 1994; **23**: 1541–6.

36. Verrier RL, Nearing BD. T wave alternans as a harbinger of ischemia-induced sudden cardiac death. In: Zipes DP, Jalife J (eds), *Cardiac Electrophysiology: From Cell to Bedside* (2nd edn). Philadelphia: W.B. Saunders, 1994: 467–77.

37. Rosenbaum MB, Acunzo RS. Pseudo 2:1 atrioventricular block and T wave alternans in the long QT syndromes. *JACC* 1991; **18**: 1363–6.

38. Han J, Millet D, Chizzonitti B, Moe GK. Temporal dispersion of recovery of excitability in atrium and ventricle as a function of heart rate. *Am Heart J* 1966; **71**: 481–7.

39. Leenhardt A, Glaser E, Burguera M, Nurnberg M, Maison-Blanche P, Coumel P. Short-coupled variant of torsade de pointes: a new electrocardiographic entity in the spectrum of idiopathic ventricular tachyarrhythmias. *Circulation* 1994; **89**: 206–15.

40. Locati EH, Maison-Blanche P, Bozza F, Dejode P, Coumel P. Probability of ventricular arrhythmias following stereotyped short–long sequences. In: *Computers in Cardiology*, Los Alamitos, CA: IEEE Comp. Soc. Press, 1993: 883–6.

6

Sudden Cardiac Death

A. Bayés de Luna, J. Guindo, X. Viñolas,
A. Bayés Genís and J. Sobral

Cardiac disease is the most frequent cause of death in the western world. Sudden cardiac death is dramatic in its presentation and its social and economic repercussions.

The term 'sudden death' has been used in different ways by epidemiologists, clinicians, forensic pathologists, and others.[1] There is no consensus regarding the precise definition of 'sudden' in terms of the duration of the time interval from the onset of symptoms to death. From a clinical point of view, sudden death generally is considered to be due to natural causes (thus excluding accidents, suicides, poisoning, and so on) and complete within an hour of the onset of symptoms. Sudden death may be caused by arrhythmias (90% of cases in the Hinkle and Thaler series[2]) or by irreversible heart failure (the remaining 10%). Sudden death due to arrhythmia is characterized by loss of consciousness and absence of an arterial pulse, without prior circulatory collapse, whereas sudden death due to heart failure involves progressive failure and leads to circulatory collapse before cardiac arrest occurs. If the patient is found dead, death is considered sudden if the subject was seen alive and well in the preceding 24 hours.

In this chapter we will discuss the epidemiology, associated diseases, final events, markers, and trigger mechanisms of sudden death, as well as the detection of patients at risk. Special emphasis will be placed on the value of Holter ambulatory ECG recordings in the study of these subjects.

Epidemiology

The worldwide incidence of sudden death is difficult to estimate because it varies with the prevalence of coronary artery disease in different countries. According to a study by the WHO,[3] the annual incidence of sudden death in the industrialized countries ranges from 19 to 159 cases per 100 000 males and from 35 to 64 per 100 000 females. Sudden death represents 12–32% of all natural deaths, depending on the time allotted to the interval from the onset of symptoms to death. In the Spanish sudden death study,[4] the percentage of sudden deaths was less than 10% of natural deaths. Sudden death is the most common form of death of cardiac origin. About 50% of patients with ischemic heart disease die suddenly.

In the USA and in other industrialized populations,[5] sudden death has decreased notably, probably because of the reduction in the number of new cases of ischemic heart disease produced by changes in diet and lifestyle. Nonetheless, the incidence of sudden death is still high and can be considered one of the foremost challenges in modern cardiology.

Sudden death shows a clear *circadian rhythm*, occurring most frequently between 7 am and 11 am.[6] This concurs with the higher incidence at that time of various clinical manifestations of ischemic heart disease (infarction, coronary spasm, and so on).

As regards *age*, there are two peaks in the incidence of sudden death. The first peak is from birth to 6 months of life (infantile sudden death syndrome), sudden death being the most important cause of death in the first year of life in the USA (8000 deaths per year). The second peak, which is much larger, occurs from 45 to 75 years and is characterized by an increasingly greater frequency of ischemic heart disease after the age of 40.

Coronary risk factors increase the incidence of sudden death just as they influence the presentation of ischemic heart disease.[4,7] In the Spanish study of sudden death, hypertension was the risk factor most often associated with sudden death in both sexes.[4] However, normalization of blood pressure levels in postinfarction patients who have a history of hypertension is a factor of poor prognosis, as shown by the Framingham study.[7] This is not a contradiction of the earlier statement, because normalization of blood pressure in postinfarction patients is due to deterioration of left ventricular function. In the Coronary Drug Project[8] and the aforementioned Spanish study, hypercholesterolemia was associated with both sudden death and increased total mortality. When *multivariant logistical analysis* is done on the Framingham study, including all coronary risk factors, it is found that age, systolic pressure, cigarette consumption, and relative body weight are all risk factors independently related with the incidence of sudden death.[9] In females, aside from age, only cholesterolemia and vital capacity are associated independently with increased risk of sudden death. Based on these parameters, 42% of sudden deaths in males and 53% in females occur in the 10% of the population situated in the highest percentile of multivariant risk.

Pathophysiology

The pathophysiology of sudden death must be viewed as a multifactorial problem[1] that is inseparable from the associated diseases and that includes the final evidence responsible for sudden death as well as the markers and trigger mechanisms of this event.

Associated Diseases

In about 90% of cases, sudden death occurs in persons with heart disease. In a small number of cases (<5%), sudden death is accompanied by a noncardiac catastrophe, such as massive cerebral or digestive hemorrhage. In other cases, no associated disease of any type is found.

Most heart diseases can produce sudden death (Table 6.1). However, ischemic heart disease is, by far, the one most frequently responsible for sudden death and is present in more than 80% of the subjects who die suddenly, particularly among patients over 35–40 years of age. Some of them die suddenly in the course of an acute coronary accident, with or without a known history of the disease, and others have chronic ischemic heart disease (particularly old acute myocardial infarction), in which sudden death often occurs in the absence of an evident acute ischemic crisis. This difference is not purely academic because the trigger mechanisms as well as the final arrhythmia and their potential prevention and treatment may differ.

From a pathological vantage point, it has been demonstrated[10] that the incidence of coronary atherosclerotic lesions is high in patients who die suddenly, whether or not preceded by symptoms, and that it is similar in the two groups. On the other hand, it has been reported[11] that the incidence of acute arterial lesions, including coronary thrombosis, is very high in patients who die suddenly. Fornes *et al.*[12] conducted a study of patients

Table 6.1 Principal causes of sudden death*

1. Ischemic heart disease

2. Cardiomyopathies
     idiopathic dilated cardiomyopathy
     hypertrophic cardiomyopathy
     arrhythmogenic right ventricular dysplasia

3. Valvular heart disease
     aortic stenosis
     mitral valve prolapse

4. Electrophysiological abnormalities
     pre-excitation syndromes
     long QT syndrome
     conduction system abnormalities

5. Congenital cardiac abnormalities (e.g. tetralogy of Fallot, abnormal coronary origin)

6. Other cardiovascular diseases (e.g. pulmonary embolism, dissecting aneurysm of the aorta)

7. Sudden death without apparent structural heart disease (e.g. idiopathic ventricular fibrillation)

8. Non-cardiac diseases (e.g. massive gastrointestinal bleeding, cerebral hemorrhage)

9. Sudden infant death syndrome

*Heart failure is frequently present.

with out-of-hospital sudden death, with or without known heart disease. Although these patients had a high incidence of significant coronary atherosclerotic lesions, the incidence of coronary thrombosis was low, in both the patients with and those without known heart disease (13% and 15% respectively). The findings of this study concur with those of clinical studies of patients who died out of hospital while wearing a Holter recorder[13] (see below), in which evidence of a new ischemic episode before sudden death was found in only a third of all patients but was very frequent (>80%) in the 20% of cases in whom sudden death was due to bradyarrhythmia, and was infrequent (12%) when the final arrhythmia that produced sudden death was classic ventricular fibrillation (>60%) (see below). Therefore, it seems evident that, although acute clinical manifestations of coronary atherosclerosis are usually caused by plaque rupture and subsequent thrombus formation,[18] the incidence of thrombosis varies greatly in different subsets of patients who die suddenly: it is very high in acute coronary syndromes and low in ambulatory sudden death without clinical evidence of acute myocardial ischemia. Undoubtedly, the presence on the plaque of components with a greater or a lesser thrombogenic capacity influences thrombus formation. Plaques that have a large atheromatous core content are at high risk of leading to acute coronary syndromes after spontaneously or mechanically induced rupture because of the increased thrombogenicity of plaque content.[18]

In subjects under 35–40 years, sudden death is relatively common in patients with hypertrophic cardiomyopathy, particularly in young athletes[15] and in subjects with valvular disease, above all aortic valve disease. Other associated diseases in this age group are Wolff–Parkinson–White type pre-excitation,[16] arrhythmogenic dysplasia of the right ventricle,[17] mitral prolapse,[18] congenital anomalies of the coronaries,[19] and others.

Regardless of age and associated disease, sudden death occurs more often in the presence of left ventricular hypertrophy and/or heart failure.[20]

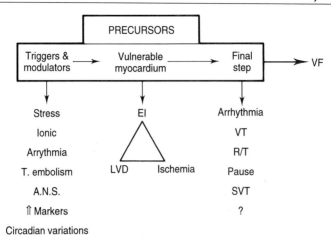

Figure 6.1 Cascade of factors leading to ventricular fibrillation (VF). ANS = autonomic nervous system; EI = electrical instability; LVD = left ventricular dysfunction; VT = ventricular tachycardia; R/T = R-on-T phenomenon; SVT = supraventricular tachyarrhythmias.

The Concept of Cardiac Arrest Cascade

Cardiac sudden death occurs as a result of cardiac arrest due to earlier ventricular fibrillation or secondary malignant bradycardia. In both cases, a series of trigger mechanisms can act on a vulnerable myocardium to precipitate the appearance of the final steps that terminate in either ventricular fibrillation or, less frequently, cardiac arrest due to bradyarrhythmia. The sequence of precursor events which act on a vulnerable myocardium to precipitate ventricular fibrillation can be called the 'ventricular fibrillation cascade'[21] (Figure 6.1). Similarly, the term 'cardiac arrest cascade' can be used to describe the events leading to bradyarrhythmia. We will remark on the most interesting of these phenomena below.

Final Events[1,13]

These include not only the final arrhythmia responsible for sudden death (ventricular fibrillation or severe bradyarrhythmia), but also the electrophysiological events that often precede sudden death. Continuous ECG recording, usually by means of the Holter technique, has thrown light on the final arrhythmia as well as on the characteristics of the 'final step' and some of the other precursors of these malignant arrhythmias in different groups of patients.

In this chapter we describe the arrhythmias and events preceding them in the following situations: (1) the pre-hospital phase of acute myocardial infarction; (2) ambulatory patients who suffer out-of-hospital sudden death; (3) patients with congestive heart failure; (4) patients with electrophysiological disorders; and (5) patients in terminal stages of noncardiac disease.

Pre-hospital phase of acute myocardial infarction

In patients whose sudden death is related to an acute ischemic event, records taken in mobile coronary units showed that the most frequent final arrhythmia[22] was primary ventricular fibrillation; that is, ventricular fibrillation not preceded by ventricular tachycardia (82%). In these patients, an R-on-T phenomenon was observed in 70% of cases

(Figure 6.2). Characteristically, an increased heart rate was seen before the lethal arrhythmia in patients with sudden death related to acute myocardial infarction as well as in ambulatory patients;[13] logically, this is related to an increase in sympathetic activity.

Ambulatory patients with out-of-hospital sudden death

Since the first case described by Gradman *et al.*,[23] several isolated cases and a small series of patients who have died while wearing a Holter recorder have been reported.[13] We have published the results of a worldwide survey including 233 such cases.[24] The most important conclusions of these studies seem to be the following (see Figures 6.3–6.7).

1. The causes of sudden death are ventricular tachyarrhythmia in 80% of cases and severe bradyarrhythmia in the remaining cases (10–20%).
2. Ventricular fibrillation (VF) starts abruptly in 10% of the cases; in the rest it is triggered by classical VT or less often a torsades de pointes arrhythmia. The clinical characteristics of these patients are summarized in Table 6.2.[13]
3. The VT leading to VF was often preceded by sinus tachycardia or new supraventricular tachyarrhythmia.

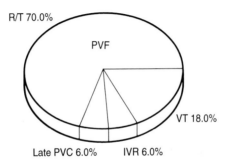

Figure 6.2 Proportions of final events in patients with ventricular fibrillation during the acute phase of myocardial infarction. R/T = R-on-T phenomenon; PVC = premature ventricular contractions; IVR = idioventricular rhythm; VT = ventricular tachycardia; PVF = primary ventricular fibrillation. (Modified from reference 22)

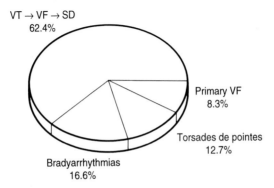

Figure 6.3 Causes of ambulatory sudden death recorded by Holter electrocardiography. VT = ventricular tachycardia. (Modified from reference 24)

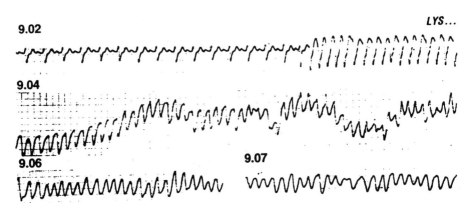

Figure 6.4 Ambulatory sudden death by ventricular fibrillation in a coronary patient treated with amiodarone for complex premature ventricular contraction. A monomorphic sustained ventricular tachycardia occurred at 9.02 am and ventricular fibrillation ensued at 9.04 am after an increase of ventricular tachycardia rate and QRS width. (Reproduced with permission from reference 13)

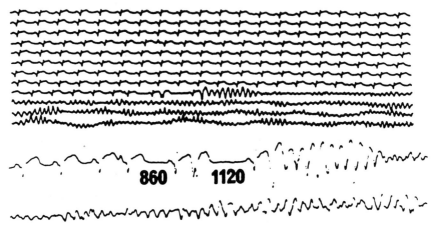

Figure 6.5 Ambulatory sudden death by primary ventricular fibrillation initiated by a ventricular extrasystole with short coupling interval occurring after a postextrasystolic pause (1120 ms). (Reproduced with permission from reference 13)

4. In the group of patients with VF, only 12% of patients presented ischemic ST changes prior to the final event. Therefore, the number of patients who die suddenly from acute infarction is probably lower than is usually assumed.
5. In patients who died suddenly from bradyarrhythmia, the cause was more often sinus depression then atrioventricular block, and the incidence of previous ST changes was surprisingly high (>80%).

Several conclusions can be drawn from our study. First, to prevent VF, sustained VT must be prevented. This may be achieved by preventing the sinus tachycardia or rapid heart rate that accompanies rapid supraventricular arrhythmia, an expression of the adrenergic mechanisms of lethal arrhythmia, and by suppressing premature ventricular complexes. It is possible that in some situations eliminating sinus tachycardia could help to suppress premature ventricular complexes.

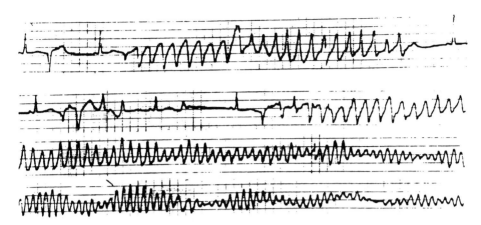

Figure 6.6 Typical pattern of torsades de pointes in a woman treated with quinidine for nonsustained ventricular tachycardia in the absence of heart disease. A long sequence of torsades de pointes induces ventricular fibrillation. (Reproduced with permission from reference 13)

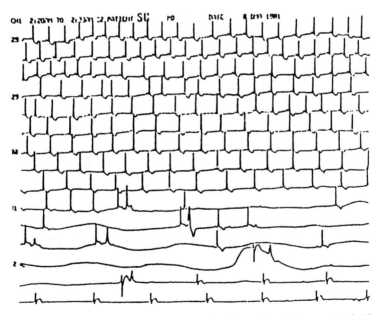

Figure 6.7 Ambulatory sudden death due to a progressive depression of sinus and subsidiary automatism in a postmyocardial infarction patient in the subacute phase. The primary cause of death was cardiac rupture with electromechanical dissociation.

Second, in cases of VF, the increase in basal heart rate before death can be reduced with beta-blockers – the best method of controlling the adrenergic mechanisms of lethal arrhythmia. This may explain the preventive effect these drugs have on sudden death after myocardial infarction.

Third, in some cases the final arrhythmia is triggered by a pause that is often postextrasystolic. Conceivably, pacing could prevent sudden death in these patients.

Table 6.2 Clinical characteristics of patients with Holter-recorded cardiac arrest

| | Ventricular tachyarrhythmias | | |
	Group I: VT or VF $n = 143$	Group II: Torsades de pointes $n = 42$	Group III: Bradyarrhythmias $n = 48$
Mean age (years)	70	60	70
Sex (males)	76%	40%	39%
Coronary patients	84%	50%	70%
No known heart disease	4%	22%	10%
Resuscitated	20%	28.5%	4%
Prior antiarrhythmic treatment	64%	76%	—

VT = sustained monomorphic ventricular tachycardia; VF = ventricular fibrillation.

These two important determinants (sympathetic tone and cardiac pause) are independent, but may have additive effects.

Fourth, certain patients sense palpitations when VT appears, and because these episodes can sometimes be interrupted by coughing, it is not too farfetched to hypothesize that a few hard, dry coughs at the onset of palpitations could save the patient's life.

Fifth, acute ischemia, manifested as ST segment changes on the ECG, with or without chest pain, was once considered a fundamental mechanism of sudden death. In view of the new findings this does not seem to be as important today. However, the incidence of ST segment alterations is higher in patients dying with bradyarrhythmia, probably because of the ischemic origin in these cases of the electromechanical dissociation leading to death. The higher incidence of ST segment depression before the final arrhythmia found by Pepine et al.[25] is probably related to a higher number of patients who died of bradyarrhythmia in their series.

Sixth, sudden death is sometimes due to the arrhythmogenic effect of antiarrhythmic drugs, even in patients without heart disease. This is especially true in the torsades de pointes group (Table 6.2) and physician awareness could limit sudden death especially in this group. For this reason, we feel that antiarrhythmic agents should be prescribed only when arrhythmia carries a significant risk. The possible arrhythmogenic effects of these drugs[26] may be studied by Holter ECG, and Holter parameters for existence of proarrhythmia are listed in Table 6.3.[27]

Seventh, future Holter studies of the mechanisms of production of ambulatory sudden death should be prospective and should use uniform methods. The subjects studied should have malignant or potentially malignant ventricular arrhythmias, and certainly not a 'general population'. The ECG mechanisms of sudden unexpected death in the

Table 6.3 Proposed definition of proarrhythmia based on change in frequency of ventricular premature complexes (VPC)

Mean VPC/hour frequency at baseline	Increase required for proarrhythmia
1–50	× 10
51–100	× 5
101–300	× 4
>301	× 3

general population are unknown, but are probably related to an acute myocardial infarction in a person who was asymptomatic and therefore went undiagnosed.

Finally, the incidence of ischemic ST alterations requires further study using Holter instruments equipped with three leads or more, and including observations on disturbances in the autonomic nervous system (such as heart rate variability).

Patients with congestive heart failure

In patients who die suddenly in the presence of advanced congestive heart failure, Luu *et al.*[28] have demonstrated that the incidence of ventricular tachyarrhythmias as the final arrhythmia is much lower (40%) than the incidence obtained in ambulatory patients in our series (approximately 80%) (Figure 6.8). Interestingly, all patients who died of VT/VF had a previous myocardial infarction, but previous myocardial infarction was present in fewer than half of the cases of the bradyarrhythmia/electromechanical dissociation group. This finding, and hyponatremia in the latter group, were the only two parameters that differentiated between the bradyarrhythmia and tachyarrhythmia groups (Table 6.4).

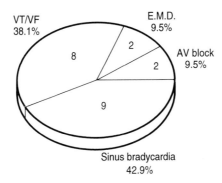

Figure 6.8   Final events in patients with advanced heart failure who died suddenly. VT = ventricular tachycardia; VF = ventricular fibrillation; EMD = electromechanical dissociation; AV = atrioventricular. (Reproduced with permission from reference 28)

Table 6.4   Comparison of sudden death victims in relation to the final event (bradyarrhythmia versus tachyarrhythmia)

Characteristic	BA/EMD $n = 13$	VT/VF $n = 8$	p
Age (years)	46 ± 16	54 ± 5	
Prior MI	6	8	0.02
History of sustained VT	2	2	
History of nonsustained VT	6	2	
Antiarrhythmic treatment	9	5	
Bundle branch block	4	2	
PR > 200 ms	3	1	
LV ejection fraction (%)	19 ± 9	15 ± 13	
Na (meq/l)	129 ± 3	133 ± 4	0.02
K (meq/l)	4.6 ± 1.2	4.4 ± 1.1	
Mg (meq/l)	2.1 ± 0.7	1.8 ± 0.1	
Resuscited	5	4	

Modified from Luu *et al.*[28]

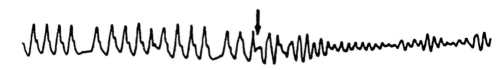

Figure 6.9   Atrial fibrillation leading to ventricular fibrillation in a patient with Wolff–Parkinson–White syndrome.

Other electrical causes

In patients with Wolff–Parkinson–White syndrome who die suddenly, it has been shown[16] that the final trigger of VF leading to sudden death is a supraventricular tachyarrhythmia, usually atrial fibrillation with a very rapid ventricular rate (Figure 6.9).

In patients with long QT syndrome, there is evidence that adrenergic hyperactivity produced by physical and/or mental stress may be responsible for triggering malignant ventricular tachycardia of the torsades de pointes type.[29]

On rare occasions, sudden death can be produced by primary bradyarrhythmia outside the context of heart failure. In these cases, sudden death from bradyarrhythmia is often due to electromechanical dissociation.[45]

Patients with terminal noncardiac disease

Wang *et al.*[30] studied terminal cardiac activity in adults who died without apparent heart disease, generally as a consequence of terminal malignancy. These patients were wearing Holter recorders and the final cause of death was confirmed to be bradyarrhythmia in 87% of the patients and ventricular tachyarrhythmia in 17%. Agonal ST segment elevation was often observed; the exact explanation of this phenomenon is unclear.

Markers and Trigger Mechanisms of Sudden Death[1,21,31,32]

The majority of patients who die suddenly present a vulnerable myocardium, for which different markers exist. Trigger factors act on this vulnerable myocardium to precipitate sudden death.

In the group of patients who die of ventricular tachyarrhythmia, postinfarction patients are the most numerous group, so we will give them particular attention. The risk of sudden death is related especially to the presence of electrical instability and to its interaction with left ventricular dysfunction and ischemia. These three factors form the imaginary triangle of risk of postinfarction complications[33] (Figure 6.10). As can be seen in Figure 6.11, the presence of markers of electrical instability (i.e. ischemia and left ventricular dysfunction) should alert us to the possible onset of a serious complication of myocardial infarction (sudden death, new coronary accident, and evident heart failure) that directly or indirectly potentiates the possibility of triggering sudden death. Different morphofunctional parameters (postinfarction scar, left ventricular hypertrophy, reduced ejection fraction), autonomic nervous system parameters (heart rate variability, QT interval, baroreflex sensitivity), and clinical and electrocardiographic findings (anamnesis and number and nature of the ventricular arrhythmias) can be considered as markers of electrical instability and, therefore, of myocardial vulnerability for sudden death. The markers of ischemia and left ventricular dysfunction are also shown in Figure 6.11.

The five most important trigger factors which act on a vulnerable myocardium are:

1. Physical or mental stress.
2. Ionic or metabolic disorders.

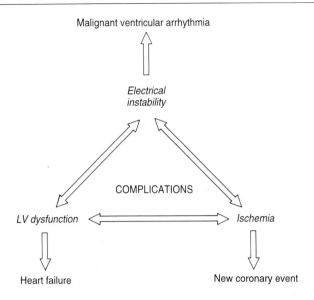

Figure 6.10   Triangle of risk factors for malignant ventricular arrhythmias in postmyocardial infarction patients. LV = left ventricular.

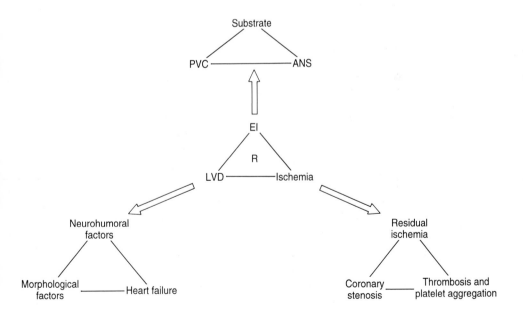

Figure 6.11   Triangle of risk factors for malignant ventricular arrhythmias in postmyocardial infarction patients. R = risk; ANS = autonomic nervous system; PVC = premature ventricular contraction; EI = electrical instability; LVD = left ventricular dysfunction.

3. Acceleration of sinus rhythm or appearance of a supraventricular arrhythmia or a pause.
4. The arrhythmogenic effect of certain drugs as demonstrated in the CAST study.[26]
5. Interaction of electrical instability with ischemia and/or left ventricular dysfunction due to multiple causes.[34]

The relationship between ischemia and sudden death depends to a great extent on the duration and severity of ischemia.[32] It is evident that persistent and severe transmural ischemia can induce sudden death in acute infarction. However, in transitory transmural ischemia, as Prinzmetal's angina[35] and during PTCA,[36] the relationship between ischemia and malignant ventricular arrhythmias is less definite. During moderate subendocardial ischemia, in our opinion[37] malignant ventricular arrhythmias are only infrequently induced.

In ambulatory patients,[12] ischemia probably precipitates ventricular tachyarrhythmias and sudden death only in a small number (12%) of patients.

Holter ECG was recorded in four patients during evolving acute infarction, by Turitto *et al.*, who demonstrated a significant time delay between the onset of ST elevation and the occurrence of ventricular arrhythmias in all four patients studied.[38] Only in one of the four patients studied was a VT seen to degenerate into VF. As in most cases who die from classic VF, sustained VT precedes this event, we believe strongly that acute thrombosis is not responsible for the majority of sudden deaths. Thus, it appears that although an ischemic milieu is present in most patients who die suddenly, and that a new episode of acute ischemia contributes to sudden death in the course of acute myocardial infarction, acute ischemia is usually not responsible for ambulatory sudden death in patients with chronic coronary disease.

Sudden death that occurs in patients with noncoronary heart disease[15–17] also is conditioned by a vulnerable myocardium and certain triggering factors. Heart failure, left ventricular hypertrophy and electrical instability (ventricular arrhythmias, autonomic nervous system dysfunction) are usually the most important markers of vulnerable myocardium, while other factors such as physical or mental stress, ionic or metabolic disturbances, drug administration, etc., may also act as triggers.

The presence of either wall motion or ECG abnormalities define patients with a several-fold higher risk of recurrent cardiac arrest compared with subjects without such abnormalities.[39] The risk of recurrent cardiac arrest within 5 years was 30% (versus 5% without) in subjects with an abnormal ECG ($p < 0.03$). Age also was an independent predictor of recurrent cardiac arrest in this group ($p < 0.03$), but surprisingly, recurrent cardiac arrest occurred more frequently among younger patients.

Identification of High-Risk Candidates

Patients at the highest risk of sudden death (Table 6.5) are those who have previously experienced a malignant ventricular arrhythmia (sustained ventricular tachycardia or out-of-hospital cardiac arrest). In patients without previous malignant ventricular arrhythmias, the risk of sudden death is related to the presence of different markers and

Table 6.5 Patients at high risk of sudden death

---

1. History of malignant ventricular arrhythmia (sustained ventricular tachycardia or out-of-hospital cardiac arrest)
2. Heart disease with markers of a vulnerable myocardium for malignant ventricular arrhythmias (depressed contractility, ischemia, electrical instability)
3. Severe bradyarrhythmias

Table 6.6   Methods to identify a high-risk patient

1. Clinical history and physical examination (syncope, angina, etc.)
2. Surface ECG (Q waves, ventricular enlargement, QT interval, arrhythmias, etc.)
3. Exercise testing (ST segment abnormalities, poor hemodynamic response, arrhythmias, etc.)
4. Ambulatory Holter ECG (arrhythmias, ischemia, autonomic tone, ventricular late potentials, etc.)
5. Electrophysiological studies (induction of sustained ventricular tachyarrhythmias, anomalous pathways, sinus node dysfunction, etc.)
6. Signal-averaged ECG (ventricular late potentials)
7. Echocardiography–Doppler (ventricular function, aneurysm, ischemia, valvular dysfunction, etc.)
8. Nuclear studies (ventricular function, aneurysm, ischemia, etc.)
9. Cardiac angiography (coronary artery lesions, ventricular function, aneurysm, cardiac biopsy, valvular abnormalities, etc.)

trigger factors, described earlier. These latter patients usually have advanced heart disease (postinfarction cardiomyopathy), frequently with heart failure, acute-stage of coronary insufficiency and/or other markers. Various techniques and clinical findings are used to detect them (Table 6.6).

We can emphasize that clinical data are still very useful both for stratifying risk in patients who have presented severe arrhythmias[40] and for the general study of postinfarction patients.[41] Nonetheless, complementary studies must be made to obtain more information.

In postinfarction patients, simple surface ECG[42] and an exercise test[43,44] and an echocardiogram[45] may suffice for evaluating the risk of complications. However, the realization of a Holter ECG using currently available techniques reveals many markers of electrical instability[46–49] (number and characteristics of the premature ventricular complexes, heart rate variability, dynamic behavior of the QT) and permits the study of late potentials and the evaluation of residual ischemia.[50–52] We address this later.

The Value of the Holter Technique

Studies in the early 1980s[47,53] showed that postinfarction patients with more premature ventricular complexes had a worse prognosis. These studies highlighted two interesting findings: (1) that the prognosis was not related to the Lown grade, but was related to the number and presence of repetitive forms; and (2) that the prognosis was poor, especially if the ventricular function was depressed. These suggested that premature ventricular complexes were of minor importance and that the only important consideration was ventricular function.[54] However, different studies[55,56] have shown that premature ventricular complexes are an independent factor of poor prognosis. The BHAT study[55] showed in a group without beta-blocker treatment that the incidence of sudden death was much greater in the patients who had ventricular arrhythmias, regardless of the presence or absence of other risk factors. Moreover, it has been reported recently[56] that patients with heart failure who died suddenly had significantly longer ($p = 0.003$) and faster ($p = 0.029$) ventricular tachycardias in their baseline ambulatory ECG than survivors. This association was not observed in patients who died of progressive pump failure. Therefore, a low left ventricular ejection fraction and ventricular tachycardia on the 24-hour ECG recording predict an increased risk of cardiac mortality. These results also suggest that longer and faster ventricular tachycardias recorded by 24-hour ECG may identify patients at risk of sudden death, a finding which may have therapeutic implications.

It is not yet known whether the prognosis will improve if premature ventricular complexes are suppressed pharmacologically. It seems clear that the class I drugs are harmful,[34] but we now are awaiting the results of large-scale trials with class III drugs (the amiodarone [EMIAT] and the solatol [SWORD] studies) to see if the good preliminary results of pilot studies are confirmed.

Abnormalities of autonomic input to the heart, as indicated by a decreased heart rate variability (HRV), are associated with increased susceptibility to ventricular arrhythmia. Lower HRV indices are also associated with congestive heart failure, diabetes, and alcoholic cardiomyopathy. It has been reported[38] that, in spite of evidence that HRV is significantly depressed in patients with heart failure, the analysis of HRV (with the signal-averaged electrocardiogram and electrophysiological studies) is not helpful in identifying patients with heart failure at risk of sudden cardiac death. On the other hand, patients with advanced heart failure of similar functional class, ejection fraction and disease etiology may show marked differences in beat-to-beat HRV detected in Poincaré plots but not necessarily in standard deviation measures of HRV. Complex Poincaré plots are associated with higher norepinephrine levels, suggesting more severe heart failure than that suggested by torpedo-shaped patterns. Nevertheless, further investigation is warranted to determine whether Poincaré plots can provide additional prognostic information and insight into autonomic disorders and sudden cardiac death in patients with heart failure.

Decreased HRV (CLV > 50 ms) was reported to be an independent risk factor for postmyocardial infarction mortality by the Multicenter Post Infarction Project (MPIP) in 1987.[59] Since then, other investigators have corroborated this finding.[60] In addition, among survivors of acute myocardial infarction, both Bigger et al.[61] and Farrell et al.[62] have shown that decreased HRV predicted both death and arrhythmic events with more sensitivity and specificity than conventional predictors, such as left ventricular ejection fraction. Moreover, HRV parameters are markedly lower in survivors of sudden cardiac death with inducible VT in the electrophysiology laboratory than in controls.[63] Low HRV also has been reported to predict mortality among patients undergoing coronary angiography. It has been reported[64] that in 100 stable patients who had previous elective angiography (none had myocardial infarction within 4 weeks, nonischemic cardiomyopathy, or valvular disease), SDNN below 50 ms was associated with greater one-year mortality compared with patients who had SDNN above 50 ms. In patients awaiting cardiac transplantation, SDNN below 55 ms identified patients at a 20-fold greater risk of mortality.[65]

The dynamic behavior of the QT interval throughout a Holter recording is a reliable marker for malignant ventricular arrhythmias, as our preliminary studies using manual measurements suggest.[48,66] A rapid, automatic readout on the incidence of the R-on-T phenomenon would also be helpful, as well as information on different variables related to this phenomenon (heart rate, QT interval, and ST change). This would help to elucidate the factors that contribute to conversion of the R-on-T phenomenon into a trigger mechanism for fatal arrhythmia. It would also be interesting to find out if sudden death is preceded by changes in blood pressure and cardiac function.

Recently, the Holter technique has been used to study late potentials and a good correlation with conventional techniques has been encountered.[67] However, there is no evidence that changes in HRV or QT trigger sudden death. These two parameters thus are markers but not triggers of sudden death.

The Holter technique may also be useful for stratifying prognosis in hypertrophic cardiomyopathy, according to the experience of McKenna.[68] However, results have been inconclusive.[69] Holter ECG is not very useful in patients with Wolff–Parkinson–White syndrome. Electrophysiological studies are needed to determine the prognosis and stratify the risk.[16]

The usefulness of the Holter technique has also been studied after repair of Fallot tetralogy. Ventricular arrhythmia is common after repair of tetralogy of Fallot and has been proposed as an indicator of risk of late sudden death. Recently, Deanfield's group have reported[70] that late ventricular arrhythmias are rare in patients with successful early

Table 6.7 Sensitivity, specificity and predictive value of ventricular late potentials in postmyocardial infarction patients

Cardiac events	LP ($n = 49$)	No LP ($n = 161$)	
MVA ($n = 10$)	9	1	Sensitivity = 90% (1/10)
No MVA ($n = 200$)	40	160	Specificity = 80% (40/200)
	PPV = 18% (9/49)	NPV = 99% (1/161)	

LP = ventricular late potentials; MVA = malignant ventricular arrhythmias; PPV = positive predictive value; NPV = negative predictive value.

correction of tetralogy of Fallot, unless complex or multiple operations are performed, and that nonsustained ventricular arrhythmia on ambulatory ECG does not identify patients at high risk for sudden death after repair of tetralogy of Fallot.[71] There does not appear to be any advantage in potentially dangerous long-term antiarrhythmic therapy for asymptomatic postoperative patients.

Most of the procedures used for stratifying the risk of sudden death are of limited value, whether they are used to evaluate electrical instability (any of its markers), ischemia, or left ventricular dysfunction. This is due to the fact that, while specificity and sensitivity usually are high, the positive predictive value for malignant arrhythmia or sudden death is low (<20%). An example of the value of the presence of late potentials for stratifying risk of malignant arrhythmias in postinfarction patients is shown in Table 6.7. It can be seen how even with a high sensitivity (90%) and a fairly high specificity (80%), epidemiological reality (the majority of postinfarction patients do not present malignant arrhythmias) dictates a low positive predictive value (20%). This means that out of 100 patients with positive late potentials, only about 20 will present a malignant arrhythmia. In contrast, the negative predictive value is very high (>99%), which means that postinfarction patients who do not present late potentials have a good prognosis in relation to sudden death. It is thus evident that we should use a multifactorial approach to increase positive predictive value. For this reason, it is advisable to evaluate different parameters for studying factors related with the multifactorial problem of sudden death.[72,73] To date, the association that has the highest positive predictive value (about 50%) is the sum of RR variability, late potentials, and runs of ventricular tachycardia in the Holter recording. In the future, we should aim to raise the positive predictive value by adding new parameters to those that have been studied to identify high-risk patients more clearly.

In carriers of severe bradyarrhythmia (sinus node disease and/or atrioventricular block), the risk of sudden death can be detected[31] by symptoms (syncope), by the Holter technique (pauses), and by intracavitary electrophysiological studies.

Prognostic Stratification in the Thrombolytic Era

There are indications that the prognosis of patients with or without fibrinolytic therapy following an acute myocardial infarction differs. In a study by Farrell *et al.*[74] in nonthrombolyzed patients, the presence in the Holter recording of VPBs decreased RR variability, and late ventricular potentials, and the results of the exercise test and an ejection fraction below 40% discriminated the patients at high risk of future arrhythmic events. However, in thrombolyzed patients only the diminished RR variability discriminated between the two groups. In this study, the incidence of risk markers (late ventricular potentials, low

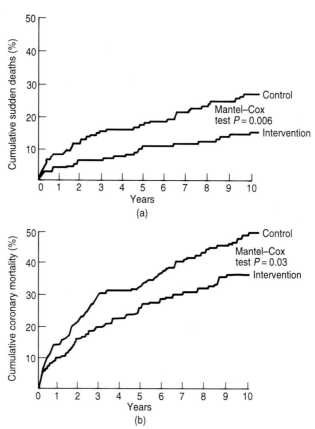

Figure 6.12 Effect of multifactorial intervention on mortality of postmyocardial infarction patients. (Reproduced with permission from reference 79)

ejection fraction, positive exercise test, and absence of RR variability) did not differ in the two groups. Other authors found variations in some markers after thrombolysis. Although our series of patients[75] and that of Turitto et al.[76] disclosed a similar incidence of late potentials in thrombolyzed and nonthrombolyzed patients, most studies have found a significant relationship with the incidence of late potentials.[77,78] Moreover, the reduction of the incidence of late ventricular potentials seems to be independent of ejection fraction.

Pedretti et al.[80] investigated postmyocardial infarction thrombolyzed patients with electrophysiological, 48-hour Holter, signal-averaged ECG and 2-D echo studies. They demonstrated that thrombolysis significantly reduced the occurrence of arrhythmic events. The GISSI-2 study[81] showed that frequent premature ventricular beats, studied by Holter monitoring, remained even in the fibrinolytic era, an independent risk factor of total and sudden death in the first 6 months following an acute myocardial infarction.

However, it should be emphasized that, although it is evident that thrombolytic treatment produces a substantial reduction in postinfarction mortality, it cannot be forgotten that a global cardioprotective approach may be the key to reducing postinfarction mortality, particularly in the post-hospital phase. Undoubtedly, thrombolytic treatment is an important, perhaps even the single most important short-term factor, but other factors such as ventricular arrhythmias and decreased heart rate variability that were important in the prethrombolytic era have not ceased to be important. The study of Hämäläinen *et al.*[79] evaluated the effectiveness of a long-term multifactorial intervention program, to reduce sudden death by medication, cessation of smoking, physical exercise, diet, psychosocial support and optimal medical care. The patients included in the intervention group had an incidence of sudden death of 12.6% at 10 years versus 23% in the group that received no standardized intervention (Figure 6.12).

Thus it seems to be evident that, in the overall approach to patients with heart disease and potential risk of sudden death, the Holter technique is a low-cost option that can be used to study more parameters than any other technique. Its value does not seem to have diminished in postinfarction patients even in the thrombolytic era.

References

1. Goldstein S, Bayés de Luna A, Guindo Soldevila J. *Sudden Cardiac Death.* Armonk, NY: Futura, 1994.
2. Hinkle LE, Thaler HT. Clinical classification of cardiac deaths. *Circulation* 1982; **63**: 457–64.
3. WHO Technical Report. *Sudden Cardiac Death.* Geneva: WHO, 1985: 726.
4. Cosin J. Out-of-hospital sudden death in Spain. In: Bayés de Luna A, Brugada P, Cosin J, Navarro Lopez F (eds), *Sudden Cardiac Death.* Dordrecht: Kluwer Academic, 1991, 19–30.
5. Goldberg RJ. Declining out-of-hospital sudden coronary death rates: additional pieces of the epidemiologic puzzle. *Circulation* 1989; **79**: 1396–73.
6. Muller JE, Lubner PL, Willich SN, Tofler GH, Aylmer G, Klangos I, Stone PH. Circadian variation in the frequency of sudden cardiac death. *Circulation* 1987; **75**: 131–8.
7. Kannel WB, Thomas HE. Sudden coronary death: the Framingham study. *Ann NY Acad Sci* 1982; **382**: 3–21.
8. Coronary Drug Project Research Group. Natural history of myocardial infarction in the Coronary Drug Project: long-term prognostic importance of serum lipid levels. *Am J Cardiol* 1978; **42**: 489.
9. Kannel WB, McGee DL, Scharzkin A. An epidemiological perspective of sudden death: 26-year follow-up in the Framingham study. *Drugs* 1984; **28** (Suppl 1): 1–16.
10. Warnes C, Roberts W. Sudden coronary death: relation of amount and distribution of coronary narrowing at necropsy to previous symptoms of myocardial ischemia, left ventricular scarring and heart weight. *Am J Cardiol* 1984; **54**: 65–73.
11. Davies MJ, Thomas A. Thrombosis and acute coronary artery lesions in sudden cardiac death. *N Engl J Med* 1984; **310**: 1137–40.
12. Fornes F, Lecomte D, Nicolas G. Mort subite coronaire extrahospitalière: étude autopsique comparative netre des sujeys avec et sans antécédents cardiovasculaires. *Arch Mal Coeur* 1994; **87**: 319–24.
13. Bayés de Luna A, Coumel P, Leclercq JF. Ambulatory sudden death: mechanisms of production of fatal arrhythmia on the basis of data from 157 cases. *Am Heart J* 1989; **117**: 151–59.
14. Fuster V, Badimon L, Badimon JJ, Chesebro JH. The pathogenesis of coronary artery disease and the acute coronary syndromes. *New Engl J Med* 1992; **326**: 242,310–18.
15. Maron BJ, Fananapazir L. Sudden cardiac death in hypertrophic cardiomyopathy. *Circulation* 1992; **85**: I57–63.
16. Torner P, Brugada P, Smeets J, *et al.* Ventricular fibrillation in the Wolff–Parkinson–White syndrome. *Eur Heart J* 1991; **12**: 144–50.
17. Thiene G, Nava A, Conando D, Rossi L, Pennelli N. Right ventricular cardiomyopathy and sudden death in young people. *New Engl J Med* 1988; **328**: 129–33.
18. Kligfield P, Levy D, Devereux RB, Savage DD. Arrhythmias and sudden death in mitral valve prolapse. *Am Heart J* 1987; **113**: 1298–307.
19. Cheitlin MD, DeCastro CM, McAllister HA. Sudden death as a complication of anomalous left coronary origin from the anterior sinus of Valsalva: a not so minor congenital anomaly. *Circulation* 1974; **50**: 780.
20. Bayés de Luna A, Viñolas X, Guindo J, *et al.* Ventricular arrhythmias in left ventricular hypertrophy and heart failure. *Eur Heart J* 1993; **14**: J62–64.
21. Bayés de Luna A, Viñolas X, Guindo J, Bayés Genis A. The concept of ventricular fibrillation cascade. *J Cardiovasc Electrophysiol* (in press).
22. Adgey AA, Devlin JE, Webb SW, Mulholland HC. Initiation of ventricular fibrillation outside hospital in patients with acute ischemic heart disease. *Br Heart J* 1982; **47**: 55–61.
23. Gradman AH, Bell PA, DeBusj RF. Sudden death during ambulatory monitoring: clinical and electrocardiographic correlations: report of a case. *Circulation* 1977; **55**: 210.
24. Bayés de Luna A, Guindo J, Rivera J. Ambulatory sudden death in patients wearing Holter devices. *J. Ambulat Monitor* 1989; **2**: 3–13.
25. Pepine C, Morganroth J, McDonald JT, Gottlieb SO. Sudden death during ambulatory ECG monitoring. *Am J Cardiol* 1991; **68**: 785–8.
26. CAST investigators' preliminary report. Effect of encainide and flecainide on mortality in a randomised trial of arrhythmia suppression after myocardial infarction. *New Engl J Med* 1989; **321**: 406–12.

27. Morganroth J, Borland M, Chao G. Application of a frequency definition of ventricular proarrhythmia. *Am J Cardiol* 1987; **59**: 97-9.
28. Luu M, Stevenson WG, Stevenson LW, Baron K, Walden J. Diverse mechanisms of unexpected cardiac arrest in advanced heart failure. *Circulation* 1989; **80**: 1675-80.
29. Moss AJ, Schwartz PJ, Crampton RS, *et al*. The long QT syndrome: prospective longitudinal study of 328 families. *Circulation* 1991; **84**: 1136-44.
30. Wang F, Lien W, Fong T, *et al*. Terminal cardiac electrical activity in adults who die without apparent cardiac disease. *Am J Cardiol* 1986; **58**: 491-5.
31. Bayés de Luna A, Guindo J, Fiol M, Dominguez de Rozas JM. Sudden cardiac death. In: Fisch C, Surawicz B (eds), *Cardiac Electrophysiology and Arrhythmias*. New York: Elsevier, 1991.
32. Bayés de Luna A, Guindo Soldevila J, Viñolas X. Do silent myocardial ischemia and ventricular arrhythmias interact to result in sudden death? *Cardiol Clin* 1992; **10**: 449-59.
33. Bayés de Luna A. (ed.). *Prevención Secundaria del Infarto de Miocardio*. Barcelona: Ed. MCR, 1994.
34. Bayés de Luna A, Viñolas X, Guindo J, Bayés Genis A. Risk stratification after myocardial infarction: role of electrical instability, ischemia, and left ventricular function. *Cardiovasc Drug Ther* 1994; **8**: 335-43.
35. Báyes de Luna A, Carreras F, Cladellas M, Oca F, Sagués F, García Moll M. Holter ECG study of the electrocardiographic phenomena in Prinzmetal angina attacks with emphasis on the study of ventricular arrhythmias. *J Electrocardiol* 1985; **18**: 267-76.
36. Meinertz T, Zeheder M, Hohnloser S, Just H. Prevalence of ventricular arrhythmias during silent myocardial ischemia. *Cardiovasc Rev Rep* 1988; (Suppl A): 34-7.
37. Camacho AM, Guindo J, Bayés de Luna A. Usefulness of silent myocardial ischemia detected by ST segment depression in postmyocardial infarction patients as a predictor of ventricular arrhythmias. *Am J Cardiol* 1992; **69**: 1243-4.
38. Turitto G, Zanchi E, Prati P. Acute myocardial infarction during Holter recording. *Am J Cardiol* 1989; **63**: 364-6.
39. Kudenchuck PJ, Cobb LA, Greene HL, Fahrenbruch CE, Sheehan FH. Late outcome of survivors of out-of-hospital cardiac arrest with left ventricular ejection fraction >50% and without significant coronary arterial narrowing. *Am J Cardiol* 1991; **67**: 704-8.
40. Brugada P, Talajic M, Smeets J, Mulleneers R, Wellens HJJ. The value of clinical history to assess prognosis of patients with ventricular tachycardia or ventricular fibrillation after myocardial infarction. *Eur Heart J* 1989; **10**: 747-52.
41. Arnold AER, Simoons ML, Deetry JM, *et al*. Prediction of mortality following hospital discharge after thrombolysis for acute myocardial infarction: is there a need for coronary angiography? *Eur Heart J* 1993; **14**: 306-15.
42. Fisch C. Role of the electrocardiogram in identifying the patient at increased risk for sudden death. *J Am Coll Cardiol* 1985; **5**(Suppl B): 6-8.
43. Waters DD, Bosch X, Bouchard A, Moise A, Roy D, Pelletier G, Theroux P. Comparison of clinical variables derived from a limited predischarge exercise testing as predictors of early and late mortality after myocardial infarction. *J Am Coll Cardiol* 1985; **5**: 1-8.
44. Theroux P, Waters D, Halphenm C, Debaisieux JC, Mizgala H. Prognostic value of exercise testing soon after myocardial infarction. *New Engl J Med* 1979; **301**: 341-5.
45. Shiina A, Tajik AJ, Smith HC, Lengyel M, Seward JB. Prognostic significance of regional motion abnormality in patients with prior myocardial infarction: a prospective correlative study of two-dimensional echocardiography and angiography. *Mayo Clin Proc* 1986; **61**: 254-62.
46. Bigger JT, Fleiss JL, Kleiger R, Miller P, Kolnitzky. The relationship among ventricular arrhythmias, left ventricular dysfunction, and mortality in the 2 years after myocardial infarction. *Circulation* 1984; **69**: 250-8.
47. Kleiger RE, Miller JP, Bigger JT, Moss AJ. Decreased heart rate variability and its association with increased mortality after acute myocardial infarction. *Am J Cardiol* 1987; **59**: 256-62.
48. Martí V, Guindo J, Homs E, Viñolas X, Bayés de Luna A. Peaks of QTc lengthening measures in Holter recordings as a marker of life-threatening arrhythmias in postmyocardial infarction patients. *Am Heart J* 1992; **124**: 234-5.
49. La Rovere MT, Specchia G, Mortara A, Schwartz PJ. Barorelex sensitivity, clinical correlates, and cardiovascular mortality among patients with first myocardial infarction: a prospective study. *Circulation* 1988; **78**: 816-24.
50. Tzivoni D, Gavish A, Gottlieb S, Moriel M, Keren A, Banai S, Stern S. Prognostic significance of ischemic episodes in postinfarction patients. *Am J Cardiol* 1988; **62**: 661-4.
51. Rocco MB, Nabel EG, Campbell S, Goldman L, Barry J, Mead K, Selwyn AP. Prognostic importance of myocardial ischemia detected by ambulatory monitoring in patients with stable coronary artery disease. *Circulation* 1988; **78**: 877-84.
52. Gottlieb LS, Weisfeldt M, Ouyang P, Mellits D, Gertenblinth G. Silent ischemia as a marker for early unfavorable outcomes in patients with unstable angina. *New Engl J Med* 1986; **314**: 1.214-19.
53. Ruberman W, Weinblatt E, Golberg J. Ventricular premature complexes and sudden death after myocardial infarction. *Circulation* 1981; **64**: 297-305.
54. Ahnve S, Gilpin E, Henning H, Curtis G, Ross J. Limitations and advantages of the ejection fraction for defining high risk after acute myocardial infarction. *Am J Cardiol* 1986; **58**: 872-8.
55. Kostis JB, Byington R, Friedman LM, Goldstein S, Furberg C, and the BHAT study group. Prognostic significance of ventricular ectopic activity in survivors of acute myocardial infarction. *J Am Coll Cardiol* 1987; **10**: 231-42.
56. Szabó BN, Nan Veldhuisen DJ, Crijns HJGM, Wiesfeld ACP, Hillege HL, Lie KI. Value of ambulatory electrocardiographic monitoring to identify increased risk of sudden death in patients with left ventricular dysfunction and heart failure. *Eur Heart J* 1994; **15**: 928-33.

57. Stein PK, Bosner MS, Kleiger RE, Conger BM. Heart rate variability: a measure of cardiac autonomic tone. *Am Heart J* 1994; **127**: 1376–81.
58. Woo MA, Stevenson WG, Moser DK, Middlekauff HR. Complex heart rate variability and serum noreprinephine levels in patients with advanced heart failure. *J Am Coll Cardiol* 1994; **23**: 565–9.
59. Kleiger RE, Miller JP, Bigger JT, Moss AJ and the Multicenter Post-Infarction Research Group. Decreased heart rate variability and its association with increased mortality after acute myocardial infarction. *Am J Cardiol* 1987; **59**: 256–62.
60. Cripps TR, Malik M, Farrell TS, Camm AJ. Prognostic value of reduced heart rate variability after acute myocardial infarction: clinical evaluation of a new analysis method. *Br Heart J* 1991; **65**: 14–19.
61. Bigger JT, Fleiss J, Steinman RC, Rolnitzky LM, Kleiger RE, Rottman JN. Frequency domain measures of heart period variability and mortality after myocardial infarction. *Circulation* 1992; **85**: 164–71.
62. Farrell TG, Bashir Y, Cripps T, Malik M, Poloniecki J, Bennett ED, Ward DE, Camm AJ. Risk stratification for arrhythmic events in postinfarction patients based on heart rate variability, ambulatory electrocardiographic variables and the signal-averaged electrocardiogram *J Am Coll Cardiol* 1991; **18**: 687–97.
63. Singer DH, Martin GL, Magid L, *et al.* Low heart rate variability and sudden cardiac death. *J Electrocardiol* 1988; **21**: S46–55.
64. Rich MW, Saini JS, Kleiger RE, Carney RM, Tevelde A, Freedland KE. Correlation of heart rate variability with clinical and angiographic variables and late mortality after coronary angiography. *Am J Cardiol* 1988; **62**: 714–17.
65. Binder T, Frey B, Porenta G, *et al.* Prognostic value of heart rate variability in patients awaiting cardiac transplantation. *PACE* 1992; **15**: 2215–20.
66. Laguna P, Thakor NV, Caminal P, Jané R, Yoon HR, Bayés de Luna A, Marti V, Guindo J. New algorithm for QT interval analysis in 24-hour Holter ECG: performance and applications. *Med Biol Eng Comput* 1990; **28**: 67–73.
67. Kelen GJ, Henkin R, Lannon M, Bloonsield D, El-Sherif N. Correlation between the signal-averaged electrocardiogram from Holter tapes and from real-time recordings. *Am J Cardiol* 1989; **63**: 1321.
68. McKenna WJ, England D, Doi YL, Deanfield JE, Oakley C, Goodwin JF. Arrhythmia in hypertrophic cardiomyopathy. I: Influence on prognosis. *Br Heart J* 1981; **46**: 168–72.
69. Fananapazir L, Tracy CM, Leon MB, *et al.* Electrophysiologic abnormalities in patients with hypertrophic cardiomyopathy: a consecutive analysis in 155 patients. *Circulation* 1989; **80**: 1259–68.
70. Joffe H, Gergakopoulos D, Celemajer DS, Sullivan ID, Deanfield JE. Late ventricular arrhythmia is rare after early repair of tetralogy of Fallot. *J Am Coll Cardiol* 1994; **23**: 1146–50.
71. Cullen S, Celermajer DS, Franklin RCG, Hallidie-Smith A, Deanfield JE. Prognostic significance of ventricular arrhythmia after repair of tetralogy of Fallot: 12-year prospective study. *J Am Coll Cardiol* 1994; **23**: 1151–5.
72. Kuchar DL, Thorburn CW, Sammel NL. Prediction of serious arrhythmic events after myocardial infarction: signal-averaged electrocardiogram, Holter monitoring and radionuclide ventriculography. *J Am Coll Cardiol* 1987; **9**: 531–8.
73. Cripps T, Bennett D, Camm J, Ward D. Prospective evaluation of clinical assessment, exercise testing and signal-averaged electrocardiogram in predicting outcome after acute myocardial infarction. *Am J Cardiol* 1988; **62**: 995–9.
74. Farrell T, Bashir Y, Poloniecki J, Ward D, Camm AJ. The effects of thrombolysis on risk stratification for arrhythmic events in post infarction patients. *J Am Coll Cardiol* 1991; **17**: 17A.
75. Madoery C, Guindo J, Lousada N, *et al.* Incidencia de los potenciales ventriculares tardios en pacientes postinfarto de miocardio. *Rev Argentina Cardiol* 1991; **59**: 67–75.
76. Turitto G, Risa AL, Zanchi E, Prati PL. The signal-averaged electrocardiogram and ventricular arrhythmias after thrombolysis for acute myocardial infarction. *J Am Coll Cardiol* 1990; **15**: 1270–6.
77. Gang ES, Lew AS, Hong M, Wang FZ, Siebert CA, Peter T. Decreased incidence of ventricular late potentials after successful thrombolytic therapy for acute myocardial infarction. *New Engl J Med* 1989; **321**: 712–16.
78. Moreno FL, Karagounis L, Ipsen S, Marshall H, Anderson JL. Thrombolysis-related early reperfusion reduces ECG late potentials after acute myocardial infarction. *J Am Coll Cardiol* 1991; **17**: 312A.
79. Hämäläinen H, Luurila OJ, Kallio V, Knuts LR, Arstila M, Hakkila J. Long-term reduction in sudden death after a multifactorial intervention program in patients with myocardial infarction: 10-year results of a controlled investigation. *Eur Heart J* 1989; **10**: 55–62.
80. Pedretti RFE, Colombo E, Braza SS, Caru B. Effect of thrombolysis on heart rate variability and life-threatening ventricular arrhythmias in survivors of acute myocardial infarction. *J Am Coll Cardiol* 1994; **23**: 19–26.
81. Maggioni AP, Zuanetti G, Franzosi MG, Rovelli F, Santoro E, Staszewsky L, Tavazzi L, Tognoni G. Prevalence and prognostic significance of ventricular arrhythmias after acute myocardial infarction in the fibrinolytic era: GISSI-2 results. *Circulation* 1993; **87**: 312–22.

7

Arrhythmias Detected With Implantable Cardioverter– Defibrillators

Marc Roelke and Jeremy N. Ruskin

Introduction

Historically, ambulatory rhythm monitoring has been limited to Holter and other surface electrocardiographic recording systems. The insertion of the first implantable pacemaker in 1958[1] followed by QRS sensing circuitry in 1964[2] heralded a new era in which cardiac rhythm (albeit only rate) could be monitored continuously by an implantable device. Although pacemaker sensing circuitry has improved significantly since that time, more sophisticated rhythm analyses and storage capabilities have not been a priority in bradycardia pacing and have been slow to develop. Future pulse generators, however, may offer Holter capabilities.

With the advent of the implantable cardioverter–defibrillator (ICD) in the late 1970s it soon became apparent that with antitachycardia devices monitoring the heart rate alone was not sufficiently specific. Discrimination between different types of tachycardia became important to avoid inappropriate therapies for supraventricular tachycardias. Initial ICDs monitored rate and delivered therapy when the arrhythmia rate exceeded a programmed interval. The physician had to rely on patient symptomatology (e.g. palpitations, syncope) to determine whether ICD therapy was appropriate. Ventricular tachyarrhythmias which trigger ICD therapy may be asymptomatic[3–5] and symptoms associated with supraventricular tachyarrhythmias may mimic those associated with ventricular arrhythmias. This lack of specificity in arrhythmia recognition spurred the development of improved algorithms for arrhythmia detection and enhanced data storage retrieval capabilities. With such features, the ICD becomes analogous to a self-triggering event recorder, automatically storing intracardiac electrograms during arrhythmias which satisfy ICD detection criteria.

Rate, RR Intervals and Algorithms to Enhance Diagnostic Specificity

Currently, all ICDs use rate counters to diagnose tachyarrhythmias. When the tachycardia cycle length becomes shorter than the programmed detection interval (for a pre-programmed number of intervals), ICD therapy is delivered. Generally, depending on the specific device, the pulse generator stores a detailed history of delivered therapies. This may include identification of the therapy zone (e.g. 'fast' or 'slow' tachycardia zones), the type of therapy delivered (e.g. defibrillation, cardioversion, or antitachycardia pacing), whether therapy was aborted or delivered, the time of the episode, and the average rate of the triggering tachycardia. The device may also report whether therapy was successful or not, based on the rate detected immediately following therapy.

Because rate alone is a highly nonspecific feature of an arrhythmia, many ICDs also report a specific number of RR intervals prior to and following therapy (usually approximately 15 intervals). Rapid irregular RR intervals are suggestive of atrial fibrillation, whereas regular RR intervals in a tachycardia that begins abruptly are suggestive of ventricular tachycardia. Exceptions are frequent. Constant or nearly constant RR intervals are also observed during atrial fibrillation with a more regular ventricular response, supraventricular tachycardias, and marked sinus tachycardia. Furthermore, ventricular tachycardia cycle length may vary, particularly at slower rates and early after the onset of the arrhythmias[6] as well as during polymorphic ventricular tachycardia. Consequently, recorded RR intervals during ventricular tachycardia may simulate atrial fibrillation.

To improve the diagnostic accuracy of the ICD, various algorithms have been developed examining features of tachycardia which may aid in distinguishing supraventricular from ventricular tachyarrhythmias. 'Probability density function' (PDF) was an early attempt at defining arrhythmias by morphology. During sinus rhythm and supraventricular tachycardias, a large portion of the ventricular electrogram is isoelectric, whereas the electrogram during ventricular tachycardia is not. PDF has been found to be inaccurate and is rarely used.[7] 'Turning point morphology' is another morphology criterion which identifies ventricular tachycardias by slew rate and isoelectric time. 'Stability' determines the regularity of a triggering arrhythmia to prevent inappropriate therapy for atrial fibrillation. 'Sudden onset' measures the rate of transition of cycle lengths between baseline rhythm and tachycardia. Paroxysmal tachyarrhythmias, unlike sinus tachycardia, tend to begin abruptly. 'Sustained rate duration' allows therapy to be delivered if an arrythmia has exceeded the programmed elapsed time period, regardless of whether sudden-onset or stability criteria have been satisfied. Similarly, when arrhythmias exceed an 'extended high rate' interval, the device can be programmed to deliver a high energy defibrillation shock. To avoid therapy for nonsustained arrhythmias, 'noncommitted' ICDs confirm the presence of an arrhythmia during charging and/ or prior to shock therapy. Therapy is withheld if the tachycardia no longer satisfies detection criteria.

Although such algorithms improve the specificity of ICD therapy, they do not provide the physician with the ability to verify the appropriateness of such therapy. The storage of RR intervals provides some useful diagnostic information but, for reasons previously cited, discrimination between supraventricular and ventricular tachycardia may be difficult or impossible.

Stored Electrograms

Stored intracardiac electrograms allow the physician to validate with greater specificity the events which trigger ICD therapy. In a manner akin to event recorders, intracardiac electrograms during arrhythmias which meet tachycardia detection criteria are automatically stored by the device and become available for later retrieval. By allowing confirmation of appropriate device therapy, stored electrograms mark a major advance in ICD technology. Electrograms may be recorded from a variety of leads and electrode pairs. Bipolar electrograms may be recorded from the ring and tip electrodes of the pacing/

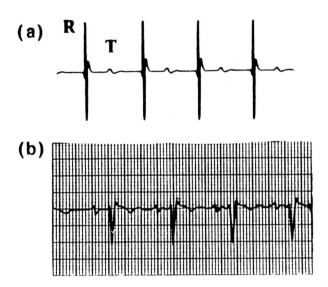

Figure 7.1 Real-time recordings from (a) the Ventritex Cadence ICD and (b) the CPI P-2 ICD during sinus rhythm. Ventricular depolarizations (R) and repolarizations (T) are recorded. With the CPI ICD the electrogram is recorded from the defibrillation electrodes from which right atrial electrograms may also be recorded.

sensing lead (Ventritex Cadence V-100, Telectronics Guardian 4211, Medtronic Jewel 7219) or from the coils and/or patches used for shock delivery (CPI P-2 1625 and CPI PRX-II 1715). Bipolar transvenous lead electrodes are generally placed in the right ventricular apex and they record right ventricular apical electrograms. If necessary, leads with active fixation can be placed in the right ventricular outflow tract, which may be necessary when a lead from a separate pacemaker is positioned in the right ventricular apex. During sinus rhythm, ventricular depolarizations and repolarizations are recorded (Figure 7.1(a)). Not infrequently, with the CPI system, right atrial intracardiac electrograms are recorded as well (Figure 7.1(b)). Documentation of atrial activity can facilitate discrimination between sinus rhythm, supraventricular tachycardia, and ventricular tachycardia. Although stored electrograms do not enhance the specificity of arrhythmia detection by the ICD, they do allow the physician to retrospectively validate the events which trigger ICD therapy.

Rhythm Diagnosis with Stored Electrograms

At the time of device interrogation, stored intracardiac electrograms may be retrieved for analysis. The number and duration of electrograms which may be stored are limited by the memory capacity of the device. For example, with the Ventritex Cadence ICD, ventricular electrograms may be stored in batches of seven events (16 s per event), three events (32 s per event), or one event (64 s). Electrograms of arrhythmias which meet detection criteria are stored, regardless of whether therapy was delivered or aborted. Once storage capacity is full, the most recent event displaces the oldest event stored in memory.

During the analysis of intracardiac electrograms, the classification of arrhythmias is often self-evident. At times, however, it is helpful to compare the stored episode with

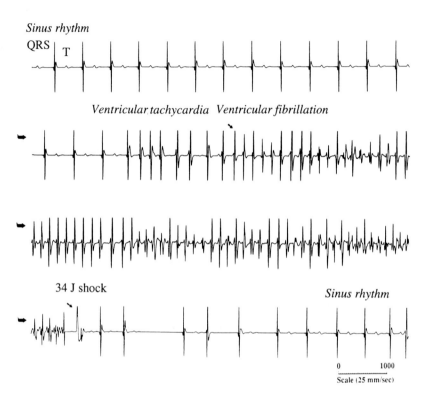

Figure 7.2 Intracardiac electrograms recorded from the right ventricular rate-sensing lead (continuous) during an episode of ventricular fibrillation. Following baseline sinus rhythm, rapid ventricular tachycardia develops, which evolves into ventricular fibrillation. Ventricular fibrillation is terminated by a single 34 J countershock.

real-time recordings during sinus rhythm and/or recordings of ventricular tachyarrhythmias induced during noninvasive programmed ventricular stimulation. Clinical information (e.g. symptomatology) may reinforce the diagnosis.

Ventricular fibrillation is readily identifiable by stored electrograms. Very rapid, chaotic ventricular depolarizations of varying amplitudes and cycle length are recorded. The arrhythmia usually starts abruptly, but may be preceded by slower ventricular tachycardia (Figure 7.2).

Ventricular tachycardia may be recognized by a sudden change in rate and local electrogram morphology with a constant or near-constant cycle length and uniform morphology during tachycardia[8] (Figure 7.3). Although most episodes of ventricular tachycardia are associated with a distinct change in electrogram morphology, this does not occur in 8% of ventricular tachycardias.[9] Thus, at times supraventricular tachycardias with regular rates (with or without aberrancy) and sinus tachycardia may be difficult to distinguish from ventricular tachycardia. Furthermore, caution must be used in interpreting ventricular tachycardia as monomorphic or polymorphic since electrograms are recorded from a single bipolar lead.[8,10]

Tachycardia with the same morphology as sinus but with varying cycle lengths generally represents atrial fibrillation (Figure 7.4), although sinus rhythm with frequent premature atrial beats may mimic atrial fibrillation. Variability in cycle lengths of more than 60 ms for three or more of 10 consecutive intervals has been used to diagnose atrial fibrillation.[5,11] Ventricular tachycardia with irregular cycle lengths may be mistaken for

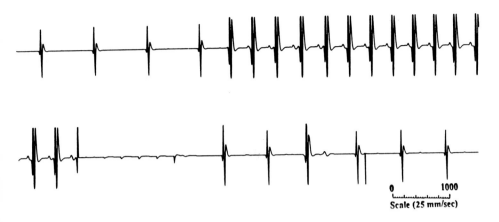

Figure 7.3 Intracardiac electrograms recorded during an episode of ventricular tachycardia. Ventricular tachycardia is recognized by its sudden onset and the abrupt change in rate and electrogram morphology. The tachycardia is terminated by a brief burst of antitachycardia pacing.

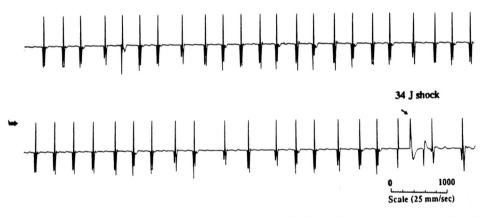

Figure 7.4 Intracardiac electrograms recorded during atrial fibrillation. The electrogram morphology is identical to sinus rhythm but with varying cycle lengths. The ventricular response was rapid enough to satisfy rate detection and duration criteria, leading to an inappropriate ICD countershock.

atrial fibrillation, especially if the morphology is similar to sinus. Fortunately, intracardiac electrogram morphology generally changes with ventricular tachycardia[9] but not during supraventricular tachycardias.[12] Morphology during atrial fibrillation and other supraventricular tachycardias are generally similar or identical to the electrogram morphology during sinus rhythm. The development of bundle branch block during supraventricular tachycardia alters electrogram morphology if the block is ipsilateral to the recording electrode, but not if the block is contralateral to the recording site.[13] Despite their regularity, in most cases, supraventricular tachycardias with constant cycle lengths (e.g. atrial flutter, atrioventricular nodal re-entrant tachycardia) can be distinguished from ventricular tachycardia by the lack of change in electrogram morphology. In some cases, atrial electrograms may be recorded during supraventricular tachycardias by the CPI system which further facilitates correct rhythm diagnosis. Marchlinski[14] has proposed a method of classifying arrhythmias triggering ICD therapy based on tachycardia cycle length, cycle length variability, and the presence or absence of changes in electrogram morphology (Table 7.1).

Table 7.1 Classification of rhythms triggering ICD therapy

Diagnosis	EGM morphology same as baseline*	Mean CL (ms)	Cycle length variability†
Probable VT	No	>260	No
Rapid VT/VF	No	≤260	No/yes
Prob reg SVT	Yes	>260	No
AF	Yes	>260	Yes

*During some ventricular tachycardias the electrogram morphology may be very similar to baseline rhythm, and with the development of bundle branch block ipsilateral to the site of the recording leads a change in electrogram morphology may occur during supraventricular tachycardias.

†Cycle length variability is present if there is greater than 60 ms difference in cycle length for 3/10 intervals.

Reproduced with permission from reference 14.

Utility of Stored Electrograms

Stored ventricular electrograms are a useful and accurate tool in diagnosing arrhythmias and/or electrical events preceding ICD therapy. There is little interobserver variability in classifying arrhythmias using stored ventricular electrograms.[15] In reviewing 595 stored electrograms, we found that 92% of episodes can be classified by the physician.[16] The 8% of indeterminate episodes represented tachycardias with either regular or slightly irregular cycle lengths with the same electrogram morphology as baseline rhythm and with either slowing or termination by ICD therapy.[16] During such cases, electrogram morphology may be very similar to sinus rhythm, making it difficult to distinguish between ventricular tachycardia and supraventricular tachycardia.

In contrast, only 72% of episodes which triggered ICD therapy were due to ventricular tachycardia or ventricular fibrillation. The remainder of therapies were delivered for nonventricular arrhythmias. This emphasizes the need for improved ICD algorithms to achieve more specific arrhythmia classification as well as the value of stored electrograms for confirming arrhythmia diagnoses retrospectively. The largest subset of arrhythmias which were properly diagnosed by the device included ventricular tachycardia (with ATP or cardioversion therapy) and ventricular fibrillation. Episodes of ventricular tachycardia with unsuccessful outcomes, such as failed ATP and pseudotermination of ventricular tachycardia, were also properly recognized. Pseudotermination of rhythms, defined as transient slowing (below rate detection) by ATP, occurs most commonly with atrial fibrillation (Figure 7.5) but is also observed with sinus tachycardia and some ventricular tachycardias.[16] Pseudotermination may lead to slowing of the ventricular response due to concealed retrograde conduction during antitachycardia pacing. Appropriate therapy also includes nonsustained events which are correctly recognized by the device and where therapy is properly withheld (Figure 7.6). These include both arrhythmias (nonsustained ventricular tachycardia, atrial fibrillation, sinus tachycardia) and electrical events (e.g. lead noise).

Unnecessary ICD shocks and ATP therapy may result from failure of the ICD to distinguish supraventricular from ventricular arrhythmias. Atrial fibrillation is the rhythm most commonly responsible for inappropriate shocks (Figure 7.4), representing 58% of unnecessary shocks in our series.[16] The incidence of therapy for atrial fibrillation can be decreased by slowing the ventricular response with negatively dromotropic medications and/or by increasing the cutoff rate and number of intervals required to satisfy detection criteria. Sinus tachycardia and supraventricular tachycardias cause approximately 10% of unnecessary shocks.[16]

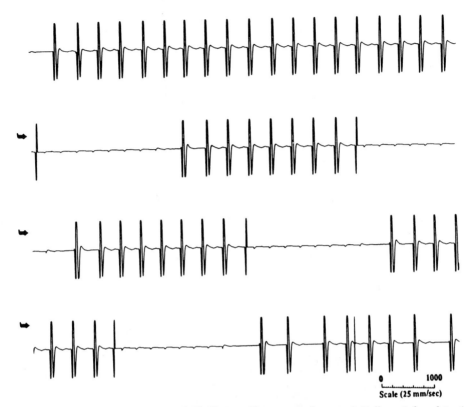

Figure 7.5 Pseudotermination of atrial fibrillation. The ventricular rate initially satisfies detection criteria in the 'slow ventricular tachycardia zone' leading to attempts at termination with antitachycardia pacing (ATP). Following ATP, there is transient slowing of the ventricular response and the rate no longer meets detection criteria.

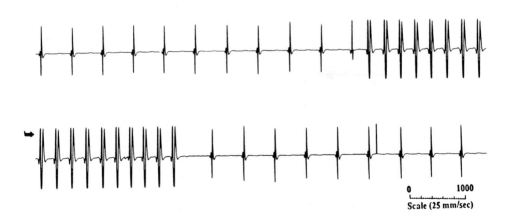

Figure 7.6 Nonsustained ventricular tachycardia. The noncommited ICD takes a 'second look' to reconfirm the presence of the triggering arrhythmia. When the rhythm is no longer present, therapy is withheld.

Stored Electrograms as an Aid in Troubleshooting

Unnecessary shocks may also result from electrical events and illustrate the value of stored electrograms in troubleshooting. Mechanical disruptions such as adaptor or sensing lead fractures and loose set screws may produce electrical artifacts which are generally high-frequency, high-amplitude signals which may mimic ventricular tachyarrhythmias. Such artifacts may be of sufficient amplitude to satisfy detection criteria and lead to spurious shocks.[17] Not infrequently, the signals are intermittent and therapy is appropriately withheld (the event is treated by the ICD as a nonsustained arrhythmia). The diagnosis may be confirmed by chest X-ray demonstrating fractures or displaced set screws, by measurement of abnormal impedance values in the rate-sensing lead, and/or by reproducing the artifact during manipulation of the device during real-time electrogram recordings. In our series, lead noise was responsible for 18% of unnecessary shocks, but the series included early ICD recipients with epicardial rate-sensing leads as well as patients who required adaptors for some lead configuration. With the development and widespread use of nonthoracotomy lead systems and endocardial rate-sensing leads, the incidence of lead noise has decreased substantially. Spurious shocks may still result from damaged rate-sensing leads, as can occur with lead compression in the 'subclavian crush syndrome', a consequence of percutaneous subclavian venipuncture (Figures 7.7 and 7.8).[17]

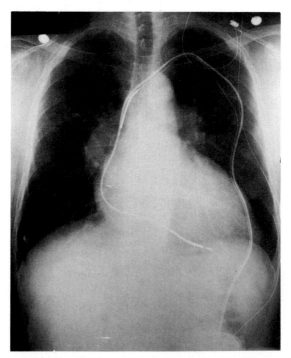

Figure 7.7 A posteroanterior chest X-ray of a transvenous lead system implanted via the percutaneous subclavian technique. 'Subclavian crush syndrome' is present causing compression of the lead between the left first rib and clavicle. Spurious shocks resulted from electrical 'noise' which was interpreted by the ICD as a ventricular tachyarrhythmia.

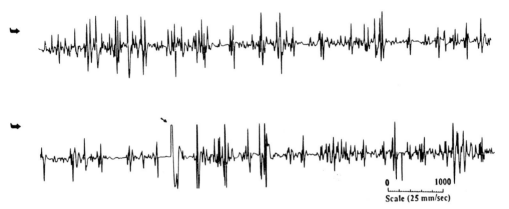

Figure 7.8 High-frequency electrical artifacts from a lead fracture results in an inappropriate ICD shock.

The availability of stored intracardiac electrograms facilitates the recognition and diagnosis of sensing errors, which occur in approximately 20% of tiered therapy ICDs with bradycardia pacing capabilities.[18] Sensing errors may lead to delivery of unnecessary therapy or inhibition of appropriate therapy. Unnecessary ICD shocks may occur from T wave oversensing during both sinus and ventricular paced rhythms. To avoid undersensing of ventricular fibrillation, ICDs differ from pacemakers and do not have fixed programmable sensitivity settings. Instead, sensitivity is automatically adjusted based on the amplitude of previously sensed beats. One consequence of such an approach is the potential for T wave oversensing if the sensitivity has been adjusted at too high a level. Oversensing may lead to multiple counting of the P–QRS–T complex (or a paced beat as well) and trigger ICD therapy (Figure 7.9). In one series, 8% of patients who were ICD recipients were reported to have experienced unnecessary shocks due to T wave oversensing.[19] Oversensing of P waves is unusual but has been described. In one pacer-dependent patient, P wave oversensing led to inhibition of VVI pacing and subsequent asystole.[20] The amplitude of a sinus beat following a premature ventricular beat may be lower than sinus beats during baseline rhythm[21] and thus not be sensed. If competitive ventricular pacing then occurs, ventricular tachycardia may be initiated.[22] Transient ventricular undersensing following an abrupt decrease in the autogain sensitivity (e.g. following nonsustained ventricular tachycardia) may also lead to competitive ventricular pacing and possibly ventricular tachycardia. In addition to inappropriate shocks, oversensing of T waves may lead to inappropriate inhibition of bradycardia pacing or antitachycardia pacing therapy.[18]

Stored Electrograms as a Tool in Understanding the Initiation and Termination of Ventricular Tachycardia

In addition to their value in arrhythmia diagnosis and ICD troubleshooting, stored electrograms act as an intracardiac analog to an event recorder and may be useful in studying the initiation and termination of spontaneous ventricular tachycardia.

In an analysis of 73 sets of electrograms from 22 postinfarction patients, we found all episodes of VT to be preceded by late coupled premature complexes,[8] refuting the 'R-on-T' hypothesis. This is consistent with recent evidence from Holter ECG studies demonstrating the frequent initiation of ventricular tachycardia by late-coupled premature ventricular complexes in ambulatory patients with nonsustained and sustained ventricular tachycardia.[23–25] In 14% of cases, short–long–short sequences occurred immediately

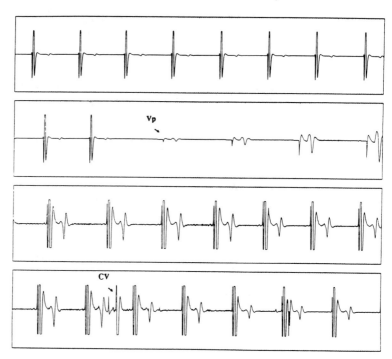

Figure 7.9   VVI pacing (Vp) with automatic increases in sensitivity leading to multiple counting and inappropriate ICD countershock. CV = cardioversion.

prior to the onset of ventricular tachycardia.[8] These sequences result from a premature beat (producing a short cycle), followed by a pause (the long cycle) and then another premature beat (another short cycle). A similar sequence has been noted to precede both monomorphic ventricular tachycardia and torsade de pointes.[14,26,27] Long–short sequences increase the dispersion of repolarization and may facilitate re-entry.[28] Experimentally, abrupt short-to-long changes in cycle length have been shown to increase the incidence of initiation of sustained ventricular tachycardia by ventricular extrastimuli.[29] Rapid supraventricular rhythms such as atrial fibrillation may alter refractoriness, making the ventricle more prone to VT, and have been noted to precede VT for 5–20% of the time.[8,14] Alternatively, the pause of the short–long–short sequence may induce ventricular tachycardia by generating early afterdepolarizations.[30] Such sequences occur more frequently prior to polymorphic ventricular tachycardia,[27] raising the possibility that some ventricular tachycardias which appear monomorphic during intracardiac electrogram recordings from a single ventricular site, might prove to be polymorphic if multiple recording sites were available.[8]

Appropriate bradycardia (VVI) pacing has been observed to precede VT in 8% of stored episodes.[31] VT was triggered by a noncompetitive pacing stimulus which occurred late in diastole after an appropriately timed ventricular escape interval (Figure 7.10). The mechanism of pacing-induced VT in these patients is most likely re-entry. Sudden changes in cycle length (ICDs were programmed to long bradycardia escape intervals of 1500 ms) may increase the dispersion of refractoriness and facilitate re-entry.[31]

Analysis of stored electrograms during VT in postinfarction patients reveals the onset of VT (not preceded by ventricular pacing) and is most commonly marked by single

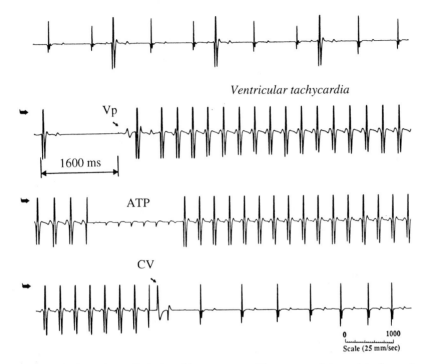

Ventricular tachycardia

Figure 7.10 Ventricular tachycardia induced by noncompetitive, appropriate ventricular pacing (Vp). ATP fails to terminate the tachycardia and cardioversion (CV) is required to restore sinus rhythm.

premature beats (45% of episodes). The premature beats are frequently morphologically similar to VT (48% of episodes).[8] Studies using Holter monitor recordings and electrophysiologic testing have also shown that premature complexes and the first nonpaced beat of induced monomorphic VT are often morphologically similar to the ensuing tachycardia.[25,32] Similar morphologies between premature beats and the ensuing VT suggest the possibility of a common origin. Premature beats with the same morphology as VT may be due to concealed decremental conduction of the prior sinus beat.[25] A sinus impulse may conduct slowly through an area of diseased ventricular tissue and, if unidirectional block is present in an adjacent area, re-entry may occur. The first beat exiting the circuit is the premature depolarization, which would be late-coupled (having traversed the circuit) and of the same morphology as the VT (assuming the same exit site). On the other hand, premature beats with a morphology dissimilar to VT occur earlier in the cardiac cycle than those with a morphology similar to that of the tachycardia[8] and may reflect a more classical model for the initiation of re-entry. The premature beat presumably originates from a site different from that of the VT and occurs earlier in the cardiac cycle because it is entering rather than exiting the circuit. The pattern of initiation of VT in an individual patient tends to be relatively constant. There is similar consistency in both the number and morphology of premature beats preceding spontaneous VT.[33]

Stored electrograms provide objective documentation of ICD termination of tachyarrhythmias as well. The use of antitachycardia pacing and, to a lesser extent, low-energy cardioversion, has decreased symptomatology during ICD therapy. The response to either therapy is unpredictable; a given patient with VT responding to ATP may not respond to low-energy cardioversion. Conversely, only low-energy cardioversion may be successful in some patients.[34] Stored electrograms provide confirmation of the response to therapy and, hence, may aid in optimal programming of a device.

Limitations of Stored Electrograms

Interpretations of stored electrograms are based on local bipolar electrograms recorded from a single lead, usually positioned in the right ventricular apex. Caution must be used in arrhythmia diagnoses from a single recording site. The diagnosis of ventricular tachycardia is based on a change in electrogram morphology, which although frequently present,[35] may not be observed on a recording from a single lead. Supraventricular tachycardia with aberration may also produce a change in electrogram morphology and be mistaken for VT. Atrial electrograms, which would aid in differentiating supraventricular from ventricular arrhythmias, are not universally or reliably recorded. Finally, in investigating the properties of spontaneous VT, it is possible that VT which appears monomorphic in a single lead may in fact be polymorphic on multiple-lead recordings.

References

1. Senning A. Discussion. *J Thoracic Surg* 1959; **38**: 639.
2. Castellanos A, Lemberg L, Berkovitz B. The 'demand' cardiac pacemakers: a new instrument for the treatment of AV conduction disturbances. Presented at the Inter-American College of Cardiology Meeting, Montreal, Canada, 1964.
3. Maloney J, Masterson M, Khoury D. Clinical performance of the implantable cardiovascular defibrillator: electrocardiographic documentation of 101 spontaneous discharges. *PACE* 1991; **14**(II): 280–5.
4. Steinberg J, Sugalski J. Cardiac rhythm precipitating automatic implantable cardioverter–defibrillator discharge in outpatients as detected from transtelephonic electrocardiographic recordings. *Am J Cardiol* 1991; **67**: 95–7.
5. Hook B, Callans D, Kleiman R, Flores B, Marchlinski F. Implantable cardioverter–defibrillator therapy in the absence of significant symptoms: rhythm diagnosis and management aided by stored electrogram analysis. *Circulation* 1993; **87**: 1897–906.
6. Volosin K, Beauregard L, Fabiszewski R. Spontaneous changes in ventricular tachycardia cycle length. *J Am Coll Cardiol* 1991; **17**: 409–14.
7. Furman S, Kim S. The present status of implantable cardioverter defibrillator therapy. *J Cardiovasc Electrophysiol* 1992; **3**: 602–25.
8. Roelke M, Garan H, McGovern B, Ruskin J. Analysis of the initiation of spontaneous monomorphic ventricular tachycardia by stored intracardiac electrograms. *J Am Coll Cardiol* 1994; **23**: 117–22.
9. Callans D, Hook B, Marchlinski F. Use of bipolar recordings from patch–patch and rate sensing leads to distinguish ventricular tachycardia from supraventricular rhythms in patients with implantable cardioverter–defibrillators. *PACE* 1991; **14**(II): 1917–22.
10. Berger M, Waxman H, Buxton A, Marchlinski F, Josephson M. Spontaneous compared with induced onset of sustained ventricular tachycardia. *Circulation* 1988; **78**: 885–92.
11. Olson W, Bardy G, Mehra R, *et al.* Onset and stability for ventricular tachyarrhythmia detection in an implantable pacer–cardioverter–defibrillator. *Comp Cardiol* 1986: 167–170.
12. Callans D, Hook B, Marchlinski F. Magnitude of R wave amplitude variability in permanent ventricular sensing lead systems. *Circulation* 1991; **84**: 608.
13. Sarter B, Hook B, Callans D, *et al.* Effect of bundle branch block on local electrogram morphology: potential cause of arrhythmia misdiagnosis (abstract). *PACE* 1992; **15**: 562.
14. Marchlinski F, Gottlieb C, Sarter B, *et al.* ICD data storage: value in arrhythmia management. *PACE* 1993; **16**(II): 527–34.
15. Marchlinski F, Hook B. Local ventricular electrograms for diagnosis of arrhythmia leading to cardioverter defibrillator shock. *Circulation* 1990; **82**(Suppl III): 661.
16. Roelke M, O'Nunain S, Osswald S, Garan H, Harthorne J, Garan H. The clinical utility and limitations of stored electrograms in determining the appropriateness of implantable cardioverter–defibrillator therapy. *J Am Coll Cardiol* 1994: 419A.
17. Roelke M, O'Nunain S, Osswald S, Garan H, Harthorne J, Ruskin J. 'Subclavian crush syndrome' complicating transvenous cardioverter defibrillator systems. *PACE* (in press).
18. Callans D, Hook B, Kleiman R, Mitra R, Flores B, Marchlinski F. Unique sensing errors in third-generation implantable cardioverter–defibrillators. *J Am Coll Cardiol* 1993; **22**: 1135–40.
19. Singer I, Veltri E, Griffith L, *et al.* Diastolic T wave sensing in the new generation automatic defibrillator: a source of asymptomatic discharges (abstract). *PACE* 1988; **11**: 485.

20. Curwin J, Roelke M, Ruskin J. Inhibition of bradycardic pacing related to autogain in a third-generation defibrillator. *PACE* (in press).
21. Callans D, Hook B, Marchlinski F. Magnitude of R wave amplitude variability in permanent ventricular sensing lead systems (abstract). *Circulation* 1991; **84**(Suppl II): 608.
22. Callans D, Hook B, Marchlinski F. Paced beats following single non-sensed complexes in a 'codependent' cardioverter defibrillator and bradycardia pacing system: potential for ventricular tachycardia induction. *PACE* 1991; **14**: 1281–7.
23. Qi W, Fineberg N, Surawicz B. The timing of ventricular premature complexes initiating chronic ventricular tachycardia. *J Electrocardiol* 1984; **17**: 377–84.
24. Winkle R, Derrington D, Schroeder J. Characteristics of ventricular tachycardia in ambulatory patients. *Am J Cardiol* 1977; **39**: 487–92.
25. Berger M, Waxman H, Buxton A, Marchlinski F, Josephson M. Spontaneous compared with induced onset of sustained ventricular tachycardia. *Circulation* 1988; **78**: 885–92.
26. Kay G, Plumb V, Arciniegas J, Henthorn R, Waldo A. Torsade de pointes: the long–short initiating sequence and other clinical features: observations in 32 patients. *J Am Coll Cardiol* 1983; **2**: 806–17.
27. Gomes J, Alexopoulos D, Winters S, Deshmukh P, Fuster V, Suh K. The role of silent ischemia, the arrhythmic substrate and the short–long sequence in the genesis of sudden cardiac death. *J Am Coll Cardiol* 1989; **14**: 1618–25.
28. Han J, Moe G. Nonuniform recovery of excitability of ventricular muscle. *Circ Res* 1964; **54**: 44–59.
29. Denker S, Lehmann M, Mahmud R, Gilbert C, Akhtar M. Facilitation of ventricular tachycardia induction with abrupt changes in ventricular cycle length. *Am J Cardiol* 1984; **53**: 508–15.
30. Cranefield P, Aronson R. Torsade de pointes and other pause-induced ventricular tachycardia: the short–long–short sequence and early afterdepolarizations. *PACE* 1988; **11**: 670–8.
31. Roelke M, O'Nunain S, Osswald S, *et al.* Ventricular pacing-induced ventricular tachycardia in patients with implantable cardioverter–defibrillators. *PACE* (in press).
32. Moroe K, Coelho A, Chun Y, Gosselin. Observations on the initiation of sustained ventricular tachycardia by programmed stimulation. *PACE* 1991; **14**: 452–9.
33. Roelke M, Garan H, McGovern B, Ruskin J. Intra-patient variability in the initiation of ventricular tachycardia by analysis of stored ventricular electrograms (abstract). *J Am Coll Cardiol* 1993; **21**(Suppl A): 405A.
34. Bardy G, Poole J, Kudenchuk P, Dolack G, Kelso K, Mitchell R. A prospective randomized repeat-crossover comparison of antitachycardia pacing with low-energy cardioversion. *Circulation* 1993; **87**: 1889–96.
35. Hook B, Marchlinski F. Value of ventricular electrogram recordings for diagnosis of arrhythmia leading to cardioverter defibrillator shock. *J Am Coll Cardiol* 1991; **17**: 985–90.

8

Evaluation of Pacemaker Function by Holter Recordings

S. Serge Barold

Introduction

The value of Holter electrocardiography in patients with pacemakers was first suggested by Iyengar *et al.*[1] in 1971 by documenting pacemaker failure. Although the 1973 report of Mymin *et al.*[2] describing symptomatic myopotential interference in unipolar ventricular demand (VVI) pacemakers did not involve Holter recordings, the observations suggested that such disturbances of pacemaker function could also be detected by Holter electrocardiography. In 1974, Bleifer *et al.*[3] reported pacemaker malfunction (presumably in VVI devices) by Holter recordings in 18% of patients thought to have normal pacemaker function at the time of routine follow-up and recommended that all patients with newly implanted pacemakers should have Holter recordings before leaving the hospital. Most of the literature on Holter electrocardiography in pacemaker patients involves relatively simple single-chamber devices, mostly in the VVI mode.[4–19] The few publications describing patients with dual-chamber pacemakers have focused on relatively narrow or specific issues of pacemaker function.[8,19–21]

In the days of single-chamber devices, an astute physician could interpret Holter recordings in pacemaker patients by deriving the fundamental timing cycles with a pair of calipers. Today one can no longer analyze a Holter recording with only a rudimentary knowledge of pacemaker function because contemporary pacemakers have become complex and dual-chamber devices now constitute about 50% of all new implantations in the USA. The interpretation of Holter recordings now requires a knowledge of pacemaker timing cycles and their interrelationships, types of lower rate timing, a large variety of programmable parameters or functions, behavior of the nonatrial sensor in rate-adaptive systems, device-specific responses to protect the system from a variety of undesirable situations and pacemaker eccentricities.

Recording Technology for Pacemaker Evaluation

Holter recordings in pacemaker patients, especially those with dual-chamber (DDD) pacemakers, may be difficult or impossible to interpret because of pauses, shortening of intervals, and inapparent or concealed pacemaker stimuli. Conventional commercial Holter recorder/scanner systems can faithfully reproduce ECG waveforms, but they attenuate the high-frequency signal produced by pacemaker stimuli (typically 0.5 ms with a very rapid rise time). The limited frequency response (0.05–100.0 Hz) of traditional tape-recorders and the relatively low sampling or digitizing rate of such systems (conventionally 128 samples/s) cause unreliable reproduction of pacemaker stimuli. Technology introduced in the early 1980s has facilitated recognition of the pacemaker stimulus in a second dedicated channel that amplifies the stimulus artifact and presents it alone. Such Holter recorders with a special marker channel have proven invaluable in the understanding of pacemaker function.[7,8,10,18,21–26]

The marker channel merely indicates that the pacemaker stimulus was detected. Traditional pacemaker channels do not reflect the amplitude or pulse width of pacemaker stimuli and give no detail whether they are atrial or ventricular, bipolar or unipolar. In some Holter systems, the pacemaker channel can differentiate between atrial and ventricular stimuli only when the programmed pulse durations are different.[25] A Holter pacemaker system may occasionally generate electrostatic charges that produce deflections resembling pacemaker stimuli (pseudopacemaker spikes), occasionally arising from a loose electrode, crushed tape, or a dirty recording head.[10,25] False positive spikes or spurious marker deflections in Holter pacemaker channels are relatively uncommon and occasionally challenging in the interpretation of complex tracings (Figures 8.1 and 8.2). Sole reliance on the pacemaker channel can be misleading when the system identifies signals unrelated to the pacemaker as a pacemaker output or fails to detect occasional tiny bipolar stimuli (Figure 8.3). Multichannel recordings have simplified the recognition of various artifacts (Figure 8.4).

In multiple-channel recorders, skewing of the recording heads may lead to timing errors when one of the ECG or pacemaker channels lags behind others, producing asynchrony or malalignment in simultaneously recorded tracings.[27–29] Indeed, some of the recordings in this chapter show this problem to some extent (e.g. Figures 8.4 and 8.5). VanGelder *et al.*[27] recently published puzzling Holter recordings from a system that eliminates the pacemaker stimulus from the ECG channel. Malalignment of the recorder head produced a puzzling ECG because pacemaker stimuli were delivered well beyond the onset of depolarization actually initiated by the stimuli in question.

Current technology using dedicated pacemaker channels can automatically provide information concerning failure to capture, failure to sense, failure to generate an impulse, number of pacemaker stimuli, and percentage of beats paced for single-chamber ventricular pacemakers.[18,30] Automatic analysis of atrial demand (AAI) pacemakers is less reliable because detection of spontaneous and paced P waves is difficult and at times impossible (especially when a large unipolar stimulus masks depolarization) because they are so much smaller than ventricular complexes. Thus, the complexity of dual-chamber devices has made automatic Holter evaluation difficult and not yet significantly refined for routine clinical application.[30]

Indications for Holter Recordings

In 1989 the American College of Cardiology and the American Heart Association published guidelines for the use of ambulatory electrocardiography in pacemaker patients[30] (Table 8.1 on page 113). In practice, the greatest utility of Holter recordings is in the correlation of arrhythmias with symptoms.

Timing Cycles and Basic Operational Characteristics of Dual-Chamber Pacemakers

According to Furman,[31] all comprehension of pacemaker electrocardiography depends on the interpretation of pacemaker timing cycles. Consequently, a review of the timing

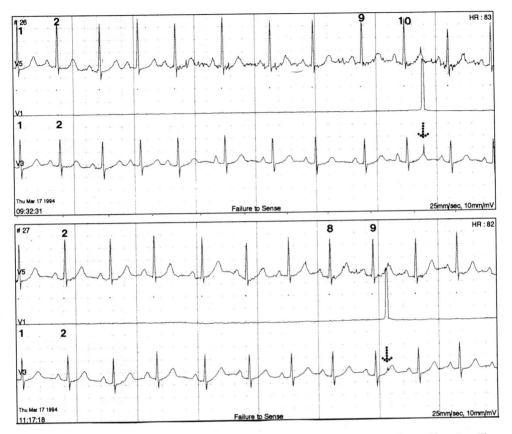

Figure 8.1 Holter recording during VVI pacing with artifacts simulating pacemaker malfunction. The pacemaker channel interprets the artifacts as stimuli (arrows). Lower rate interval = 857 ms. (rate = 70/min). In the top panel it appears superficially that the pacemaker senses beat 9, but not beat 10. In the bottom panel it also appears that the pacemaker senses beat 8, but not 9. By measuring the timing cycles it becomes evident that beat 9 (top) and beat 8 (bottom) do not initiate escape intervals of 857 ms terminating with ventricular stimuli (arrows).

cycles of complex (mostly DDD) pacemakers is presented here as a basis for the understanding of normal and abnormal pacemaker function as it pertains to ambulatory electrocardiography. The following abbreviations are used in the text: Ap = atrial paced event; As = atrial sensed event; Vp = ventricular paced event; Vs = ventricular sensed event; VPC = ventricular premature contraction or extrasystole; APC = atrial premature contraction or extrasystole.

The lower rate interval

In contemporary devices, either atrial or ventricular events control the lower rate (corresponding to the lower rate interval) of a dual-chamber pulse generator. In the past, comprehension of lower rate timing was relatively easy when virtually all pacemakers were designed with ventricular-based lower rate timing. The recent release of pacemakers with atrial-based lower rate timing and hybrid systems (with either atrial- or

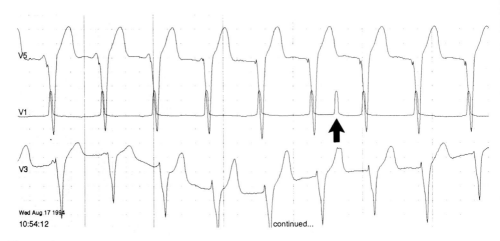

Figure 8.2   Holter recording during VVI pacing showing a spurious marker (in the pacemaker channel) suggesting an additional stimulus. The ECG on top shows no abnormality. Without the bottom recording, this ECG could be misinterpreted as pacemaker malfunction. The bottom channel shows flattening of the top of the T wave, suggesting that this artifact is associated with the false stimulus in the pacemaker channel.

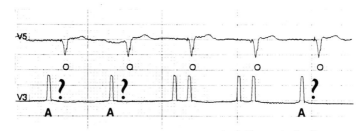

Figure 8.3   Holter recording showing apparent absence of ventricular stimuli in a patient with a DDD pacemaker. Lower rate interval = 857 ms, AV interval = 200 ms, atrial escape interval = 657 ms. The pacemaker channel detects the bipolar atrial stimuli (A), but only some of the bipolar ventricular stimuli. Atrial capture cannot be determined from this tracing. Ventricular stimuli following the first, second and fifth atrial stimuli are not represented by the pacemaker channel. This tracing illustrates the limitations of the pacemaker channel in detecting tiny bipolar stimuli and does not represent malfunction of the Holter system.

ventricular-based lower rate timing according to circumstances) has introduced new complexity to the evaluation of pacemaker function.[32]

  Ventricular-based lower rate timing. Traditional and many contemporary dual-chamber pacemakers are designed with ventricular-based lower rate timing (LRT) or simply V-V timing.[31,32] With ventricular-based LRT, the lower rate interval (corresponding to the lower rate) is initiated (and therefore controlled) by a ventricular event (Vp or Vs) and is the longest Vp–Vp or Vs–Vp interval (without intervening atrial and ventricular sensed events). Similarly the atrial escape interval (Vp–Ap or Vs–Ap) always remains constant provided there are no intervening atrial or ventricular sensed events. A ventricular sensed event either in the AV interval or during the atrial escape interval (AEI) resets both the lower rate interval (LRI) and the AEI so that both start again. Constancy of the AEI is the cardinal feature of ventricular-based LRT.[31,32] All tracings in this chapter come from devices with ventricular-based LRT unless specified otherwise.

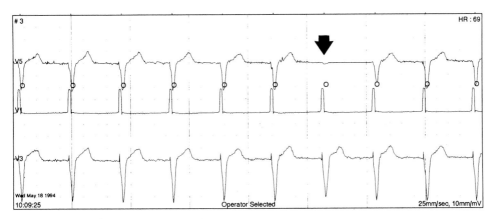

Figure 8.4 Three-channel Holter recording showing VVI pacing with a recording artifact (probably from a loose electrode) simulating pacemaker failure. If only the top two channels had been recorded, the ECG could have been interpreted as showing lack of capture by a bipolar stimulus (arrow). The lower channel confirms successful ventricular capture. This tracing illustrates the importance of recording multiple channels for pacemaker evaluation.

The AV interval

The AV interval is the programmed interval from the atrial stimulus to the ventricular stimulus or the interval between the point at which a P wave is sensed to the following ventricular stimulus. The AV interval is the electronic analog of the PR interval. Some DDD pulse generators have different AV intervals according to initiation by a sensed or paced atrial event. In such a case, the AV interval after atrial sensing is shorter than the one initiated by an atrial stimulus. The AV interval can also shorten on exercise according to the sensed atrial rate and/or according to the activity of a nonatrial sensor in rate-adaptive devices.

The atrial escape interval

The atrial escape interval starts with a ventricular pacing stimulus (Vp) or sensed ventricular signal (Vs) and terminates with the release of the atrial stimulus (Ap) provided there are no intervening sensed events (As or Vs). The atrial escape interval is derived by subtracting the paced AV interval (Ap–Vp) from the programmed lower rate interval.

The ventricular refractory period

The ventricular refractory period is traditionally defined as the interval following a paced or sensed event (Vp or Vs) during which the ventricular amplifier becomes insensitive to incoming signals. Because some contemporary pulse generators can sense signals during part of the refractory period, the refractory period is best defined as the period during which the lower rate interval cannot be reset (and reinitiated) by any signal regardless of its detection by the pulse generator.

The postventricular atrial refractory period

The pacemaker initiates the postventricular atrial refractory period (PVARP) with the emission of a ventricular stimulus or upon sensing of a ventricular signal. An atrial signal

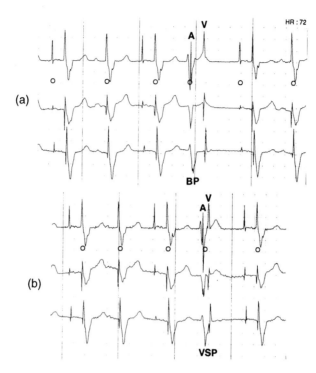

Figure 8.5 Holter recording of DDD pacemaker showing the effect of crosstalk timing cycles. (a) The fourth beat is a ventricular premature contraction (VPC) deformed by an atrial stimulus (A). The effective electrogram of the VPC occurs within the ventricular blanking period (BP) initiated by the atrial stimulus. The VPC is therefore unsensed by the ventricular channel of the pacemaker. The delivery of the atrial stimulus within the QRS complex (capable of being sensed) is called a pseudopseudofusion beat, as explained later in the text. (b) The ventricular electrogram of the VPC (fourth beat) is of sufficient amplitude to be sensed. The VPC is deformed by an atrial stimulus as in panel (a). However, the atrial stimulus occurs earlier than in (a), thereby allowing the pacemaker to sense the effective electrogram beyond the ventricular blanking period, but still within the ventricular safety pacing (VSP) period (this feature is discussed later in the text). The abbreviated Ap–Vp interval provides proof that the VPC is sensed in the ventricular safety pacing period.

that falls within the PVARP cannot initiate an AV interval. The PVARP prevents the atrial channel from sensing undesirable signals such as the ventricular pacing stimulus, the farfield QRS complex in the atrial electrogram, retrograde P waves, and early atrial ectopic beats. The PVARP should be programmed to a value longer than the retrograde ventriculoatrial (VA) conduction time to prevent sensing of retrograde atrial depolarization by the atrial channel. Some pacemakers provide automatic prolongation of the PVARP after a sensed VPC to contain retrograde VA conduction that may initiate endless-loop tachycardia.[31,32]

The total atrial refractory period

The total atrial refractory period (TARP) consists of two components. The first part begins with an atrial event paced or sensed and lasts for the duration of the AV interval (Ap–Vs, Ap–Vp, As–Vp, As–Vs). The AV interval must terminate with a ventricular event (Vp or Vs) which immediately restarts (or continues) the atrial refractory period as the PVARP that forms the second part of the TARP. The atrial channel of a DDD pulse generator

Table 8.1 Indications for ambulatory electrocardiography to assess pacemaker function (American College of Cardiology/American Heart Association 1989)

Class I
  a. Evaluation of paroxysmal symptoms in patients with pacemakers
  b. Detection of myocardial inhibition
  c. Detection of pacemaker-mediated tachycardia
  d. Evaluation of antitachycardia pacing device functioning
  e. Evaluation of rate-responsive physiologic pacing function

Class II
  a. Routine pacemaker follow-up evaluation
  b. Evaluation of atrial and/or ventricular sensing and pacing immediately after implantation of either dual- or single-chamber pacing devices
  c. Evaluation of percentage of time pacemaker is functioning and utilized in a 24-hour day
  d. Evaluation of rate and supraventricular arrhythmias in patients with implanted defibrillators

Class III
Evaluation of pacemaker failure identified by standard ECG or pacing surveillance instrumentation or both

Class I: Conditions for which (or patients for whom) there is general agreement that an ambulatory ECG is a useful and reliable test.
Class II: Conditions for which (or patients for whom) an ambulatory ECG is frequently used but there is a divergence of opinion with respect to its utility.
Class III: Conditions for which (or patients for whom) there is general agreement that an ambulatory ECG is not a useful test.

must remain refractory during the entire AV interval (initiated by Ap or As) to prevent initiation of a new AV interval while one is already in progress. TARP = AV interval + PVARP. The duration of the TARP defines the shortest upper rate interval or the fastest ventricular pacing rate.

Crosstalk intervals. Crosstalk with self-inhibition refers to the inappropriate detection of the atrial stimulus by the ventricular channel.[32] It occurs more commonly in unipolar than bipolar dual-chamber pacemakers. In patients without an underlying ventricular rhythm, inhibition of the ventricular channel by crosstalk could be catastrophic by causing ventricular asystole.

The prevention of crosstalk requires at least one timing interval, called the 'ventricular blanking period', a brief absolute ventricular refractory period that starts coincidentally with release of the atrial stimulus. The duration of the ventricular blanking period ranges usually from 10 to 60 ms. A QRS occurring within the ventricular blanking period soon after Ap will be unsensed and the pulse generator will release a competitive ventricular stimulus (Figure 8.5(a)). Thus, if the programmed AV interval is relatively long, such a competitive ventricular stimulus can fall on the T wave of the unsensed ventricular beat (whose QRS falls within the ventricular blanking period).

In pulse generators (ventricular-based lower rate timing) without a ventricular safety pacing mechanism, crosstalk produces distinctive electrocardiographic manifestations:

1. Unexpected prolongation of the interval between the atrial stimulus and the succeeding conducted (spontaneous) QRS complex to a value greater than the programmed AV interval (Figure 8.6). If there is no AV conduction, ventricular asystole will occur. Myopotential interference sensed during the AV interval of unipolar DDD pulse generators can superficially resemble crosstalk.
2. Increase in the rate of atrial pacing compared with the programmed free-running AV sequential (lower) rate in DDD (or DDI) systems with ventricular-based lower rate timing. There is no paced QRS complex. The atrial stimulus (sensed by the ventricular

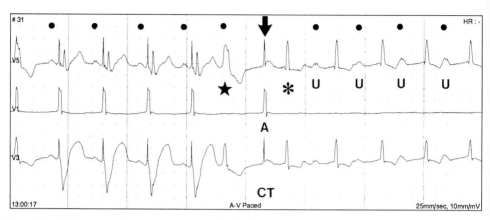

Figure 8.6 Holter recording showing crosstalk of a Pacesetter–Siemens Synchrony II DDDR unipolar pacemaker programmed to the DDD mode. Ventricular safety pacing was programmed off. Lower rate interval (LRI) = 857 ms, AV = 200 ms, PVARP = 250 ms. Solid black circles indicate P waves. The pacemaker senses the first four P waves and triggers a corresponding ventricular stimulus. The atrial stimulus (A) at the arrow induces crosstalk. The ventricular channel senses the voltage related to the atrial stimulus just beyond the ventricular blanking period. The pacemaker therefore completes its electronic AV interval prematurely. Thus the Ap–Vs interval (starting at the arrow) is longer than the programmed Ap–Vp interval, a characteristic feature of crosstalk in pulse generators that function without a ventricular safety pacing mechanism. The VPC depicted by the star initiates an atrial escape interval of 657 ms. This device is designed with an automatic extension of the postventricular atrial refractory period (PVARP) upon sensing a VPC. This function is called '+PVARP on VPC' and also causes prolongation of the escape interval initiated by a VPC to 830 ms. In this case the pacemaker senses a sinus P wave (note timing depicted by black circle) before it senses the ventricular electrogram of the VPC. Consequently the pacemaker does not define the QRS complex (star) as a VPC. In contrast, the P wave initiated by the atrial stimulus A (arrow) that causes crosstalk, is conducted to the ventricle with prolonged AV conduction. The pacemaker interprets this conducted QRS (asterisk) as a VPC because it is preceded by a ventricular event (the sensed atrial stimulus detected by the ventricular channel) without an intervening sensed P wave. Thus the +PVARP on VPC features goes into effect and the PVARP lengthens to 480 ms. Consequently the P wave depicted by the first U (after the spontaneous beat depicted by an asterisk) is unsensed. This arrangement promotes the emergence of sinus rhythm with a long PR interval. The pacemaker interprets all the QRS complexes as VPCs so that the PVARP continually extends to 480 ms. The long PVARP perpetuates atrial undersensing because sinus P waves continually fall within the automatically extended PVARP. Such a 'locked' rhythm can continue until an RR interval exceeds 830 ms (an atrial stimulus is then delivered at the completion of the extended atrial escape interval) or the pacemaker senses a P wave beyond the PVARP. The 'locked' rhythm simulates pacemaker malfunction because Ap is not released at the end of the programmed basic atrial escape interval (657 ms).

channel) initiates a new atrial escape interval. Consequently, the interval between two consecutive atrial stimuli becomes equal to the atrial escape interval (ignoring the negligible duration of the blanking period).

Ventricular safety pacing

In many dual-chamber pulse generators, the AV interval initiated by Ap contains an additional safety mechanism to prevent the potentially serious consequences of crosstalk. The AV delay initiated by an atrial stimulus is divided into two parts. The first part is called the 'ventricular safety pacing' (VSP) period (also known as the 'nonphysiologic AV delay' or 'ventricular triggering period'). The VSP period encompasses the first 100–120 ms of the AV interval. During the VSP period, a signal (atrial stimulus, QRS, etc.) sensed by the ventricular channel does not inhibit a dual-chamber pulse generator. Rather, the signal initiates or triggers a ventricular stimulus delivered prematurely only

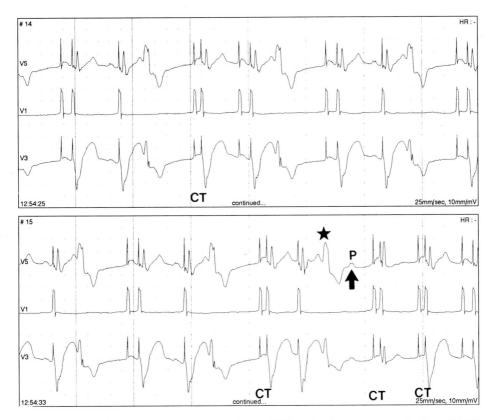

Figure 8.7 Holter recordings showing crosstalk during DDD pacing (same patient as in Figure 8.6). The pacemaker parameters are unchanged except that ventricular safety pacing was programmed on. Intermittent abbreviation of the Ap–Vp interval to 120 ms (CT) indicates the presence of crosstalk (atrial stimulus sensed by the ventricular channel). When the pacemaker senses crosstalk beyond the ventricular blanking period, it triggers a premature ventricular output at the end of the ventricular safety pacing period (120 ms). In this device, the +PVARP on VPC feature increases the PVARP to 480 ms and the atrial escape interval to 830 ms (regardless of the programmed rate) after a sensed VPC (in contrast to its basic value of 657 ms). All the VPCs in the recording initiate extended atrial escape intervals. In the bottom panel the last VPC (star) initiates a PVARP of 480 ms that prevents the atrial channel from sensing a succeeding sinus P wave (arrow). The paced ventricular beat before the last VPC (at the arrow) is triggered by an atrial premature beat (APC), producing a Vp–Vp interval equal to the programmed upper rate interval. The first paced ventricular beat after the last VPC (star) is a fusion beat.

at the completion of the VSP period, producing characteristic abbreviation of the paced AV (Ap–Vp) interval (usually 100–120 ms). (For a variation on the same theme, see Figure 8.16). If the ventricular channel detects crosstalk beyond the ventricular blanking period, activation of the VSP mechanism prevents ventricular asystole by delivering an early Vp (Figure 8.7). Consequently, during continual crosstalk in pacemakers with ventricular-based lower rate timing, the AV sequential pacing rate becomes faster than the programmed lower rate because the AV interval shortens, but the atrial escape interval remains constant. When a QRS complex is sensed during the VSP period, the early triggered ventricular stimulus is supposed to fall harmlessly during the absolute refractory period of the myocardium because of the abbreviated AV interval.

Although the duration of the VSP period is generally described as beginning from the atrial stimulus, obviously ventricular sensing cannot occur until termination of the initial ventricular blanking period. A sensed ventricular signal beyond the VSP in the second part of the AV interval inhibits rather than triggers the ventricular output. Consequently, VSP provides a 'backup' mechanism to deal with crosstalk and allows the use of relatively short ventricular blanking periods to optimize ventricular sensing.

Fusion, Pseudofusion and Pseudopseudofusion Beats

A *ventricular fusion* beat occurs when the ventricles are depolarized simultaneously by spontaneous (intrinsic) and pacemaker-induced activity. A ventricular fusion beat is often narrower than a pure ventricular paced beat and can exhibit various morphologies depending on the relative contribution of the two sources to ventricular depolarization (Figure 8.8(a)). Ventricular fusion can mimic lack of capture if it produces an isoelectric complex in a single ECG lead.

A ventricular *pseudofusion* beat consists of the superimposition of an ineffectual pacemaker stimulus on the surface QRS complex originating from a single focus and represents a normal manifestation of VVI pacing.[32] A substantial portion of the *surface* QRS complex can be inscribed before *intracardiac* electrical activity or the electrogram monitored by the ventricular lead generates the required voltage or signal to inhibit the output circuit of a VVI pacemaker. Therefore, a normally functioning VVI pacemaker

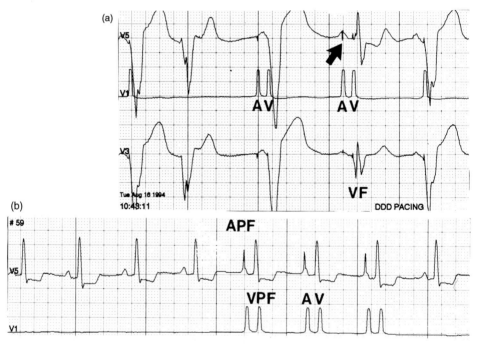

Figure 8.8 (a) Holter recording of a DDD pacemaker showing ventricular fusion. AV = 150 ms. The arrow points to an unsensed P wave deformed by an ineffectual atrial stimulus delivered within the atrial myocardial refractory period. Spontaneous AV conduction causes fusion with a paced ventricular beat (VF). (b) Atrial and ventricular pseudofusion beats in another patient. P wave sensing was normal in the 24-hour Holter recording. The atrial stimuli never occurred beyond the peak of the P wave. Consequently the atrial stimuli deform the P waves, producing atrial pseudofusion (APF) beats. Similarly all the QRS complexes were sensed in the 24-hour recording and the ventricular stimuli within the spontaneous QRS complexes produce ventricular pseudofusion beats (VPF).

according to its programmed timing mechanism can deliver its impulse within a spontaneous surface QRS complex (mimicking undersensing) before the pulse generator has the opportunity to sense the 'delayed' *intracardiac* signal or electrogram at the right ventricular apex (Figure 8.8(b)). In a pseudofusion beat, the pacemaker stimulus falls within the absolute refractory period of the myocardium. In the presence of normal ventricular sensing, striking examples of ventricular pseudofusion beats with pacemaker stimuli released late within the surface QRS complex can occur with right bundle branch block, left ventricular extrasystoles or intraventricular conduction delay because all these conditions cause late arrival of activation at the sensing electrode(s) at the right ventricular apex. Pacemaker stimuli falling clearly beyond the surface QRS complex indicate undersensing. Fusion and pseudofusion atrial beats can also occur with atrial pacing, but are more difficult to recognize in view of the smaller size of the P wave in the ECG (Figure 8.8(b)).

A dual-chamber pacemaker delivers an atrial stimulus at the completion of the atrial escape interval (AEI) unless a sensed atrial or ventricular signal aborts the AEI and inhibits the atrial output. Consequently a dual-chamber pacemaker that detects no atrial or ventricular signal in its AEI can deliver its atrial stimulus within a spontaneous QRS complex whenever the ventricular electrogram has not yet generated sufficient intracardiac voltage to inhibit the atrial channel (Figures 8.5(a) and (b)). The QRS complex that contains such an atrial stimulus may be called a *pseudopseudofusion* beat because different chambers are involved in contrast to one chamber in the case of pseudofusion beats.[32]

Atrial or Ventricular Stimulus?

The origin of a pacemaker stimulus within a QRS complex can be puzzling in a Holter system without different markers for atrial and ventricular outputs. To determine the origin of the stimulus in a dual-chamber pacemaker with ventricular-based LRT, first measure the atrial escape interval (AEI) starting with any Vp. Then measure the interval from the preceding ventricular event to the stimulus in question. If the latter occurs earlier (common situation) or later than the anticipated release of Ap (according to the AEI), the stimulus in question is ventricular (Figure 8.9(a) and (b)). This rule is accurate when the previous ventricular event is Vp. If the previous event is Vs, the electronic AEI starts at the time of intracardiac sensing. Consequently the AEI measured from the onset of Vs must be slightly longer than the electronic AEI. The rule is invalid for rate-responsive DDD (DDDR) devices that increase their pacing rate with activity or in dual-chamber devices with atrial-based LRT (controlled by atrial events – discussed later).

Upper Rate Response of DDD Pacemakers

The *upper rate interval* (corresponds to the upper rate) is the shortest interval between two consecutive ventricular stimuli or from a sensed ventricular event to the succeeding ventricular stimulus while maintaining 1:1 AV synchrony with the sensed atrial rate.[32]

No separately programmable upper rate interval

In a DDD pacemaker without a separately programmable upper rate interval (URI), the TARP is equal to the (ventricular) URI and provides a simple way of controlling the paced ventricular response to a fast atrial rate. This upper rate response is often called 'fixed-ratio AV block'. The TARP defines the fastest atrial rate associated with 1:1 AV pacemaker response or the fastest paced ventricular rate associated with 1:1 AV synchrony. As the atrial rate increases, any P wave falling within the PVARP is unsensed. The degree of

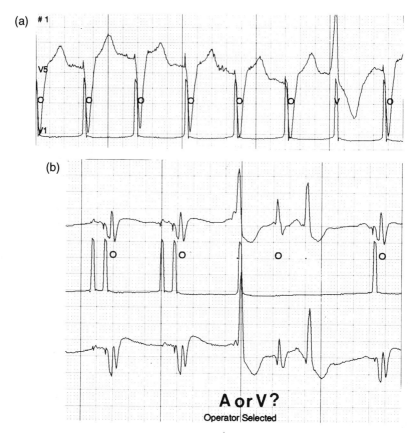

Figure 8.9 Atrial or ventricular stimulus? (a) Holter recording from a DDD pacemaker. LRI = 857 ms, AV = 150 ms. The second to last beat is a VPC deformed by a ventricular stimulus triggered by a P wave occurring on time according to the sinus rate. The pacemaker releases its stimulus before the VPC can generate sufficient voltage to inhibit the ventricular channel of the pacemaker, i.e. pseudofusion beat. Note that the interval from the preceding Vp to the stimulus with the VPC is shorter than the atrial escape interval, a finding that rules out an atrial stimulus issued into the VPC. (b) The third beat is a VPC. The pacemaker channel shows delivery of a stimulus within the first VPC. The atrial escape interval from the first ventricular stimulus to the second atrial stimulus measured 720 ms. However, the interval from the second ventricular stimulus to the next stimulus (within the first VPC) is *longer* than the atrial escape interval (720 ms). Consequently the stimulus within the VPC cannot originate from the atrial channel because the atrial escape interval always remains constant with ventricular-based lower rate timing during DDD pacing. Scrutiny of the electrogram shows a deflection just before the first VPC consistent with a P wave. The P wave inhibits the atrial output and aborts the atrial escape interval. Consequently the stimulus within the first VPC is ventricular.

block depends on the atrial rate and where the P waves occur in the pacemaker cycle. The AV interval (As–Vp) always remains constant and equal to its programmed value. As the atrial rate increases, more P waves fall within the TARP and the degree of block increases.

Wenckebach upper rate response

Only DDD pulse generators with an independently programmable upper rate (interval) produce a Wenckebach (or pseudo-Wenckebach block) response to faster atrial rates.[31,32] In order for a Wenckebach response to occur with *prolongation* of the AV interval (As–Vp), the URI must be *longer* than the TARP. The maximal prolongation of the AV interval during a Wenckebach sequence represents the difference between these two intervals. If As–Vp as programmed is less than Ap–Vp as programmed, the maximum extension of the basic As–Vp interval will be equal to $[(Ap–Vp) - (As–Vp)] + [URI - TARP]$, where TARP = PVARP + Ap–Vp as programmed; i.e. maximum AV extension = URI − (PVARP + As–Vp). When the separately programmable URI becomes equal to the TARP, a Wenckebach block response cannot occur, and the URI becomes a function of the programmed TARP, thereby creating fixed-ratio AV block. With a progressive increase in the atrial rate, the Wenckebach response of a pacemaker with URI > TARP eventually switches to (2:1) fixed-ratio AV block when the PP interval becomes shorter than the TARP.

During the Wenckebach response, the pacemaker synchronizes its ventricular stimulus to sensed atrial activity (Figures 8.10(a) and (b)). The ventricular stimulus can be released only at the completion of the URI because the pacemaker cannot violate its (ventricular) URI. The AV delay (initiated by a sensed P wave) becomes progressively longer because the ventricular channel waits to deliver its stimulus until the URI has timed out. The atrial channel remains refractory and therefore insensitive to incoming signals through the entire duration of the AV interval, regardless of its duration. Eventually a P wave falling within the PVARP is not followed by a ventricular output, and a pause occurs. The pacemaker Wenckebach upper rate response exhibits variability of the AV (As–Vp) interval, a sustained fast paced ventricular rate (the programmed upper rate) and an occasional abrupt change in the ventricular beat-to-beat interval. Should a P wave not occur before the end of the atrial escape interval, the Vp–Vp interval in the pause will be maximal and equal to the LRI and the pacemaker will release Ap. The Wenckebach upper rate response is often recognized by the behavior of the pacing intervals because P waves are often not clearly discernible. Basically a pacemaker Wenckebach sequence contains only two ventricular intervals: (1) Vp–Vp pacing at the URI, and (2) the pause following the undetected P wave in the PVARP when Vp–Vp or $V_p–V_s$ > URI. Figure 8.10(b) shows that in special circumstances the pause in a Wenckebach upper rate response can produce two different intervals longer than the URI.

Types of pacemaker response when the upper rate interval is longer than the total atrial refractory period

When URI > TARP, the upper rate response of a DDD pulse generator depends on the duration of three variables: TARP, URI, and PP interval (corresponding to the atrial rate).

PP interval < URI. When the PP interval becomes shorter than the URI but remains longer than the TARP (i.e. URI > PP interval > TARP), the pulse generator responds with Wenckebach pacemaker AV block.

PP interval < TARP. When the PP interval is shorter than TARP (and therefore also shorter than URI), a Wenckebach upper rate response cannot occur and the upper rate response consists of only a fixed-ratio pacemaker AV block. Therefore, when the URI > TARP, a progressive increase in the atrial rate (shortening of the PP interval) causes first a pacemaker Wenckebach upper rate response (when PP < URI); when the PP interval becomes equal or shorter than the TARP, the upper rate response then switches from Wenckebach AV block to fixed-ratio AV block.

Sufficiently premature single APCs trigger a ventricular stimulus only after the URI has timed out in the form of Vs–Vp or Vp–Vp intervals, thereby causing extension of the As–Vp interval beyond its programmed value. Holter monitoring often records single ventricular cycles equal in duration to the URI (Figure 8.11). This form of upper rate response is usually due to sensed APCs that may be concealed within the T wave of the previous ventricular beat.

Capture

Ventricular capture is usually easy to determine (Figure 8.12) except when it produces isoelectric fusion beats or tiny bipolar stimuli either invisible or not detected by the Holter pacemaker channel. In a VVI system, the rate of the wide QRS complexes at the programmed lower rate provides indirect proof of ventricular capture. In contrast, confirmation of atrial capture can occasionally be difficult, especially unipolar devices. Modern Holter systems with laser printers have enhanced recognition of paced atrial depolarization, in contrast to the old heated stylus mechanism of ECG printers that often obscured spontaneous and paced atrial activity. Nevertheless, in probably 20–30% of cases, a modern Holter system cannot register clearcut paced atrial depolarization partly because it may be isoelectric in the leads used for recording. In some cases, Holter

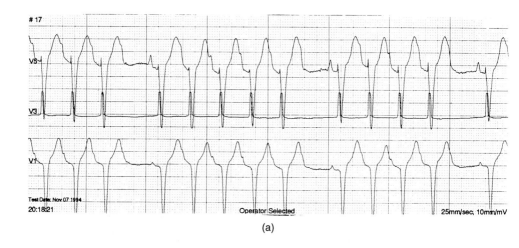

(a)

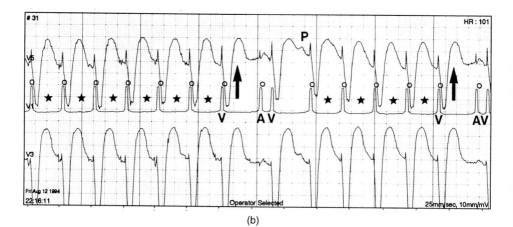

(b)

recordings provide indirect evidence of lack of atrial capture by registering retrograde P waves (Figure 8.13). When faced with questionable atrial depolarization related to Ap (barring hyperkalemia identifiable because of widening of the QRS complexes and its acute setting), the following causes should be excluded:

1. High threshold situation or lead displacement.
2. Isoelectric P waves.
3. Atrial fibrillation (often overlooked during continuous pacing).
4. Atrial fusion beats with isoelectric activity.
5. Latency or delayed interatrial conduction, especially if the programmed AV interval is relatively short so that most or all of the P wave occurs beyond the ventricular stimulus.
6. Atrial stimulus falling in the atrial myocardial refractory period of a preceding atrial depolarization (from sinus, ectopic, or retrograde atrial activation), i.e. atrial stimuli occurring too close to an unsensed P wave.

Some workers have used Holter systems to record the esophageal electrocardiogram simultaneously with the surface electrocardiogram to enhance atrial activity, but this technique is unlikely to become popular.[33,34]

Sensing

The evaluation of sensing is straightforward in single-lead ventricular pacing systems if one knows the ventricular refractory period (Figure 8.14). In normally functioning dual-chamber devices, short Vs–Vp intervals can superficially resemble ventricular under-sensing (Figure 8.15). Atrial undersensing is one of the commonest problems in dual-chamber pacing (Figure 8.16). Atrial sensing in dual-chamber pacemakers can remain concealed if the RR interval of the spontaneous ventricular rate is shorter than the atrial

---

Figure 8.10   (a) Holter recording showing upper rate response of a Medtronic Minuet DDD pacemaker the day after implantation in a patient with AV block and no retrograde VA conduction. Nominal settings were retained (LRI =1000 ms, AV = 150 ms, PVARP = 320 ms, URI = 500 ms). The maximum extension of the As–Vp interval (*W*) is equal to URI − TARP = 500 − (150 + 320) = 30 ms. This set of values in effect cannot produce a significant Wenckebach upper rate response. The sinus rate is slightly faster than the programmed upper rate. Individual sinus P waves deform the descending part of the T wave. Because *W* = 30 ms, the P waves do not appear to initiate progressively longer As–Vp intervals. The Vp–Vp intervals remain constant at the URI except in the cycle where a P wave falls in the PVARP and a pause occurs. As terminates the pause by triggering Vp. The very small increments of the As–Vp intervals produce an upper rate response essentially like fixed-ratio AV block. Consequently the PVARP was shortened to 225 ms to produce a better Wenckebach upper rate response with maximum As–Vp extension of 500 − (225 + 150) = 125 ms aimed at avoiding sudden fixed-ratio AV block that may not be tolerated hemodynamically with activity.

(b) Holter recordings of DDD pacemaker showing atypical Wenckebach upper rate response. LRI = 857 ms, AV = 200 ms, URI = 545 ms (rate = 110/min). PVARP = 250 ms. Individual P waves are rarely seen clearly in Holter recordings of a Wenckebach upper response unless the URI is long. The diagnosis depends on finding a sequence of Vp–Vp intervals equal to the URI with occasional pauses longer than the URI. In this recording the sinus rate is faster than the programmed upper rate. The P waves (assumed to occur at the time depicted by the stars) initiate progressively longer As–Vp intervals (keeping Vp–Vp constant at the URI) until the pacemaker fails to sense a P wave in the PVARP (first arrow) and a pause occurs. Ap resets the sinus rhythm so that the next spontaneous P wave (marked P) occurs relatively late and therefore triggers a ventricular output beyond the URI. The next P wave reinitiates the Wenckebach upper rate response (Vp–Vp interval = URI). The maximum extension of the As–Vp interval (*W*) is equal to 545 − (200 + 250) = 95 ms. This Wenckebach upper rate response is somewhat atypical because the pause consists of two successive intervals longer than the URI.

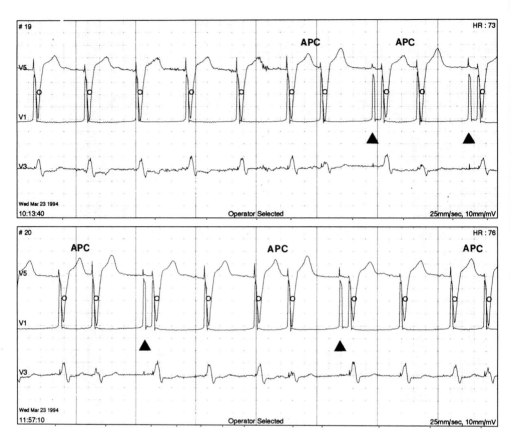

Figure 8.11 Three-channel Holter recording of a DDD pacemaker showing that isolated Vp–Vp intervals equal to the URI are often due to atrial premature contractions (APC) not discernible electrocardiographically (URI = 545 ms). Other early atrial signals capable of triggering a ventricular stimulus cannot be ruled out, but a sensed APC is by far the commonest cause of ventricular pacing at the URI for one cycle only. In this tracing, all APCs trigger a ventricular output at the completion of the URI except for the second APC in the top panel because it occurs later in relation to the previous ventricular paced beat.

escape interval (Figure 8.17). Random infrequent loss of atrial sensing is not uncommon and rarely of any clinical significance in chronic atrial-based (single-chamber atrial or dual-chamber) pacing systems.[20] Changes in body position and exercise influence atrial sensing.[35,36] Holter recordings are particularly useful to characterize atrial sensing under a variety of circumstances in patients with a low-amplitude atrial signal registered by pacemaker telemetry. However, atrial sensing problems soon after implantation should be interpreted with caution. In this respect, Byrd et al.[27] reported that the loss of atrial sensing was the most prevalent problem during the follow-up of 466 patients with DDD pacemakers over a period of 44 months. In this population there was an overall 7.5% loss of atrial sensing. Temporary loss of atrial sensing during lead maturation occurred in 5.8% (4.7% were corrected by reprogramming and 1.1% returned spontaneously with time). Thus there was a 1.7% permanent loss of atrial sensing.

Atrial undersensing can occur when an adequate signal falls within an extended or reinitiated postventricular atrial refractory period.[32] The diagnosis of this form of

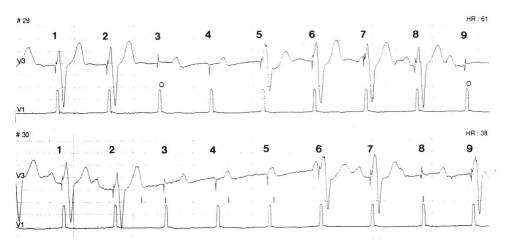

Figure 8.12 Holter recording with pacemaker channel showing lack of capture by a VVI pacemaker. Stimuli 3, 4 and 9 in the top panel and 3, 4, 5 and 8 in the lower panel are ineffectual. Note that the pauses between the ventricular paced beats are multiples (×3, ×4, ×2) of the automatic interval. When bipolar stimuli are not discernible electrocardiographically and undetected by the pacemaker channel, such pauses could be misinterpreted as oversensing. The regularity of pauses as multiples of the automatic interval in *single*-chamber (but not dual-chamber) pacing suggests that the pacemaker delivers stimuli to the heart according to its programmed rate (or lower rate interval).

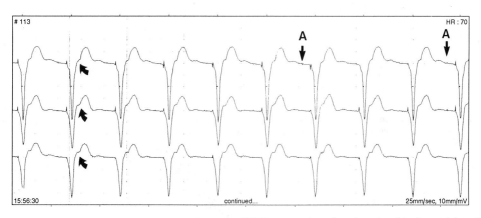

Figure 8.13 Three-channel Holter recording of a DDD pacemaker showing tiny bipolar atrial and ventricular stimuli. LRI = 857 ms, AV = 150 ms. A depicts atrial stimuli that produce no visible atrial depolarization. Continual notching of the ST segment suggests the presence of retrograde P waves and therefore lack of atrial capture by the preceding atrial stimulus. The atrial stimuli are sufficiently removed from the preceding retrograde P waves to occur beyond the atrial myocardial refractory period generated by retrograde atrial depolarization. (Compare with Figure 8.33.)

undersensing and other causes of apparent lack of atrial tracking requires a knowledge of pacemaker timing cycles (Figure 8.6).

Pacemaker Pauses

Oversensing is the most common cause of pacemaker pauses and a common clinical problem during follow-up of patients with implanted pacemakers.[37] With a defective

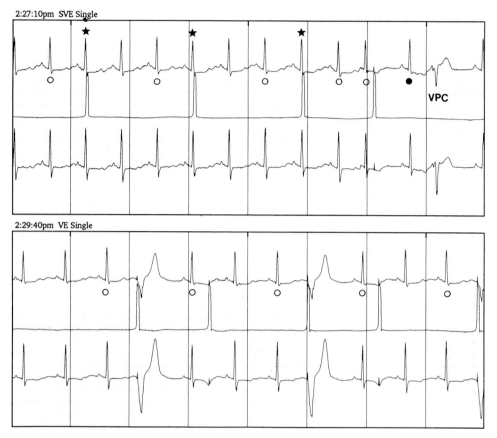

Figure 8.14 Holter recording showing undersensing by a VVI pacemaker. LRI = 1200 ms. *Top panel*: The first three ventricular stimuli (stars) fall within the spontaneous QRS complexes and could be interpreted as pseudofusion beats. The pacemaker senses the first (only terminal portion recorded), fourth, and seventh QRS complexes because they reset the pacemaker with an escape interval of about 1200 ms. The tenth and eleventh ventricular beats (following third star) are unsensed. It is impossible to determine whether the pacemaker senses the QRS complex depicted by a solid black circle because the succeeding VPC occurs before completion of the escape interval initiated by the last ventricular stimulus. If a pacemaker stimulus had occurred just beyond the VPC, it would have indicated undersensing of both the narrow QRS (black circle) and the VPC. The pacemaker senses the VPC for the following reasons. (1) Assume that the pacemaker senses the preceding supraventricular QRS complex (black circle). The RR interval of the last two supraventricular beats exceeds 1200 ms (and contains the VPC). Consequently the VPC is sensed because it inhibits release of Vp otherwise expected to occur just beyond the last supraventricular QRS complex. (2) Assume that the pacemaker does not sense the preceding supraventricular QRS (black circle). In this situation the pacemaker should release VP just beyond the VPC, 1200 ms after the preceding Vp (last open circle). Consequently the VPC is sensed because it inhibits release of Vp otherwise expected to occur shortly after the VPC. *Bottom panel*: Intermittent ventricular undersensing with occasional ventricular capture when the stimuli occur beyond the ventricular myocardial refractory period.

lead or connector system (e.g. partial fracture), pacemaker pauses may be due to a combination of oversensing and failure of the lead to transmit an otherwise effectual pacemaker stimulus at a time when the system (pacing) impedance is high. Apart from undersensing secondary to oversensing (discussed later), a faulty lead system may also cause undersensing by attenuation of the electrogram detected by the sensing circuit.[38]

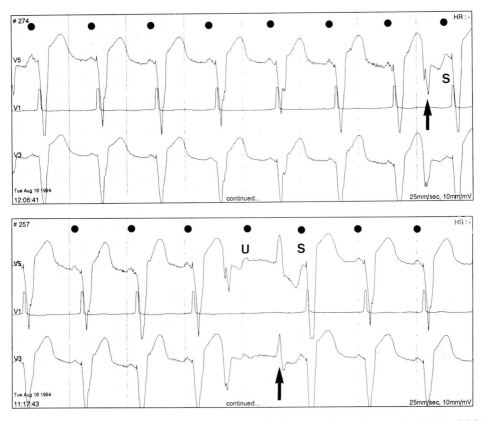

Figure 8.15 Holter recording showing apparent atrial and ventricular undersensing during DDD pacing. The solid black circles indicate sinus P waves. PVARP = 300 ms – automatic PVARP extension was programmed off. *Top panel:* The VPC at the arrow appears unsensed because the Vp–Vp interval between the last two ventricular paced beats remains unchanged. The VPC does not affect the sinus rate so that the succeeding P wave (S) is sensed by the atrial channel and the pacemaker delivers a ventricular stimulus that maintains a constant ventricular pacing rate. One cannot categorically state that the VPC is either sensed or unsensed. If the pacemaker senses the VPC, the PVARP initiated by the VPC would have to terminate before the sensed P wave at S. If the pacemaker had been programmed with a long automatic PVARP extension, sensing the VPC would have prevented sensing of the ensuing P wave falling within the extended PVARP. This discussion illustrates that the evaluation of pacemaker arrhythmias requires a thorough knowledge of timing cycles. *Bottom panel:* The pacemaker senses the second VPC (arrow) because the interval from the first VPC to the succeeding ventricular stimulus (triggered by the P wave labeled S) is longer than the LRI of the pacemaker (1050 ms). Note that the morphology of the first VPC is identical to that in the upper panel, suggesting that in the upper panel the pacemaker senses the VPC at the arrow. The atrial channel does not sense the P wave (U) that follows the first VPC because it falls within the PVARP and earlier after the onset of the VPC than the sensed P wave (S) beyond the PVARP in the upper panel.

Pacemaker pauses should not be confused with *hysteresis* in which the escape interval is intentionally longer than the automatic interval. Barring extracorporeal interference such as distant electromagnetic fields, unwanted signals causing oversensing arise from three main sources: (1) skeletal muscle potentials, by far the commonest cause; (2) voltages generated in the pacing system itself independent of cardiac activity; and (3) physiologic voltages such as the P or T wave.[38] Other causes of pacemaker pauses in Holter recordings include pure pacemaker component failure (with or without intermittent

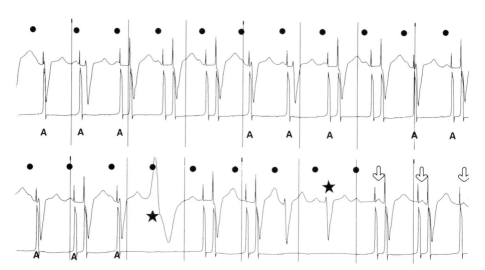

Figure 8.16 Holter recording of a patient with a Pacesetter–Siemens Synchrony II DDDR pulse generator (programmed to the DDD mode) showing intermittent atrial undersensing (lower rate timing is ventricular-based). LRI = 750 ms, AV = 175 ms, A = atrial stimuli. Solid black circles indicate sinus P waves. Atrial stimuli are ineffectual when they occur in the atrial myocardial refractory period of a preceding unsensed atrial depolarization. Only the last three atrial stimuli in the bottom panel capture the atrium. The first effective atrial stimulus (first arrow) close to the previous spontaneous P wave proves the efficacy of atrial capture and rules out the coincidental occurrence of an ineffectual stimulus followed by a spontaneous P wave (i.e. apparent atrial pacing). The pacemaker senses only the second last P wave in the upper panel and the third P wave in the bottom panel. In the bottom panel, the atrial escape interval initiated by the first VPC (star) measures 830 ms, substantially longer than the atrial escape interval initiated by the succeeding ventricular paced beat. In this pacemaker, a sensed VPC (defined as two successive ventricular events without an intervening sensed P wave) initiates a fixed atrial escape interval of 830 ms (regardless of the programmed value) and automatic prolongation of the PVARP to 480 ms (+PVARP on VPC). This feature was designed to prevent sensing of a VPC-related retrograde P wave and the initiation of endless loop tachycardia (discussed later). The longer atrial escape interval after VPC promotes AV synchrony (and prevents competitive atrial pacing) by delaying the atrial stimulus from unsensed atrial activity in the PVARP. A spontaneous QRS complex preceded by a sensed P wave initiates an atrial escape interval equal to the programmed value. *Bottom panel:* The star on the right refers to a conducted QRS complex preceded by a P wave. The pacemaker interprets this QRS as a VPC because it fails to sense the preceding P wave. Consequently the QRS initiates an atrial escape interval of 830 ms. In the bottom panel it appears that the pacemaker senses the first P wave and triggers a ventricular stimulus with apparent ventricular capture. However, the first stimulus is atrial and the QRS is spontaneous and not paced. The pacemaker does *not* identify the first QRS complex as a VPC because it is preceded by Ap. This pacemaker functions with ventricular-based lower rate timing so that the atrial escape interval remains constant except after a pacemaker-defined VPC. The first spike-to-spike interval is longer than the atrial escape interval so that the first stimulus cannot be ventricular because the second one is atrial. The pacemaker actually senses the first QRS complex beyond the 64 ms crosstalk window (measured from the atrial stimulus and including the ventricular blanking period), but before termination of the ventricular safety pacing (VSP) period (120 ms). The VSP feature of this device is uncommitted so that ventricular sensing in the VSP beyond the first 64 ms inhibits the ventricular channel rather than triggers a ventricular stimulus at the completion of the entire VSP interval as in many other devices. Other Ap–Ap intervals (without an intervening Vp) behave similarly (top panel).

increase in the pacing rate – the runaway phenomenon)[39] (Figure 8.18), algorithms for endless-loop tachycardia prevention or termination, and automatic mode switching as a response to a sensed supraventricular tachyarrhythmia. Artifactual pauses can be due to invisible isoelectric electrical activity, intermittent signal attenuation (malfunction of the recording electrodes) (Figure 8.4) or system malfunction with regard to the speed of the

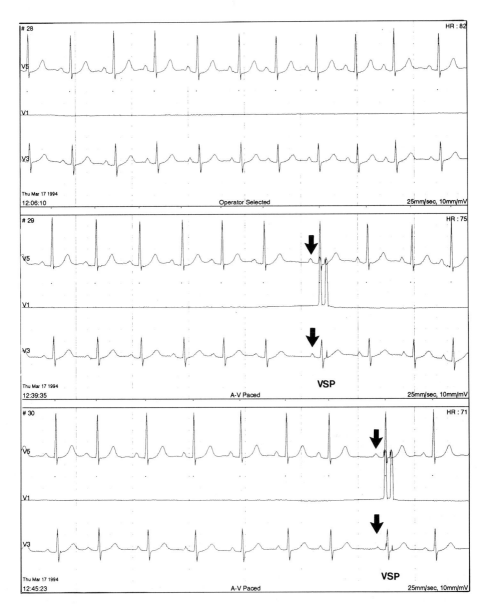

Figure 8.17 Holter recording showing concealed P wave undersensing unmasked by slowing of the sinus rate. LRI = 1200 ms, AV = 200 ms. Atrial undersensing remains concealed until the RR interval lengthens to a value exceeding the atrial escape interval (1000 ms). Slowing of the spontaneous rhythm permits the atrial escape interval to time out with the release of Ap within a QRS complex (arrows). The QRS falls within the VSP period initiated by the atrial stimulus and is therefore sensed by the ventricular channel. The latter therefore triggers a ventricular stimulus with an abbreviated Ap–Vp interval of 100 ms.

Holter recording. Occasionally failure to capture by tiny bipolar stimuli can simulate pacemaker pauses (lengthening of the pacemaker interval) if the Holter pacemaker channel cannot reproduce the stimuli. In single-lead atrial pacemakers, oversensing of the farfield QRS complex can also cause pauses.[32]

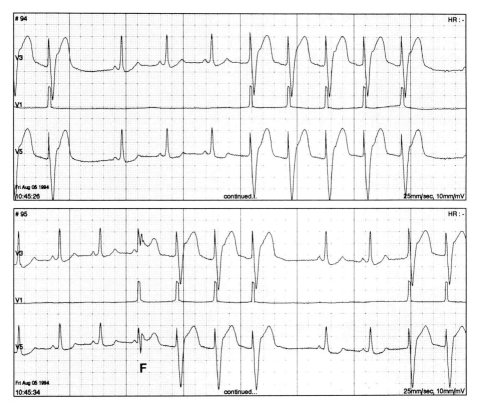

Figure 8.18 Holter recording of a 15-year-old lithium powered VVI pacemaker programmed to a rate of 50/min, implanted in a patient with rare episodes of sinus bradycardia. The patient complained of palpitations and pacemaker evaluation was unremarkable. Holter recordings show malfunction with (1) intermittent runaway behavior at 90/min, and (2) pauses longer than 1200 ms. F = ventricular fusion beat. The sequence represents pacemaker component malfunction with potentially serious consequences should the runaway rate increase unpredictably to nonphysiological levels.

Myopotentials

In 1972, Wirzfeld and coworkers[40] first described the inhibition of unipolar VVI pulse generators by skeletal muscle potentials. Many reports have since documented this form of inhibition by appropriate provocative maneuvers in unipolar single- and dual-chamber pacemakers, with an incidence varying from 12 to 85%.[41–50]

No unipolar pacemaker is totally immune to myopotential oversensing. The advent of unipolar dual-chamber pacemakers and the need for high sensitivity to sense atrial activity have not reduced the incidence of myopotential oversensing seen with earlier generations of unipolar single-chamber pacemakers.[4–8,10–17] In this respect, Gross et al.[44] recently demonstrated a high incidence of myopotential atrial oversensing (61%) in unipolar DDD pacemakers programmed with an atrial sensitivity of 0.4–1.0 mV, a range commonly used to achieve adequate atrial sensing. Although myopotential oversensing is the most common cause of oversensing in unipolar systems, its real clinical significance remains controversial because most patients do not describe concomitant symptoms. Probably only 10% of patients with demonstrable myopotential interference will actually be symptomatic and require an intervention such as reprogramming of the pacemaker (Figure 8.19) or rarely replacement with a bipolar device.

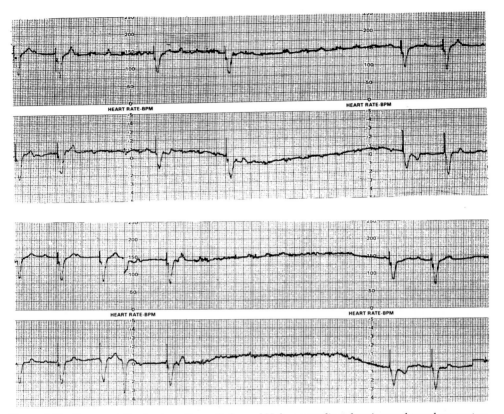

Figure 8.19 Representative tracings from a 2-channel Holter recording showing prolonged myopotential inhibition of a unipolar VVI pulse generator in a patient who presented with near syncope. The pauses were eliminated by reducing the sensitivity of the pacemaker. (Reproduced with permission from reference 76.)

The varying incidence of myopotential inhibition reported in the literature may be related to implantation technique, different characteristics of sensing circuits, programmed sensitivity, size and type of pulse generator, coating, method of provocation or detection, and patient population. Myopotential signals may vary according to the patient, proximity of the pacemaker to the active muscle group, site of implant, and depth of the pocket. The amplitude of myopotential signals decreases rapidly with distance and is also influenced by fatigue occurring during the testing procedure. Pectoralis major myopotentials have been traditionally considered as the main source of pacemaker inhibition, but the rectus abdominis, diaphragm, intercostal muscles may also generate or contribute to myopotentials capable of being sensed by a pacemaker.[38,48,50,51] Muscle artifacts are readily registered in two- or three-channel Holter recordings so that the source of interference by myopotentials is usually apparent.

Myopotential sensing during bipolar pacing

Skeletal myopotential interference in bipolar pacing systems cannot be demonstrated under ordinary circumstances, and the geometry of the sensing electrodes makes its occurrence difficult to understand. However, myopotential sensing by a bipolar device may occur in the following situations:[38,50]

1. Diaphragmatic inhibition of the ventricular channel of single- or dual-chamber devices programmed at high sensitivity.
2. Insulation defect of a bipolar system. An insulation defect of the pacing lead relatively close to a pulse generator may detect myopotentials and inhibit a bipolar pulse generator that functions as to a unipolar–bipolar system.
3. Intercostal myopotentials sensed by a J lead in the atrial appendage if the pacemaker is programmed at high sensitivity.[51]

The occasional occurrence of myopotential inhibition in otherwise normally function-ing bipolar (sensing) systems (unrelated to the above causes) reported by some workers remains intriguing, but unfortunately poorly characterized in terms of source and mechanisms.[5,8,52,53] In this respect, marked myopotential interference of the baseline especially in a single-channel Holter recording can obscure the presence of spontaneous ventricular beats and could be misinterpreted as myopotential inhibition.[54]

Undersensing secondary to oversensing

Myopotential oversensing by unipolar devices and other causes of oversensing can cause various combinations of oversensing and undersensing (Figures 8.20 and 8.21). Under-sensing occurs secondary to oversensing in the absence of other causes of undersensing

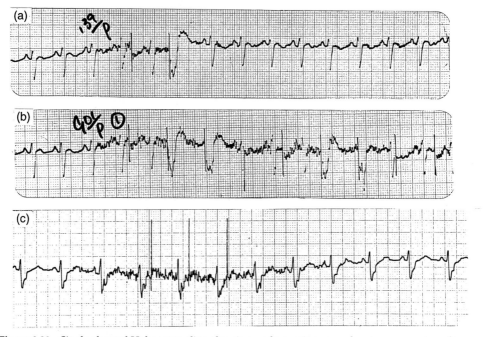

Figure 8.20 Single-channel Holter recording showing undersensing secondary to oversensing of myo-potentials by a unipolar multiprogrammable VVI pulse generator. The pulse generator was implanted in a patient who survived an anteroseptal myocardial infarction complicated by transient complete AV block. The largest ventricular electrographic signal was 2 mV. The sensitivity of the pacemaker was programmed to 0.8 mV, and the rate to 50/min. (a) and (b) are representative Holter ECG strips showing that oversensing of myopotential causes undersensing of the QRS complex. Oversensing of myopotentials (note disturbance of baseline) causes reversion to the VOO interference mode at a rate of 90/min, with competitive pacing (equal to the magnet rate of this particular pacemaker). (c) Myopotential interference was reproduced in the Pacemaker Clinic with isometric exercise of the arm on the side of the pacemaker, but only at sensitivities of 0.6 and 0.8 mV. (Reproduced with permission from reference 77)

such as a low-voltage electrographic signal or pacemaker malfunction. Undersensing due to oversensing is caused by one of two mechanisms:[14,50]

1. A sensed myopotential signal generates a new pacemaker refractory period. In the case of a VVI pacemaker, the QRS complex then falls within the newly generated refractory period and undersensing occurs.
2. Repetitive signals may cause reversion of the pacemaker to its interference (noise) asynchronous mode. The reversion circuit requires continual and frequent sensing of signals for activation of the interference (noise) mode. A QRS complex in a cycle controlled by the interference function of a pacemaker will not be sensed (Figure 8.21). In a unipolar system, intermittent reversion to the interference mode may produce a complex response if the amplitude of myopotentials changes rapidly. Inhibition occurs rather than asynchronous pacing if the rate of the repetitive signals falls below the interference reversion threshold.

Myopotential oversensing by a VVI pacemaker does not cause pauses when the spontaneous rate exceeds the programmed lower rate. In such a case, myopotential oversensing remains masked unless the disturbance activates the interference mode, whereupon the pacemaker will deliver ventricular stimuli asynchronously, resulting in competitive pacing.[14] This situation mimics pure undersensing, but is correctable by decreasing the sensitivity of the ventricular channel (Figure 8.21).

Myopotential interference in dual-chamber pacemakers

According to the programmed atrial and ventricular sensitivities, the following manifestations may occur[50] (Figure 8.21):

1. Inhibition of the ventricular channel.
2. Increase in the ventricular pacing rate because the atrial channel triggers a ventricular stimulus when it senses myopotentials. The resultant pacemaker tachycardia may be regular or irregular and often at or near the programmed upper rate of the pulse generator. Rapid pacing for more than a brief period may cause uncomfortable palpitations, angina, dyspnea, and hypotension.
3. Mixed response with alternating ventricular triggering and ventricular inhibition.
4. Reversion to interference asynchronous pacing, for one or more cycles. Various combinations of atrial and ventricular undersensing can occur with oversensing.
5. Precipitation of endless-loop tachycardia by myopotential sensing by the atrial channel (or inhibition of the ventricular channel, allowing ventricular escape beats to conduct retrogradely to the atrium) – see Figure 8.21.
6. Single missing stimulus. A ventricular stimulus may not follow Ap if myopotential sensing occurs during the AV interval, a situation that mimics crosstalk.
7. Abbreviation of the AV interval if myopotentials are sensed in the ventricular safety pacing period of a pulse generator possessing this form of protection against crosstalk.

Some workers have claimed that Holter documentation of myopotential inhibition correlates more closely than other methods (including demonstrable interference by a variety of maneuvers) with the likelihood of symptoms from this type of interference.[5,17] In this respect Secemsky *et al.*[17] evaluated the performance of 228 unipolar VVI pacing systems. Eighty-six patients (38%) exhibited oversensing of myopotentials with pectoral muscle exercises, or with 24-hour Holter recordings, or both. Twelve of these 86 patients (14%) or about 5% of all the patients had symptoms ranging from mild dizziness to syncope during one or more episodes of myopotential inhibition. Only 7% of the patients with myopotential inhibition during pectoral muscle exercise alone were symptomatic, while symptoms were present in 25% of patients who had oversensing during Holter monitoring. Moreover, four of five (80%) patients with myopotential inhibition during both pectoral muscle exercise and Holter recordings were symptomatic. Oka et al.[5] compared Holter recordings with provocative maneuvers in 16 patients with unipolar VVI pulse generators. The study of Oka et al.[5] revealed 13 cases of Holter-detected myopotential inhibition in 25 patients with unipolar VVI pacemakers. In eight of the 25 patients, myopotential inhibition was provoked with arm exercise. Oka et al.[5] documented two patients in whom both provocation and Holter recordings were positive, four patients in whom provocation was negative and Holter recordings were positive, six patients in whom provocation was positive and Holter recordings negative, and four patients in whom both Holter recordings and provocation were negative. Unfortunately,

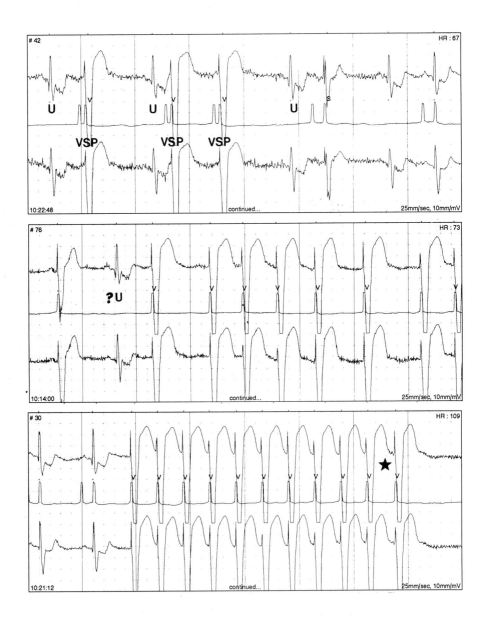

Oka *et al.* performed limited testing for myopotentials because it involved only pressing the hands, a maneuver far less effective than others in reproducing myopotential interference.[43] Thus the incidence of demonstrable myopotential inhibition was almost certainly underestimated.

In contrast to the above observations,[5,17] other investigators comparing the efficacy of 24-hour Holter recordings and provocative maneuvers for the detection of myopotential inhibitions have shown that Holter recordings offer few advantages over routine provocative tests for the detection of myopotential inhibition and likelihood of symptoms.[16,42] Despite these findings, Holter recordings provide the advantage of assessing patients during their ordinary activities including sleep, situations not always reproducible during provocative testing for myopotential interference.[5]

Other Causes of Oversensing

Oversensing of the pacemaker afterpotential (polarization voltage at the electrode–myocardial interface) by the ventricular channel of a pacemaker is now rare. Afterpotential oversensing resembles T wave oversensing and should be suspected whenever the interval between two consecutive pacemaker stimuli always lengthens to a value approximately equal to the sum of the one automatic interval and the refractory period of the pacemaker.[38] So-called T-wave oversensing occurs more often after paced beats than after spontaneous beats because the polarization (afterpotential) voltage related to the stimulus combines with the natural T wave of repolarization to create a signal capable of being sensed under certain circumstances by the ventricular channel of a pacemaker (Figure 8.22).

Figure 8.21 Holter recording of a unipolar DDD pacemaker showing myopotential oversensing. LRI = 857 ms, AV = 250 ms, URI = 480 ms, PVARP = 200 ms. *Top panel*: Myopotential oversensing (with visible interference of the baseline) by the ventricular channel causes pauses between ventricular events longer than the LRI. Undersensing occurs secondary to oversensing. The pacemaker does not sense the QRS complexes labeled U because the intervals from these complexes to the succeeding Ap events are shorter than the programmed atrial escape interval (857 − 250 = 607 ms). The pacemaker appears to sense the second to last QRS complex. According to the timing cycles and pacemaker behavior, there are two explanations for undersensing of the three QRS complexes labeled U. (1) The QRS complexes occur within asynchronous cycles at the interference rate (same as programmed rate for this particular device) because of repetitive oversensing. (2) The unsensed QRS complexes occur within the ventricular refractory period (200 ms) generated by a preceding sensed myopotential signal. In terms of timing cycles, the second possibility cannot apply to the second unsensed beat. When the ventricular channel senses a myopotential signal within the ventricular safety pacing (VSP) period, the pacemaker triggers a ventricular stimulus at the termination of the VSP period, leading to abbreviation of the Ap–Vp interval to 100 ms. *Middle panel*: The sinus rate is about 60/min. It is impossible to determine whether the pacemaker actually senses the spontaneous QRS complex (?U) because an entire atrial escape interval does not time out. Myopotential oversensing by the atrial channel triggers the second ventricular stimulus. There are pauses from myopotential oversensing by the ventricular channel and an irregular increase in the ventricular pacing rate (faster than sinus rhythm) secondary to myopotential oversensing by the atrial channel. *Bottom panel*: The first two beats show normal sinus rhythm at a rate of about 60/min. Following the second beat, the atrial channel senses a myopotential signal. The triggered ventricular paced beat initiates a pacemaker tachycardia at the upper rate of 125/min. The regularity of the tachycardia suggests endless-loop tachycardia rather than continual myopotential triggering of ventricular paced beats. The last cycle of the tachycardia lengthens abruptly (star) because of (1) VA conduction block freeing the atrial channel to sense a myopotential signal that triggers a delayed ventricular response, or (2) delayed and sensed retrograde VA conduction. However, subsequent myopotential oversensing by the ventricular channel prevents reinitiation of endless-loop tachycardia. Initiation of the regular tachycardia at the upper rate was prevented by lengthening the PVARP without changing the other parameters.

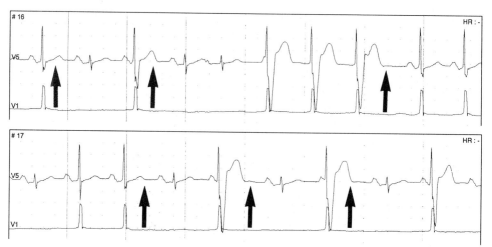

Figure 8.22 Holter recording during VVI pacing with apparent T wave oversensing (arrows). *Top panel*: The first and the last two beats are pseudofusion beats, and the third beat is a ventricular fusion beat. *Bottom panel*: The second and third beats are pseudofusion beats and the last beat is a ventricular fusion beat. The differential diagnosis of this abnormality includes oversensing of (1) T wave of paced ventricular beats, (2) afterpotential sensing (with or without T wave contribution), (3) false signals from a defective lead causing make and break signals close to the T wave according to mechanical activity during a particular time of the cardiac cycle, (4) component failure (rare). Only the first two possibilities are benign and treatable by reprogramming the pacemaker. The abnormality was corrected by decreasing the sensitivity of the pacemaker, suggesting elimination of the first two possibilities. Oversensing related to pseudofusion beats favors the diagnosis of afterpotential oversensing because T wave oversensing of spontaneous ventricular beats is rare.

False signals (electrical transients)

Varying pacemaker pauses with a chaotic pattern during single chamber pacing suggests the presence of false signals.[38] Abrupt changes in resistance within a pacing system can produce corresponding voltage changes between the anode and the cathode and generate relatively large signals. Sudden and large changes in resistance (and therefore voltage) generate false signals responsible for the sensing problems seen with brief derangement of the pacemaker circuit such as intermittent loose connections, wire fractures with otherwise well-apposed ends, short-circuits, and insulation defects (Figure 8.23). False signals can also produce pauses of varying duration during DDD pacing. However, during DDD pacing the pauses between ventricular stimuli can become exact multiples of the PP interval related to sinus rhythm (provided the sinus rate remains constant and faster than the lower rate of the pacemaker) and P waves continually trigger ventricular stimuli before and after the pauses.

The characteristic occurrence of false signals *late* in the cardiac cycle (determined by the timing of the pacemaker escape interval) permits the exclusion of T-wave oversensing (and P wave oversensing in VVI devices) by simple scrutiny of the electrocardiogram. An intermittent wire fracture may present as a pure sensing problem if its timing always allows the fractured ends to be in contact whenever the pacemaker delivers its impulse. The defective lead may induce rhythmic recycling of the pacemaker if mechanical systole consistently creates make-and-break signals. Such an abnormality can be indistinguishable from T-wave and/or afterpotential sensing. The differential diagnosis is important because T-wave or afterpotential sensing is relatively harmless and leads only to pacemaker bradycardia, whereas oversensing of false signals may be the earliest manifestation of a potentially catastrophic lead disruption.

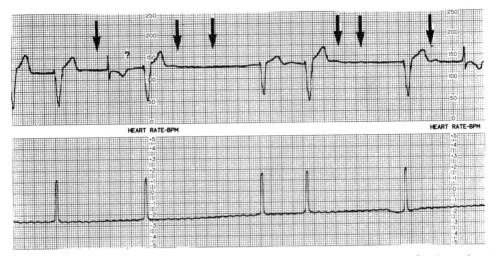

Figure 8.23 Holter recording from a patient with a VVI pacemaker (LRI = 857 ms) and an intermittent lead fracture. The underlying rhythm is atrial fibrillation. The intermittent lead fracture creates false signals and oversensing. The arrows indicate the presumed time of oversensing according to the timing cycles of the VVI pacemaker. The first spontaneous QRS complex (3rd beat) is unsensed because it occurs in the pacemaker refractory period generated by the preceding sensed false signal (arrow) that recycles the pacemaker according to its automatic (or escape) interval.

P wave oversensing

P wave oversensing is rare with conventional VVI pacemakers because a well-wedged lead at the right ventricular apex never registers sufficient P wave voltage to reach the sensitivity of the sensing circuit.[38,55] P wave oversensing with preservation of ventricular pacing can occur during VVI pacing if the lead is displaced towards the tricuspid valve, because the largest P wave voltage occurs in the right ventricular inflow tract. P wave oversensing can mimic T wave oversensing. In some cases the pacemaker oversenses the combination of P and T wave voltage[56] (Figures 8.24 and 8.25).

Pacemaker Tachycardias

Endless-loop tachycardia

Endless-loop tachycardia (sometimes called 'pacemaker-mediated tachycardia') is a well-known complication of DDD (DDDR, VDD) pacing and represents a form of ventriculoatrial (VA) synchrony.[31,32] Any circumstance causing AV dissociation with separation of the P wave away from the paced or spontaneous QRS complex coupled with the capability of retrograde VA conduction can initiate endless-loop tachycardia. The most common initiating mechanism is a ventricular extrasystole with retrograde VA conduction. Figure 8.21 shows how myopotential oversensing by the atrial channel can initiate endless-loop tachycardia.[57] Occasionally Holter recordings cannot delineate the initiating mechanism of endless-loop tachycardia (Figure 8.26).

When the atrial channel senses a retrograde P wave, a ventricular pacing stimulus is issued at the completion of the programmed AV interval. The pulse generator itself provides the anterograde limb of the macro re-entrant loop because it functions as an artificial AV junction. Retrograde VA conduction following ventricular pacing provides the retrograde limb of the re-entrant loop. The pulse generator again senses the

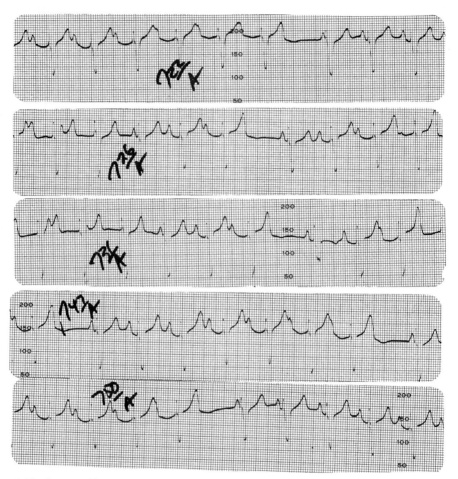

Figure 8.24 Apparent T wave oversensing in single-channel Holter recording obtained for investigation of lightheadedness in a patient with a VVI pacemaker (LRI = 750 ms, rate = 80/min). No pauses longer than those shown were recorded over 24 hours and no symptoms occurred during the recording. Consequently another 24-hour Holter recording was obtained and the diagnosis of P wave oversensing was confirmed (see Figure 8.25). This figure therefore demonstrates oversensing of combined voltage arising from P and T waves (with a possible contribution from the afterpotential).

retrograde P and the process perpetuates itself. Endless-loop tachycardia often occurs at the same rate as the programmed upper rate, but it can be slower than the upper rate when the sum of the VA conduction time and the programmed AV interval is longer than the upper rate interval. Prevention of endless-loop tachycardia requires programming of the PVARP beyond the VA conduction time.

Approximately 80% of patients with sick sinus syndrome and 35% of patients with AV block exhibit retrograde VA conduction. Consequently over 50% of patients receiving dual-chamber pacemakers are susceptible to endless-loop tachycardia.[32] Retrograde VA conduction is influenced by various circumstances, including the resting heart rate, level of activity, changes in autonomic tone, pacing rate, catecholamines, and concurrent drug therapy.[32] In some patients, measurements made at the time of pacemaker implantation may have little bearing on future VA conduction patterns because improvement in VA

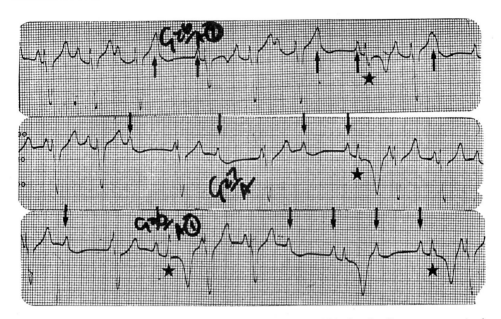

Figure 8.25 Holter recording from the same patient as in Figure 8.24, showing P wave oversensing by VVI pacemaker (LRI = 750 ms). In the pauses, the interval from the onset of a P wave to the subsequent ventricular paced beat is equal to the escape or automatic interval of 750 ms. Oversensing of the P wave causes undersensing of the QRS complex (stars) because the QRS complexes fall within the ventricular refractory period generated by the preceding ventricular sensed event (a P wave in this particular case). The bipolar pacing catheter was displaced towards the tricuspid valve, allowing oversensing of the P wave with preservation of ventricular pacing.

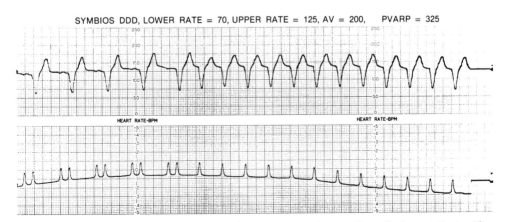

Figure 8.26 Holter recording showing 'spontaneous' endless-loop tachycardia in a patient with a bipolar DDD pacemaker. The initiating mechanism cannot be determined from this recording. Myopotential triggering can be ruled out in a bipolar system without any baseline interference. The tachycardia was probably initiated by an APC. The cycle length of the tachycardia is approximately 540–560 ms. (Reproduced with permission from reference 78)

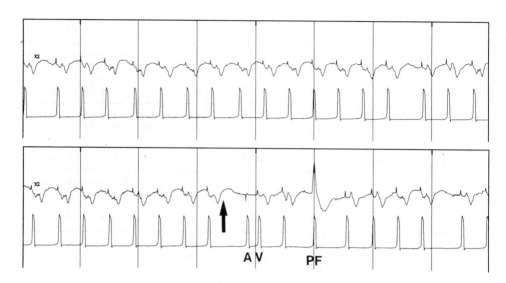

Figure 8.27 Holter recording showing atrial fibrillation with rapid and irregular ventricular pacing by a DDD pacemaker. LRI = 857 ms, AV = 200 ms, URI = 429 ms, PF = ventricular pseudofusion beat. The most frequent Vp–Vp intervals are the shortest ones that are equal to the URI. When the f waves are unsensed (arrows), the pacemaker delivers an atrial stimulus at the completion of the atrial escape interval, but the stimulus is ineffectual. The diagnosis of atrial fibrillation was confirmed by programming the pacemaker to the VVI mode at a lower rate.

conduction may occur with ambulation and may indeed return when it was absent at the time of implantation. However, only a minority of patients (5–10%) with no VA conduction at the time of implantation will subsequently develop VA conduction.[32]

Supraventricular tachycardia versus sinus tachycardia

A pacemaker upper rate Wenckebach response indicates that the atrial rate is faster than the programmed upper rate of the pacemaker, but it does not differentiate between supraventricular tachycardia and sinus tachycardia, particularly if the programmed upper rate is relatively slow. P or f waves may not be discernible, especially with a long programmed AV interval, because the preceding T wave often conceals atrial activity. A Wenckebach upper rate response effectively rules out endless-loop tachycardia. In this respect, a pause related to an algorithm designed to terminate endless-loop tachycardia automatically should not be interpreted as a pause terminating a Wenckebach upper rate response.

Atrial flutter and fibrillation

In both atrial flutter and atrial fibrillation, varying amplitude of the atrial f waves may cause intermittent loss of atrial sensing, with the occasional delivery of atrial stimuli at the completion of the atrial escape interval. When associated with periods of rapid and irregular ventricular pacing, the combination produces a chaotic pattern virtually diagnostic of underlying atrial flutter or fibrillation[32] (Figure 8.27). Supraventricular tachycardia or atrial flutter (even atrial fibrillation) can occasionally produce regular rapid ventricular pacing, sometimes at the programmed upper rate, thereby mimicking endless-loop tachycardia with retrograde VA conduction.

Myopotential triggering

In unipolar dual-chamber pacemakers, tachycardia triggered by myopotential sensing by the atrial channel can be regular or irregular and is often associated with periods of myopotential inhibition of the ventricular channel and/or asynchronous pacing at the interference rate. The disturbances are easily reproducible by a variety of provocative maneuvers. Occasionally two different responses to myopotentials alternate from one to the other. For example, myopotential triggering may precipitate endless-loop tachycardia which in turn can be terminated by myopotential oversensing by the ventricular channel and again restarted by myopotential oversensing by the atrial channel.

Crosstalk tachycardia

In pulse generators with a VSP period, continual crosstalk can induce tachycardia if the pulse generator utilizes ventricular-based lower rate timing.[32] For example, with a lower rate of 80 ppm (lower rate interval = 750 ms) and an AV interval of 300 ms, the atrial escape interval is equal to 450 ms. During crosstalk with a VSP interval of 100 ms, the Ap–Vp interval shortens to 100 ms. Consequently the interval between two consecutive ventricular paced beats (Vp–Vp) becomes equal to 450 + 100 = 550 ms, corresponding to a rate of 109 ppm. The continual abbreviation of the paced AV intervals immediately identifies this tachycardia.

False signals sensed by the atrial channel

When a defective atrial electrode produces irregular false signals sensed by the atrial channel, the resultant irregular and rapid ventricular response resembles that produced by atrial fibrillation. In the case of false signals, the occasional presence of sinus and/or retrograde P waves excludes the diagnosis of atrial fibrillation.

Atrial-Based Lower Rate Timing

Despite the well-established performance of dual-chamber pacemakers with ventricular-based LRT, recently a number of manufacturers introduced dual-chamber pulse generators with atrial-based LRT (AA timing) designed to avoid cycle-to-cycle fluctuations or beat-to-beat oscillations.[32] With atrial-based LRT, the LRI is initiated and therefore controlled by atrial (As or Ap) rather than ventricular events. In atrial-based LRT, the LRI is the longest Ap–Ap or As–Ap interval (without an intervening atrial sensed event or VPC). The basic definition of the AEI as the interval from Vp or Vs to the succeeding Ap remains identical for all lower rate timing mechanisms.

In a DDD pulse generator with atrial-based LRT, the duration of the AEI must adapt to preserve constancy of the atrial-based LRI or AA interval (As–Ap, Ap–Ap) (Figures 8.28 and 8.29). The actual AEI of a given pacing cycle becomes equal to the sum of the basic AEI (as defined above) plus an extension equal to the difference of the programmed AV delay (Ap–Vp) and the actual PR interval (Ap–Vs, As–Vs, As–Vp, or Ap–Vp) that immediately precedes the AEI. Alternatively, the duration of the AEI can be calculated as the LRI less than AV interval immediately preceding the particular AEI. The AEI may therefore change by a positive value, zero, or even a negative value. This response assures that the atrial-based LRI or AA interval (As–Ap or Ap–Ap) remains constant under all circumstances, even when the sensed AV interval (As–Vp) and the paced AV interval (Ap–Vp) are different. During AA timing in pacing sequences consisting of As–Vs–Ap–Vp, Ap–Vs–Ap–Vp or As–Vp–Ap–Vp (when As–Vp < Ap–Vp), the interventricu-

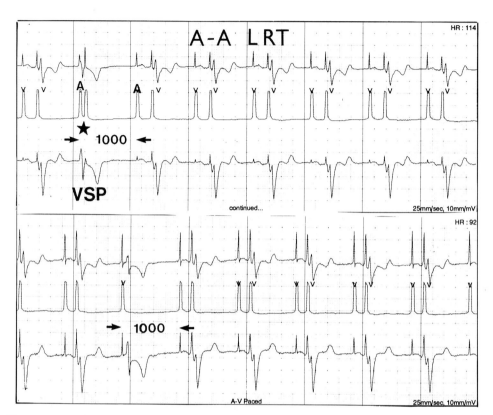

Figure 8.28 Holter recording showing normal function of a DDD pacemaker with atrial-based lower rate timing. LRI = 1000 ms, AV = 250 ms. *Top panel*: The second QRS (star) is deformed by an atrial stimulus (pseudopseudofusion beat). The pacemaker senses the QRS complex within the ventricular safety pacing (VSP) period, thereby shortening the AV delay to 100 ms and delivering Vp within the QRS. The second Vp–Ap interval measures 900 ms to conform to the constancy of the Ap–Ap interval equal to the LRI. *Bottom panel*: The second Ap is closely followed by a spontaneous QRS complex that inhibits Vp. The Ap–Ap interval containing the spontaneous QRS complex measures 1000 ms and is equal to the atrial-based LRI. The atrial escape interval initiated by the spontaneous QRS complex is longer than the basic value of 800 ms during continual AV sequential pacing.

lar (or VV) interval (Vs–Vp or Vp–Vp) can be longer than the programmed atrial-based LRI (Figure 8.28). When a pulse generator with atrial-based LRT senses a late QRS preceded by a (nonconducted) spontaneous or paced P wave (i.e. very short PR interval), it actually detects a short AV interval (i.e. Ap–Vs or As–Vs). In this situation, constancy of the atrial-based LRI mandates delay of the subsequent Ap. The AEI initiated by such a sensed ventricular event lengthens and produces a form of hysteresis related to the interval between the spontaneous QRS and the subsequent Vp output (Figure 28.9). Other forms of lower rate timing include a variety of hybrids with either atrial or ventricular LRT according to circumstances. For example, some pulse generators function with atrial-based LRT only in response to all AV intervals shorter than the programmed Ap–Vp interval, while others exhibit atrial-based LRT only in response to AV intervals initiated by Ap (not As), provided they are shorter than the programmed Ap–Vp interval. Finally, most contemporary pulse generators with pure atrial-based hybrid LRT systems exhibit ventricular-based LRT in response to VPCs (not preceded by a sensed P wave).

Rate-Adaptive Pacemakers

In the rate-responsive VVIR and DDDR modes, the LRI is variable and changes according to the activity of the sensor (that monitors activity in terms of body vibration, minute ventilation volume, temperature, etc.) designed to increase the pacing rate with effort. The ECG does not show sensor activity except for its effect on the timing cycles. At any given time, the duration of the LRI can either be its basic programmed value or the constantly changing sensor-controlled LRI, whichever is shorter. The shortest sensor-driven LRI is equal to the programmed sensor-driven URI.[32] The duration of the sensor-driven AEI represents the difference of the sensor-driven LRI and the rate-adaptive (shorter) Ap–Vp interval at a given time.

Control of the upper rate of DDDR pacemakers is complex and involves four intervals (TARP, PP interval, atrial-driven URI, and sensor-driven URI). The last two intervals can be identical or different. DDDR devices have added a new and complex dimension to the interpretation of Holter recordings of pacemaker patients[32] (Figure 8.30). Holter recordings of patients with minute ventilation rate-adaptive DDDR pacemakers can show characteristic interference of the baseline produced by the continual electrical activity used to measure transthoracic impedance[58] (Figure 8.31).

In patients with rate-adaptive devices, Holter recordings can be useful in the following circumstances:

1. In the DDD mode for the characterization of atrial chronotropic incompetence to optimize the benefit of rate-adaptive function with activity.[20,59]
2. Optimal programming of the pacemaker with activity if the implanted pacemaker does not possess a sophisticated implanted 'Holter' system.
3. Evaluation of symptoms such as palpitations, chest pain, etc., to rule out pacemaker tachycardia from an oversensitive rate-adaptive response by the non-atrial sensor.
4. Evaluation of non-atrial sensor idiosyncrasies.[60]
5. Spontaneous ventricular arrhythmias precipitated by rapid ventricular pacing[59,61,62] and/or atrial arrhythmias precipitated by competitive atrial pacing (when the atrial stimulus is close to a preceding unsensed P wave in the PVARP).
6. Evaluation of various fallback and automatic mode switching functions for the control of the ventricular pacing rate during supraventricular tachyarrhythmias.[63]

Pacemaker Syndrome

The pacemaker syndrome is best defined according to Schuller and Brandt as 'symptoms and signs present in the pacemaker patient which are caused by inadequate timing of atrial and ventricular contractions'.[64] This broader definition is more appropriate to contemporary pacemaker practice because the introduction of pacing modes more physiologic than the VVI or VVIR mode have not entirely eliminated the pacemaker syndrome which can also occur under certain circumstances with atrial-based pacing in the presence of 'inadequate timing of atrial and ventricular contractions'. The diagnosis of pacemaker syndrome during VVI or VVIR pacing may require Holter recordings to exclude pacemaker malfunction and correlate continual ventricular pacing and retrograde VA conduction (less commonly AV dissociation) with symptoms[65] (Figure 8.32). Additionally, the relief of symptoms with restoration of AV synchrony when the pacemaker is inhibited by spontaneous activity supports the diagnosis of pacemaker syndrome.

A recent review addressed the causes of pacemaker syndrome during atrial-based pacing.[66] One example involves repetitive non-reentrant VA synchrony that occurs when a paced ventricular beat engenders an unsensed retrograde P wave falling within

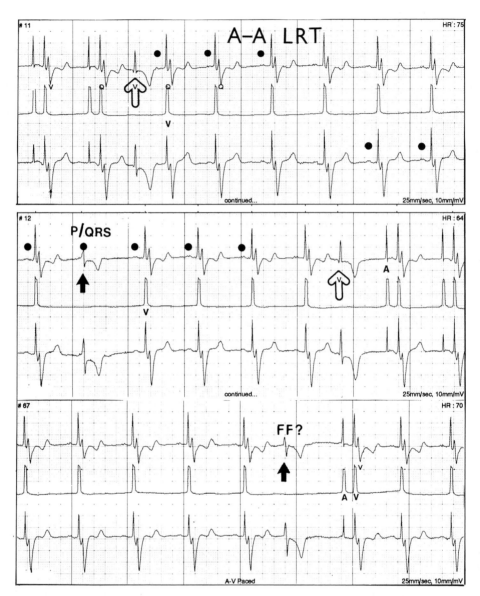

Figure 8.29 Holter recording showing DDD pacing with atrial-based lower rate timing. LRI = 1000 ms, AV = 200 ms. Solid black circles depict sinus P waves. *Top panel*: The open arrow points to a sensed QRS complex followed by a sensed P wave that triggers the third Vp. The early P wave (first black circle) aborts the atrial escape interval. *Middle panel*: The second QRS complex is a spontaneous beat that initiates a Vs–Vp interval longer than the LRI of 1000 ms. According to the sinus rate, it appears that a P wave occurs coincidentally with the second QRS complex (black arrow). The pacemaker senses the concealed P wave before the QRS complex. Because of atrial-based lower rate timing, the pacemaker initiates the LRI from the sensed P wave. Thus the atrial escape interval from the sensed ventricular event lengthens beyond the basic value of 800 ms to maintain constancy of the atrial-based LRI. The open arrow points to a QRS complex (without a preceding sensed P wave) that initiates an atrial escape interval corresponding to the basic value of 800 ms. *Bottom panel*: The QRS at the arrow (FF?) seems to initiate an atrial escape interval of 920–940 ms that cannot be explained in terms of late sensing of a narrow QRS complex. The prolonged

the PVARP (in contrast, endless-loop tachycardia produces repetitive reentrant VA synchrony[66]). This process may become self-perpetuating because the pacemaker continually delivers ineffectual atrial stimulation during the atrial *myocardial* refractory period generated by the preceding retrograde atrial depolarization (Figure 8.33). Loss of atrial capture occurs despite a low atrial pacing threshold during normal AV sequential pacing. The predisposing factors for the development of repetitive non-reentrant VA synchrony include a prolonged retrograde VA conduction time, relatively fast programmed lower rate, and relatively long AV delay. When sustained, it may cause the pacemaker syndrome during normal function of a DDD, DDI, DDDR, or DDIR pulse generator. Repetitive non-reentrant VA synchrony should not be misinterpreted as primary failure of atrial capture.

Holter Recordings in Symptomatic Patients

Bianconi *et al.*[12] evaluated 40 patients with syncope or presyncope presenting 1–32 months (mean 14) after pacemaker implantation. This group constituted 6.9% of all the patients who received pacemakers during 1980–82 at their institution. After 48-hour Holter recordings, Bianconi *et al.* separated their patients into two groups: *Group I:* Twenty patients (50%) were *symptomatic* during Holter recordings (2 had syncope and 18 presyncope). In this group, the symptoms were related to a cardiac cause in 15 patients (37.5% of all patients in Groups I and II). The causes included (a) myopotential inhibition in 3, (b) pacing rate too low in 2 (40/min), (c) failure to capture in 1 (syncope), (d) paroxysmal supraventricular tachycardia in 2, and (e) ventricular tachycardia in 7 (1 with syncope). In the other 5 patients with symptoms, Holter recordings were negative (12.5% of the total number of patients in Groups I and II) and a cardiac etiology was excluded. Thus, Holter recordings provided a diagnosis for the symptomatic patients in Group I: tachycardia unrelated to pacemaker 45%, malfunction or misprogramming of pacemaker 30%, and noncardiac causes 25%. *Group II:* Twenty patients (50%) were *asymptomatic* during Holter recording. (a) In 6 patients (15% of the total number of patients), Holter recordings were negative, and (b) in 14 patients (35% of the total number of patients), Holter recordings were abnormal, suggesting a cardiac cause for symptoms: 7 showed pacemaker malfunction (1 sensing failure during AAI, 2 failures to capture, 4 myopotential inhibition) and 7 exhibited ventricular arrhythmias (Lown classes IV and V), including 2 with ventricular tachycardia. These abnormalities were not correlated with symptoms in Group II, although they did suggest a diagnosis in cases of serious spontaneous arrhythmias or pacemaker lack of capture.

Hoffman *et al.*[19] reported an incidence of 8.6% (49 patients) of persisting symptoms (palpitations, dizziness, or syncope) in 570 consecutively followed patients with implanted pacemakers during a mean follow-up of 10 months. *Group I* (VVI pacemakers): 43 patients (8%) were symptomatic among a total of 540 patients (19 patients had syncope and 24 had dizziness). *Group II* (dual chamber pacemakers): 6 patients (20%) were symptomatic among a total of 30 patients (5 had palpitations and 1 had dizziness). In the 49 patients (Group I and Group II), symptoms were pacemaker-related in 17, caused by tachyarrhythmias in 12, noncardiac in origin in 16, and of unknown cause in 4. No Holter

---

[**Figure 8.29** continued] atrial escape interval represents a manifestation of atrial-based lower rate timing due to either a P wave sensed by the pacemaker before it senses the QRS complex, or more likely a farfield phenomenon whereby the atrial channel by sensing the QRS deflection in the atrial electrogram initiates the LRI. These normal manifestations of atrial-based lower rate timing should not be misinterpreted as T wave or other forms of oversensing, programmed hysteresis, or malfunction.

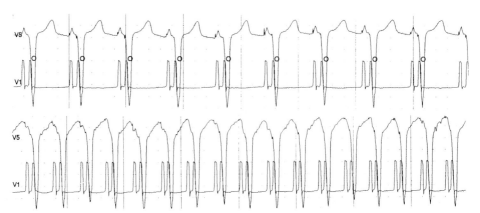

Figure 8.30 Holter recording in a patient with a rate-adaptive DDDR pacemaker. *Upper panel:* Normal AV sequential pacing. *Lower panel:* On exercise, the AV sequential pacing rate increases and the Ap–Vp interval shortens according to sensor activity. Note that atrial capture, obvious in the upper panel, is not discernible in the lower panel.

recordings were necessary to identify the causes of symptoms in 13 of the 49 symptomatic patients (27%). Holter recordings were obtained in the other 36 patients (73%) and the procedure was diagnostic in 32 patients (89%); i.e. positive ECG findings or symptoms during negative Holter recordings. (Seven patients were symptomatic with a negative Holter recording, thereby ruling out a pacemaker etiology, while 25 exhibited an abnormal Holter recording: tachyarrhythmias unrelated to the pacemaker in 12 and pacemaker-related abnormalities in 13.) Thus, in 49 symptomatic patients (Groups I and II), a pacemaker-related cause was found in 17 patients (27%) (13 of whom had Holter recordings). The pacemaker-related causes included: endless-loop tachycardia in 6 (all DDD), myopotential oversensing in 3, oversensing of T wave in 1, lead dislodgement in 3, lead fracture in 1, battery exhaustion in 2, and pacemaker syndrome (symptomatic drop of systolic blood pressure when the pacemaker took over) in 1. Non-pacemaker-related tachyarrhythmias occurred in 25% of the 49 symptomatic patients.

Kaul *et al.*[11] evaluated 56 pacemaker patients who presented with symptoms of palpitations in 26 (46.5%), lightheadedness in 20 (35.7%), syncope in 7 (12.4%) and chest pain in 3 (5.4%). The patients were followed in a Pacemaker Clinic from one month to 8 years (mean 4 years). Thirty-five patients received bipolar VVI pacemakers, 18 unipolar VVI pacemakers, and 2 bipolar AAI devices. All patients exhibited normal pacemaker function when seen in Pacemaker Clinic. No specific testing for myopotential interference was performed. In 11 patients (19.7%), pacemaker malfunction was detected with Holter recordings. Loss of sensing occurred in 7 (3 of these showed loss of sensing of only 3–4 beats in 24 hours), loss of capture in 1, battery failure in 2, myopotential inhibition in 1. Paroxysmal ventricular tachycardia was reported in 3 patients, causing syncope in 2 and lightheadedness in 1, while 11 patients complained of palpitations when ventricular premature beats were recorded. Four patients (7%) demonstrated paroxysmal atrial fibrillation at a rate of 100–125/min. Frequent change of sinus rhythm to paced rhythm or vice versa was a common cause of palpitations in 21 symptomatic patients (37%).

Djordjevic *et al.*[39] presented in abstract form data concerning 186 patients with 'intensive' complaints after pacemaker implantation. Holter recordings were abnormal in 61% (oversensing 24%, undersensing 2%, arrhythmias 15%, tachycardias 4%, exit block 2%, lead dislodgement 2%, pacemaker syndrome 9%, pacemaker runaway phenomenon 0.5%). No details were given about specific symptoms, characteristics of

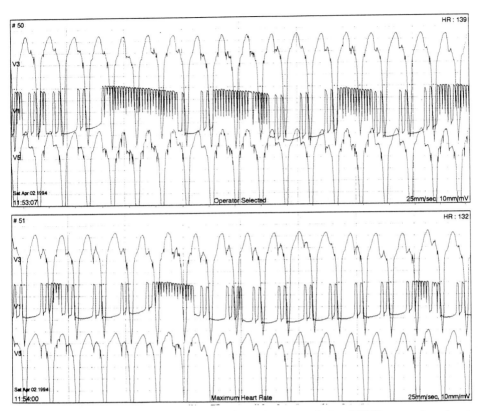

Figure 8.31 Holter recordings of a patient with a minute ventilation DDDR pacemaker showing interference of the ECG and the pacemaker channels. This system delivers frequent short-duration low-amplitude pulses (considerably smaller than the level required to stimulate the heart) to determine the changes in intrathoracic impedance that correlate with minute ventilation. These tiny pulses cause the interference in the ECG and pacemaker channels.

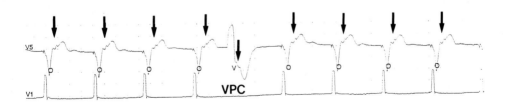

Figure 8.32 Holter recording from a patient with a VVI pacemaker implanted because of sick sinus syndrome. The patient complained of intermittent lightheadedness and dyspnea. The recording obtained during a symptomatic period shows ventricular pacing followed by retrograde P waves (arrows). A sensed VPC also generates a retrograde P wave. The patient was asymptomatic when the Holter recording showed restoration of AV synchrony and sinus rhythm faster than the programmed rate of the pacemaker. These observations confirmed the diagnosis of pacemaker syndrome.

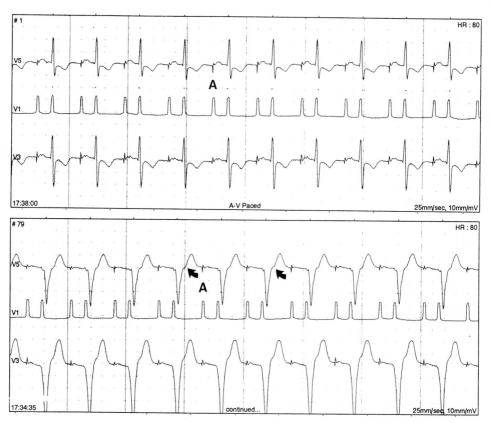

Figure 8.33 Holter recording showing repetitive non-reentrant ventriculoatrial (VA) synchrony during DDD pacing. LRI = 750 ms, AV = 250 ms. *Top panel*: Each atrial stimulus (A) produces clearly visible atrial depolarization. The ventricular stimulus produces either ventricular fusion or pseudofusion. (The mechanism deforming the QRS complex can only be determined by comparison with a spontaneous QRS complex free of a ventricular stimulus.) *Bottom panel*: Representative tracings from the same Holter recording as in the top panel. The atrial stimulus (A) no longer produces visible atrial depolarization. Notching of the ST segment (arrows) suggests retrograde atrial depolarization. The pacemaker does not sense the retrograde P wave because it falls within the PVARP. The atrial stimulus is ineffective because it occurs in the atrial myocardial refractory period generated by the preceding retrograde atrial depolarization. This process perpetuates itself in the form of a repetitive non-reentrant VA synchrony, an arrhythmia often initiated by a VPC with retrograde VA conduction. Note how a relatively fast lower rate (short LRI) and long AV interval can produce VA synchrony that may if sustained cause the pacemaker syndrome. (Compare with Figure 8.13.)

pacemakers and pacing mode, time since implantation, and number of noninvasive or invasive interventions to correct the abnormalities.

Pavlovic *et al.*[9] who followed 2500 patients with VVI pacemakers found 46 patients complaining of syncope after pacemaker implantation (1.8%). The patients presented from two months to 12 years after implantation with a mean of 3.4 ± 4.2 years. Holter monitoring showed exit block (high pacing threshold) in 2 patients (4.3%) and under-sensing in 1 (2.1%). Presumably all pacemakers were bipolar because no myopotential inhibition was documented. This study, published in December 1991, indicates that pacemaker malfunction is no longer a major cause of syncope in pacemaker patients, but vasovagal syncope demonstrable by headup tilt testing seems to be the most common cause.

Prospective Studies with Holter Recordings

Only three prospective studies have been conducted to evaluate the usefulness of routine Holter recordings in pacemaker patients. Janosik *et al.*[8] studied the value of Holter recordings in a prospective study involving 100 patients (35 VVI, 8 VVIR, 7 AAI, 47 DDD, 3 VDD) a mean of 1.2 days after pacemaker implantation (range 0–5). One type of pacemaker malfunction was detected in 35% of patients, while routine telemetry identified pacemaker malfunction in only 8% ($p < 0.001$). Exercise maneuvers for the evaluation of myopotential interference were not conducted because of pain from recent surgery. Pacemaker malfunction was found in 42% of patients with dual-chamber devices and 27% of those with single-chamber devices (difference not significant). A total of 50 instances of pacemaker malfunction was detected in 35 patients. Failure of atrial capture occurred in 2% of patients, failure of atrial sensing in 9%, and failure of atrial output in 1%, failure of ventricular capture in 8%, failure of ventricular sensing in 14%, failure of ventricular output due to myopotential inhibition in 11% (9% with unipolar and 2% with bipolar systems), myopotential inhibition of output in an AAI device in 1%, and pacemaker-mediated (endless-loop) tachycardia in 5%. Only 2 of the 35 patients with pacemaker malfunction were symptomatic (one with intermittent capture and one with endless-loop tachycardia). Of the 14 with intermittent ventricular undersensing, 5 failed to sense intrinsic QRS complexes, 5 failed to sense VPCs, and 4 failed to sense both types of QRS complexes. Many of the problems were corrected by reprogramming, while the authors considered that infrequent ventricular undersensing and some of the cases of myopotential oversensing were not significant enough to warrant reprogramming or another invasive intervention. Pacemakers were initially programmed for at least 2- to 3-fold safety factor for both output and sensitivity.[8] The outputs for ventricular pacing were programmed too low, especially if the safety factor for pacing was calculated in terms of energy (microjoules) rather than voltage. The 8% incidence of failure to capture the ventricle would be unacceptable today and it was probably due to the way the pacemakers were programmed before Holter recording.

Bethge *et al.*[4] conducted a prospective study of the diagnostic usefulness of 24-hour ambulatory electrocardiography in 100 consecutive patients with VVI pacemakers regardless of symptoms (0.1–95 months after implantation, mean 23.3 ± 25.4 months). The patients were not tested for myopotential interference by standard exercise before Holter recordings. Only one patient showed pacemaker malfunction with the use of standard techniques. Yet Holter recordings detected transient pacemaker malfunction in 74 patients while analysis with a special computer-aided module increased the yield to 83 patients with pacemaker malfunction. Pacemaker malfunction could not be correlated with the presence or absence of symptoms or the time from implantation to Holter recording. Malfunctions consisted of inappropriate inhibition in 73% of abnormal episodes (presumably due to myopotential inhibition, though a number of patients with unipolar devices was unspecified) and failure to sense in 23% of the abnormal episodes. No single case revealed failure to capture.

Oka *et al.*[5] performed Holter monitoring about four years after pacemaker implantation in 27 patients with VVI devices selected at random from a Pacemaker Clinic and presumably asymptomatic. These workers found undersensing in 5 patients (19%), not previously discovered during routine follow-up.

Overview

Most Holter studies in pacemaker patients are outdated and were conducted with relatively simple single-chamber (occasionally nonprogrammable) VVI devices. Complex dual-chamber devices now account for about 50% of all pacemakers implanted in the USA. Consequently the spectrum of pacemaker arrhythmias in Holter recordings has changed dramatically from the early years of VVI devices.

Previous causes of symptoms such as failure to capture by a ventricular lead (displacement or high threshold with normal lead impedance) and battery exhaustion are now rare. The incidence of Holter-detected pacemaker malfunction reported in the literature varies widely and appears related to the following factors: varying proportions of single- and dual-chamber devices in any given study, a large variety of devices from different manufacturers, presence or absence of symptoms, unipolar versus bipolar systems, inconsistent methodology to test for myopotentials, extent of programmability if any, and the frequency of appropriate testing and programming of devices *before* or after Holter recordings.

In many of the older studies, the commonest abnormality detected by Holter monitoring consisted of myopotential inhibition of unipolar VVI pacemakers. The incidence of myopotential interference is diminishing because unipolar devices are less popular than in the past[68] (bipolar devices are affected by myopotentials only in exceptional circumstances). Some of the Holter studies showing a high incidence of myopotential interference failed to correlate the findings with the results of various maneuvers commonly utilized to provoke myopotential interference in the Pacemaker Clinic. Failure to correlate appropriate provocation versus recorded myopotential interference negates the value of the observations during Holter monitoring.

Undersensing reported in some of the older studies was often intermittent and not always specified as affecting only VPCs or a few spontaneously conducted beats. A number of undersensing observations may have involved only a few beats and some may have resulted from oversensing myopotentials. Furthermore, some cases of undersensing occurred as a result of limited pacemaker technology, because many cases can now be corrected by reprogramming sensitivity, though atrial undersensing remains an important clinical problem.

A number of pacemaker arrhythmias are not clinically important. Symptoms should not be automatically attributed to myopotential oversensing which is often asymptomatic. Correlation between symptoms and occasional abnormality of pacemaker function during Holter monitoring remains poorly characterized. For example, in one series of 157 unselected patients (119 VVI, 5 AAI, 13 DDD, 5 DVI, 1 VAT, 14 VVIR), 60% of patients exhibited Holter abnormalities (19% failure to capture), but there was no significant correlation between pacemaker function and reported symptoms.[10] In current pacemaker practice, failure to capture in an appropriately programmed pacemaker system should occur in no more than 1–2% for ventricular pacing and up to 5% for atrial pacing. On the other hand, component failure with runaway behavior is now a rare but still serious pacemaker arrhythmia that can occur unpredictably, especially in older devices.

Holter recordings are useful in asymptomatic patients showing a potential lead problem when telemetry indicates a high or low lead impedance (fracture or insulation defect respectively) with otherwise normal pacemaker function. Although ambulatory electrocardiography can occasionally demonstrate previously unsuspected asymptomatic pacemaker malfunction such as intermittent undersensing, intermittent loss of atrial capture, or myopotential oversensing, Holter recordings uncommonly discover unsuspected pacemaker arrhythmias or malfunction after an unrevealing thorough evaluation in the Pacemaker Clinic.[54] The real value of Holter recordings is in symptomatic patients when symptoms occur during the recording period.[18] In 10–20% of symptomatic patients after pacemaker implantation, normal Holter recordings during symptoms exclude a cardiac cause.[12,19,39,69] Indeed the cause of symptoms is frequently unrelated to the pacemaker system.[19] In about 4–30% of symptomatic patients, supraventricular or ventricular tachyarrhythmias are documented,[11,12] but coexisting arrhythmias may not be the cause of symptoms.[9]

Has the Diagnostic Function of Pacemakers Eliminated the Need for Conventional Holter Recordings?

A modern pacing system can keep track of the number of times it releases a pacemaker stimulus or senses a native depolarization. These data provide information on how the pacemaker is being used.[70] Event counters can record data such as the percentage time of atrial or ventricular pacing, number of VPCs, the number of times the pacemaker reaches the upper rate, the amount of time spent in the upper rate, or the number of times the algorithm for the termination of endless-loop tachycardia is activated. Such event counters have been called diagnostic data, implanted Holter systems, or event histograms.[70]

Sensor-indicated rate histograms (rate distribution) can provide short-term or long-term data (many days). If the monitoring period is short, the sensor-indicated rate counters reflect the response of the system to a specific activity and therefore facilitate programming of rate-adaptive devices. In some systems, such data can also be obtained when the pacemaker is inhibited by a faster native rhythm or when the sensor function is programmed to a passive state, thereby providing theoretical rates that would have been achieved had the sensor been controlling the pacing system.[70] Time-based event counters require extensive memory to store the pacing state (Ap–Vp, Ap–Vs, As–Vs, As–Vp, and VPC events), rate and time because every cardiac event must have a time reference. This form of memory, currently available in some advanced pacemakers, is useful for short-term (one hour) monitoring as in Pacemaker Clinic evaluation.[70]

As yet, memory systems of pacemakers cannot retrospectively identify an intermittent problem or provide an explanation for a variety of symptoms. One cannot characterize the present memory logging function of pacemakers as an implanted Holter system because continuous ECG rhythm strips, the hallmark of Holter recordings, are not retained in memory. Indeed, pacemakers with extensive ECG or event marker memory are not yet a reality. It is to be hoped that in the future a portable device could be used by a patient to activate an implanted pacemaker at the time of symptoms instructing the system to store a relatively short segment of the electrogram and/or event markers to clarify the etiology of a variety of symptoms. Subsequent interrogation of the device could then retrieve the memorized data.

Holter Recordings of Event Markers and Electrograms

One pacemaker manufacturer has developed special instrumentation to record telemetry data from implanted pacemakers[71] and defibrillators[72] simultaneously with ambulatory electrocardiography. Such a telemetry system utilizes a magnet (in its programming head) to close a reed switch within the implanted pacemaker to instruct it to be ready to receive programming orders or issue telemetry signals. This system is easy to use for routine pacemaker follow-up, but for ambulatory recordings the heavy and cumbersome magnet represents a major limitation. A system was therefore developed for one specific family of pacemakers to allow ambulatory recordings of telemetry without a magnet. In this way, telemetry remains effective up to 24 hours after removal of the programming head. A battery-powered adaptor and lightweight antenna were also developed to transmit marker channel signals and/or electrograms from an implanted pacemaker to a Holter recorder.

Figure 8.34 shows the Holter telemetry adaptor and Figure 8.35 shows a block diagram of the arrangement. The antenna receives telemetry from the implanted pacemaker. A light-emitting diode (LED) serves as an indicator for positioning the antenna over the pacemaker to ensure that the system is receiving the telemetry signal. The ECG

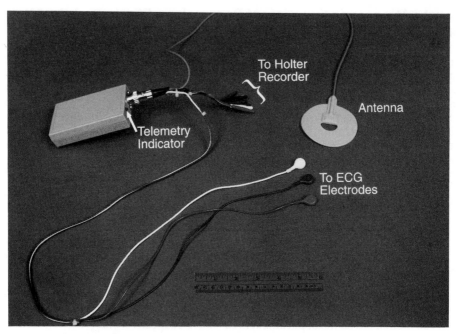

Figure 8.34 Holter telemetry adaptor developed by Medtronic for ambulatory recording of ECG and telemetry from an implanted pacemaker.

electrodes are connected to the adaptor and then passed to the Holter recorder. This arrangement may be used with a multichannel Holter recorder wherein one channel serves to record the electrocardiogram and the other channel(s) record telemetry signals from the implanted pacemaker. Nineteen different markers were created to represent various aspects of pacemaker function. Figure 8.36 shows a simple example of ECG and telemetry data (markers) recorded simultaneously by a Holter system.

Holter recordings of telemetry data will undoubtedly facilitate interpretation of the ambulatory ECGs from complex pacemakers. However, disclosure of pacemaker behavior by event recorders has limitations because the marker corresponding to a pacemaker stimulus indicates that the pacemaker has issued an output, but it does not confirm whether the stimulus has reached the heart or captured the appropriate chamber. A marker of a sensed event indicates that sensing has occurred, but gives no information about the source of the signal or whether the pacemaker responds to appropriate or inappropriate signals. Holter recordings of the ECG and the telemetered electrogram by characterizing the sensed signals (with or without event markers on another channel) partially overcomes the limitations of event markers. Transmission of the atrial electrogram to a Holter recorder would be invaluable in situations where the ECG does not clearly delineate spontaneous atrial depolarization.

Determination of Atrial Capture by Telemetry of Evoked Response

Conventional recordings of the electrogram of paced beats from the same electrodes used for pacing provide no useful information because the huge polarization voltage (afterpotential) of the released stimulus obscures the paced evoked response. It is not

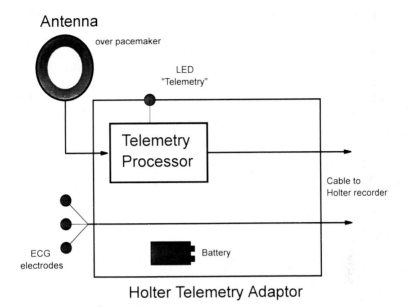

Figure 8.35   Block diagram of the Medtronic Holter telemetry system shown in Figure 8.34.

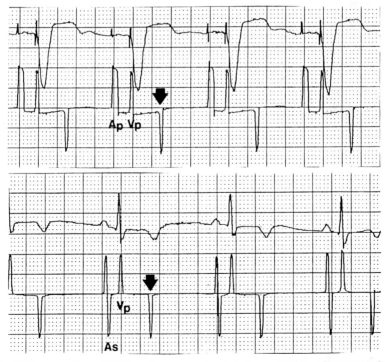

Figure 8.36   Holter recordings of ECG and event marker data transmitted by telemetry in the arrangement shown in Figures 8.34 and 8.35. An Ap event is represented by an upward marker wider than Vp, also an upward but more narrow marker. An As event is represented as a narrow biphasic deflection. The arrows point to a downward marker indicating the end of the PVARP. The ventricular beats in the lower panel are pseudofusion beats.

possible to filter the large polarization voltages because their frequency spectra overlap those of cardiac activity. The afterpotential of the pacing pulse must be eliminated to reliably identify the presence or absence of the *paced depolarization*. Recent advances in electrode material, special circuitry with active recharge techniques, and refined algorithms have minimized the polarization voltage enough to detect the electrogram produced by *paced atrial or ventricular depolarization* from the same electrodes that provide the pacemaker stimulus.[73,74] Detection of the early paced endocardial depolarization signal has become reliable so that capture and noncapture (and fusion beats at least in the case of ventricular activity) can now be differentiated. Conceivably this technology could be used in the future to transmit the paced atrial electrogram to a Holter recorder (for a programmable period). Alternatively, atrial capture could be confirmed indirectly by continuous telemetry of the evoked mechanical response to atrial systole determined by sensor(s) based on fluctuations of intracardiac impedance or other physiologic variables.[75] As yet, little clinical experience is available concerning the usefulness of such intracardiac data for capture recognition.

References

1. Iyengar R, Castellanos A, Spence M. Continuous monitoring of ambulatory patients with coronary disease. *Prog Cardiovasc Dis* 1971; **13**: 392–404.
2. Mymin D, Cuddy TE, Sinha SD, Winter DA. Inhibition of demand pacemakers by skeletal muscle potentials. *JAMA* 1973; **223**: 527–9.
3. Bleifer SB, Bleifer DJ, Hansmann DR, Sheppard JJ, Karpman HL. Diagnosis of occult arrhythmias by Holter electrocardiography. *Prog Cardiovasc Dis* 1974; **16**: 569–99.
4. Bethge KP, Brandes A, Gonska BD. Diagnostic sensitivity of Holter monitoring in pacemaker patients. *J Ambul Monitor* 1989; **2**: 79–89.
5. Oka Y, Ito T, Sada T, Sekine I, Naito A, Okabe F, Matsumoto S. Ambulatory electrocardiograms obtained by Holter monitoring systems in patients with permanent pacemakers. *Jpn Heart J* 1985; **26**: 23–32.
6. Casella G, Pavia L, Buttafarro A, Casella F, Consolo G. Evaluation by Holter monitoring in patients with implanted VVI pacemaker presenting syncope (abstract). *PACE* 1985; **8**: A47.
7. Famularo MA, Kennedy HL. Ambulatory electrocardiography in the assessment of pacemaker function. *Am Heart J* 1982; **104**: 1086–94.
8. Janosik DL, Redd RM, Buckingham TA, Blum RI, Wiens RD, Kennedy HL. Utility of ambulatory electrocardiography in detecting pacemaker dysfunction in the early postimplantation period. *Am J Cardiol* 1987; **60**: 1030–5.
9. Pavlovic SU, Kocovic D, Djordjevic M, Belkie K, Kostic D, Velimirovic D. The etiology of syncope in pacemaker patients. *PACE* 1991; **14**: 2086–91.
10. Höher M, Winter UJ, Behrenbeck DW, Vonderbank E, Verhoeven HW, Hombach V, Hilger HH. Pacemaker Holter ECG: value and limitations in follow-up of pacemaker patients. In: Behrenbeck DW, Sowton E, Fontaine G, Winter UJ (eds), *Cardiac Pacemakers*. New York: Springer-Verlag, 1985: 68–77.
11. Kaul UA, Balachander J, Khalilullah M. Ambulatory monitoring in patients with implanted pacemakers. *Indian Heart J* 1984; **36**: 23–6.
12. Bianconi L, Ambrosini M, Serdoz R, Greco S, Saba G, Mennuni M, Pistolese M. Syncope in pacemaker patients: diagnostic value of dynamic electrocardiography. In: Steinbach K, Glogar D, Laszkowicz A, Scheibelhofer W, Weber H (eds), *Cardiac Pacing* (Proceedings of the VIIIth World Symposium on Cardiac Pacing). Darmstadt: Steinkopff Verlag, 1983: 567–75.
13. Jacobs LJ, Kerzner JS, Diamond MA, Berlin HF, Sprung CL. Pacemaker inhibition by myopotentials detected by Holter monitoring. *PACE* 1982; **5**: 30–3.
14. VanGelder LM, ElGamal MIH. Undersensing in VVI pacemakers detected by Holter monitoring. *PACE* 1988; **11**: 1507–11.
15. Breivik K, Ohm OJ. Myopotential inhibition of unipolar QRS-inhibited (VVI) pacemakers, assessed by ambulatory Holter monitoring of the electrocardiogram. *PACE* 1980; **3**: 470–8.
16. Gaita F, Asteggiano R, Bocchiardo M, Commodo E, diLeo M, Gobbi G, Grande A, Rosettani E, Brusca A. Holter monitoring and provocative maneuvers in assessment of unipolar demand pacemaker myopotential inhibition. *Am Heart J* 1984; **107**: 925–8.
17. Secemsky SI, Hauser RG, Denes P, Edwards LM. Unipolar sensing abnormalities: incidence and clinical significance of skeletal muscle interference and undersensing in 228 patients. *PACE* 1982; **5**: 10–19.
18. Kennedy HL. Ambulatory (Holter) electrocardiography technology. *Cardiol Clin* 1992; **10**: 341–59.
19. Hoffman A, Jost M, Pfisterer M, Burkart F, Burckhardt D. Persisting symptoms despite permanent pacing: incidence, causes, and follow-up. *Chest* 1984; **85**: 207–10.

20. Kristensson BE, Karlsson O, Ryden L. Holter-monitored heart rhythm during atrioventricular synchronous and fixed-rate ventricular pacing. *PACE* 1986; **9**: 511–18.
21. Janosik DL, Redd RM, Kennedy HL. Crosstalk inhibition of a dual chamber pacemaker diagnosed by ambulatory electrocardiography. *Am Heart J* 1990; **120**: 435–8.
22. Tranesjö J, Fåhraeus T, Nygårds ME, Wigertz O. Automatic detection of pacemaker pulses in ambulatory ECG recording. *PACE* 1982; **5**: 120–3.
23. Kelen GJ, Bloomfield DA, Hardage M, Gomes JA, Khan R, Gopalaswany C, El-Sherif N. A clinical evaluation of an improved Holter monitoring technique for artificial pacemaker function. *PACE* 1980; **3**: 192–7.
24. Fontaine JM, Ursell S, El-Sherif N. Electrocardiography of single chamber pacemakers. In: El-Sherif N, Samet P (eds), *Cardiac Pacing and Electrophysiology* (3rd edn). Philadelphia: W.B. Saunders, 1991: 568–98.
25. Casey TP, Miyasaki P, Rylaarsdam A, Evans K, Casey SS, Li CK, Messenger JC. Holter monitoring of pacemaker patients. *Cardio* 1988; January: 47–52.
26. Murray A, Jordan RS, Gold RG. Pacemaker assessment in the ambulant patients. *Br Heart J* 1981; **46**: 531–8.
27. VanGelder LM, Bracke FALE, El Gamal MIH. Fusion or confusion on Holter recording. *PACE* 1991; **14**: 760–3.
28. Lesh MD, Langberg JJ, Griffin JC, Scheinman MM, Witherell CL. Pacemaker generator malfunction: an artifact of Holter monitoring. *PACE* 1991; **14**: 854–7.
29. Feldman CL. Letter to the Editor. *PACE* 1982; **15**: 245.
30. Knoebel SB, Hutter AM, Crawford MH, Kennedy HL, Dunn MI, Lux RL, Fisch C, Sheffield LT, Forrester JS. Guidelines for ambulatory electrocardiography: a report of the American College of Cardiology/American Heart Association Task Force on Assessment of Diagnostic and Therapeutic Cardiovascular Procedures Subcommittee on Ambulatory Electrocardiography. *J Am Coll Cardiol* 1989; **13**: 249–58.
31. Furman S. Comprehension of pacemaker timing cycles. In: Furman S, Hayes DL, Holmes DR (eds), *A Practice in Cardiac Pacing* (3rd edn). Mt Kisco, NY: Futura, 1993: 135–94.
32. Barold SS. Timing cycles and operational characteristics of pacemakers. In: Ellenbogen KA, Kay GN, Wilkoff BL (eds), *Clinical Cardiac Pacing*. Philadelphia: W.B. Saunders, 1995: 567–638.
33. Grille W, Holst T, Laessing C, Schröder E, Asbeck F. Detection of atrial fusion systole in patients with dual chamber pacemakers by 24-hour esophagus ECG. *PACE* 1994; **17**: 331–6.
34. Bongiorni MG, Soldati E, Paperini L, Pozzolini A, Levorato D, Arena G, Pistelli P, Quirino G, Biagini A, Contini C. Evaluation of rate-responsive pacemakers by transesophageal Holter monitoring of spontaneous atrial rate. *PACE* 1990; **13**: 1755–60.
35. Lagenfeld H, Maisch B, Kochsiek K. Variations of the intraatrial potential in patients with a DDD pacemaker. In: Belhassen B, Feldman S, Cooperman Y (eds). *Cardiac Pacing and Electrophysiology* (Proceedings of the VIIth World Symposium on Cardiac Pacing and Electrophysiology). Jerusalem: R & L Creative Communications, 1987: 185–9.
36. Fröhlig G, Schwerdt H, Schieffer H, Bette L. Atrial signal variations and pacemaker malsensing during exercise: a study in the time and frequency domain. *J Am Coll Cardiol* 1988; **11**: 806–13.
37. Byrd CL, Schwartz SJ, Gonzales M, Byrd CB, Ciraldo RJ, Sivina M, Yaht WZ, Greenberg JJ. DDD pacemakers maximize hemodynamic benefits and minimize complications for most patients. *PACE* 1988; **11**: 1911–16.
38. Barold SS, Falkoff MD, Ong LS, Heinle RA. Oversensing by single-chamber pacemakers: mechanisms, diagnosis, and treatment. *Cardiol Clin* 1986; **4**: 565–85.
39. Djordjevic M, Jelic V, Velimirovic D. The usefulness of Holter monitoring in pacemaker patients (abstract). *PACE* 1985; **8**: A23.
40. Wirtzfeld S, Lampadius M, Ruprecht EO. Underdruckung von demand-schrittmacher in durch muskelpotentials. *Dtsch Med Wochenschr* 1972; **97**: 61–6.
41. Watson WS. Myopotential sensing in cardiac pacemakers. In: Barold SS (ed), *Modern Cardiac Pacing*. Mt. Kisco, NY: Futura, 1985, 813–37.
42. Rosenqvist M, Norlander R, Andersson M, Edhag O. Reduced incidence of myopotential pacemaker inhibition by abdominal generator implantation. *PACE* 1986; **9**: 417–21.
43. Jain P, Kaul U, Wasir HS. Myopotential inhibition of unipolar demand pacemakers: utility of provocative manoeuvres in assessment and management. *Intern J Cardiol* 1992; **34**: 33–9.
44. Gross JN, Platt S, Ritacco R, Andrews C, Furman S. The clinical relevance of electromyopotential oversensing in current unipolar devices. *PACE* 1992; **15**: 2023–7.
45. Lau CP, Linker NJ, Butros GS, Ward DE, Camm AJ. Myopotential interference in unipolar rate responsive pacemakers. *PACE* 1989; **12**: 1324–30.
46. Zimmern SH, Clark MF, Austin WK, Fedor JM, Gallagher JJ, Svenson RH, Duncan JL. Characteristics and clinical effects of myopotential signals in a unipolar DDD pacemaker population. *PACE* 1986; **9**: 1019–25.
47. Fetter J, Hall DM, Hoff GL, Reeder JT. The effects of myopotential interference on unipolar and bipolar dual chamber pacemakers in the DDD mode. *Clin Prog Electrophysiol Pacing* 1985; **3**: 368–79.
48. Gialofos J, Maillis A, Kalogeropoulos C, Kalikazaros J, Basiakos L, Avgoustakis D. Inhibition of demand pacemakers by myopotentials. *Am Heart J* 1985; **109**: 984–91.
49. Gabry MD, Behrens M, Andrews C, Wanliss M, Klementowicz PT, Furman S. Comparison of myocardial interference in unipolar–bipolar programmable DDD pacemakers. *PACE* 1987; **10**: 1322–30.
50. Barold SS, Falkoff MD, Ong LS, Heinle RA. Interference in cardiac pacemakers: endogenous sources. In: El-Sherif N, Samet P (eds), *Cardiac Pacing and Electrophysiology* (3rd edn). Philadelphia: W.B. Saunders, 1991: 634–51.

51. Furman S. Sensing and timing the cardiac electrogram. In: Furman S, Hayes DL, Holmes DR (eds), *A Practice of Cardiac Pacing* (3rd edn). Mt. Kisco, NY: Futura, 1993: 89–133.
52. Binner L, Richter P, Wieshammer S, Oertel F, Stauch M. Bipolar versus unipolar mode in dual chamber pacing: comparison of myopotential interference, acute and long-term pacing and sensing thresholds (abstract). *PACE* 1987; **10**: 646.
53. Midei MG, Levine JH, Walford GD, Brinker JA. Incidence of myopotential interference in unipolar and bipolar dual chamber pacemakers (abstract). *PACE* 1987; **10**: 1010.
54. Goldschlager N, Ludmer P, Creamer C. Follow-up of the paced patient. In: Ellenbogen KA, Kay GN, Wilkoff BL (eds), *Clinical Cardiac Pacing*. Philadelphia: W.B. Saunders, 1995: 780–808.
55. Strasberg B, Erdman S, Agmon J. P-wave oversensing and pseudo-QRS undersensing by a programmable ventricular demand pacemaker. *Clin Prog Pacing Electrophysiol* 1985; **3**: 25–8.
56. Fernandez PO. Disfuncion de marcapasos: caso especial de sobrepercepcion de T+P. *Revista Espan Cardiol* 1982; **35**: 477–9.
57. Rozanski JJ, Blankstein RL, Lister JW. Pacemaker arrhythmias: myopotential triggering of pacemaker mediated tachycardia. *PACE* 1983; **6**: 795–7.
58. Maloney JD, Vanerio G, Pashkow FJ. Single-chamber rate-modulated pacing, AAIR–VVIR: follow-up and complications. In: Barold SS, Mugica J (eds), *New Perspectives in Cardiac Pacing 2*. Mt. Kisco, NY: Futura, 1991: 429–58.
59. Sulke N, Pipilis A, Bucknall C, Sowton E. Quantitative analysis of contribution of rate response in three different ventricular rate-responsive pacemakers during out of hospital activity. *PACE* 1990; **13**: 37–44.
60. Barold SS. Limitations and adverse effects of rate-adaptive pacemakers. In: Benditt DG (ed.), *Rate-adaptive Pacing*. Cambridge, MA: Blackwell, 1993: 233–63.
61. Himbert C, Lascault G, Tonet J, Coutte R, Busquet P, Frank R, Grosgogeat Y. Tachycardie ventriculaire chez un porteur de stimulateur cardiaque a frequence asservie. *Arch Mal Coeur* 1992; **85**: 1605–8.
62. Lefroy DC, Crake T, Davies DW. Ventricular tachycardia: an unusual pacemaker-mediated tachycardia. *Br Heart J* 1994; **71**: 481–3.
63. Mond HG, Barold SS. Dual chamber rate-adaptive pacing in patients with paroxysmal supraventricular tachyarrhythmias: protective measures for rate control. *PACE* 1993; **16**: 2168–85.
64. Schuller H, Brandt J. The pacemaker syndrome: old and new causes. *Clin Cardiol* 1991; **14**: 336–40.
65. Ellenbogen KA, Stambler BS. Pacemaker syndrome. In: Ellenbogen KA, Kay GN, Wilkoff BL (eds), *Clinical Cardiac Pacing*. Philadelphia: W.B. Saunders, 1995: 419–31.
66. Barold SS. Pacemaker syndrome during atrial-based pacing. In: Aubert AE, Ector H, Stroobandt R (eds), *Cardiac Pacing and Electrophysiology: A Bridge to the 21st Century*. Dordrecht: Kluwer Academic, 1994: 251–67.
67. Barold SS. Repetitive reentrant and non-reentrant ventriculoatrial synchrony in dual-chamber pacing. *Clin Cardiol* 1991; **14**: 754–63.
68. Mond HG. Unipolar versus bipolar pacing – poles apart. *PACE* 1991; **14**: 1411–24.
69. Strathmore NF, Mond HG. Noninvasive monitoring and testing of pacemaker function. *PACE* 1987; **10**: 1359–70.
70. Levine PA, Sanders R, Markowitz HT. Pacemaker diagnostics: measured data, event marker, electrogram and event counter telemetry. In: Ellenbogen KA, Kay GN, Wilkoff BL (eds), *Clinical Cardiac Pacing*. Philadelphia: W.B. Saunders, 1995: 639–55.
71. Markowitz TW. Personal communication. Medtronic Inc., Minneapolis, MN, 1994.
72. Feldman CL, Olson WH, Hubbelbank M, Mitchell R, Kelso D, Bardy GH. Identification of an implantable defibrillator lead fracture with a new Holter system. *PACE* 1993; **16**: 1342–4.
73. Curtis AB, Vance F, Quist SM, Domijan A, Keim SG, Duran A, Miller K. A new algorithm for minimizing pacemaker polarization artifact: universally applicable in permanent pacing system. *PACE* 1991; **14**: 1803–8.
74. Curtis AB, Maas SM, Domijan A, Keim SG, Duran A. A method for analysis of the local atrial evoked response for determination of atrial capture in permanent pacing systems. *PACE* 1991; **14**: 1576–81.
75. Wortel HJJ, Ruiter JH, De Boer HGA, Heemels JP, VanMechelen R. Impedance measurements in the human right ventricle using a new pacing system. *PACE* 1991; **14**: 1336–42.
76. Barold SS, Falkoff MD, Ong LS, Heinle RA. Differential diagnosis of pacemaker pauses. In: Barold SS (ed.), *Modern Cardiac Pacing*. Mt Kisco, NY: Futura, 1985: 587–613.
77. Barold SS, Falkoff MD, Ong LS, Heinle RA. Programmable pacemakers: clinical indications, complications and future directions. In: Barold SS, Mugica J (eds), *The Third Decade of Cardiac Pacing*. Mt Kisco, NY: Futura, 1982: 27–76.
78. Barold SS, Falkoff MD, Ong LS, Heinle RA. Electrocardiology of contemporary DDD pacemakers. In: Saksena S, Goldschlager N (eds), *Electrical Therapy for Cardiac Arrhythmias, Pacing and Antitachycardia Devices, Catheter Ablation*. Philadelphia: W.B. Saunders, 1990: 225–64.

SECTION III

RR Interval Monitoring

*Introduction by Thomas J. Mullen and
Richard J. Cohen*

Cardiovascular variables such as heart rate and blood pressure vary on a beat-to-beat basis. This variability is due to dynamic interactions between ongoing perturbations to the cardiovascular system and the response of control mechanisms which serve to regulate cardiovascular function. Recognition of cardiovascular variability, and in particular RR interval variability, is not new. In fact, in the early 18th century, when Stephen Hales made the first quantitative measurements of arterial blood pressure, he noted a relationship between the respiratory cycle, the interbeat interval and blood pressure levels.[1] The fluctuation in RR interval associated with respiration became known as the respiratory sinus arrhythmia and clinicians have generally accepted its presence as a sign of good health. However, it was not until the latter part of the 20th century that Hon and Lee first demonstrated a well-defined clinical application of RR interval variability in the area of fetal monitoring.[2]

One of the earliest attempts to investigate RR interval variability quantitatively was made by Sayers. He applied power spectral estimation to characterize fluctuations in the RR interval[3] and found that, not only was there a significant fluctuation at the respiratory frequency but there was also significant variability at lower frequencies, which was later associated with vasomotor regulation. In 1981, Akselrod *et al.* demonstrated the role of the autonomic nervous system in mediating these RR interval fluctuations.[4] As a result, RR interval variability was soon recognized as a quantitative tool to investigate autonomic function. The clinical relevance of RR interval variability was re-emphasized in 1987 when Kleiger *et al.* reported that the degree of RR variability served as a significant, independent predictor of mortality after myocardial infarction.[5] Over the last decade, there has been an explosive growth of interest in the study of RR interval variability and its potential as a powerful, noninvasive clinical tool has been widely recognized.

The objective of this section of the book is to introduce current concepts in the study of RR interval variability. First, to avoid possible confusion, one should recognize that many researchers and clinicians analyze sequences of RR intervals while others analyze a derived instantaneous heart rate signal. Although there are subtle differences in the specifics of these two approaches, the underlying information content is essentially the same. The term 'heart rate variability' (HRV) is widely used to encompass both approaches to quantify the variability. A second important point is that the study of heart rate variability generally involves only normal beats and thus researchers often refer to the analysis of normal-to-normal (NN) intervals. Therefore, in this respect, events such as ectopic or nonconducted beats interfere with HRV analyses.

There are two broad classes of techniques for investigating heart rate variability: time-domain and frequency-domain techniques. Time-domain techniques are perhaps the most straightforward. HRV can be quantified in terms of changes in mean heart rate or RR interval in response to interventions such as Valsalva maneuver or body tilt. It can also be quantified in terms of statistical measures such as the variance of rate or interval or by ratios involving the variance and the mean. For example, one widely used parameter for characterizing HRV is the standard deviation of normal intervals (SDNN) which is calculated as the square-root of the variance over a specified time duration. A wide variety of similar parameters have been proposed and applied in laboratory and clinical investigations.

The second broad class of techniques for the analysis of HRV is based in the frequency domain. The most common frequency-domain approach involves estimation of power spectra of short (minutes) segments of heart rate time series. A representative power spectrum of heart rate is shown in Figure III.1(a). In this spectrum three discrete peaks are discernible. The high-frequency peak is located at the respiratory frequency. The low- and mid-frequency peaks are generally located between 0.05 and 0.15 Hz and often overlap. Akselrod *et al.* demonstrated the effects of autonomic blockade on the structure of the heart rate power spectrum. Figure III.1(b) reveals that during parasympathetic blockade essentially all fluctuations in heart rate above 0.1 Hz are abolished. Further-more, during combined parasympathetic and sympathetic (beta-adrenergic) blockade, the SA node is chemically denervated and all HRV is effectively abolished. This study demonstrated that the parasympathetic system can mediate HRV over a wide range of frequencies but the sympathetic system can mediate fluctuations only below approximately 0.1 Hz.

Both time-domain and frequency-domain techniques provide tools for investigating cardiovascular regulatory mechanisms. Heart rate variability is normally mediated by the

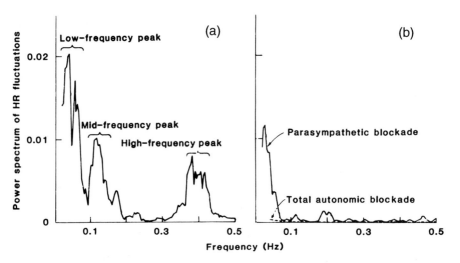

Figure III.1 (a) Power spectrum of heart rate in an adult conscious dog, demonstrating three discrete spectral peaks. The low- and mid-frequency peaks are often not distinct. The high-frequency peak is associated with respiration. (b) Power spectrum of heart rate fluctuations under parasympathetic blockade and combined parasympathetic and sympathetic (beta-adrenergic) blockade. (Reproduced with permission from reference 4: © American Association for the Advancement of Science)

two branches of the autonomic nervous system. It is important to recognize, however, that HRV reflects modulations of heart rate related to changes in autonomic activity. That is, mean levels of autonomic tone do not determine HRV; fluctuations in autonomic tone determine HRV. Only by empirical associations under specific conditions, in which an alteration in fluctuations of autonomic tone accompanies an alteration in mean autonomic tone, can one infer mean levels of autonomic tone from HRV.

One can also analyze HRV over longer periods of time ranging from hours to days. However, far fewer such long-term investigations have been performed. One approach to analysis of long-term HRV is to separate the long data segment into short epochs and determine how the statistical properties of HRV change with each epoch. Time-domain analyses of this type have revealed reproducible circadian rhythms in HRV. For example, changes in variability seem to be associated with wake/sleep cycles. In the frequency domain, such an approach leads to plots such as those shown in Figure III.2(a). The long data segment is separated into a series of short epochs and the power spectrum of each epoch is calculated and plotted in sequence. Note in Figure III.2(a) that the magnitude and location of the respiratory frequency peak and other spectral peaks vary from epoch to epoch. In general there is a trend towards an increase in the magnitude of the respiratory frequency peak during sleep as a result of an increase in heart rate modulation at this frequency by the parasympathetic nervous system.

An alternative approach to analysis of long-term HRV is to treat the entire heart rate or interval sequence as a single data epoch. For example, in the time domain one can calculate a long-term standard deviation of normal intervals. Such parameters calculated from longer data segments will incorporate longer-term variability and therefore reflect information somewhat different from the same parameters calculated from short-term data. In the frequency domain one can, for example, calculate a long-term power spectrum. Kobayashi and Musha were the first to demonstrate the characteristic shape of the power spectrum of a 24-hour heart rate record. They reported that over a number of decades the power spectrum decays as an inverse power law of frequency, $1/f^{\alpha}$, where α is approximately equal to unity.[6] On a log–log scale, a $1/f^{\alpha}$ spectrum appears as a straight line with a slope of $-\alpha$ (see Figure III.2(b)). This spectral characteristic of heart rate variability is remarkable and undoubtedly has important implications regarding the mechanisms of intermediate- and long-term HRV. One implication which is important to analyses of HRV is that the variance of heart rate is not well defined at least for measurement times less than 24 hours. In fact, at least for data epochs less than 24 hours, longer data epochs will lead to a larger estimate of the heart rate variance.

Analysis of heart rate variability is a very powerful tool for investigating the function of underlying regulatory mechanisms and, in particular, the autonomic nervous system. However, it is also subject to a number of limitations. Heart rate can be viewed as one output from an extremely complex regulated system. The system responds to a wide range of inputs and perturbations. In general, from the measurement of only one system output, it is impossible to independently characterize both the system and its inputs. That is, a change in a system output could be due to a change in a system input or to a change in a regulatory mechanism. For example, an increase in respiratory effort will lead to an increase in the respiratory peak in the heart rate power spectrum, as will an increase in the gain of the parasympathetically mediated coupling of respiration to heart rate. In order to eliminate some of the uncertainty associated with analysis of HRV, techniques are being developed to employ multisignal analyses which can more directly characterize the underlying regulatory system.

One such approach is nonparametric transfer function estimation. This technique is used to characterize the transfer function of a system relating an input and output signal. Saul *et al.* applied this approach to investigate the respiratory sinus arrhythmia.[7] Figure III.3 shows two instantaneous lung volume (ILV) to heart rate transfer functions which were estimated from recordings of lung volume and heart rate made during a 'vagal' state

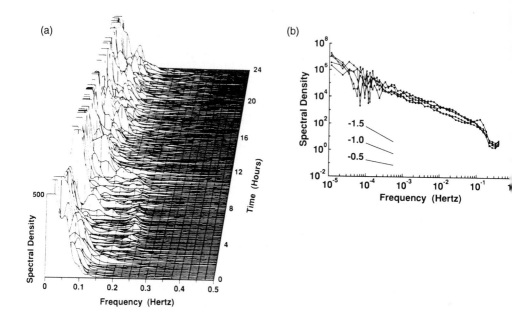

Figure III.2 (a) Consecutive 5-minute heart rate power spectra over a 24-hour period. (b) Smoothed spectra of 24-hour heart rate records for five subjects. The negative numbers below the spectra indicate slopes of the adjacent lines. (Reproduced with permission from reference 9: © IEEE)

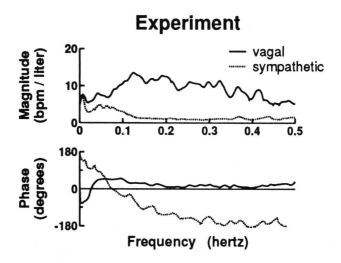

Figure III.3 Group average magnitude and phase of the instantaneous lung volume to heart rate transfer function (estimated nonparametrically) under conditions of selective autonomic blockade. Vagal = blockade of beta-adrenergic system with subject supine; sympathetic = blockade of parasympathetic system with subject standing. (Reproduced with permission from reference 7)

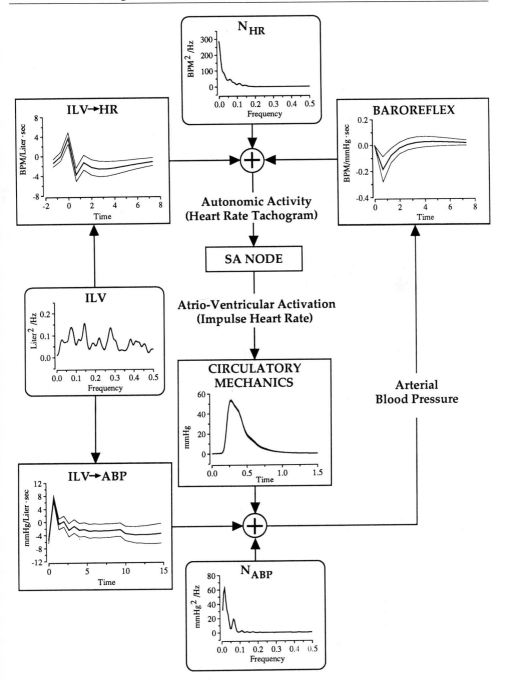

Figure III.4 System identification results relating instantaneous lung volume (ILV), arterial blood pressure (ABP) and heart rate (HR) for one healthy subject. The ILV→HR, ILV→ABP, CIRCULATORY MECHANICS and BAROREFLEX blocks represent the transfer relations from ILV to HR, ILV to ABP, impulse HR to BP and BP to HR, respectively. N_{HR} and N_{ABP} represent physiological perturbations to HR and ABP not otherwise explicitly represented in the model. Square boxes represent transfer relations expressed as impulse responses with confidence bounds and rounded boxes represent power spectra.
(Figure provided courtesy of Ramakrishna Mukkamala)

(subject supine, beta-adrenergic blockade) and during a 'sympathetic' state (subject standing, parasympathetic blockade). These data were obtained during random interval breathing, which serves to broaden the frequency content of the ILV signal and thus make it suitable for transfer function analysis over the 0–0.5 Hz frequency band. The transfer function corresponding to the 'vagal' state maintains a relatively large gain across a wide passband. In contrast, the transfer function corresponding to the 'sympathetic' state has a narrow passband with a cutoff frequency near 0.1 Hz. Nonparametric transfer function estimation provides more consistent and sensitive means of quantifying cardiovascular regulatory function than does analysis of heart rate fluctuations alone. However, it also suffers from limitations. In particular, nonparametric transfer function analysis does not allow one to distinguish between feedforward and feedback couplings of signals. Such a coupling exists, for example, in the cardiovascular regulatory system between heart rate and blood pressure. Heart rate influences blood pressure through the mechanical effects of the heart and vasculature. Blood pressure in turn affects heart rate through the baroreceptor reflex. Nonparametric transfer function estimation mathematically intertwines these very distinct physiological mechanisms.

Parametric system identification approaches are currently under development in order to overcome this limitation.[8] In parametric system identification, each transfer relation in a system may be parameterized as a causal relation. Figure III.4 presents system identification results superimposed on a simple block diagram model relating heart rate, arterial blood pressure (ABP) and ILV. These data were obtained during random interval breathing to enrich the frequency content of the signals. There are four transfer relations which can be independently identified. In particular, the closed-loop feedback relationship between blood pressure and heart rate can be dissected into two blocks, one representing a feedforward and the other a feedback pathway. All transfer functions and noise sources in the model are identifiable from simultaneous records of lung volume, heart rate and blood pressure. The system identification approach provides a more detailed representation of cardiovascular regulatory mechanisms.

The analysis of heart rate variability, and more generally of cardiovascular signal variability, promises to provide a powerful and noninvasive tool for cardiovascular and physiological research, and for clinical diagnosis and treatment.

Acknowledgement

The authors would like to acknowledge the support of NASA grant NAGW-3927 and NIH grant 5-RO1-HL39291.

References

1. Hales S. Haemastaticks. In: *Statistical Essays, Vol 2*. London: Innings & Manby, 1733.
2. Hon EH, Lee ST. Electronic evaluation of the fetal heart rate. VIII: Patterns preceding fetal death, further observations. *Am J Obst Gynec* 1963; **87**: 814–26.
3. Sayers BMcA. Analysis of heart rate variability. *Ergonomics* 1973; **16**: 17–32.
4. Akselrod S, Gordon D, Ubel FA, Shannon DC, Barger AC, Cohen RJ. Power spectrum analysis of heart rate fluctuation: a quantitative probe of beat-to-beat cardiovascular control. *Science* 1981; **213**(4504): 220–2.
5. Kleiger RE, Miller JP, Bigger JT, Moss AJ and the Multicenter Post-Infarction Research Group. Decreased heart rate variability and its association with increased mortality after acute myocardial infarction. *Am J Cardiol* 1987; **59**: 256–62.
6. Kobayashi M, Musha T. 1/f fluctuation of heart period. *IEEE Trans Biomed Eng* 1982; **29**(6): 456–7.
7. Saul JP, Berger RD, Albrecht P, Stein SP, Chen MH, Cohen RJ. Transfer function analysis of the circulation: unique insights into cardiovascular regulation. *Am J Physiol* 1991; **261**(4 Pt 2): H1231–45.
8. Appel ML, Saul JP, Berger RD, Cohen RJ. Closed-loop identification of cardiovascular regulatory mechanisms. *Comp Cardiol* 1990; 3–7.
9. Saul JP, Albrecht P, Berger RD, Cohen RJ. Analysis of long-term heart rate variability: 1/f sealing and implications. *Comp Cardiol* 1988; 419–22.

9

Heart Rate Variability: Time Domain

Marek Malik

Introduction

In principle, there are numerous ways of expressing the variability of heart rate and heart periods. The initial methods which were predominantly applied to the assessment of fetal rate variability were, for understandable practical reasons, oriented to processing of short-term tachograms and periodograms and involved rather simple arithmetic formulas in order to express the variability in numerical terms.

As the measurements of heart rate variability was being applied to wider groups of laboratory investigations and clinical conditions, the need emerged for developing methods based on a more solid mathematical basis, and the so-called statistical methods appeared. These methods treat the sequence of RR intervals or of pairs of adjacent RR intervals as a set of unordered data and express its variability by conventional statistical approaches; e.g. by applying the formula for calculating standard deviation.

Later, detailed physiological studies required the distinction of different components of heart rate variability which are attributable to individual regulatory mechanisms. This need led to the application of spectral methods to series of RR intervals in which their original order was carefully recorded.

Statistical and spectral methods both require a high precision and a reliable quality of RR interval data, which is difficult to maintain when analyzing long-term ECGs recorded under conventional clinical conditions. This difficulty led to the introduction of the so-called 'geometrical methods' which were developed in order to provide approximate assessment of heart rate variability even when applied to RR interval data containing low levels of errors and artifacts.

The physiologic and pathophysiologic mechanisms governing heart rate and its oscillations are not only complex but also substantially irregular in their periodicity. Methods of nonlinear dynamics are currently under investigation for the analysis of heart rate variability. However, practical experience with these methods is limited.

Thus, apart from complex nonlinear methods which may play a role in the future, there are in principle two broad categories of methods for heart rate variability measurement. The spectral methods treat the RR interval data as a time-ordered series, and the nonspectral methods process the sequence of RR intervals or their pairs without paying any attention to the original order and timing of individual intervals.

Substantial numbers of nonspectral methods (but not all of them) report the results of heart rate variability in units of time; e.g. in milliseconds. For this reason, the whole group of nonspectral methods is frequently called 'time-domain methods'.

Simple Approaches

Variability of RR intervals during a short recording can be approximated by a number of simple methods; e.g. by the difference between the longest and the shortest interval, or by the proportion of the shortest versus the longest interval. Simple methods like these were once popular for the assessment of RR variations, especially when the individual RR intervals were measured manually in paper-recorded ECGs. Then finding, for instance, the shortest and the longest interval was by far less time-consuming than an accurate measurement of all intervals in the record. Whole catalogues of simple methods ranging from very basic ones to moderately advanced approaches have been published[1] but are probably of little importance now.

Advances in recording technologies led to the possibility of converting an ECG into a sequence of RR interval durations automatically or almost automatically. This means that more complex methods which take into account the whole series of RR intervals and not only its extremes can be applied equally easily. Thus the value of simple approaches for the assessment of heart rate and RR interval variability is currently limited. Simple assessments are only used when quantifying the effects of uncomplicated provocative maneuvers; e.g. the Valsava ratio.

Statistical Methods

The task of expressing numerically the variability of a series of data is a standard requirement of descriptive statistics. Thus, having the data on the durations of individual RR intervals or on heart rate in consecutive segments of an ECG, the application of the formula for calculating standard deviation is an obvious choice, at least from a mathematical or statistical point of view.

Understandably, a solely mathematical approach such as the application of the standard deviation formula does not reflect any physiological or pathophysiological facets of heart rate variations. Because of this conceptual limitation, some possibilities of how to analyze a continuous series of RR interval durations have been based on simple physiological reasoning. However, the concepts derived in this way resemble to a certain degree the purely mathematical approaches. Therefore, all these possibilities of a numerical manipulation of the RR intervals sequence are frequently grouped together under the term 'statistical methods'.

Data Analyzed by Statistical Methods

Before describing individual methods, the contents and character of data analysed by them have to be specified in more detail. Indeed, with the original simple approaches, the character of data did not deserve special attention. The minimum, maximum, and other specific RR intervals were clearly understood as belonging to sinus rhythm – that is, coupling intervals and compensatory pauses of atrial and ventricular ectopics were excluded, and manual analysis of short paper-recorded ECGs was hardly a source of any errors in terms of measurement or R wave localization.

In order to provide meaningful results, similar quality and contents of data are required by the statistical methods. However, the automatic or semiautomatic way of obtaining data from electronically recorded ECGs, and especially long-term ECGs, is not as robust and error-free as the manual analysis of paper-recorded ECGs. Thus before applying any statistical method to the data of RR interval durations of consecutive heart rates, visual checks and manual corrections of the automatic ECG analysis or other additional data preparation phase has to ensure that all coupling intervals and compensatory pauses of premature cycles have been excluded and that, on the other hand, all sinus rhythm QRS complexes were correctly recognized and included into the data stream. In order to specify this character of intervals included into the analyzed data stream and to postulate that extra care has been given to the quality of the data stream, the term 'normal-to-normal' intervals (or NN intervals) has been proposed and widely accepted.

In principle, the formulas of statistical methods can be applied to sequences of both individual RR interval durations and consecutive heart rate samples. Nevertheless, heart rate samples are also calculated from individual RR interval durations. Thus, application of any statistical method to heart rate samples is merely an application of a slightly modified method to the RR interval series. Moreover, the series of RR interval durations rather than heart rate samples are a more direct result of an automatic ECG analysis. For these reasons, the use of heart rate samples in statistical methods has practically been abandoned in recent studies.

Standard-Deviation Based Methods in Short-Term Recordings

In NN interval series obtained from short-term recordings, the formula of standard deviation can be applied either to durations of individual intervals or to the differences between the neighboring intervals. The first possibility leads to the so-called *SDNN* measure of heart rate variability, the numerical value defined as:

$$SDNN = \sqrt{\frac{1}{n} \sum_{i=1}^{n} (NN_i - m)^2}$$

and usually computed according to an equivalent formula:

$$SDNN = \sqrt{\frac{1}{n} \sum_{i=1}^{n} (NN_i)^2 - \left(\frac{1}{n} \sum_{i=1}^{n} NN_i\right)^2}$$

where NN_i is the duration of the ith NN interval in the analysed ECG, n is the number of all NN intervals, and m is their mean duration. The true standard deviation of all NN intervals is being used rather than its estimate; however, the difference is negligible for large values of n which are common in all practical applications of *SDNN*.[2,3]

Although the true standard deviation of differences between neighboring intervals has also been used in some studies, much more frequently is its application based on the assumption that the mean of differences between neighboring intervals is zero (which is approximately true in practically all ECG that are recorded for at least tens of seconds – the mean of differences between successive NN intervals is substantially different from zero only during individual phases of respiratory arrhythmia and during similarly fast adaptations of heart rate). To avoid a zero value, the mean of the differences is squared, averaged and the square-root obtained. The formula which results is the so-called *RMSSD* measure (*R*oot *M*ean *S*quare of *S*uccessive *D*ifferences) defined as:

$$RMSSD = \sqrt{\frac{1}{n-1} \sum_{i=1}^{n-1} (NN_{i+1} = NN_i)^2}$$

where NN_i is again the duration of the ith NN interval in the analyzed ECG, and n is the number of all NN intervals.[4] This simple form of the formula assumes that there are no ectopic beats in the ECG which would lead to the omission of some RR intervals. If there are some, the difference between NN intervals which are not immediately successive is omitted from the calculation and the number n is decreased accordingly.

Standard-Deviation Based Methods in Long-Term Recordings

When assessing heart rate variability in long-term recordings, there are more possibilities for applying statistical formulas. First of all, both *SDNN* and *RMSSD* can be used as such; that is, with all the NN intervals and pairs of NN intervals found in the recording.

In addition, there are two other principal possibilities. First, the methods may be used with shorter segments of the whole recordings (e.g. segments of 1, 5 or 30 minutes) and the results obtained from such segments averaged in order to characterize the total period of recording. Second, the mean NN interval may be found for individual segments (in other words, the reciprocal of the heart rate may be calculated in each segment) and statistical formulas applied to the resulting series of samples of the mean NN interval.

In practice, both these possibilities are being used with the formula of standard deviation of NN interval durations when the long-term recording is divided into segments of 5 minutes. Calculating the *SDNN* value for each 5-minute segment and averaging the result for the whole recording leads to the so-called *SDNN index* measure. On the other hand, calculating standard deviation of 5-minute means of NN intervals results in the so-called *SDANN* measure (Standard Deviation of Averaged NN intervals).

The 5-minute duration of individual segments into which the long-term recording is subdivided has historical rather than physiological or valid practical justification. Indeed, the observations of more recent physiological studies might possibly be interpreted as suggesting that a division of long-term recording into much shorter segments (e.g. of 10 or 20 seconds) might perhaps lead to more physiologically related measures of heart rate variability. Thus far, however, no systematic investigation has been performed analyzing the effect of different segment durations on the practical value of the *SNNN index* and the *SDANN* measures.

Surprisingly, the approach of breaking long-term recordings into segments has never been attempted with the *RMSSD* method. Hence, although theoretically possible and physiologically no less appropriate than the *SDANN* and *SDNN index* measures, the methods *RMSSD index* and *RMSSDA* do not really exist, at least in terms of general acceptance or practical experience.

Counts and Relative Counts

From a physiological point of view, the fastest changes of heart rate can be attributed to the changes in the parasympathetic tone and to fast-acting neurohumoral regulation. Indeed, release of acetylcholine from the vagal fibers is associated with marked prolongation of RR intervals that can create large differences between two consecutive cardiac cycles. Similarly, neurohumoral regulation is responsible for immediate increases in heart rate, such as those associated with sudden fright.

The degree and frequency of these marked changes of RR intervals contributes naturally to the mathematically defined measures of heart rate variability such as *SDNN* or *RMSSD*. However, these changes can be masked by the extent of slower regulatory mechanisms and external stimuli; e.g. by thermoregulation and by psychosomatic responses to the environment. This led to the concept of measuring the immediate changes in heart rate separately from the more gradually acting regulations.

The principle of these methods is simple. For a selected threshold t of RR interval prolongation or shortening, we can count the number of cases in which an NN interval is prolonged or shortened by more than t within one cardiac cycle; that is the number of NN intervals which are longer than $NN'-t$ or longer than $NN'+t$, where NN' is the duration of the immediately preceding NN interval. Alternatively, both such counts can be merged together by counting all NN intervals which differ from the immediately preceding NN interval by more than *t*.

The performance of such a method naturally depends on the value of the threshold *t*. The method has been proposed with a threshold of 50 ms. The heart rate variability measures $NN + 50$ (count of prolongation of NN intervals), $NN - 50$ (count of shortening of NN intervals) and *NN50* (both counts together) are defined in this way.[5] Whether such a value is the optimum has never been systemically investigated, but it seems that the optimum threshold depends also on the goal of the study in which the method of counts is used to measure heart rate variability. In some practical studies, the original proposal of 50 ms has been challenged.[6]

The numerical values of $NN + 50$, $NN - 50$ and *NN50* crucially depend on the length of the recording. This is a serious disadvantage because to standardize the length of recording absolutely is not practicable, especially with long-term recordings performed in a clinical setting (nominal 24-hour recording frequently varies between, say, 22 and 25 hours and such a variation may on its own lead to differences in counts of more than 10%). For this reason, the concept of *relative counts* has been proposed. The value of heart variability measure *pNN50* (and similarly $pNN + 50$ and $pNN - 50$) is defined as the relative numbers of NN intervals differing by more than 50 ms from the immediately preceding NN interval; in other words *pNN50* equals *NN50* divided by the number of NN intervals in the whole analyzed ECG.

Although it may seem to be smart, the concept of relative counts (that is of the *pNN threshold* method) is to a certain degree illogical and contradicts the original idea behind the introduction of the method of counts. If the goal is to measure the frequency of occurrences of strong vagal and neurohumoral discharges, the counts should be normalized by the duration of the whole recording rather than by a number of all NN intervals which makes the method dependent on the underlying heart rate. More precisely, if each efferent vagal stimulus produces a marked increase of the RR interval, slow underlying heart rate will result in higher, and fast underlying heart rate in lower, values of *pNN50* even when the absolute number or frequency of vagal discharges remains the same. This is because the number of all NN intervals which is used as the normalizer in the formula of *pNN50* is lower for slow heart rate and higher for fast heart rate. Unfortunately, the measurement of the duration of recording is also not straightforward as it should exclude intervals surrounding ectopic beats, episodes of invalid data, etc. Perhaps this is the reason why normalization of counts by the recording duration has never been seriously attempted.

It is also possible that manifestation of the suddenly acting regulatory mechanisms depends on the underlying heart rate. Should this be the case, the absolute threshold of 50 ms would create a bias between episodes of slow and fast heart rate which can both be present during a longer recording. Having this in mind, a proportional threshold has been proposed. Such a proportional count enumerates the instances in which an NN interval differs from the immediately previous NN interval by more than *q* percent. Specifically, a threshold *q* of 6.25% has been proposed (this corresponds to a 50 ms difference at a heart rate of 75 beats per minute). However, there is very little experience in comparison of such counts of proportional differences with the more common counts of absolute differences, and the argument for counting the proportional differences is at present only theoretical.

Unfortunately, independently of whether the absolute or the proportional threshold is used, the method of counts is bound to suffer from peculiar statistical properties of its results. From a point of view of statistical robustness, this is not really surprising as the statistical properties of the results are related to the discrete nature of the method of counts (in spite of the huge difference, NN interval prolongations by 1 and 49 ms are treated equally whilst, in spite of the negligible difference, NN interval prolongations of

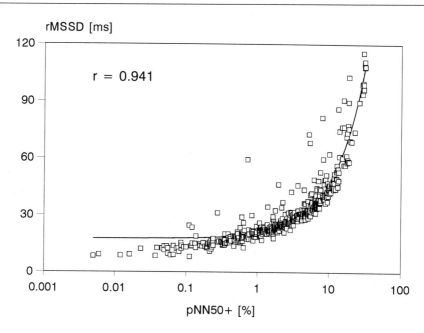

Figure 9.1 Scatter diagram showing pairs of *RMSSD* and *pNN+50* values measured in predischarge 24-hour ECGs of 542 survivors of the acute phase of myocardial infarction (data of St George's Hospital Post-Infarction Research Survey). The figure also shows a linear regression line between both measures (note that the *pNN+50* values are plotted on a logarithmic scale) and Pearson correlation coefficient between both measures.

49 and 51 ms are treated differently). This makes the method rather sensitive to the precision with which the sequence of RR intervals is obtained. The discrete nature of the method is also bound to contribute to poor reproducibility of the counts and to hugely abnormal distributions of their values in clinical populations. Moreover, the numerical results of counts have been observed to correlate reasonably with the values of *RMSSD* in larger sets of clinical recordings (Figure 9.1). Thus, although no systematic comparison of both approaches is available at present, the advantages of the method of counts over the more stable and more regularly behaving *RMSSD* measure are questionable.

Geometric Methods

The major practical limitation of the statistical methods is their dependency on the quality of data of RR interval series. This dependency was fully appreciated when the conventional statistical methods were applied to RR data obtained by an automatic analysis of long-term electrocardiograms. Although a high quality of long-term (e.g. 24-hour) electrocardiograms is in principle achievable, it requires not only careful mainten-ance of the recording equipment and appropriate subject-specific positioning of the electrodes, but also a high degree of cooperation from the patient who is the subject of the recording in respect of the electrode contact, lead stability, etc. This makes high quality long-term electrocardiograms difficult to sustain in clinical settings.

In principle, there are two practical methods for assessing heart rate variability from imperfect long-term records. First, the RR interval sequence obtained from such records can be 'filtered' using different physiologically based requirements of the data. For instance, it has been proposed that the durations of neighboring RR intervals of sinus rhythm should never differ by more than 20%.[3] Only the subset of RR intervals which satisfy the logical 'filter' are then used in the statistical formulas. Unfortunately, this logical filtering is not always successful and in some cases makes the sequence of RR intervals even less valid.[7] This leads to a second possibility for processing imperfect records using completely different methods which are substantially less affected by the quality of the data. In searching for such techniques, the so-called geometric methods were invented.

Principles of Geometric Methods

As the name suggests, the geometric methods use the sequence of RR intervals to construct a geometric form and extract a heart rate variability measure from this form. The geometric forms used in different methods vary; in most cases, the methods are based on the sample density histogram of NN interval durations, on the sample density histogram of differences between successive NN intervals, or on the so-called Lorenz plots or Poincaré maps which plot the duration of each NN or RR interval against the duration of the immediately preceding NN or RR interval.

The way in which the heart rate variability measure is extracted from the geometric form varies from method to method. In general, three approaches are used. First, some measurements of the geometric form are taken (e.g. the baseline width or the height of a sample density histogram) and the measure is derived from these values. Second, the geometric pattern is approximated by a mathematically defined shape and heart rate variability measures are derived from the parameters of this shape. Finally, the general pattern of the geometric form can be classified into one of several predefined categories, and a heart rate variability measure or characteristic is derived from the selected category.

Methods based on the RR interval histogram

The most studied geometric methods include the sample density histogram of NN interval durations. The incorrect NN intervals are usually either substantially shorter or substantially longer than the population of correct NN intervals. The short incorrect intervals are frequently obtained when the computerized analysis of a long-term electrocardiogram recognizes a tall T wave or recording noise as a QRS complex; the long incorrect intervals are most frequently acquired when the analysis fails to identify one or several QRS complexes and measures an RR interval which is in reality composed of two or even more interbeat intervals. Such incorrect measurements of RR interval fall outside the major peak of the distribution histogram and can frequently be clearly identified (Figure 9.2).

The geometric methods processing the histogram reduce the effect of the incorrect NN intervals by concentrating on the major (e.g. the highest) peak of the sample density curve. The simplest method is the co-called *HRV triangular index* which is based on the idea that, if the major peak of the histogram were a triangle, its baseline width would be equal to its area divided by one half of its height.[8] The height H of the histogram can easily be obtained as the number of RR intervals with modal duration, whilst the area A of the histogram equals the number of all RR intervals used to construct it. Thus the HRV triangular index approximates the baseline width of the histogram by a simple fraction A/H. The numerical value of the index depends on the sampling applied to construct the histogram; that is, on the discrete scale used to measure the NN intervals. Most experience with the method has been obtained with a sampling rate of 128 Hz; i.e. when measuring the NN intervals on a scale with steps of approximately 8 ms (precisely 7.8125 ms).[9] However, slight departures from this sampling frequency do not affect the results of the method greatly.

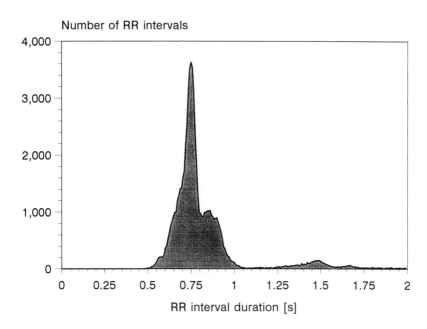

Figure 9.2 Example of RR interval histograms obtained from 24-hour Holter recordings when automatic analysis of the recordings was not working satisfactorily. The figure shows a histogram obtained when the analysis failed to identify several thousands of QRS complexes. Note that the secondary peak of the histogram appears at an RR interval duration which equals approximately double the RR intervals of the main peak of the histogram. In reality, these measured RR intervals were composed of two cardiac cycles in which the middle QRS complex was not recognized.

The so-called *triangular interpolation* of NN interval histogram (the *TINN* method) is a modification of the HRV triangular index method which is less dependent on (but not completely independent of) the sampling frequency. Using the method of minimum-square-difference interpolation, the highest peak of the sample density histogram is approximated by a triangle and heart rate variability is expressed as the length of the base of this triangle (Figure 9.3).[10]

Both these methods are particularly suited when the NN interval histogram contains only one dominant peak. This is frequent in recordings obtained from subjects exposed to a stable environment without physical and mental excesses. Such an environment is often present during inhospital recordings which makes these geometric methods easily applicable to many clinical studies. On the other hand, 24-hour recordings of normally active healthy individuals frequently register two distinct populations of RR intervals corresponding to active day and resting night periods. In such situations, the geometric algorithms concentrate on the most dominant peak of the histogram and lead to underestimation of global value of heart rate variability.

In addition to these 'triangular' methods, other approaches have been suggested (e.g. assessment of the sharpness of the dominant peak of the histogram). However, little is known about the practical value of these proposals.

Methods based on the histogram of successive differences

Approaches similar to those used to process the histograms of NN interval durations can be applied to the histograms of differences between successive intervals. However, the

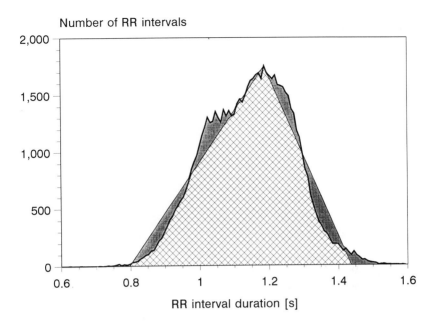

Figure 9.3 The triangular interpolation method interpolates the RR interval histogram by a triangle which has its base on the horizontal axis of the histogram and the peak on the maximum point of the histogram. Computation of the method identifies such a triangle for which the sum of the squares of the differences between the histogram and the triangle is the minimum among all possible triangles. The length of the base of such a triangle is taken as the measure of HRV.

differential histograms are much narrower than the interval histograms and their approximation by triangles is not as appropriate as in the case of interval histograms. Thus those geometric methods which are proposed for the processing of differential histograms concentrate on the sharpness of the peak of the differential histogram.

A very simple method for such an assessment proposes to measure the width of the histogram at two selected heights (e.g. at the level of 1000 and 10 000 pairs of intervals – Figure 9.4) and to express heart rate variability as the difference between, or the proportion of these widths.[11] Understandably, the width of the histogram at a selected height depends not only on the sampling frequency of NN intervals, but also on the absolute duration of the recording. The experience with the method shows that when analyzing recordings of standardized length (e.g. nominal 24-hour electrocardiograms) and using the usual sampling frequency of 128 Hz (which is currently the most common precision of commercial Holter systems), the method provides applicable results.

Interpolation of differential histograms by a mathematically defined curve has also been proposed. For this purpose, the histogram composed of absolute values of interinterval differences is used. The method expects that in such a histogram, the variability of the genuine sinus rhythm will create a smooth, sharply falling curve while errors in the assessment of the NN intervals and premature beats will lead to additional secondary peaks of the tail of the histogram. The dominant curve of the histogram can be extracted by a negative exponential interpolation. The degree of heart rate variability is then characterized by the slope of such an interpolation.[12] This method is potentially suitable for fully automatic assessment of heart rate variability in long-term recordings. However, its performance has not been investigated in sufficiently large sets of ECGs.

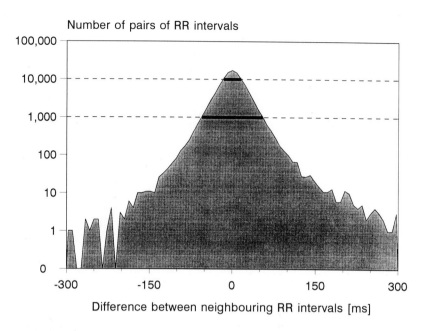

Figure 9.4   The width of a histogram of absolute differences between successive RR intervals measured at two specified levels of histogram height. The histogram is plotted on a semi-logarithmic scale which enhances the outliers caused by errors in the analysis of a long-term electrocardiogram.

Lorenz plots

Simple visual judgment of heart rate variability in a long-term ECG is perhaps best facilitated by the Lorenz plot, which is a map of dots in Cartesian coordinates. Each pair of successive RR or NN intervals is plotted as a dot with coordinates [duration R_iR_{i+1}, duration $R_{i+1}R_{i+2}$].

Incorrectly measured RR intervals or coupling intervals and the compensatory pauses of atrial and ventricular premature beats lead to clear outliers in the map of the plot which are easily visible. Thus, compared with the histograms of RR durations, Lorenz plots are even more appropriate to judge the quality of the RR intervals that were identified in a long-term electrocardiogram, although such a possibility is not frequently exploited in commercial Holter systems.

Preserved physiologic RR interval variations lead to a wide-spreading Lorenz plot while a record with markedly reduced heart rate variability produces a compact pattern of the plot (Figure 9.5). Based on such a visual judgment, some studies have led to proposals for classification of patterns of Lorenz plots and distinguished, for instance, 'comet' and 'torpedo' shapes[13] (note the shapes shown in Figure 9.5). While such approaches are valid for initial visual judgment, they lack a precise definition of each category and, as different plots create a continuous spectrum between the 'comet' and 'torpedo' shapes, are subject to a significant operator bias. Thus these simple classifications of the shape of the plots are not very well suited for systematic studies of large clinical populations, and therefore the practical experience with them is limited. More complex and mathematically precise classifications of Lorenz plots have also been proposed, usually based on computing several parameters of the plot and classifying the

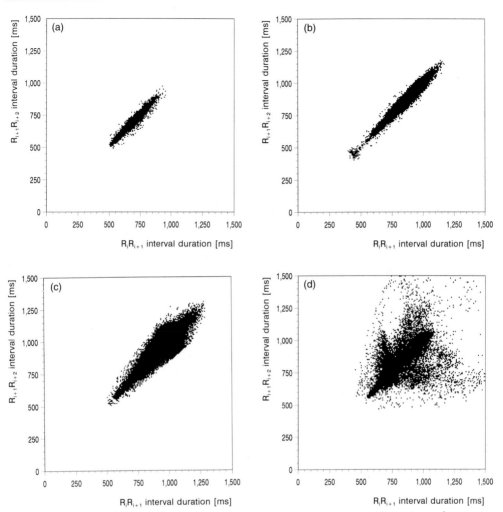

Figure 9.5 A series of Lorenz plot patterns, ordered from (a) minimum to (d) maximum heart rate variability.

shape of the plot according to these indices. However, this means that the Lorenz plot is used only as an additional graphics expression of the results of the time-domain methods and does not have any superiority over the NN sequence processing methods used on their own.

Recent investigations have also disputed a direct link between heart rate variability of long-term ECGs and the two-dimensional pattern of the corresponding Lorenz plots.[14] It has been suggested that 'height' of the plot – that is the number of pairs of RR intervals corresponding to the same dot of the plot – should be considered. Indeed, it is possible to find recordings with markedly different heart rate variability which lead to almost identical patterns of the plot. The more complex analyses of the plots which have been proposed following these observations are both typical geometric methods (e.g. interpolation of the plots with the height used as the third dimension by mathematically defined shapes) and methods which are a mixture of geometric and nonlinear approaches.

Advantages and Disadvantages of Individual Methods

Statistical methods

Statistical methods, especially those based on the standard deviation formula, can be applied to any recording ranging from the very short ones to 24- or 48-hour or possibly even longer ECGs. The results provided are stable and have suitable statistical properties.

For processing of short-term recordings, the statistical measures are the method of choice in cases which are not suitable for processing by spectral methods. Thus, *SDNN* and/or *RMSSD* are valuable also for physiological studies (which are otherwise best served by spectral methods) when the tachogram of the recorded ECG is not stationary; e.g. during dynamic phases of provocative maneuvers. Similarly, statistical methods are preferential for the analysis of short-term recordings that contain too many premature beats, the interpolation around which would invalidate the more detailed spectral analysis. For example, heart rate variability during the sinus rhythm episodes in patients with paroxysmal atrial fibrillation is difficult to assess spectrally because of the high level of atrial ectopic activity. High quality of data extracted from short-term recordings can easily be maintained as it is not impractical to review the record for each cardiac cycle visually and to localize ectopic beats manually. If the frequency methods are excluded for the abovementioned or other reasons, the statistical methods are the only possibility for heart rate variability measurement.

In cases of long-term ECGs, statistical methods should be used when the quality of the NN interval data is guaranteed. In such recordings, the *SDNN* measure characterizes the overall variability of heart rate while the *RMSSD* measure assesses the fast components. The *SDANN* measure using 5-minute averages is believed to be a measure of the very slow components of heart rate variability, although physiological understanding of such components is lacking – it is not even obvious whether an exactly defined physiological correlate of such very slow components exists. The *SDNN index* measure integrates the fast and intermediate components of heart rate variability. However, evident practical advantages of *SDANN* and *SDNN index* over *SDNN* and *RMSSD* have never been clearly demonstrated.

The major disadvantage of the statistical methods, especially when they are used for processing of long-term ECGs, is their sensitivity to the quality of NN interval data. This is a significant obstacle to the use of statistical methods in a number of clinical studies (e.g. assessment of heart rate variability in patients with frequent ventricular arrhythmias). The need for having high-fidelity NN data applies to all statistical methods. Unfortunately, the occasional theoretically derived claims that the *SDANN* method is almost as robust as the geometric methods are unfounded.[15]

Geometric methods

The geometric methods are capable of providing a reasonable assessment of heart rate variability even when the quality of data does not permit the use of conventional statistical and spectral methods. This does not mean that the geometric methods can replace the other methods entirely. Their results are only approximate and they are not as precise as the more exact statistical and spectral analyses.

The approximate nature of the results of geometrical methods is, of course, their limitation. Another important limitation of the methods lies in the fact that, in general, a substantial number of RR or NN intervals is needed to construct a representative geometrical pattern. Experience shows that at least 20-minute recordings are needed to create a valid histogram of RR interval durations and an even longer record is needed to obtain a satisfactory shape of the Lorenz plot. Naturally, the longer the recording the better is the definition of the derived geometric pattern. Thus, it is optimal to apply geometric methods to 24-hour or even longer recordings.

The need to record a sufficient number of cardiac cycles excludes the geometric methods from being used in physiological studies which investigate short-term recordings made under specific conditions. However, the accuracy and quality of recordings obtained during such studies in usually high and careful manual editing of short records can easily be performed. In principle, this removes the need to use geometric methods in physiological studies and makes the statistical and spectral methods more appropriate.

Thus the application of geometric methods should be restricted to clinical investigations and to cases in which obtaining an error-free sequence of RR intervals is impractical. Those geometric methods which analyze the histogram of RR durations provide assessment of overall heart rate variability and for error-free sequences of RR intervals without clear bimodal distribution provide results comparable with the *SDNN* results. The methods of processing the histogram of differences between successive RR intervals assess short-term HRV comparable to the *RMSSD* and *pNN50* statistical methods. It has been proposed that some measurements taken from Lorenz plots are able to approximate both overall and short-term HRV (e.g. the length and the width of the pattern of the plot, respectively), but no systematic investigation involving a sufficient number of recordings has provided confirmation. At present, sufficient experience exists only with the methods analyzing histograms of RR interval durations. Clinical studies which employed these methods demonstrated that the practical value of their assessment of global heart rate variability is not inferior to that of the statistical and spectral methods.

References

1. Parer WJ, Parer JT. Validity of mathematical methods of quantitating fetal heart rate variability. *Am J Obstet Gynecol* 1985; **153**: 402–9.
2. Wolf MM, Varigos GA, Hunt D, Sloman JG. Sinus arrhythmia in acute myocardial infarction. *Med J Austr* 1978; **2**: 52–3.
3. Kleiger RE, Miller JP, Bigger JT, Moss AJ, and the Multicenter Post-Infarction Research Group. Decreased heart rate variability and its association with increased mortality after acute myocardial infarction. *Am J Cardiol* 1987; **59**: 256–62.
4. Bigger JT, Kleiger RE, Fleiss JL, Rolnitzky LM, Steinman RC, Miller JP, and the Multicenter Post-Infarction Research Group. Components of heart rate variability measured during healing of acute myocardial infarction. *Am J Cardiol* 1988; **61**: 208–15.
5. Ewing DJ, Neilson JMM, Traus P. New method for assessing cardiac parasympathetic activity using 24-hour electrocardiograms. *Br Heart J* 1984; **52**: 396–402.
6. Malik M, Odemuyiwa O, Poloniecki J, Staunton A, Camm AJ. Time-domain measurement of vagal components of heart rate variability in automatically analysed long term electrocardiograms: prognostic power of different indices for identification of post-infarction patients at high risk of arrhythmic events. *J Ambul Monit* 1991; **4**: 235–44.
7. Malik M, Cripps T, Farrell T, Camm AJ. Prognostic value of heart rate variability after myocardial infarction: a comparison of different data processing methods. *Med Biol Eng Comput* 1989; **27**: 603–11.
8. Malik M, Farrell T, Cripps T, Camm AJ. Heart rate variability in relation to prognosis after myocardial infarction: selection of optimal processing techniques. *Eur Heart J* 1989; **10**: 1060–74.
9. Cripps TR, Malik M, Farrell TG, Camm AJ. Prognostic value of reduced heart rate variability after myocardial infarction: clinical evaluation of a new analysis method. *Br Heart J* 1991; **65**: 14–19.
10. Farrell TG, Bashir Y, Cripps T, Malik M, Poloniecki J, Bennett ED, Ward DE, Camm AJ. A simple method of risk stratification for arrhythmic events in post-infarction patients based on heart rate variability and signal averaged ECG. *J Am Coll Cardiol* 1991; **18**: 687–97.
11. Björkander I, Held C, Forslund L, Erikson S, Billing E, Hjemdahl P, Rehnqvist N. Heart rate variability in patients with stable angina pectoris. *Eur Heart J* 1992; **13**(abstr suppl): 379.
12. Scherer P, Ohler JP, Hirche H, Höpp H-W. Definition of a new beat-to-beat parameter of heart rate variability (abstract). *Pacing Clin Electrophys* 1993; **16**: 939.
13. Woo MA, Stevenson WG, Moser DK, Middlekauff HR. Complex heart rate variability and serum norepinephrine levels in patients with advanced heart failure. *J Am Coll Cardiol* 1994; **23**: 565–9.
14. Hnatkova K, Staunton A, Camm AJ, Malik M. Numerical processing of Lorenz plots of RR intervals is superior to conventional time-domain measures of heart rate variability for risk stratification after acute myocardial infarction (abstract). *Pacing Clin Electrophys* 1994; **17**: 767.
15. Malik M. Effect of ECG recognition artefact on time-domain measurement of heart rate variability. In: Malik M, Camm AJ (eds), *Heart Rate Variability*. Armonk: Futura, 1995.

10

Heart Rate Variability: Frequency Domain

J. Thomas Bigger Jr

Overview of RR Variability

RR variability has been used lately to study the physiology and the pharmacology of the cardiovascular system. In patients after a myocardial infarction, RR variability has proven useful for predicting death or arrhythmic events and is being used for detecting and assessing the severity of autonomic neuropathy in patients with diabetes mellitus. Spectral analysis is commonly used to quantify RR variability because this method provides mutually exclusive and all-inclusive measures of RR variability and some measures provide mechanistic insight. For prediction of death, time- and frequency-domain measures of RR variability are equivalent. For physiological and pharmacological studies, frequency-domain measures of RR variability resolve parasympathetic/sympathetic influences better than time-domain measures.

Power spectral measures of the RR time series (read below) can delineate cyclic fluctuations in the RR intervals in terms of their frequency and amplitude. Physiological perturbations and pharmacological interventions help to define physiological systems responsible for cyclic fluctuations in the RR intervals. Studies of this kind have shown that high-frequency power (0.15–0.40 Hz) represents a pure vagal efferent signal that is modulated by ventilation (respiratory sinus arrhythmia). Low-frequency power (0.04–0.15 Hz) has contributions from vagal and sympathetic modulation of RR intervals. Although somewhat crude, high- and low-frequency power in a power spectrum of the RR time series can provide important information about the autonomic nervous system. Power spectral analysis can be done noninvasively and inexpensively, making large-scale use feasible.

Methods for Power Spectral Analysis

Power spectral analysis of RR interval data can identify periodic components and estimate their frequency and power.[1] There is no single best way to accomplish this task. Methods are chosen based on the characteristics of the data set and the information sought. Technical aspects of frequency-domain analysis importantly affect the quality and interpretability of results.

QRS Labeling

Power spectral analysis can be used as a tool to quantify modulation of sinus node activity by neural or hormonal inputs. Thus, a series of normal sinus RR intervals is the desired object for study. If artifact or R waves of ectopic origin are included in the RR time series, they can confound the analysis. It is much more important to properly annotate QRS complexes when RR variability is small because, under these conditions, large errors in the spectrum can be produced by very few misclassified QRS complexes. Even a single mislabeled ventricular premature complex (VPC) can produce most of the variance in a recording that has little variability of RR intervals.[2] Mislabeled QRS complexes affect all forms of power spectral analysis, e.g. FFT or autoregression analysis.

Unfortunately, the Holter recordings that require the most careful annotation also are most likely to contain frequent ectopic complexes. Current algorithms for automated QRS labeling are more accurate for VPC than for atrial premature complexes (APC) detection. Recognition of APCs by morphology alone is not possible, and, consequently, template-based algorithms may miss them. It is hoped that clinical use of RR variability will stimulate development of improved algorithms for QRS annotation.

Recorder Artifacts

Wow and flutter due to tape transport errors can produce artifactual peaks and increase the power in the high-frquency region of the RR interval power spectrum. This problem can be overcome by using Holter recorders that have a phase-locked timing track. When calculating RR variability from Holter tapes that do not have a phase-locked loop, it is important to evaluate the wow and flutter issue. Often, wow and flutter error is so minor that it can be ignored. In other cases, the spectral pattern of wow and flutter permits correction of the data.[3]

Dealing with Missing Data and Ectopic Complexes

Missing (undetected) QRS complexes, VPC and APC pose a problem for power spectral analysis because it is important to maintain the order and intervals of the RR interval time series. Albrecht and Cohen[4] compared two methods of dealing with missing values or ectopic complexes in the sequence of RR intervals, a sophisticated and a 'naive' method. The sophisticated method computed the autocorrelation functions without making explicit assumptions about the missing RR intervals. The 'naive' method used simple linear splines to fill in the sampled RR sequence when there was missing data. They compared the ability of these two methods to provide estimates of the low- and high-frequency power when variable (0–45%) amounts of the RR data were missing. Surprisingly, the simple splining approach substantially outperformed the autocorrelation method in their simulation studies. Splining across missing data produces an RR time series that is suitable for efficient fast fourier transform (FFT) computational methods. Linear splining selectively reduces high-frequency power without affecting low-frequency components. The amount by which high-frequency power is attenuated is quite small in most cases.

Sampling the RR Interval Sequence

Berger *et al.*[5] discuss approaches for converting the sequence of RR intervals into data suitable for subsequent frequency-domain analysis. The simplest approach is to use the actual sequence of RR intervals. However, this approach distorts the power spectrum, over-representing short RR intervals and under-representing longer RR intervals, and it also produces harmonics at multiples of the fundamental frequencies. Sampling a continuous function of the RR intervals at fixed time intervals generates an unbiased time series. In practice, it is reasonable to use a sampling interval of 250–330 ms, with the instantaneous RR interval based on an interval twice the sampling interval. To avoid artifacts from the sampling process, it is advisable to use a 'boxcar' filter with a boxcar width exceeding that of the sampling interval. Sampling a function at a constant interval convolves the RR interval series with the rectangular sampling window and can attenuate high-frequency power (about 5–8% at 0.40 Hz). However, this frequency-dependent attenuation can be corrected accurately.[5,6]

Stationarity

A process has *wide-sense stationarity* if its mean is constant for all starting points and its autocorrelation function depends only on lag.[7] Wide-sense stationarity is a nominal requirement for much of the mathematical theory that underlies time series analysis. However, stationarity is hardly ever present in biological systems. When the mean RR interval changes slowly with respect to the time periods under consideration (say 5 minutes), it is common and reasonable to ignore this violation. However, when analyses are to be performed on a sequence of RR intervals in which a strong trend is evident, the trend should be removed prior to frequency-domain analysis. The practical limits on stationarity requirements for power spectral analysis of RR intervals are not yet defined.

Methods of Spectral Estimation

Extracting periodic components from time-domain data corresponds statistically to *spectral estimation*. There are several methods of spectral estimation; each has its pros and cons.

The Fourier Transform

The Fourier transform represents the RR time series as a sum of periodic functions and yields a specific energy or power for a discrete set of uniformly distributed frequencies called the *periodogram*.[8] The total power of the periodogram equals the variance of the original RR sequence. The Fourier transform decomposes the variance of the input data into the variance attributable to specific frequencies. Techniques for estimating periodic components have been used with experimental data since the 19th century, but the popularity of these techniques increased substantially when efficient algorithms for computing Fourier transforms were developed by Cooley and Tukey.[9] The discrete Fourier transform is the most commonly used method for frequency-domain analysis of RR interval data. Factors contributing to the dominance of FFT methods include: (1) simple theoretical basis, (2) efficient and standard computational techniques, and (3) complete statistical theory for analyzing the distribution characteristics of the FFT estimates. Two periodograms computed from 5-minute segments of RR data are illustrated in Figure 10.1(a). A peak in the 'low-frequency range' can be appreciated at 0.08 Hz, and a 'high-frequency peak' representing respiratory modulation is centered at 0.20 Hz.

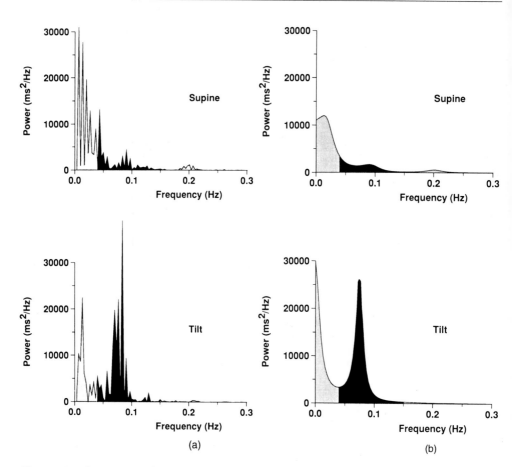

Figure 10.1 Power spectral analysis of RR interval time series. (a) FFT analysis of two 5-minute recordings of RR intervals. The upper panel shows the FFT of a recording made in a resting supine healthy 50-year-old man; the lower panel shows the FFT of a recording made during 60° head-up tilt. (b) The results of autoregression analysis for the same two 5-minute recordings. The autoregression algorithm smooths the data, but gives almost identical areas under the curves in the frequency bands of interest. In the supine recording, there is a peak at about 0.20 Hz in the high-frequency (HF) power band (0.15–0.40 Hz), and a peak at about 0.08 Hz in the low-frequency (LF) power band (0.04–0.15 Hz). More than half the power is in the very-low-frequency (VLF) power band (below 0.04 Hz). Both methods show a decrease in HF power and a marked increase in LF power during head-up tilt, reflecting baroreflex activity. (Reprinted with permission from reference 57)

Averaging or Smoothing the Periodogram

One major shortcoming with classical spectral analysis is that the fluctuations in the periodogram introduced by noise can have a magnitude similar to those caused by cyclic physiological phenomena. Bartlett[10] suggested averaging sequential periodograms to obtain better statistical estimates, and this approach is now widely used.[11,12] Also, for spectral estimation of RR interval data, it is usually necessary only to know the power within a few frequency bands. If the bands of interest encompass a sufficient number of discrete points at which the Fourier transform is computed, the power present in the band is statistically well-behaved,[7] making estimation of RR frequency domain information reasonably precise even on single windows. Periodogram data is inherently 'spiky', and, although statistically valid, can be difficult to appreciate visually. The periodogram can be 'smoothed' to improve its appearance without degrading its statistical properties.[8]

Parametric Identification Techniques (Autoregression)

Yule developed an alternative approach to spectral analysis, consisting of fitting linear predictive models to time-series data.[13] For analysis of RR variability, regression techniques are used to predict an RR interval from a linear combination of the immediately previous RR intervals.[14] Parametric identification techniques represent the RR time series as the sum of a small number of periodic components chosen at specific frequencies at which power is maximal. This simple frequency decomposition facilitates cross-spectral analysis of RR interval data with other physiologic time series such as blood pressure.[15]

The power spectral density function computed using such an approach from two 5-minute segments of RR data is illustrated in Figure 10.1(b). Because the spectrum is constructed from a mathematical function, it is smooth and the high-frequency peak resulting from respiratory (vagal) modulation is clearly visible at 0.20 Hz. The parametric identification process identified another peak at 0.08 Hz. About half of the power in the 5-minute recording of RR intervals is in very-low-frequency power (Figure 10.1(b)). (Some authors subtract very-low-frequency power from the power spectral density and display only peaks in the low- and high-frequency ranges.)

Complex Demodulation

Complex demodulation is another technique for spectral analysis of RR interval data.[8] In this technique, power is continuously estimated in the vicinity of a small number of discrete frequencies. Complex demodulation is free from the theoretical requirement of stationarity, and the filter parameters can be adjusted to separate the centers of the high- and low-frequency bands while maintaining a time resolution of less than one minute. Such an approach can be used, for example, to track the high-frequency component representing vagal activity over a variety of conditions.[16,17]

Hypothesis-Driven Signal Processing

The art of frequency-domain analysis lies as much in extracting the biological information from the power spectrum as in producing a spectral estimate. Several spectral techniques are available to investigate specific problems of interest to investigators. In publications of work using power spectral methods, the full details of spectral analysis should be presented or cited, because they determine the final results and interpretation.

Conventions for Power Spectral Analysis of RR Interval Data

Power spectral methods for physiological or pharmacological studies

Several conventions have evolved for power spectral analysis of RR interval data. For investigations that explore physiological or pharmacological issues, recordings of about 5 minutes are used. Investigators who employ FFT techniques usually analyze a 5-minute or a 256-second recording of RR intervals. Investigators who use parametric identification methods (autoregression) often use recordings that are 256 or 512 RR intervals in duration. Usually, the components of interest in physiological or pharmacological studies are high-frequency power, low-frequency power, and the ratio of low- to high-frequency power. For stability in the estimates of spectral components, between three and five cycles of the oscillation under study are required. In a 5-minute segment, there will be about 30 cycles of low-frequency oscillations and 75 cycles of high-frequency oscillations. Thus, the conventional 5-minute recording estimates the power components of interest with considerable precision. Even a 2-minute segment is sufficient to estimate low- and high-frequency power. To obtain a spectral component for an interval of interest (e.g. a 6-hour dosing interval), a single periodogram can be computed for the 6 hours as a single unit, or the power in 72 five-minute intervals can be averaged. The two methods give essentially the same results.[6]

Power spectral measures of RR variability for predicting outcomes

For investigations that aim to predict death or arrhythmic events, a 24-hour continuous ECG recording is standard. Either time- or frequency-domain measures of RR variability can be computed over the 24-hour interval. These two approaches have equivalent predictive value. The time-domain measures are discussed in Chapter 9. Power spectra have been computed in two ways. First, a power spectrum can be computed for the entire 24 hours as a single FFT.[5,6] This method permits total power and its components to be estimated over the 24 hours. Since total power is equal to the total variance over the 24 hours, total power will equal the square of *SDNN* if no distortions have been introduced by the power spectral calculations; e.g. correction for windowing errors, etc.[18] Second, a power spectrum can be computed for each of the 288 five-minute intervals in a 24-hour period.[6] This procedure permits power spectral measures to be averaged over any subinterval of the 24 hours. For example, the average low- and high-frequency power for daytime and nighttime can be compared. The average LF or HF power for a 24-hour period can be calculated from a single 24-hour power spectrum or by averaging the values found in 288 five-minute power spectra in a day; these two methods of calculating give equivalent values for LF and HF power.[6]

Standard frequency bands for RR interval power spectra

The definitions of frequency-domain measures of RR variability are simpler than the definitions of time-domain measures:

1. For 5-minute power spectra, three power spectral bands are usually reported: high-frequency (0.15–0.40 Hz), low-frequency (0.04–0.15 Hz) and very-low-frequency (<0.04 Hz). The low- to high-frequency power ratio has also been used as an index of vagosympathetic balance.
2. For the 24-hour power spectra, total power (i.e. power below 0.40 Hz) is reported along with four component bands: high-frequency (as above), low-frequency (as above), very-low-frequency (0.0033–0.04 Hz) and ultra-low-frequency (<0.0033 Hz).[6]

Below 0.04 Hz, power increases a log unit as frequency decreases a log unit, so that the value for power is the reciprocal of the value for frequency – the so-called 1/f relationship (Figure 10.2).[2,19] It would be logical then to report all power below 0.04 Hz as a single band. Why then are two bands, very-low-frequency power and ultra-low-frequency power, reported? The two bands are calculated in 24-hour spectra to maintain coherence with 5-minute spectra where very-low-frequency power is the lowest component that can be estimated.[6] The 24-hour power spectrum provides an all-inclusive description of RR variability over a 24-hour period. The four frequency bands that comprise total power are mutually exclusive; i.e. they resolve the frequency of fluctuation more precisely than time-domain measures.

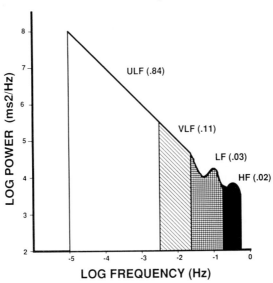

24-Hour RR Power Spectrum - 1/f

Figure 10.2 The relationship between power and frequency in the 24-hour RR interval power spectrum. Power in units of ms^2/Hz is plotted on the y axis as a function of frequency in Hz on the x axis. The x and y axes have common logarithmic scales. As frequency decreases a log unit, power increases a log unit so that the slope of the line is -1. This is the so-called 1/f relationship. The shading under the 1/f curve shows the standard power bands used for predicting mortality and for physiological and pharmacological studies. ULF = ultra-low-frequency; VLF = very-low-frequency; LF = low-frequency, HF = high-frequency. The numbers in parentheses indicate the fraction of total power found in each of the four power bands.

Physiological correlates of power spectral bands

The physiological correlates of power spectral bands are summarized in Table 10.1. The physiological modulators of ULF power are unknown. The renin–angiotensin system and temperature regulation have been suggested as physiological systems that may regulate ULF power.[20,21]

VLF power shows a relative increase in patients with congestive heart failure[22] and is the lowest frequency band that can be estimated by our 5-minute method.[6] VLF power is influenced substantially by rhythmic changes in posture or physical activity.[23]

Table 10.1 Power spectral measures of RR interval variability

Power component	Frequency band (Hz)	Efferent nerve(s)	Physiologic modulator
ULF	<0.003	Vagus Sympathetic	Renin–angiotensin system?
VLF	0.003–0.04	?	?
LF	0.04–0.15	Vagus Sympathetic	Baroreflexes
HF	0.15–0.40	Vagus	Ventilation
HF/LF	—	Vagus Sympathetic	Baroreflexes

LF power reflects modulation of sympathetic and parasympathetic tone by baroreflex activity [24] and seems to modulate on spontaneous cycling of arterial blood pressure; i.e. the Mayer waves.[25]

HF power reflects modulation of vagal tone, primarily by breathing.[26,27] The frequency of HF power is determined by the frequency of breathing.[25,28] The amplitude of HF power is measurably influenced by the tidal volume and frequency of breathing.[29] The ratio of low- to high-frequency power (LF/HF ratio) is an indicator of sympathovagal balance.[28] High values for the ratio suggest predominance of sympathetic nervous activity.

The simple act of standing up evokes dynamic changes in power spectral measures of RR variability that reflect the cardiovascular reflex adjustments to maintain blood pressure. On standing, HF power decreases to about 25% of its supine value; LF power shows a variable response ranging from a small decrease to a moderate increase (see Figure 10.1). As a result of changes in HF and LF power, LF/HF increases about 4-fold on standing up. Supine HF and LF power decrease markedly after treatment with atropine, indicating the substantial vagal contribution to these frequency bands in the supine position.[25,28] The increase in LF/HF ratio on standing is decreased substantially after beta-adrenergic blockade, indicating a beta-adrenergic contribution to this response.[25,28]

If the LF/HF ratio is being calculated for a period of time that involves several periodograms, the ratio can be computed in each periodogram and then averaged across the intervals or average LF can be divided by average HF power. These two methods give similar results and there is no compelling reason to prefer one method over the other.

Spectral Analysis of RR Variability to Predict Death or Arrhythmic Events

RR variability decreases during acute myocardial infarction and then recovers during convalescence. The recovery of RR variability after infarction complicates its use for risk prediction. Happily, studies have been done to clarify how to use RR variability for assessing risk at various stages of coronary heart disease. Power spectral measures of RR variability can identify patients who have a high risk of dying or developing malignant ventricular arrhythmias. RR variability has higher positive predictive accuracy than most other postinfarction risk predictors and adds independent predictive information to traditional risk predictors.

Effect of Myocardial Ischemia and Infarction on RR Variability

Episodes of asymptomatic ST depression are associated with transient decreases in high- and low-frequency power.[30] Transient occlusion of the anterior descending coronary artery in the dog causes a transient decrease in high-frequency power. Table 10.2 shows that two to three weeks after myocardial infarction, total power is reduced to less than 40% of the values found in a healthy age- and sex-matched control group.[31]

The decreases in RR variability caused by myocardial infarction are much larger than differences due to age, sex, or the habitual level of physical activity. The mean values are decreased because the distribution of frequency-domain measures of RR variability broadens and shifts to the left after acute myocardial infarction (Figure 10.3).

Despite the drastic reduction in total power after myocardial infarction, the fractional distribution of total power into its four component bands is similar to the distribution found in healthy age- and sex-matched controls (Figure 10.4).

Table 10.2 Comparison of frequency-domain measures of RR variability for healthy middle-aged subjects with patients with chronic coronary heart disease (CAPS), and patients with recent acute myocardial infarction (MPIP)

Measure	Healthy subjects ($n = 274$)	CAPS patients ($n = 278$)	MPIP patients ($n = 684$)
Duration of ECG recording (h)	23.8 ± 0.43	22.5 ± 1.62	22.9 ± 1.51
Total (<0.40 Hz) power (ms²)†	$21,222 \pm 11,663$	$14,303 \pm 10,353$	$7,323 \pm 5,720$
Ln (total power)	9.83 ± 0.51	$9.31 \pm 0.77**$	$8.62 \pm 0.78**$
ULF (<0.0033 Hz) power (ms²)†	$18,420 \pm 10,639$	$12,130 \pm 9,241$	$6,067 \pm 4,861$
Ln (ULF power)	9.68 ± 0.54	$9.13 \pm 0.79**$	$8.43 \pm 0.79**$
VLF (0.0033–0.04 Hz) power (ms²)†	$1,782 \pm 965$	$1,460 \pm 1,090$	850 ± 800
Ln (VLF power)	7.35 ± 0.53	$6.97 \pm 0.87**$	$6.32 \pm 1.02**$
LF (0.04–0.15 Hz) power (ms²)†	791 ± 563	511 ± 538	277 ± 335
Ln (LF power)	6.45 ± 0.68	$5.75 \pm 1.07**$	$5.01 \pm 1.19**$
HF (0.15–0.40 Hz) power (ms²)†	229 ± 282	201 ± 324	129 ± 203
Ln (HF power)	5.05 ± 0.83	$4.69 \pm 1.08**$	$4.28 \pm 1.06**$
LF power/HF power†	4.61 ± 2.33	3.60 ± 2.43	2.75 ± 2.13
Ln (LF power/HF power)	1.41 ± 0.51	$1.07 \pm 0.67**$	$0.73 \pm 0.79**$

CAPS: Cardiac Arrhythmia Pilot Study, baseline recordings made 404 ± 21 days after myocardial infarction. MPIP: Multicenter Post Infarction Program, recordings made 11 ± 6 days after myocardial infarction.
Ln stands for natural logarithm, and values in the table are means ± standard deviations.
*$p < 0.05$ after adjustment for multiple comparisons using the method of Bonferroni.
**$p < 0.01$ after adjustment for multiple comparisons using the method of Bonferroni.
†Skewness coefficient was greater than 1.0; therefore, statistical tests were done only after logarithmic transformation.
Reproduced from reference 31 with permission.

The decrease in cardiac vagal activity seen in anterior infarction may be caused by an increase in afferent cardiac sympathetic nerve impulses due to wall motion abnormalities.[32] It is not yet known whether RR variability is normal or somewhat reduced in patients with coronary atherosclerosis prior to angina pectoris or myocardial infarction. Similarly, it is not known whether an increase in the primary risk factors for coronary atherosclerosis is associated with reduced RR variability. A recent study by Bonaduce *et al.* showed that patients with single coronary artery stenoses $\geq 75\%$ had decreases in LF and HF power only if they had left ventricular segmental wall motion abnormalities in the distribution of the stenotic vessel.[33] Patients with significant stenoses but no wall motion abnormalities had LF and HF power that was significantly greater than patients with wall motion abnormalities and not different from normal age-matched control subjects. Moreover, when coronary stenosis was alleviated by percutaneous transluminal coronary angioplasty in patients with wall motion abnormality, the wall motion abnormality disappeared and LF and HF power returned to normal.[33] The authors used the same explanation as Bigger *et al.*[32] used to explain the changes in RR variability after myocardial infarction; i.e. regional contraction abnormality causes increased firing on afferent cardiac sympathetic nerves, which reduces vagal modulation of sinus node activity.[33]

Recovery of RR Variability after Myocardial Infarction

Bigger *et al.*[34] studied recovery of RR variability in the placebo cohort in the Cardiac Arrhythmia Pilot Study (CAPS). The 68 patients who had 24-hour ECG recordings at baseline, 3, 6 and 12 months after myocardial infarction were studied. The 24-hour power spectral density was computed using fast Fourier transforms. Total power was divided into the usual four components (see above). The mean baseline values (25 ± 17 days after myocardial infarction) for frequency-domain measures of RR variability in the CAPS patients were similar to those found two weeks after myocardial infarction in 715

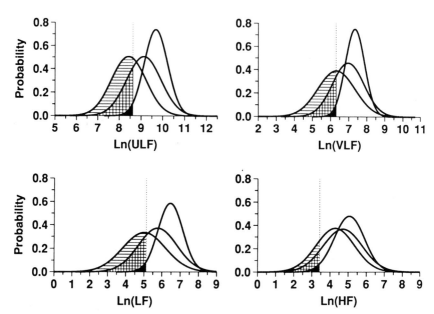

Figure 10.3   Comparison of power spectral values of RR variability for healthy subjects with patients who have subacute or chronic coronary heart disease. The curves are probability density functions calculated using the means and standard deviations for the log-transformed values of four power spectral measures of RR variability. In each panel, the rightmost curve with the tallest peak value is the distribution of healthy middle-aged subjects; the middle curve is the CAPS sample (chronic coronary heart disease); and the left curve is the MPIP sample (two weeks after myocardial infarction). In the infarct groups, the distribution is broader and shifted to the left compared with the healthy group. In each panel, a vertical line is drawn at two standard deviations below the mean for the healthy group, a traditional definition for lower limit of normal. By definition, 2.5% of the curve for healthy subjects lies below that value (black fill). The hatched areas show the fraction of the CAPS and MPIP distributions that lie below the lower limit of normal for healthy middle-aged subjects. (Reproduced with permission from reference 31)

Multicenter Post Infarction Program (MPIP) patients, indicating that the CAPS sample is generally representative of postinfarction patients with respect to these measures. The values for total power were about one-third of those found in 274 normal persons of similar age and sex (Table 10.2).[31] The fractional distribution of total power into its four component bands was similar to that found in healthy controls.

Figure 10.5 shows the time course of recovery of RR variability over the year after myocardial infaction. There was a substantial increase in all measures of RR variability between the baseline 24-hour ECG recording and the 3-month recording ($p < 0.0001$). Between 3 months and 12 months, the values were quite stable for the group as a whole as well as for individuals (intraclass correlation coefficients ≥ 0.66). Table 10.2 shows that, even at 12 months after infarction, full recovery values for the five measures of RR variability were only one-half to two-thirds the values found in the sample of 274 normal age- and sex-matched healthy persons.

Power Spectral Analysis to Predict Death after Acute Myocardial Infarction

Univariate analyses

Time-domain and frequency-domain measures of RR variability are equally predictive of death in coronary heart disease. Time-domain measures are discussed in Chapter 9.

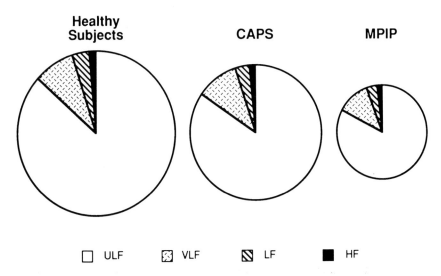

Figure 10.4 Total power and its four components for 274 healthy subjects compared with patients who have subacute (MPIP, *n* = 684) or chronic coronary heart disease (CAPS washout tapes, *n* = 278). The area of each circle is proportional to total power calculated from a 24-hour RR interval time series. Myocardial infarction causes a marked reduction in total power, but no significant change in the fractional distribution of power among the four frequency bands of interest. The percentages of total power in each component are as follows:

	ULF	VLF	LF	HF
Healthy	87	8	4	1
CAPS	85	10	4	2
MPIP	83	12	4	2

(Reproduced with permission from reference 31)

Bigger *et al.*[35] analyzed 24-hour ECG recordings from 715 patients two weeks after myocardial infarction to establish the associations between frequency-domain measures of RR period variability and mortality during four years of follow-up. Six standard power spectral measures of RR variability were calculated from spectral analysis of continuous 24-hour ECG recordings using fast Fourier transforms. Three mortality endpoints were evaluated: death from all causes, cardiac death, and arrhythmic death by the Hinkle–Thaler definition.[36] Results using all-cause mortality as the endpoint are shown in Figure 10.6.

Each power spectral measure of RR variability had a significant and at least moderately strong univariate association with all-cause mortality, cardiac death, and arrhythmic death. ULF and VLF power had stronger associations with all three mortality endpoints than did LF and HF power. 24-hour total power also had a significant and strong association with all three mortality endpoints. VLF power was the only spectral band that was more strongly associated with arrhythmic death than with cardiac death or all-cause mortality.[35] The optimum cutoff points for identifying high-risk patients early after myocardial infarction are given in Table 10.3. No healthy middle-aged person would have values below these points (see Figure 10.3). Also, it is fortunate that ULF power, the variable with the strongest association with mortality in coronary heart disease populations, does not vary significantly as a function of age or sex, as do LF and HF power.[31]

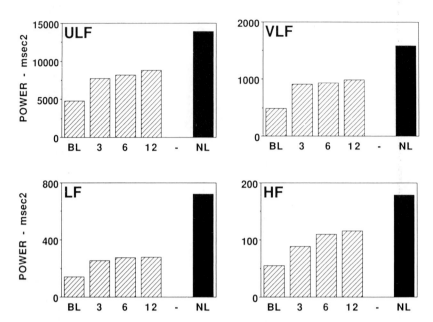

Figure 10.5   Recovery of RR variability during the year after myocardial infarction. Data are plotted for 68 patients in the placebo group of the Cardiac Arrhythmia Pilot Study who had a complete set of 24-hour ECG recordings. Because the distributions of the frequency-domain measures of heart period variability are markedly skewed, the geometric means are plotted for baseline (BL), 3, 6 and 12 months after myocardial infarction (striped bars). For comparison, the geometric means are plotted for a group of 95 normal (NL) persons of similar age and sex (black bars). On average, recovery was complete by 3 months after infarction. However, average recovery values after infarction do not reach normal. (Reproduced with permission from reference 57; data from reference 33)

Multivariate analyses

The independent associations between frequency-domain measures of RR variability and death of all causes have been evaluated using Cox regression models.[35] Using a step-up approach, ULF power was selected first; i.e. it had the strongest association with death. Adding VLF power or LF power to the Cox regression model, after ULF was entered, significantly improved the prediction of outcome. With both ULF and VLF power in the Cox regression model, the addition of the other two components, LF and HF power, singly or together, did not significantly improve the prediction of all-cause mortality.

Bigger *et al.*[35] explored the relationship between the measures of RR variability and all-cause mortality, cardiac death, and arrhythmic death after adjusting for five previously established postinfarction risk predictors using Cox regression analysis: age, New York Heart Association functional class, rales in the coronary care unit, left ventricular ejection fraction, and ventricular arrhythmias detected in a 24-hour Holter ECG recording. Measures of RR variability, especially ULF and VLF power, were significantly and strongly associated with subsequent all-cause, cardiac, and arrhythmic death after adjusting for the other five risk predictors. The tendency for VLF power to be more strongly associated with arrhythmic death than with all-cause or cardiac death was still evident after adjusting for the five covariates.

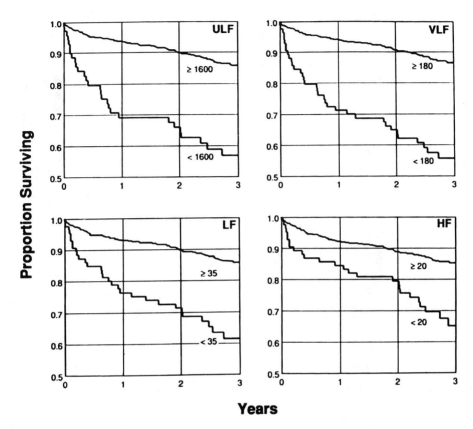

Figure 10.6 The prognostic significance of RR variability after acute myocardial infarction. Kaplan–Meier survival curves for 715 patients in the high or low categories for the four mutually exclusive frequency-domain measures of heart period variability, ULF, VLF, LF and HF power, using all-cause mortality as the endpoint. (Reproduced with permission from reference 35)

Table 10.3 Optimal cutoff points for prediction of all-cause mortality after myocardial infarction[34,40] by frequency-domain measures of heart period variability

	Optimal cutpoints	
Variable	At discharge 2 weeks after MI	After recovery from MI (>3 months)
ULF power (ms²)	1600	5000
VLF power (ms²)	180	600
LF power (ms²)	35	120
HF power (ms²)	20	35
Total power (ms²)	2000	6000
LF/HF ratio	0.95	1.6

Reproduced from reference 1 with permission.

Short ECG Recordings to Predict Death after Myocardial Infarction

Bigger et al.[37] studied 715 patients 2 weeks after myocardial infarction to test the hypothesis that short-term power spectral measures of RR variability (calculated from 2 to 15 minutes of normal RR interval data) will predict all-cause mortality or arrhythmic death. Power spectral analyses were performed on the entire 24-hour RR interval time series.

To compare with the 24-hour analysis, short segments of ECG recordings were selected for analysis from two time periods: 8am to 4pm, and 12am to 5am. The former corresponds to the time interval during which short-term measures of RR variability would most likely be obtained. The latter, during sleep, represents a period of increased vagal tone, which may simulate the conditions that exist when patients have a signal averaged ECG recorded; i.e. lying quietly in the laboratory. Four frequency-domain measures were calculated from spectral analysis of RR intervals over a 24-hour period. The 24-hour power spectral density was computed and the power within three frequency bands was calculated: (1) VLF power; (2) LF power; (3) HF power; and (4) the LF/HF ratio. These measures were also calculated for 15, 10, 5 and 2 minute segments during the day and at night. Total power and ULF power were not calculated because these measures cannot be calculated from short recordings.

Mean power spectral values from short periods during the day and night were similar to 24-hour values and the correlations between short-segment values and 24-hour values were strong (most correlations were ≥ 0.75). These findings imply that differences between patients due to disease are substantially stronger than differences due to sleep and postural changes.

Using the optimal cutoff points determined previously for the 24-hour power spectral values, the survival experience of patients with low values for RR variability in short segments of ECG recordings were compared with those with high values. Short-term power spectral measures of RR variability were excellent predictors of all-cause, cardiac, and arrhythmic mortality and of sudden death. Patients with low values were two to four times as likely to die over an average follow-up of 31 months as were patients with high values. Low-frequency power during the daytime had the strongest association with subsequent mortality. The daytime segments were selected at random without regard for posture or activity, again indicating that disease has a larger effect on RR variability than posture or activity.

This study shows that excellent prediction of postinfarction mortality can be made using power spectral analysis of a 5-minute segment of ECG recording[37] using the same cutoff points previously proposed for 24-hour recordings.[35] The power spectral measures of RR variability computed on a 5-minute segment of ECG do not predict death quite as well as ULF power computed from a full 24-hour ECG recording, but the short-term measures predict events as well or better than left ventricular ejection fraction or spontaneous ventricular arrhythmias in 24-hour ECG recordings. It has been suggested that measuring the signal-averaged ECG and RR variability on the same 5-minute segment of ECG would be an efficient and inexpensive way to stratify risk in patients with recent myocardial infarction.[37]

Adding Other Risk Predictors to Improve Prediction of Death

Correlations between time- or frequency-domain measures of RR variability and previously identified postinfarction risk predictors (e.g. left ventricular ejection fraction and ventricular arrhythmias) are remarkably weak (Table 10.4).[18] The strongest correlation is with RR interval itself ($r = 0.52$). However, Fleiss et al.[38] showed that adjusting for RR

Table 10.4 Correlation of RR variability with other post-MI risk predictors and with age ($n = 715$)

	Ln (TP)	Ln (ULF)	Ln (VLF)	Ln (LF)	Ln (HF)	Ln (LF/HF)
Age	−0.21	−0.18	−0.18	−0.31	−0.23	−0.20
NYHA class	−0.15	−0.14	−0.13	−0.14	−0.08	−0.18
Rales in CCU	−0.27	−0.25	−0.22	−0.29	−0.23	−0.18
LVEF	0.28	0.26	0.26	0.27	0.25	0.13
Ln (VPC + 1)	−0.20	−0.19	−0.17	−0.18	−0.19	−0.09
Average NN	0.56	0.52	0.50	0.59	0.57	−0.04

Reproduced from reference 18 with permission.

interval in various ways (e.g. using the coefficient of variation) did not improve the prediction of mortality.

The lack of correlation between RR variability and other risk predictors suggests that measures of RR variability could be combined with other risk predictors to improve the prediction of risk after myocardial infarction. To test this hypothesis, multivariate Cox regression models were evaluated. Adding power spectral measures of RR variability, measured about two weeks after myocardial infarction, to left ventricular ejection fraction and ventricular arrhythmias identified small subgroups with a 2.5-year mortality risk of about 50%.[35] This is a level of predictive accuracy never obtained before in attempts to predict death during long-term follow-up after acute myocardial infarction.

Predicting Arrhythmic Events after Myocardial Infarction

Farrell et al.[39] studied the ability of RR variability to predict arrhythmic events (sustained ventricular arrhythmias or arrhythmic death) in 416 patients with acute myocardial infarction. Their study group experienced 24 arrhythmic events and 47 deaths during follow-up. A 24-hour ECG and a signal-averaged ECG were performed 6 or 7 days after myocardial infarction. RR variability was measured by the RR variability index, a measure that is strongly associated with ULF power. Farrell et al. arbitrarily dichotomized the RR variability index at 20 ms, which divided their group into 113 patients (27%) with low values and 348 patients (73%) with high values.

During two years of follow-up, the arrhythmic event rate was 32 times as high in the group with a RR variability index below 20 ms. The cardiac death rate was about 7 times as high in the group with a RR variability index below 20 ms. RR variability index did not predict recurrent myocardial infarction. These results suggest that measures of RR variability predict arrhythmic events better than nonarrhythmic deaths or recurrent myocardial infarction.[39] The RR variability index was a stronger univariate predictor of arrhythmic events or cardiac death than ventricular arrhythmias, signal-averaged ECG, ejection fraction, exercise test, or coronary angiography. The best multivariate predictor for arrhythmic events was the combination of RR variability index <20 ms, a positive signal-averaged ECG, and repetitive ventricular premature complexes present in the same 24-hour ECG that was used to calculate RR variability.

Figure 10.7 shows how combinations of risk predictors improve positive predictive accuracy for arrhythmic events during long-term follow-up after myocardial infarction. The combination of these three variables had a positive predictive accuracy of 58%. This study also shows that the degree of predictive accuracy obtained using RR variability combined with other risk predictors is a major advance in postinfarction risk stratification.

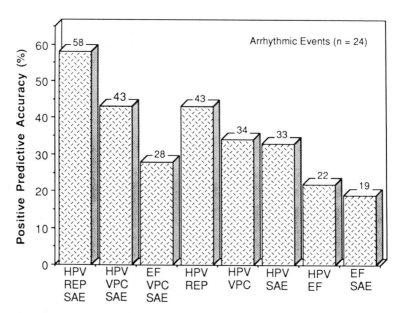

Figure 10.7 Improving positive predictive accuracy using combinations of risk predictors after myocardial infarction. Although each risk predictor has modest (<20%) positive predictive accuracy for arrhythmic events when used alone, the positive predictive accuracy is 40–60% for some of the combinations. EF = left ventricular ejection fraction; HPV = heart period variability index; REP = repetitive ventricular premature complexes; SAE = signal-averaged ECG; and VPC = ventricular premature complexes. (Reproduced with permission from reference 57; data from reference 39)

Predictive Value Late after Myocardial Infarction

To determine whether power spectral measures of RR variability predict death when measured late after infarction, Bigger et al.[40] studied the 331 patients in the Cardiac Arrhythmia Pilot Study who survived for one year, had a 24-hour ECG recording made after the CAPS drug was washed out, and were discharged on no antiarrhythmic drug therapy. Thirty deaths occurred during an average of 788 days of follow-up. Periodograms were calculated using 24-hour continuous ECG recordings and six standard power spectral measures of RR variability were calculated: total power, ULF, VLF, LF, and HF power, and the LF/HF ratio.

Because of the increase in RR variability that takes place during recovery from myocardial infarction, the optimum cutoff points for measures of RR variability in the one-year recordings were substantially higher than those previously determined for 24-hour ECG recordings made about two weeks after infarction (see Table 10.3). Fewer than 1% of healthy middle-aged persons would have values below these cutoff points (see Figure 10.3).

Each power spectral measure of RR variability had a strong and significant univariate association with 2.5-year all-cause mortality; the relative risks for these variables ranged from 2.5 to 5.6 (Figure 10.8). After adjustment for age, New York Heart Association functional class, rales in the CCU, left ventricular ejection fraction, and ventricular arrhythmias, measures of heart period variability still had a strong and significant independent association with all-cause mortality.

It is clear from this study that RR variability, measured late after infarction, predicts death independent of other important postinfarction risk predictors. Some patients recover to normal values of RR variability during the year after myocardial infarction.

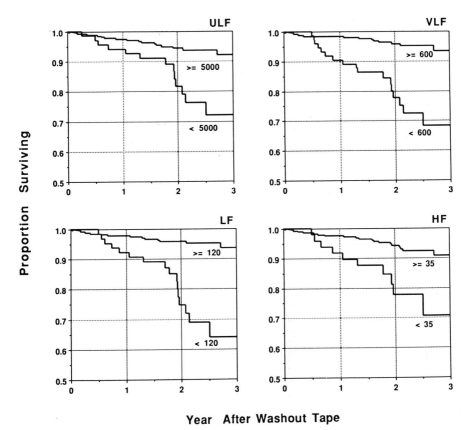

Figure 10.8 RR variability measured late (one year) after myocardial infarction predicts death during the subsequent three years. Kaplan–Meier survival curves are plotted for 331 patients in the high or low category (optimal cutoff points) for four mutually exclusive frequency domain measures of heart period variability, ULF, VLF, LF and HF power, using all-cause mortality as the endpoint. (Reproduced with permission from reference 40)

Other patients show very little recovery or actually decrease. The final recovery values for RR variability are the best predictors of subsequent events; i.e. knowledge of the recovery pattern does not improve prediction significantly.

Predictive Value of RR Variability in Other Heart Diseases

The prognostic value of RR variability in patients with coronary heart disease has been shown in several large studies. RR variability has substantial, independent predictive value in coronary heart disease when measured at the time of admission for myocardial infarction, at the time of discharge from hospital after myocardial infarction, and after full recovery from myocardial infarction.

However, it is not clear that RR variability has predictive value for nonfatal myocardial infarction or death when measured in patients who have angina pectoris without previous myocardial infarction. Similarly , it is not yet demonstrated that RR variability predicts death in patients with nonischemic, dilated cardiomyopathy, hypertrophic cardiomyopathy, valvular heart disease or congenital heart disease. On the contrary, neither frequency- nor time-domain measures of RR variability predicted mortality in hypertropic cardiomyopathy.[41] In fact, the total power in the subgroup that experienced death or cardiac arrest during follow-up was higher than in those who survived without developing sustained arrhythmias; also, the values for measures of RR variability were in the high range of normal. This finding suggests that the relationship between RR variability and outcome will have to be determined individually in each etiologic form of heart disease.

How Are Power Spectral Measures of RR Variability Related to Mortality?

A number of studies have indicated that spectral analysis of RR variability provides a robust method for measuring vagal modulation of RR intervals. Under special circumstances, spectral analysis of RR variability can provide insight into the activity of the sympathetic nervous system as well. Many authors presume that the strong predictive value of RR variability has to do with the important role the autonomic nervous system plays in the genesis of cardiac arrhythmias. A substantial argument can be made for this view.

The sympathetic nervous system and lethal cardiac arrhythmmias. Increased sympathetic nervous system activity promotes malignant ventricular arrhythmias, such as ventricular tachycardia and ventricular fibrillation.[42–47] Increased sympathetic nervous system activity during myocardial ischemia is particularly likely to cause ventricular fibrillation. The probability of ventricular fibrillation increases if a scar from previous myocardial infarction is present.

The parasympathetic nervous system and lethal cardiac arrhythmias. The parasympathetic nervous system plays a protective role, decreasing the likelihood of malignant ventricular arrhythmias. Schwarz et al. developed a dog model to study vagal protection from malignant ventricular arrhythmias.[47–50] Anterior myocardial infarction was produced by open-chest ligation of the anterior descending coronary artery and an occluder was placed around the circumflex coronary artery. A month or more after recovery, dogs were exercised on a treadmill to near maximal heart rates, about 200 per minute. At the end of the exercise period, the circumflex coronary was occluded. Coronary occlusion produced myocardial ischemia in an already scarred left ventricle and exercise decreased vagal activity and increased sympathetic activity. Under these conditions, susceptible dogs (55%) repeatedly developed ventricular fibrillation during the exercise–ischemia challenge while unsusceptible dogs (45%) did not.

Baroreflex sensitivity and RR variability predict ventricular fibrillation. The response to the exercise–ischemia challenge in the Schwartz dog model was predicted by baroreflex sensitivity, the change in RR interval as a function of the increase in systolic blood pressure after intravenous phenylephrine.[51] Dogs with low baroreflex sensitivity were susceptible to ventricular fibrillation when challenged with exercise and ischemia. Vagal measures of RR variability also predicted ventricular fibrillation during the exercise–ischemia challenge.[52,53] Susceptible dogs that were made unsusceptible by exercise training always showed increased baroreflex sensitivity and RR variability after exercise training.[54]

RR variability may not specifically predict arrhythmic death. Not all the evidence supports the theory that RR variability is an indicator of conditions that promote lethal arrhythmias. RR variability predicts all-cause mortality about as well as it predicts arrhythmic or sudden death. The autonomic nervous system responds strongly to circulatory dysfunction. When cardiac pumping action is inadequate to provide blood flow to peripheral tissues, cardiovascular reflexes cause a decrease in vagus nerve modulation of RR intervals and an increase in sympathetic nerve modulation. Also, signals from reflexogenic regions can elicit strong responses from the autonomic nervous system in the absence of circulatory failure. For example, arterial hypertension is associated with decreased vagus nerve modulation of RR intervals and increased sympathetic nerve activity. Myocardial ischemia that is too mild to cause circulatory embarrassment causes decreased vagus nerve modulation of RR intervals. Abnormal afferent signals from mechanoreceptors, including high- and low-pressure barorecep-tors, and from chemoreceptors are processed by the brain which then modulates activity in the two limbs of the autonomic nervous system. RR variability will be decreased when vagal nerve activity is decreased and/or sympathetic nerve activity is increased. Thus, decreased RR variability can be viewed as a response to circulatory distress rather than a specific arrhythmia promoter. Whatever the link between decreased RR variability and cardiac death, RR variability has a leading role to play in predicting lethal events in coronary heart disease.

Use of RR Variability to Study Disease Progression or Drug Effects

The day-to-day reproducibility of RR variability measures

Previously studied Holter variables, such as ventricular arrhythmias or ischemic epi-sodes, are quite variable from day to day. This lack of stability hampers attempts to study the effect of disease or drug therapy on arrhythmias or spontaneous episodes of myocardial ischemia. It might be expected that there would be considerable day-to-day instability in measures of RR variability as well, particularly in those components that reflect sympathetic or parasympathetic nervous activity. The amount of day-to-day stability for power spectral measures of RR variability is a strong determinant of the statistical power to separate diseased individuals from healthy persons and to establish drug effects on the autonomic nervous system. Several studies have addressed day-to-day stability of power spectral measures of RR variability. For studies of stability, the intraclass correlation coefficient is the best measure of within-subject stability. The standard error of the measurement is a statistic that quantifies the size of the difference required to declare that a change has occurred.

Stability of power spectral measures of RR variability in healthy subjects

Fourteen healthy subjects, 20 to 55 years of age, were studied by Kleiger *et al.* to determine day-to-day stability of RR variability.[55] Two 24-hour recordings were made 3 to 65 days apart (median 18 days), one under baseline conditions and the other during placebo treament in a crossover drug study.

An example of two 24-hour ECG recordings in a subject are shown in Figure 10.9. Not only are the mean values for LF and HF power virtually identical in the two 24-hour ECG recordings, but also the power spectral values are similar for any given 5-minute segment during the 24-hour period. The group data for the healthy subjects is shown in the left panel of Figure 10.10. The mean values for LF and HF power were virtually identical in the two 24-hour ECG recordings. Furthermore, the intraclass correlation coefficients (a measure of within-subject agreement) were 0.91 and 0.84 respectively for LF and HF power. The sample was divided at the median time between recordings and it was found that the intraclass correlation coefficients were 0.93 and 0.90 for recordings made less than 18 days apart and 0.88 and 0.75 for recordings made at least 18 days apart. Also, the standard errors of measurement between pairs of recordings was very small.

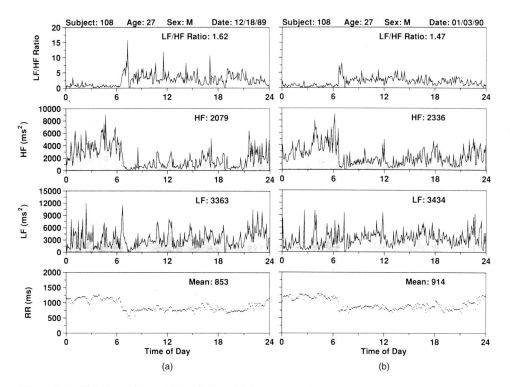

Figure 10.9 The day-to-day stability of RR variability. (a) and (b) plot RR interval, LF power, HF power, and LF/HF ratio from two 24-hour ECG recordings made 16 days apart in a normal 27-year-old man. An RR interval power spectrum is plotted for each 5-minute segment. Not only are the 24-hour average power spectral values similar for the two recordings, but also the profile of changes for each 5-minute segment are remarkably similar. (Reproduced with permission from reference 57; data from reference 57)

Thus, the power spectral measures of RR variability were essentially constant from day to day during the range of time studied (3 to 65 days). This remarkable day-to-day stability exists for the 24-hour average values for power spectral measures of RR variability despite marked differences among the 5-minute intervals during a day (see Figure 10.8). This study of healthy persons also showed a lack of any 'placebo effect'.[55] The subjects were blinded as to treatment but knew they were taking placebo, atenolol, or diltiazem. Even so, there were no differences between the values for RR variability measured during placebo treatment and those found in the baseline tape when subjects knew they were not taking any treatment. A significant 'placebo effect' can be found on blood pressure and on frequency of angina pectoris. It is interesting that no placebo effect was found for the measures of RR variability that reflect sympathetic and parasympathetic nervous activity.

Stability of power spectral measures of RR variability in patients with cardiac arrhythmias

Day-to-day stability of power spectral measures of RR variability was also studied in patients with coronary heart disease, previous myocardial infarction, left ventricular dysfunction, and ventricular arrhythmias.[56] Two groups were studied: those with unsustained, prognostically significant ventricular arrhythmias, and those with sustained ventricular arrhythmias. The sample selected to study unsustained ventricular

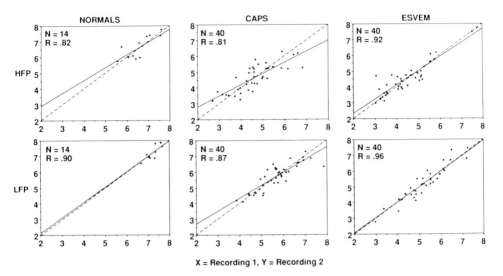

Figure 10.10 The day-to-day stability of RR variability. The natural logarithms of high-frequency power (HFP) and low-frequency power (LFP) are plotted for three groups: a group of normal subjects (left); the Cardiac Arrhythmia Pilot Study (CAPS) group (middle); and the Electrophysiologic Studies Versus Electrocardiographic Monitoring (ESVEM) group (right). From left to right, the groups are ranked for severity of cardiac disease (none, moderate, severe). The logarithms of the values for power in the first 24-hour ECG recording are plotted on the x axis and those for the second 24-hour ECG recording are plotted on the y axis. The diagonal solid lines are the lines of identity (slope = 1, intercept = 0); if the values for day 1 and day 2 were identical they would lie on this line. The diagonal dashed lines are the linear regression lines calculated for the data. The agreement between recordings is excellent for all groups.

arrhythmias was a random sample of 40 patients from the placebo group of the CAPS. The sample selected to study sustained ventricular arrhythmias was a random sample of 40 patients in the ESVEM study. The ESVEM group was much sicker than the CAPS group in terms of functional class (ESVEM functional class II–IV, 84% versus CAPS functional class II–IV, 5%), average left ventricular ejection fraction (ESVEM, 0.34 ± 0.16 versus CAPS, 0.46 ± 0.12), and median ventricular arrhythmia frequency (ESVEM, 125/hour versus CAPS, 18/hour). Total power and each of its components were lower in the ESVEM group than in the CAPS group. However, the magnitude of reduction was especially large for total and ultra-low-frequency power; the values in the ESVEM group were 51% and 56% of the values in the CAPS group ($p < 0.001$ by independent sample t-tests). The difference between the ESVEM and CAPS groups was statistically significant, but much smaller for very-low-frequency, low-frequency, and high-frequency power, where the values in the ESVEM group were 78%, 90% and 80% of those found in the CAPS group ($p < 0.01$, $p < 0.05$, and NS respectively by independent sample t-tests). There were no significant differences in measures of RR variability between the two 24-hour within-patient recording sessions in either the ESVEM or the CAPS group (see Figure 10.10). Remarkably, the two sets of mean values for the two recordings were almost identical within the ESVEM group and within the CAPS group.

Graphical examples of the paired measures for total power and for high-frequency power are shown in Figure 10.10. The agreement between the two 24-hour recordings is evident. Also, the graphs show that the agreement of paired measurements is better in the ESVEM group than in the CAPS group – the regression lines are closer to the lines of identity and the correlation coefficients are larger. The remarkable day-to-day stability of RR variability is in sharp contrast to ventricular ectopic complexes which are quite variable from day to day. Another study conducted over a year showed excellent stability for measures of RR variability at between 3 and 12 months after myocardial infarction.[34]

These studies[34,56] showed that the reproducibility of RR variability measurements in patients with previous myocardial infarction and ventricular arrhythmias is comparable with the high stability previously found in healthy subjects.[55] The stability of measures of RR variability facilitates distinguishing real changes due to progression or regression of cardiac disease or those due to drug effects from changes due to random variation. The large intraclass correlation coefficient and the small standard error of the measurement found for power spectral measures of RR variability over time make these variables sensitive for detecting and quantifying changes in disease severity or drug effects.

Effect of cardiovascular drugs on RR variability

Power spectral measures of RR variability are sensitive to drug effects, especially effects on the autonomic nervous system. Power spectral measures of RR variability have been used to gain insight into the effect of cardiovascular drugs on the autonomic nervous system and on cardiovascular reflexes. The current state of knowledge about drug effects on power spectral measures of RR variability was reviewed recently.[57] Most cardiovascular drugs have complex actions, many drugs act on several peripheral sites as well as on sites in the brain. Some act directly on cholinergic or adrenergic receptors. Such a multiplicity of actions may cloud the interpretation of changes in power spectral measures of RR variability.

Despite this problem with interpretation, power spectral analysis is proving useful to study the effects of drugs on intact human beings under conditions of normal daily living. We can expect the number and sophistication of studies that use power spectral measures of RR variability to explore drug action to increase rapidly in the near future.

Acknowledgement

This work was supported in part by NIH Grants HL-41552 from the National Heart, Lung and Blood Institute, Bethesda, MD, and RR-00645 from the Research Resources Administration, NIH; and by funds from the Bugher Foundation, the Dover Foundation, and Mrs Adelaide Segerman, New York, NY.

References

1. Bigger JT, Rottman JN. Spectral analysis of RR variability. In: Podrid PJ, Kowey PR (eds), *Cardiac Arrhythmias – Mechanism, Diagnosis, and Management*. Baltimore: William & Wilkins, 1995; 280–98.
2. Saul JP, Albrecht P, Berger RD, Cohen RJ. Analysis of long term heart rate variability: methods, $1/f$ scaling and implications. *Comp Cardiol* 1988; 419–22.
3. Pinna G, DiCesare A, Maestri R, Tangenti A. Reliability of analysis of the heart rate variability signal from a commercial Holter system. *Comp Cardiol* 1991; 429–32.
4. Albrecht P, Cohen RJ. Estimation of heart rate power spectrum bands from real-world data: dealing with ectopic beats and noisy data. *Cardiology* 1988; **15**: 311–14.
5. Berger RD, Akselrod S, Gordon D, Cohen RJ. An efficient algorithm for spectral analysis of heart rate variability. *IEEE Trans Biomed Eng* 1986; **33**: 900–4.
6. Rottman JN, Steinman RC, Albrecht P, Bigger JT, Rolnitzky LM, Fleiss JL. Efficient estimation of the heart period power spectrum suitable for physiologic or pharmacologic studies. *Am J Cardiol* 1990; **66**: 1522–4.
7. Marple SL. *Digital Spectral Analysis with Applications*. Englewood Cliffs, NJ: Prentice-Hall.
8. Bloomfield P. *Fourier Analysis of Time Series: An Introduction*. New York: John Wiley, 1976.
9. Cooley JW, Tukey JW. An algorithm for machine calculation of complex Fourier series. *Math Comput* 1965; **19**: 297–301.
10. Bartlett, MS. Smoothing periodograms from time series with continuous spectra. *Nature* (London) 1948; **161**: 686–7.

11. Myers GA, Martin GJ, Magid NM, Barnett PJ, Schaad JW, Weiss JS, Lesch M, Singer DH. Power spectral analysis of heart rate variability in sudden cardiac death: comparison to other methods. *IEEE Trans Biomed Eng* 1986; **33**: 1149–56.
12. Bigger JT, LaRovere MT, Steinman RC, Fleiss JL, Rottman JN, Rolnitzky LM, Schwartz PJ. Comparison of baroflex sensitivity and heart period variability after myocardial infarction. *J Am Coll Cardiol* 1989; **14**: 1511–18.
13. Oppenheim AV, Schafer RW. *Digital Signal Processing.* Englewood Cliffs, NJ: Prentice-Hall.
14. Burg JP. Maximum entropy spectral analysis (in Proceedings of the 37th Meeting of Society of Exploration Geophysicists, Oklahoma City, OK, 1967). Reprinted in: DG Childers (ed.), *Modern Spectral Analysis.* New York: IEEE Press Selected Reprint Series, 1978: 132–3.
15. Baselli G, Cerutti S, Civardi S, Liberati D, Lombardi F, Malliani A, Pagani M. Spectral and cross-spectral analysis of heart rate and arterial blood pressure variability signals. *Comput Biomed Res* 1986; **19**: 520–34.
16. Kiauta T, Jager F, Tapp WN. Complex demodulation of heart rate changes during orthostatic testing. *Comp Cardiol* 1990; 159–62.
17. Shin S-J. Tapp WN, Reisman SS, Natelson BH. Assessment of automatic regulation of heart rate variability by the method of complex demodulation. *IEEE Trans Biomed Eng* 1989; **36**: 277–83.
18. Bigger JT, Fleiss JL, Steinman RC, Rolnitzky LM, Kleiger RE, Rottman JN. Correlations among time and frequency domain measures of heart period variability two weeks after acute myocardial infarction. *Am J Cardiol* 1992; **69**: 891–8.
19. Kobayashi M, Musha T. 1/*f* fluctuation of heartbeat period. *IEEE Trans Biomed Eng* 1982; **29**: 456–7.
20. Akselrod S, Gordon D, Ubel FA, Shannon DC, Barger AC, Cohen RJ. Power spectrum analysis of heart rate fluctuation: a quantitative probe of beat-to-beat cardiovascular control. *Science* 1981; **213**; 220–3.
21. Kitney RI. An analysis of the nonlinear behaviour of the human thermal control system. *J Theoret Biol* 1979; **1**: 89–99.
22. Saul JP, Arai Y, Berger RD, Lilly LS, Colucci WS, Cohen RJ. Assessment of automatic regulation in chronic congestive heart failure by heart rate spectral analysis. *Am J Cardiol* 1988; **61**: 1292–9.
23. Bernardi L, Valle F, Coco M, Sleight P. Physical activity is a major determinant of heart rate variability, its 'very low' frequency component and 1/*f* (chaotic) distribution. *Eur Heart J* 1994; **15** (Suppl): 242A.
24. Koizumi K, Terui N, Kollai M. Effect of cardiac vagal and sympathetic nerve activity on heart rate in rhythmic regulations. *J Autonom Nerv Syst* 1985; **12**: 251–9.
25. Pomeranz B, Macaulay RJB, Caudill MA, Kutz I, Adam D, Gordon D, Kilborn KM, Barger AC, Shannon DC, Cohen RJ, Benson H. Assessment of automatic function in humans by heart rate spectral analysis. *Am J Physiol* 1985; **248**: H151–3.
26. Katona PG, Jih F. Respiratory sinus arrhythmia: measure of the parasympathetic cardiac control. *J Appl Physiol* 1975; **39**: 801–5.
27. Fouad FM, Tarazzi RC, Ferrario CM, Fighaly S, Alicandri C. Assessment of parasympathetic control of heart rate by a noninvasive method. *Am J Physiol* 1984; **246**: H838–42.
28. Pagani M, Lombardi, F, Guzzetti S, Rimoldi O, Furlan R, Pizzinelli P, Sandrime G, Malfatto G, dell'Orto S, Piccaluga E, Turiel M, Baselli G, Cerutti S, Malliani A. Power spectral analysis of heart rate and arterial pressure variabilities as a marker of sympatho-vagal interactions in man and conscious dog. *Circ Res* 1986; **59**: 178–93.
29. Brown TE, Beightol LA, Koh J, Eckberg DL. The important influence of respiration on RR interval power spectra is largely ignored. *J Appl Physiol* 1993; **75**: 2310–17.
30. Bigger JT, Hoover CA, Steinman RC, Rolnitzky LM, Fleiss JL, and the Multicenter Study of Silent Myocardial Ischemia investigators. Autonomic nervous system activity during myocardial ischemia in man estimated by power spectral analysis of heart period variability. *Am J Cardiol* 1990; **66**: 497–8.
31. Bigger JT, Fleiss, JL, Steinman RC, Rolnitzky LM, Schneider WJ, Stein PK. RR variability in healthy, middle-age persons compared with patients with chronic coronary heart disease or recent acute myocardial infarction. *Circulation* 1995; **91**: 1936–43.
32. Bigger JT, La Rovere MT, Steinman RC, Fleiss JL, Rottman JN, Rolnitzky LM, Schwartz PJ. Comparison of baroreflex sensitivity and heart period variability after myocardial infarction. *J Am Coll Cardiol* 1989; **14**: 215–30.
33. Bonaduce D, Petretta M, Piscione F, Indolfi C, Migaux ML, Bianchi V, Esposito N, Marciano F, Condorelli M. Influence of reversible segmental left ventricular dysfunction on heart period variability in patients with one-vessel coronary artery disease. *J Am Coll Cardiol* 1994; **24**: 399–405.
34. Bigger JT, Fleiss JL, Rolnitzky LM, Steinman RC, Schneider WJ. Time course of recovery of heart period variability after myocardial infarction. *J Am Coll Cardiol* 1991; **18**: 1643–9.
35. Bigger JT, Fleiss JL, Steinman RC, Rolnitzky LM, Kleiger RE, Rottman JN. Frequency domain measures of heart period variability and mortality after myocardial infarction. *Circulation* 1992; **85**: 164–71.
36. Hinkle LE, Thaler JT. Clinical classification of cardiac deaths. *Circulation* 1982; **65**: 457–64.
37. Bigger JT, Fleiss JL, Rolnitzky LM, Steinman RC. The ability of short term measures of RR variability to predict mortality after myocardial infarction. *Circulation* 1993; **88**: 927–34.
38. Fleiss JL, Bigger JT, Rolnitzky LM. The correlation between heart period variability and mean period length. *Statist Med* 1992; **11**: 125–9.
39. Farrell TG, Bashir Y, Cripps T, Malik M, Poloniecki J, Bennett ED, Ward DE, Camm AJ. Risk stratification for arrhythmic events based on heart rate variability, ambulatory electrocardiographic variables and the signal-averaged electrocardiogram. *J Am Coll Cardiol* 1991; **18**: 687–97.
40. Bigger JT, Fleiss J, Rolnitzky LM, Steinman RC. Frequency domain measures of heart period variability to assess risk late after myocardial infarction. *J Am Coll Cardiol* 1993; **21**: 729–36.
41. Counihan PJ, Fei L, Bashir Y, Farrell TG, Haywood GA, McKenna WJ. Assessment of heart rate variability in hypertrophic cardiomyopathy: association with clinical and prognostic features. *Circulation* 1993; **88**: 1682–90.

42. Lown B , Verrier RL. Neural activity and ventricular fibrillation. *New Engl J Med* 1976; **294**: 1165–70.
43. Schwartz PJ, Brown AM, Malliani A, Zanchetti A (eds). *Neural Mechanisms in Cardiac Arrhthmias.* New York: Raven Press, 1978.
44. Lown B. Sudden cardiac death: the major challenge confronting contemporary cardiology. *Am J Cardiol* 1979; **43**: 313–20.
45. Corr PB, Yamada KA, Witkowski FX. Mechanisms controlling cardiac autonomic function and their relation to arrhythmogenesis. In: Fozzard HA, Haber E, Jennings RB, Katz AM, Morgan HE (eds), *The Heart and Cardiovascular System, Vol. II,* New York: Raven Press, 1986, 1343–403.
46. Verrier RL, Lown B. Sympathetic–parasympathetic interactions and ventricular electrical stability. In: Schwartz PJ, Brown AM, Malliani A, Zanchetti A (eds), *Neural Mechanisms in Cardiac Arrhythmias.* New York: Raven Press, 1978: 75–85.
47. Schwartz PJ, Vanoli E. Cardiac arrhythmias elicited by interaction between acute myocardial ischemia and sympathetic hyperactivity: a new experimental model for the study of antiarrhythmic drugs. *J Cardiovasc Pharmacol* 1981; **3**: 1251–9.
48. Schwartz PJ, Stone HL. The role of the autonomic nervous system in sudden coronary death. *Ann NY Acad Sci* 1982; **382**: 162–80.
49. Schwartz PJ, Vanoli E, Stramba-Badiale M, De Ferrari GM, Billman GE, Foreman RD. Autonomic mechanisms and sudden death: new insight from the analysis of baroreceptor reflexes in conscious dogs with and without a myocardial infarction. *Circulation* 1988; **78**: 969–79.
50. Schwartz PJ, Billman GE, Stone HL. Autonomic mechanisms in ventricular fibrillation induced by myocardial ischemia during exercise in dogs with a healed myocardial infarction: an experimental preparation for sudden cardiac death. *Circulation* 1984; **69**: 790–800.
51. Billman GE, Schwartz PJ, Stone HL. Baroreceptor reflex control of heart rate: a predictor of sudden cardiac death. *Circulation* 1982; **66**: 874–80.
52. Billman GE, Hoskins RS. Time-series of heart rate variability during submaximal exercise: evidence for reduced cardiac vagal tone in animals susceptible to ventricular fibrillation. *Circulation* 1989; **80**: 146–57.
53. Hull SS, Evans AR, Vanoli E, Adamson PB, Stramba-Badiale M, Albert DE, Foreman RD, Schwartz PJ. Heart rate variability before and after myocardial infarction in conscious dogs at high and low risk of sudden death. *J Am Coll Cardiol* 1990; **16**: 978–85.
54. Billman GE, Schwartz PJ, Stone HL. The effects of daily exercise on susceptibility to sudden cardiac death. *Circulation* 1984; **69**: 1182–9.
55. Kleiger RE, Bigger JT, Bosner MS, Chung MK, Cook JR, Rolnitzky LM, Steinman RC, Fleiss JL. Stability over time of variables measuring heart rate variability in normal subjects. *Am J Cardiol* 1991; **68**: 626–30.
56. Bigger JT, Fleiss, JL, Rolnitzky, LM, Steinman RC. Stability over time of heart period variability in patients with chronic coronary heart disease and ventricular arrhythmias. *Am J Cardiol* 1992; **69**: 718–23.
57. Bigger JT. RR variability to evaluate autonomic physiology and pharmacology and to predict cardiovascular outcomes in humans. In: Zipes DP (ed.), *Cardiac Arrhythmias: From Cell to Bedside.* Philadelphia: W. B. Saunders, 1994, 1151–70.

11

Correlation of Time- and Frequency-Domain Measures of Heart Rate Variability

Robert E. Kleiger and Matthew S. Bosner

Previous chapters have discussed in detail the properties and measurement of time- and frequency-domain measures of heart rate variability (HRV). Despite the entirely different mathematical methods of calculating these variables, there is a very close relationship between the measures of HRV. This occurs because of both the physiologic bases of these measures and the purely mathematical relationships that exist between specific time- and frequency-domain measures.

This chapter briefly reviews the various measures as a basis for understanding the relationship between time- and frequency-domain measures. Time-domain analyses are conveniently divided into statistical and geometric. The former may be further subdivided into those that are calculated directly from the interval cycle lengths, and those calculated as the differences between cycle lengths or intervals.[1]

Interval Difference Measures

The two most common interval difference measures are *RMSSD* (root-mean-square successive difference)[2] and *pNN50* (proportion, in percent, of successive (NN) differences above 50 ms, or more than 6.25% of the preceding interval).[3] Often, instead of the raw counts, the proportion of interval differences greater than 50 ms over the total number of intervals is calculated. Both *RMSSD* and *pNN50* are measures of short-term variability of the cardiac cycle. Most short-term variation of heart rate is secondary to respiratory sinus arrhythmia. The typical respiratory pattern of 9–24 cycles per minute is identical to a frequency range of 0.15–0.40 Hz. In terms of spectral HRV analysis, this is commonly referred to as the high-frequency (HF) power spectrum. There are very high correlations between *RMSSD* and *pNN50* and the spectral measure of HF power. This has been validated in normal subjects,[4] in postinfarct patients,[5] and in diabetic patients.[6] There are, however, cases where this close relationship does not occur. These include patients with sinoatrial dysfunction where abrupt alterations in cardiac cycle length occur which are independent of respiratory cycle, and in certain neurologic diseases in which abrupt changes in autonomic tone occur independent of respiratory variation. It also is not a valid measure of vagal tone in atrial fibrillation. Fortunately these conditions are readily recognizable.

A small amount of HF power occurs not because of phasic alteration of autonomic outflow mediated by carotid sinus afferents, but because of mechanical changes in the lungs and chest wall during ventilation. This small amount of HF power may become an appreciable percentage of the total HF power during maximal exercise, in patients with severe congestive heart failure, and in states associated with high sympathetic drive and vagal withdrawal. However, in these cases total HF power as well as *RMSSD* and *pNN50* will all be reduced. In multiple studies in diverse subject groups, the correlations between *pNN50, RMSSD* and HF power exceed 0.9.[4]

Interval Length Measures

There are many statistical measures dependent on the NN intervals themselves. One of the most commonly utilized measures is *SDNN* (the standard deviation of the normal intervals over some recording period, also referred to as CLV, when the recording period is 24 hours). *SDNN* is the square-root of the variance of the intervals measured. But the variance of a series of time measurements during a period is equal to the spectral measure of total power in the same period. Thus the *SDNN* of a given period should equal the square-root of the total power of the same period and consequently be closely correlated with total power. Bigger *et al.*[5] demonstrated a correlation of 0.99 between *SDNN* and the square-root of total power in post-MI patients.

However, this is only true if total power and *SDNN* are calculated for precisely the same overall period. Investigation by Bigger *et al.*[7] estimated total power over 24 hours by calculating the total power of successive 5-minute periods and meaning their sum, equivalent to meaning the sum of the 5-minute variances. The result of such a process is to underestimate the true total power over 24 hours, because it fails to measure those variations associated with cycle lengths between 5 minutes and 24 hours (frequencies between 0.0033 Hz and 1.156×10^{-5} Hz); see Figures 11.1 and 11.2. The cycles between 5 minutes and 24 hours include diurnal cycles which have a major effect on 24-hour variability of heart rate. Thus in a study of the effects of atenalol and diltiazem on heart period variability, Cook *et al.*[8] demonstrated that atenalol markedly increased total power, but did not affect *SDNN*. This seeming paradox can be explained by the methods of their study. Total power was estimated by the 5-minute method, and since the cycles responsible for 5-minute variability (i.e. cycles between 0.0033 Hz and 0.4 Hz) increased, total power estimated by the 5-minute method was significantly increased. On the other hand, *SDNN* calculated over 24 hours also reflects diurnal variation which was substantially reduced by atenalol. With the exception of circumstances like these, however, total power estimated from a 5-minute method, total power calculated over the whole 24-hour period, and *SDNN* or *CLV* should and are very closely correlated.

SDANN. This index is calculated by averaging the NN intervals of some smaller period – usually 5 minutes – of the total monitoring period (usually 24 hours) and calculating the standard deviation of all the 5-minute average NN intervals. This calculation reflects the variability in mean 5-minute average NN intervals over the 24 hours. Somewhat counter-intuitively it gives no information about the variation of heart rate occurring within 5-minute periods despite being calculated over 5-minute periods.

This can be clarified by examining two very physiologically unlikely, but mathematically possible scenarios. In one case the mean 5-minute average NN is 800 ms with all intervals being exactly 800 ms. In such a case the 5-minute variation in heart rate would be 0. Conversely, a similar mean 5-minute NN interval can be obtained if half of the intervals were 1200 ms and half were 400 ms. In this case the variance over 5 minutes would be extremely high. By meaning the intervals over 5 minutes, we have thus

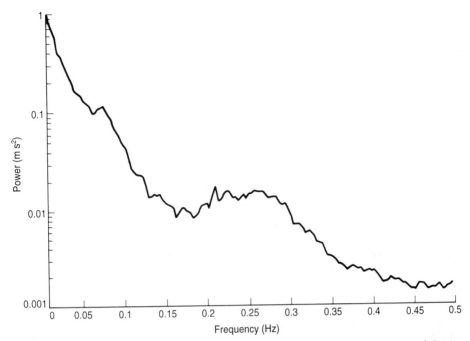

Figure 11.1 Periodogram estimate of power spectral density involving the average of 5-minute segments.

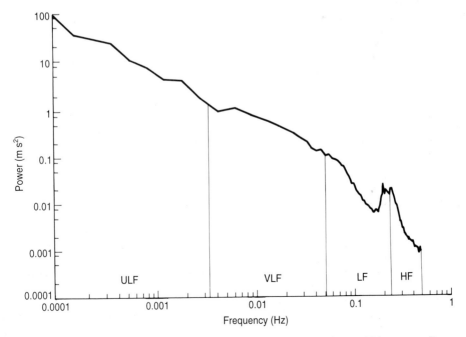

Figure 11.2 Periodogram estimate of power spectral density involving a 24-hour recording.

Table 11.1 Correlations of time and frequency intervals in normal individuals

	Total power			
	SDNN	5-min	LF power	HF power
SDNN index	0.85	1.0	0.92	0.90
Total power	0.87	1.0	0.93	0.88
	RMSSD	pMN50		
HF power	0.98	0.92		

Table 11.2 Correlation of HRV measures in the post-MI group

	Ln(TP)	Ln(ULF)	Ln(VLF)	Ln(LF)	Ln(HF)
SDNN	0.96	0.95	0.78	0.72	0.67
SDNN index	0.79	0.71	0.90	0.89	0.82
SDANN	0.94	0.96	0.68	0.61	0.57

concealed all information about variability in heart rate due to cycle variations of less than 5 minutes. However, by measuring the standard deviation of the mean 5-minute intervals we have a measure of the variability in mean heart rate due to cyclic changes between 5 minutes and 24 hours.

If, as Figure 11.1 demonstrates, most of the variability in heart rate results from cycles longer than 5 minutes, SDANN should closely correlate with total power and SDNN. It should be even more closely correlated with ULF power, the spectral density of the frequencies between 0.0033 Hz and 1.156×10^{-5} Hz (the 24-hour cycle). This is indeed the case. The correlation of SDANN and SDNN in 14 normals was above 0.9 and the correlation between SDANN and ULF power in postinfarction patients was 0.96 (see Tables 11.1 and 11.2).[4]

The relationship between SDANN and total power and ULF power can be examined in another fashion. If one creates a periodogram of the 5-minute average NN intervals, one can by the same fast Fourier transform and autoregression techniques estimate the total spectral power of this periodogram. This would be the square of SDANN and also would approximate ULF power. Since ULF power represents over 80% of total 24-hour spectral power, it would also correlate strongly with variance, total power and SDNN.

SDNN index. This index is obtained by calculating the standard deviations of the normal cardiac cycles in 5-minute periods and then obtaining the mean. As discussed above, the SDNN index, calculated in this way, is not able to measure the variability due to cycles longer than 5 minutes, but it is an estimate of the variation in heart rate due to cycle lengths less than 5 minutes. Since, as Figures 11.1 and 11.2 demonstrate, most of the variation in heart rate occurring within 5-minute periods is found in the VLF bands between 0.04 and 0.0033 Hz, SDNN index should strongly correlate with VLF power. This is indeed the case: correlations greater than 0.9 have been found both in postinfarction patients and in normals. But an even stronger correlation should be seen between SDNN index and total power estimated from 5-minute periods (correlation of 1.0 between SDNN index and total power in 5 minute intervals). The latter is the mean of total power calculated for all the 5-minute segments. This is the same as the mean of 5-minute variances. Since SDNN index is the mean of the square-roots of the 5-minute variances, the correlation should be extremely high. Indeed, Kleiger *et al.* showed a correlation of 1.0 between these variables in 14 normals.[4]

Geometric Time-Domain Measures

Malik, Camm and their coworkers have utilized several geometric measures to assess heart period variability, and this is discussed in detail in Chapter 10. In these methods the cardiac cycles are measured and then placed in bins of approximately 8 ms width. A plot is then made with the abscissa the interval length and the ordinate the number of intervals in each bin. The points are connected to create a two-dimensional area. The base of the figure is bounded by the shortest and longest cardiac interval. The height of the enclosed area is determined by the modal number of intervals. An HRV index can be measured by dividing the area subscribed by the graphic display by the height of the curve. In a patient with low variability in cardiac cycle length, there will be a very large number of intervals in the modal interval and thus the HRV index will be small since the denominator of the index, the height, will be large in relation to the area. On the other hand, a patient with the same mean NN interval but greater variability will have a more spread-out area, fewer intervals within the modal interval, shorter height in relation to total area, and hence an increased HRV index.

An alternative method proposed by Malik, Camm and coworkers is to create a triangle by fitting the sides of the triangle to minimize the difference between the plotted points and the bounds of the triangle utilizing a least-squares algorithm and then measuring the intersects of the triangle along the baseline.[9] Such a method will tend to exclude intervals much shorter and longer than the modal interval in calculating baseline width. Both baseline width and HRV index are estimates of total variability biased towards the central frequencies of the distribution. As such they would be expected to correlate strongly with total power, *SDNN* and *SDANN*. Malik, indeed, has shown very high correlation of both HRV and baseline width with *SDNN*, when *SDNN* is calculated from accurately annotated records; this strong correlation is, however, severely weakened when tapes are poorly annotated or PVCs are not excluded.

The reason for this is two-fold. If many erroneously measured intervals are included in the analysis, the mean NN interval calculated can be displaced from the true mean. Since variance has a numerator consisting of the sum of squares of each interval minus the mean interval, displacement of the mean from the true mean will markedly increase variance. Even when the mean is not displaced – as when erroneous short intervals are balanced by erroneous long intervals, such as may happen with VPC where the normal to VPC interval is short but the subsequent VPC to N interval is long – variance will increase; this is because the difference between the mean NN interval and the short and long intervals produced by the PVC will result in increased variance. Since the geometric measures weight the estimates of variability away from extreme intervals, they tend to exclude intervals produced either by artefact or PVC. In this sense they are more robust than conventional statistical measures and thus may reduce the requirement for time-consuming human editing which is needed for accurate annotation of tapes. However, even these methods will provide erroneous estimates of variability if there are very frequent VPCs or excessively poor data quality.

Frequency Domain Measures

As previously discussed, signals that vary with time in some regular fashion may, by a number of mathematical techniques, have cycle lengths and frequencies, and the density and power of their frequency components, determined. For an analysis of HRV, a tachogram consisting of either instantaneous heart rate or cycle lengths can be constructed by sampling an ECG record. Using either fast Fourier transform[10] or autoregressive[11] techniques, the frequencies responsible for the variation in heart rate can be determined.

It is vital in such a process to account for noise or ectopic beats which will grossly affect the accuracy of any analysis. In one commonly used method, a tachogram of cardiac cycles recorded over 24 hours is constructed with linear spline corrections of noise and ectopics, and then analyzed by the fast Fourier transform technique.

Two alternative methods may be used. The whole block of beats may be analyzed. The advantage of this technique is that all frequency components almost up to 1 cycle per 24 hours may be found and have their power estimated. Such an analysis allows circadian frequencies to be evaluated and also estimates the frequencies with the greatest spectral densities. On the other hand, it requires greater computer power and precludes comparison of frequency components recorded during specific smaller intervals during the 24 hours.

Another method is to break the 24 hours into small periods (e.g. 5 minutes), create the appropriate tachograms, and calculate the power of the frequency bands within each period, and then average each spectral density measured. Within intervals of 2–20 minutes, estimates of HF and LF powers are very highly correlated and virtually identical with those calculated over 24 hours. The advantages of this technique are that it requires less powerful computers, simultaneous calculations of a variety of time-domain variables can be made, and spectral densities can be compared during different intervals over the 24 hours, such as night–day, rest–activity, etc. The major drawback is the inability to estimate cycle lengths longer than the periods measured and the corresponding frequencies. Thus, a 5-minute method cannot determine the power of frequencies less than 0.0033 Hz. On the other hand, it is possible to plot some 5-minute functions such as average NN interval or high-frequency power, graph the values and, by the same fast Fourier transform or autoregressive techniques, determine whether they exhibit cyclic variation during the day. Such a technique could be useful in detecting seasonal cyclic variations of the heart rate signal (as seen in hibernating or aestivating animals).

There are no exact measures of 'pure' parasympathetic or sympathetic autonomic tones. However, it is well recognized that rapid fluctuation of heart period is a reflection primarily of parasympathetic regulatory processes.[12] Thus HRV measures derived from calculations that account for the rapid alterations in the cardiac cycle also reflect alterations in parasympathetic tone. Investigators have pointed out that short-term LF power is strongly dependent on sympathetic tone.[13] Thus, with tilt or sympathomimetic administration, LF power increases dramatically. Such short-term measurements, however, occur when parasympathetic tone either decreases or remains stable.[14] Longer-term LF power is also responsive to parasympathetic power. This is evidenced by the strong correlations between LF power and HF power (purely vagal) seen over a 24-hour period; by the marked increase in LF power that occurs after administration of beta-blockers producing sympathetic blockade and increasing vagal tone; and by the reduction in both LF and HF power in severe congestive heart failure and following infarction.

The LF/HF power ratio has also been used to assess the sympathetic/parasympathetic balance. Conceptually, this works because HF power is purely vagal in origin and because LF power is powerfully influenced by sympathetic activity. However, this variable has limitations because it is dependent on two measurements, and it may be subject to greater error than a single measurement. When either LF or HF power is close to zero, the ratio is difficult to calculate or interpret. For example, in severe congestive heart failure LF power may be totally absent, although a small residual amount of HF power remains. A high LF/HF ratio in this situation would imply a high parasympathic/sympathetic balance, a conclusion certainly incorrect.

Another method of estimating parasympathetic/sympathetic influences is to normalize LF and HF power. This is essentially performed by dividing the HF and LF components by the total power. In short monitoring periods, total power approaches the sum of LF and HF power; but in longer monitoring periods, as will be shown, total power is mainly made up of frequencies other than HF and LF power. As with the LF/HF ratio, there are problems when either of these components approaches zero.

LF power measured over a substantial period has a strong parasympathetic component. Hayano[15] has estimated that LF power is approximately two-thirds dependent on vagal tone and only one-third on nonvagal influences. Evidence to support this is the very high correlation between LF power and HF power seen in the normal population; the marked increase in LF power seen in sleep when parasympathetic tone increases and sympathetic tone decreases; and the fact that beta-blockers, despite their sympathetic blocking actions, increase LF power as well as HF power.

The contributions of spectral power bands to total power are as follows: HF, $2 \pm 2\%$; LF, $4 \pm 3\%$; VLF, $12 \pm 6\%$; and ULF, $82 \pm 8\%$. Hence most of the total power resides in the ULF and VLF spectral bands. Although the definitions of these bands are arbitrary, and the physiological determinants of their variations are not well characterized, failure to examine the ULF and VLF spectral bands would exclude important information. Since ULF power represents over 80% of total 24-hour power, it is clear that it must be highly correlated with total power, and with the time-domain measures previously described to correlate with total power, including *SDNN* and *SDANN*.

It was stated above that the definitions of ULF and VLF are arbitrary. The lower frequency of VLF (0.0033 Hz) was established because of the summation method of averaging spectral densities over 5-minute (300-second) periods. The lower limit of ULF, 1.15×10^{-5} Hz, was defined by dividing one cycle by 86 400 seconds, the total number in 24 hours. Obviously, as one attempts to measure frequencies approaching zero cycles per second, longer and longer monitoring periods are required. Although circadian intervals are practically the longest measurable in humans, there are cycles longer than circadian that influence heart rate in some animals. Examples, of course, are the profound changes in heart rate seen in hibernating or aestivating animals. Such cycles can only be estimated by repeated sampling of heart rate throughout the year.

Summary and Conclusions

In view of the physiological and mathematical relationships between time- and frequency-domain measures of HRV, and the resulting high correlations between them, a question can be posed as to the relative advantages of one analytic method over another. Spectral analysis can determine the cycle lengths and frequencies in individuals and groups having most variability. Knowing these frequencies could help determine the biological processes responsible for them. As previously noted, the factors responsible for HF and LF power are known to a large degree and they are, of course, responsible for the variation in those time-domain variables that correlate with these frequencies. The biological bases for ULF and VLF are less well known.

It is, of course, possible to divide the total power into an even larger series of mutually exclusive spectral bands and examine each band, but clearly a corresponding time-domain variable containing the same information could be constructed. Thus the choice of method depends more on personal preference and the availability of computer time and software. At present, epidemiological data do not support the superiority of one mode of analysis over another, which is not surprising given their high correlations.

References

1. Kleiger RE, Stein PK, Bosner MS, Rottman JN. Time domain measurements of heart rate variability. *Cardiol Clin* 1992; **10**: 0733–8651.

2. Von Neumann J, Kent RH, Bellinson HR *et al*. The mean square successive difference. *Ann Math Statist* 1941; **12**: 153.

3. Ewing DJ, Neilson JMM, Travis P. New method for assessing cardiac parasympathetic activity using 24 hour electrocardiograms. *Br Heart J* 1984; **52**: 416.

4. Kleiger RE, Bigger JT, Bosner MS, *et al*. Stability over time of variables measuring heart rate variability in normal subjects. *Am J Cardiol* 1991; **68**: 626.

5. Bigger JT, Albrecht P, Steinman RC, *et al*. Comparison of time- and frequency-domain based measures of cardiac parasympathetic activity in Holter recordings after myocardial infarction. *Am J Cardiol* 1989; **64**: 538.

6. Ewing DJ, Borsey DQ, Travis P, *et al*. Abnormalities of ambulatory 24-hour heart rate in diabetes mellitus. *Diabetes* 1983; **32**: 101.

7. Bigger JT, Kleiger RE, Fleiss JL, *et al*. Components of heart rate variability measured during healing of acute myocardial infarction. *Am J Cardiol* 1988; **61**: 208.

8. Cook JR, Bigger JT, Kleiger RE, *et al*. Effect of atenolol and diltiazem on heart rate variability in normal persons. *J Am Coll Cardiol* 1991; **17**: 480.

9. Malik M, Odemvyiwa O, Poloniecki J, Staunton A, Camm AJ. Time-domain measurement of vagal components of heart rate variability in automatically analyzed long-term electrocardiograms: prognostic power of different indices for identification of post-infarction patients at high risk of arrhythmia events. *J Ambulat Monit* 1991; **4**: 235–44.

10. Turiei M, Baselli G, Cerutti S, Malliani A. Power spectral analysis of heart rate and arterial pressure variabilities as a marker of sympatho-vagal interaction in man and conscious dog. *Cir Res* 1986; **59**: 178–93.

11. Rottman JN, Steinman RC, Albrecht P, Bigger JT, Rolnitzky LM, Fleiss JL. Efficient estimation of the heart period power spectrum suitable for physiologic or pharmacologic studies. *Am J Cardiol* 1990; **66**: 1522–4.

12. Eckberg DW. Parasympathetic cardiovascular control in human disease: a critical review of methods and results. *Am J Physiol* 1980; **241**: H581.

13. Lombardi F, Sandrone G, Pernproner S, *et al*. Heart rate variability as an index of sympathovagal interaction in patients after myocardial infarction. *Am J Cardiol* 1987; **60**: 1241.

14. Kaufman ES, Bosner MS, Stein PK, Kleiger RE, Bigger JT, Rolnitzky LM, Fleiss JL, Steinman R. The effect of enalapril and digoxin on heart period variability in normal subjects. *Am J Cardiol* 1993; **72**: 95–9.

15. Hayano J, Sakakibara Y, Yamada A, *et al*. Accuracy of assessment of cardiac vagal tone by heart rate variability in normal subjects. *Am J Cardiol* 1991; **67**: 199–204.

12

Influence of Sympathetic and Parasympathetic Maneuvers on Heart Rate Variability

Jeffrey J. Goldberger and Alan H. Kadish

Introduction

Beat-to-beat changes in the RR interval are predominantly due to changes in autonomic tone. Figure 12.1 demonstrates that baseline heart rate variability in a normal subject can be virtually abolished by the combined administration of propranolol (to achieve beta-adrenergic blockade) and atropine (to achieve parasympathetic blockade). The time-domain and frequency-domain techniques discussed in Chapters 9–11 have been developed to quantify this beat-to-beat heart rate variability. Our understanding of the source of this variability is still being developed. Early studies of this phenomenon identified the respiratory cycle in concert with parasympathetic tone as the source of the variability, which was therefore termed 'respiratory sinus arrhythmia'. With the advent of frequency-domain analysis, the presence of heart rate fluctuations that occur at the respiratory frequency was confirmed. In addition, heart rate fluctuations at other frequencies were noted. Several studies have suggested that the variabilities in the lower frequency ranges are due to both sympathetic and parasympathetic influences on the sinus node.

While the historical development of the field of heart rate variability assigned the oscillation in heart rate at particular frequencies to the influence of either the parasympathetic or the sympathetic nervous systems on the sinus node, more recent information suggests that these relationships are much more complex and cannot be generalized from the early studies that correctly made the initial associations. The underlying physiological issue is depicted in Figure 12.2. In the top part of the schematic of the sinus node, the parasympathetic input to the sinus node is displayed as having an intrinsic oscillation frequency, perhaps the respiratory frequency. Sinus node automaticity is then modulated based on the externally applied stimulation frequency, resulting in heart variability at the input frequency. In this case, the sinus node does not have an intrinsic predilection to oscillate at any particular frequency. In contrast, in the bottom schematic, the sinus node is depicted as having an intrinsic response to any kind of parasympathetic stimulation. Parasympathetic stimulation in this setting will also result in heart rate variability, but will not depend on the particular characteristics of the parasympathetic input. A similar depiction can be made for the sympathetic inputs to the sinus node. The discussion of the effects of autonomic stimulation and blockade will demonstrate that the first mechanism is likely to be the operative one.

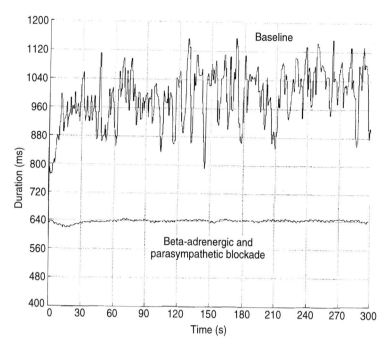

Figure 12.1 Plot of RR intervals (in milliseconds) from a normal subject over a 5-minute period during resting, supine conditions (baseline) and following combined beta-adrenergic (propranolol 0.2 mg/kg) and parasympathetic (atropine 0.04 mg/kg) blockade. During baseline conditions, significant variation in the RR intervals is noted. Following combined beta-adrenergic and parasympathetic blockade, the RR interval has significantly decreased and there is no significant variability.

When studying the effects of autonomic stimulation and blockage on heart rate variability, several technical factors must be considered. The techniques for measuring heart rate variability rely on RR interval measurement which is used as a surrogate for PP interval measurement (P waves are smaller and broader, making them more difficult to detect and align). Thus, RR interval variability is generally used to assess autonomic influences on the sinus node. The presence of ectopic atrial activation, such as may occur in subjects with a wandering atrial pacemaker, may not necessarily be detected by algorithms based on QRS detection. Thus, careful review of the electrocardiographic tracings is required to ensure that sinus node variability is being measured. It is also important to consider that the distribution of autonomic inputs is different in the atrium, AV node, and ventricles.[1,2] Therefore, the autonomic effects at these sites may differ from those at the sinus node. Finally, the techniques used to quantify heart rate variability can be applied to short-term recordings, lasting from 2 to 15 minutes, or to long-term recordings lasting hours. Typically, over a 24-hour period there may be marked changes in autonomic tone, such as typically occurs between the daytime and nighttime. Thus, heart rate variability measurements during long-term recordings may include potentially large changes in autonomic tone. In contrast, short-term recordings over a period of several minutes may be used to assess the heart rate variability associated with a particular test state. During this limited time period, the ambient level of autonomic time may not vary considerably, if conditions are stable. These types of recordings are particularly suited for assessment of the effects of sympathetic and parasympathetic stimuli in heart rate variability.

In assessing the currently available techniques for quantitating heart rate variability, criteria for identifying a particular parameter with either sympathetic or parasympathetic

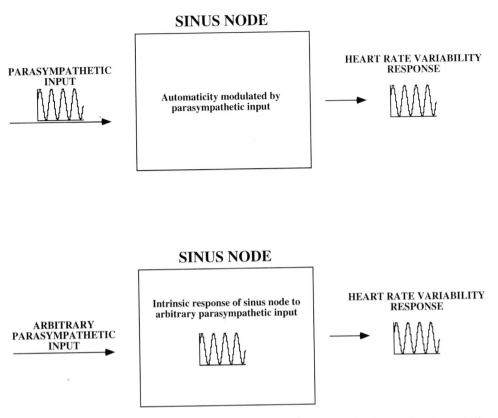

Figure 12.2 Schematic representation of parasympathetic influences on the sinus node. *Top panel*: The parasympathetic input has a characteristic frequency (i.e. the respiratory frequency) and modulates the sinus node automaticity at this frequency. *Bottom panel*: The parasympathic input has no characteristic frequency, but the sinus node is depicted as having an intrinsic response to parasympathetic stimulation. Both models may result in the same kind of heart rate variability. However, as discussed in the text, the model proposed in the upper panel is most likely the operative one.

tone need to be defined. For the purposes of this chapter, an index of heart rate variability will be considered to represent sympathetic or parasympathetic tone if it increases when sympathetic or parasympathetic tone increases and it decreases when sympathetic or parasympathetic tone decreases, respectively.

Parasympathetic Effects on Heart Rate Variability

Origin of baseline heart rate variability

It is widely accepted that respiratory sinus arrhythmia is a reflection of parasympathetic effects on the sinus node. Maneuvers such as vagotomy,[3,4] cooling of the vagi,[5] and cholinergic blockade with atropine[6,7] have been shown to eliminate sinus arrhythmia in dogs as well as in humans. Furthermore, in normal resting human subjects, the sympathetic nervous system does not contribute significantly to the baseline heart variability.[7,8] Although beta-blockers have sometimes been shown to result in an increase in heart rate variability, this has been felt to be due to a central vagotonic influence.[9,10] Thus, the resting heart rate variability in normal, resting subjects may be considered to be vagally-mediated.

The effects of the parasympathetic nervous system on the sinus node are mediated solely by efferent vagal neural stimulation. Through direct recordings of the efferent vagal nerve activity in anesthetized dogs, it has been shown[11] that during the inspiratory phase of natural respiration the activity of cardiac vagal efferent nerve fibres is greatly reduced or completely suppressed. In a further study, Katona and Jih[5] demonstrated that the degree of parasympathetic heart rate control in anesthetized dogs is directly proportional to the variations in RR intervals and suggested that the degree of respiratory sinus arrhythmia may be used as a noninvasive index of the degree of parasympathetic cardiac control. The rationale for this hypothesis is that vagal efferent discharge occurs predominantly during expiration. Thus, parasympathetic effects are maximal at this time. The effects of vagal efferent discharge on the sinus node are mediated by acetylcholine release which typically has a short duration of action due to diffusion away from the sinus node and/or hydrolysis by acetylcholinesterase. As inspiration results in suppression of vagal efferent discharge, the declining concentrations of acetylcholine at the sinus node result in less parasympathetic effect during inspiration. Thus, heart rate variability is a manifestation of the difference in parasympathetic effect between expiration and inspiration. In theory, constant parasympathetic effect during expiration and inspiration should result in no heart rate variability. Whether constant parasympathetic effect can be observed is discussed below.

The critical role of the respiratory cycle in producing the baseline heart rate variability has been studied.[12–15] A number of studies[12,13] have evaluated the effects of respiratory frequency on sinus arrhythmia. When the interval between breaths is increased, heart rate variability generally increases due to an increase in the maximum PP interval and a decrease in the minimum PP interval.[12] Interestingly, at short respiratory intervals, the minimum and maximum PP intervals approach each other, resulting in a decrease in the heart rate variability. Thus, at short respiratory intervals, the expressed difference in parasympathetic effect between expiration and inspiration is reduced, perhaps due to incomplete washout of acetylcholine. In addition, the phase relationship between the respiratory cycle and the heart rate variability changes with varying respiratory frequencies.[13] Heart rate variability may also increase with an increase in tidal volume.

Examination of the frequency spectrum of the RR intervals has identified two main peaks (Figure 12.3). The high-frequency peak (generally between 0.15 and 0.40 Hz) coincides with the respiratory frequency. The oscillation of the heart rate at this frequency follows from the preceding discussion. Parasympathectomy in dogs virtually abolishes the high-frequency heart rate variability.[16] Parasympathetic blockade with atropine in humans also results in a greater than 90% decrease in the power contained within this frequency range in both the supine and upright positions.[6,7] In contrast, beta-adrenergic blockade with propranolol does not significantly alter the high-frequency power,[7,8] even during standing, when there is heightened sympathetic tone.[7] Thus, the HF power has been considered to reflect only parasympathetic tone.

In addition to the 'high frequency' variability that occurs at the respiratory frequency, in the resting state, there is a peak in the 'low frequency' range (0.04–0.15 Hz). The power contained in this frequency band is also mediated by the parasympathetic nervous system, as atropine markedly attenuates the power in normal subjects under resting conditions, while propranolol may have no significant effect.[7,8] The power in this frequency band likely represents baroreceptor modulation of the heart rate, as described below. While heart rate variability has been reported in the VLF and ULF ranges, these measurements require longer-term recordings than those required for the HF and LF variability and their physiologic correlates are not well established.

In summary, the presence of sinus arrhythmia (which can be quantified using time-domain analysis techniques) and high (respiratory) frequency heart rate variability is a

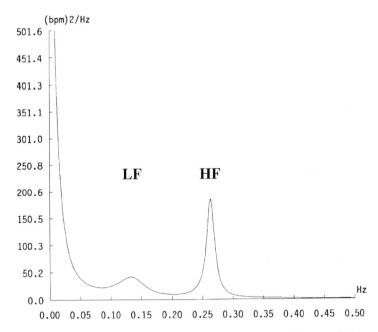

Figure 12.3 Power spectrum of heart rate variability from a normal subject. There are distinct peaks in the HF and LF ranges.

manifestation of parasympathetic effects on the sinus node, as removal of the parasympathetic effect by physical or pharmacologic vagotomy abolishes sinus arrhythmia and high-frequency heart rate variability. Many investigators have extrapolated these data to suggest that this type of analysis can be used to quantify parasympathetic tone. However, critical analysis of the data reveals that there are situations in which these extrapolations are incorrect. This implies that any extrapolations of these data must be evaluated critically.

Effects of parasympathetic stimulation

Cardiac efferent vagal activity is also sensitive to changes in blood pressure. With an increase in blood pressure, vagal discharge at a higher frequency is noted,[11,17] resulting in the well-described baroreceptor-mediated slowing of the heart rate. Katona et al.[11] demonstrated that the mean firing frequency increased from 2–6 per second at control pressures to 10–20 per second when the blood pressure was raised by norepinephrine infusion or balloon inflation in the aorta of dogs. During these experiments, it was noted that the inspiratory suppression of vagal nerve discharge continued during the increase in blood pressure. Based on this continued inspiratory suppression of vagal discharge, differential parasympathetic effects between inspiration and expiration should be observable. It would also be reasonable to postulate that the increased vagal effect during inspiration should result in an increase in heart rate variability.

Phenylephrine (an alpha-adrenergic agonist) infusion results in an elevation of the blood pressure. Baroreflex activation from this elevation in blood pressure results in a parasympathetic-mediated slowing of the heart rate.[18] As might be predicted, in conscious dogs, phenylephrine infusion has been shown to slow the heart rate significantly, accompanied by an increase in the RR variance and the high-frequency power.[19] Saul *et al.*[20] confirmed this observation in humans by performing phenylephrine infusions in ten male subjects. With a 12 mmHg increase in blood pressure, they achieved a significant baroreceptor-mediated increase in parasympathetic tone. The RR interval lengthened from 1014 ms to 1112 ms; accompanying this increase in the RR interval was an increase in the SD from 63 ± 27 ms to 83 ± 43 ms.

However, it has also been shown that parasympathetic stimulation may diminish heart rate variability. In 1936, Anrep et al.[3] demonstrated that heart rate variability in anesthetized dogs was dependent on the level of parasympathetic tone. At low levels of arterial pressure, the heart rate was fast consistent with a low degree of parasympathetic tone. In this situation, the difference between the longest and shortest RR interval was small. As the blood pressure was increased, parasympathetic tone increased. This manifested as an increase in the difference between the longest and shortest RR interval. However, beyond a pressure of 180 mmHg, the difference between the longest and shortest RR interval began to decrease. Further increases in the blood pressure resulted in further increases in parasympathetic tone, but the difference between the longest and shortest RR interval rapidly diminished. We[6] investigated the effects of parasympathetic stimulation during phenylephrine infusion in normal human subjects (titrated to increase the blood pressure by 20–30 mmHg). As alpha-adrenergic stimulation has no significant effect on the heart rate variability,[6] the observed effects on heart rate variability are due to the parasympathetic stimulation. Figure 12.4 shows a baseline electrocardiographic recording in a normal subject as well as a recording during phenylephrine infusion. The baseline recording clearly demonstrates respiratory sinus arrhythmia. The recording during phenylephrine infusion demonstrates an increase in the RR interval, consistent with the baroreflex-mediated increase in parasympathetic tone. However, the respiratory sinus arrhythmia has virtually disappeared. The group data demonstrated a marked decrease in the SD, as well as the LF and HF powers, shown in Figure 12.5. This occurred despite a dramatic lengthening of the mean RR interval from 1034 ms to 1335 ms. The suppression of heart rate variability with marked increases in parasympathetic tone is consistent with the findings of Anrep et al.[3]

Further work in our laboratory[21] investigated whether the relationship described by Anrep et al. in dogs could be identified in humans. Normal subjects were given low doses of phenylephrine (0.3 and 0.6 µg/kg/min). At a dose of 0.3 µg/kg/min, there was no significant change in heart rate variability for the group. However, there was a significant inverse relationship between the baseline heart rate variability values and the change in

BASELINE

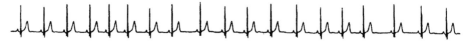

PHENYLEPHRINE

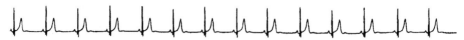

Figure 12.4 Twenty-second electrocardiographic recordings made during baseline conditions in a normal subject and during phenylephrine infusion (titrated to increase the systolic blood pressure by 20–30 mmHg). The baseline recording demonstrates normal respiratory sinus arrhythmia. During phenylephrine infusion, there is a slowing of the heart rate as well as a visible decrease in the heart rate variability. (Reproduced from reference 6 with permission of the American College of Cardiology)

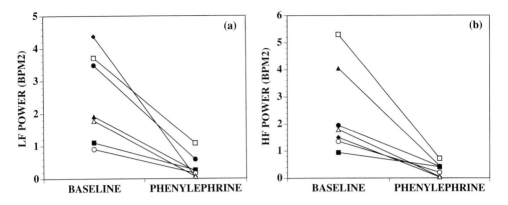

Figure 12.5 Individual results for power in the LF and HF bands during baseline conditions and during phenylephrine infusion (titrated to increase the systolic blood pressure by 20–30 mmHg). Each symbol represents a single subject. There is a consistent decrease in the LF and HF power in all subjects. (Reproduced with permission from reference 6)

heart rate variability observed with mild baroreflex parasympathetic stimulation. This implies that subjects with high heart rate variability demonstrated a decrease in heart rate variability with mild parasympathetic stimulation, while those with baseline-diminished heart rate variability had an increase in heart rate variability. Eckberg *et al.*[22] also found no significant change in respiratory peak–valley RR intervals in normal subjects during phenylephrine infusion. They concluded that respiratory sinus arrhythmia did not reflect vagal-cardiac activity when the levels of vagal traffic were greater than the baseline values of their normal subjects.

To understand the relationship between heart rate variability and parasympathetic tone, it must be appreciated that the heart rate variability measurements reflect only the difference between parasympathetic effects during expiration and inspiration. If there is no parasympathetic effect during inspiration, at a time when it has been shown that vagal efferent nerve activity in the dog is completely abolished, then this difference is directly related to parasympathetic tone. However, Kollai and Mizsei[23] have shown that, in normal humans, even the inspiratory level of cardiac parasympathetic tone is not reduced to zero. Furthermore, when parasympathetic tone is increased, the inspiratory level of cardiac parasympathetic tone likely increases. At high levels of parasympathetic stimulation, there may be minimal differences in the expiratory and inspiratory levels of parasympathetic effect, explaining the observed decrease in heart variability noted by Anrep *et al.*[3] in dogs and by our group[6] in humans.

There are two potential mechanisms by which there may be minimal differences in the expiratory and inspiratory levels of parasympathetic effect. Although it has been shown[11,24] that vagal efferent discharge remains suppressed during inspiration even with a concomitant rise in blood pressure, Kunze[17] noted a complete loss of phasic activity in cats with mean blood pressures greater than 180 mmHg. It is therefore possible that marked increases in blood pressure in humans may also result in a loss of phasic discharge. Constant vagal stimulation will result in slowing of the heart rate without significant variability.[4] Another potential mechanism relates to persistent parasympathetic effect during inspiration, despite suppression of vagal efferent discharge. Vagal effects on the sinus node are mediated by the release of acetylcholine. Typically, during inspiration, when vagal discharge is suppressed, there is less vagal effect than during expiration as the acetylcholine released during expiration diffuses away and/or is metabolized. The dose–response curve to acetylcholine in *in vitro* preparations has a rapidly rising portion and at higher concentrations is flat,[25,26] displaying a simple saturation relationship. During intense vagal stimulation in expiration, it is possible that the attainable parasympathetic effect is well on the flat portion of the curve. During inspiration, despite suppression of vagal discharges and a decline in acetylcholine concentrations in the region of the sinus node, parasympathetic effect may not decrease substantially. Either of these mechanisms will diminish the difference in parasympathetic effect between expiration and inspiration, thereby resulting in a decrease in heart rate variability.

The study of heart rate variability has gained in popularity in large part because it usually does appear to provide an index of parasympathetic activity. However, some caution must be exercised in the use of these indices. The results summarized here suggest that parasympathetic stimulation may increase or decrease the heart rate variability depending upon the strength of stimulation, the baseline level of parasympathetic tone, and the dose–response relationship between parasympathetic stimulation and inspiratory and expiratory parasympathetic effect. Although there are a number of studies that have found a good correlation between parasympathetic tone and the heart rate variability indices in selected situations, there are clearly situations where this will not be true. For example, it has been shown that endurance athletes may have lower HF power compared with nonathletic controls.[27] As correlative studies evaluating parasympathetic tone and heart rate variability have not been performed in patients with cardiac disease, it is also possible that problems may arise when data from normal individuals are extrapolated to these groups.

Alpha-Adrenergic Effects on Heart Rate Variability

Alpha-adrenergic stimulation has been reported to either increase or have no effect on the heart rate. In a study[28] of alpha-adrenergic stimulation with phenylephrine (during beta-adrenergic and parasympathetic blockade) in alpha-chloralose anesthetized dogs, a mild decrease in the mean RR interval was demonstrated. However, other investigators[6,29,30] have not noted a similar effect of alpha-adrenergic stimulation on the RR interval.

Alpha-adrenergic effects on heart rate variability have not been extensively evaluated. In our study,[6] we infused phenylephrine following complete parasympathetic blockade with atropine. Thus, the confounding effects of the baroreflex-mediated increase in parasympathetic tone that accompanies phenylephrine infusion had been eliminated. Despite a significant increase in the blood pressure, consistent with alpha-adrenergic effect, no significant change in heart rate was noted. In addition, no significant changes were noted in either the time-domain (*SD, MSSD*) or frequency-domain (low-frequency or high-frequency power) heart rate variability parameters. It is, therefore, likely that alpha-adrenergic stimulation in humans has no significant effect on heart rate variability.

Beta-Adrenergic Effects on Heart Rate Variability

Beta-adrenergic stimulation

As previously noted, resting levels of sympathetic tone are low; thus, much of the information on beta-adrenergic effects on heart rate variability arise from studies involving beta-adrenergic stimulation. While parasympathetic effects on the sinus node are mediated only through vagal efferent discharge, two sources of sympathetic input to the sinus node exist. Sympathetic stimulation in a variety of physiologic states may be mediated by neuronal stimulation, circulating epinephrine, or both.[31] It is likely that the effects of circulating catecholamines on heart rate variability differ from those due to direct neural stimulation because these inputs have different oscillation frequencies. It is therefore imperative to evaluate the effects of these stimuli individually in order to be able to better characterize the effects of beta-adrenergic stimulation on heart rate variability.

Upright tilt, or standing, is a maneuver that increases sympathetic tone predominantly owing to an increase in direct neural stimulation. This maneuver has been shown to result in a significant increase in plasma norepinephrine levels without significant changes in epinephrine levels.[8,31,32] Plasma norepinephrine levels are correlated with sympathetic nerve activity.[22,33] Thus, the absence of an increase in plasma epinephrine levels with tilt suggests that the increase in sympathetic tone results from direct neural stimulation. As upright tilt (or standing) is the best studied maneuver that results in an increase in sympathetic tone, and a variety of other physiologic sympathetic stimuli result in both neural stimulation and an increase in circulating epinephrine, upright tilt will serve as the paradigm by which to evaluate the effects of physiologic neural stimulation on heart rate variability. Only limited information is available regarding the effects of circulating beta-adrenergic agonists on heart rate variability.[8,34] This type of information can be obtained by evaluating the effects of epinephrine and/or isoproterenol infusions on heart rate variability or by using provocative maneuvers that result in primarily an adrenomedullary response (i.e. increase in plasma epinephrine) without direct neural stimulation.

Effects of beta-adrenergic neural stimulation

Studies on the change in posture from supine to standing or upright tilt have consistently demonstrated significant increases in the low-frequency power[7,8,35] and decreases in the time-domain measures of heart rate variability (SD, MSSD).[7,35–37] The LF power may increase two to ten-fold during standing or upright tilt.[7,8,35] Importantly, beta-adrenergic blockade has been shown to blunt this increase. Pomeranz *et al.*[7] demonstrated that propranolol produced a 73% reduction in the LF power induced by standing. Interestingly, parasympathetic blockade alone also produced a 72% reduction in the LF power induced by standing. Double blockade with propranolol and atropine resulted in 90% reduction in the LF power induced by standing. These findings support the concept that there is a sympathetic influence on the LF power. However, it is also clear that parasympathetic tone modulates the power in this frequency range as atropine also markedly blunted the increase in the LF power induced by standing. We[38] directly compared the effect of changing from the supine position to upright tilt in normal subjects following parasympathetic blockade. As expected, baseline heart rate variability was markedly suppressed in the supine position. With upright tilt, there was a significant 15-fold increase in the LF power. Although this 15-fold increase is of the same magnitude as that observed in the absence of parasympathetic blockade, the absolute LF power was much less than that observed in the absence of parasympathetic blockade. It can therefore be concluded that sympathetic neural stimulation increases the LF power compared with the absence of sympathetic stimulation, but there is considerable modulation of this effect by the presence of parasympathetic tone.

In order to obtain a better measure of the influence of the sympathetic nervous system on the heart rate, several methods have been proposed to correct for the dual (sympathetic and parasympathetic) influence on the absolute LF power. Pagani *et al.*[36] have employed the fractional power in the LF range. Upright tilt results in an approximately 50% increase in the fractional LF power.[36,37,39] However, upright tilt following acute beta-adrenergic blockade has also been associated with an approximately 50% increase in the fractional LF power[36] as it increased from 50.9% to 74.1%. In our study,[8] there was no significant increase in the fractional LF power with upright tilt. These findings appear to limit the usefulness of the fractional LF power as an index of sympathetic tone.

The ratio of low- to high-frequency power has also been felt to adjust for the dual contribution of the sympathetic and parasympathetic nervous systems to the LF power by dividing it by the HF power, which appears to be under the sole influence of the parasympathetic nervous system. Upright tilt has consistently demonstrated a dramatic increase in the LF/HF ratio.[8,36,37] However, after beta-blockade, Pagani et al.[36] demonstrated that the LF/HF ratio also increased from 1.74 to 7.48 with upright tilt. While these ratios were significantly lower than the ratios in the unblocked state, it is clear that stimuli other than sympathetic stimulation may increase the LF/HF ratio. These findings again limit the usefulness of the LF/HF ratio as a general index of sympathetic neural stimulation.

Effects of circulating beta-adrenergic agonists

Ahmed et al.[8] evaluated the effects of epinephrine (50 ng/kg/min) and isoproterenol (50 ng/kg/min) infusions on heart rate variability. The effects of these interventions on the time- and frequency-domain indices of heart rate variability, as well as the effects of tilt and exercise, are shown in Figures 12.6 and 12.7. As there is no significant alpha-adrenergic effect on heart rate variability, the effects of epinephrine on heart rate variability must be mediated by beta-adrenergic stimulation. Similarly, isoproterenol is an isolated beta-adrenergic agonist. As expected, these agents caused a shortening of the RR interval from 981 ms to 762 ms and 489 ms, respectively, consistent with their beta-adrenergic effects. The time-domain measures of heart rate variability (*SD, MSSD*) significantly decreased with this stimulation. Furthermore, a larger decrease was noted with isoproterenol infusion. Although it is tempting to ascribe these changes to withdrawal of parasympathetic tone, isoproterenol infusion has been associated with an increase in vagal tone.[40] In the frequency domain, the effects of epinephrine and

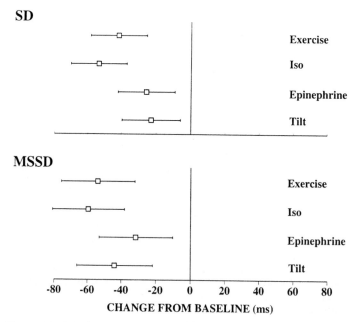

Figure 12.6 Changes in time-domain parameters of heart rate variability from baseline in 14 normal subjects following physiologic (exercise, tilt) and pharmacologic (isoproterenol, epinephrine) sympathetic stimulation. Error bars indicate 95% confidence intervals. All the changes noted are significant because the error bars do not cross the zero line. (Reproduced with permission from reference 8)

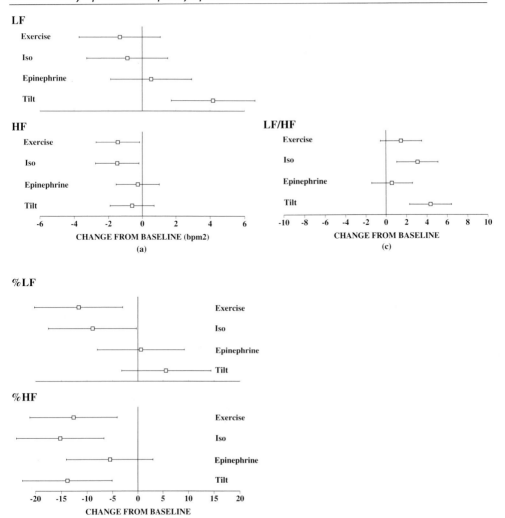

Figure 12.7 Changes in frequency-domain parameters of heart rate variability from baseline in 14 normal subjects following physiologic (exercise, tilt) and pharmacologic (isoproterenol, epinephrine) sympathetic stimulation. Error bars indicate 95% confidence intervals. When the error bars cross the zero line, the changes noted are not significant. (a) Changes in LF and HF power. (b) Changes in %LF power and %HF power. (c) Changes in LF/HF power ratio. (Reproduced with permission from reference 8)

isoproterenol infusion on the LF power were not similar to those of upright tilt. Specifically, there was no significant change in the LF power. In contrast to these findings, Binkley et al.[34] demonstrated that isoproterenol infusion at a lower dose (2 μg/kg/min) resulted in a significant increase in LF power without a significant change in the LF/HF power ratio. We have also noted that this lower dose of isoproterenol (25 ng/kg/min) does increase the LF power. These studies suggest that the intensity of stimulation may also be an important factor in determining the response of the heart rate variability to circulating beta-adrenergic agonists.

The effects of beta-adrenergic agonist infusions on the fractional LF power and the LF/HF ratio were also evaluated by Ahmed et al.[8] Although the fractional LF power remained unchanged with epinephrine infusion, it actually decreased with isoproterenol infusion.

Similarly, the LF/HF ratio increased with isoproterenol infusion, but remained unchanged with epinephrine infusion. As shown in Figure 12.7, not only were the effects of epinephrine and isoproterenol infusions on the fractional LF power different from each other, but isoproterenol infusion had the opposite effect from tilt. These findings again demonstrate the limitations of the fractional LF power and the LF/HF ratio as indices of sympathetic tone.

Although the above data suggested that the heart rate variability response to circulating beta-adrenergic agonists differed from that due to neural stimulation, the possibility remained that the differences were related to the associated level of parasympathetic tone. Further studies in our laboratory[38] have evaluated the interaction of sympathetic stimulation with parasympathetic tone by repeating the comparison of the effects of neural stimulation with upright tilt and stimulation with circulating beta-adrenergic agonists (isoproterenol) following parasympathetic blockade. Both upright tilt and isoproterenol infusion resulted in significant shortening of the RR interval prior to and following parasympathetic blockade, consistent with their beta-adrenergic effects. In the absence of parasympathetic blockade, isoproterenol (infused at a dose of 25 ng/kg/min) resulted in an increase in the LF power, resulting in a similar pattern of change in heart rate variability as that observed with upright tilt. However, following parasympathetic blockade, the pattern of heart rate variability changes associated with upright tilt were different from those associated with isoproterenol infusion. While upright tilt following parasympathetic blockade increased the LF power, isoproterenol infusion had no significant effect. These data conclusively demonstrate that the heart rate variability response of the sinus node to neural stimulation differs from the response to circulating catecholamines.

The origin of the specific increase in LF power with neural stimulation may be understood from studies that have examined the frequency spectrum of muscle sympathetic nerve activity.[20] The sympathetic nerve activity spectrum has a peak in the LF range. Saul *et al.*[20] evaluated the correlation between muscle sympathetic nerve counts and either absolute or fractional LF heart rate power in individual subjects during nitroprusside and phenylephrine infusions. They proposed that if LF power were consistently correlated with sympathetic activity, one would expect values of the correlation coefficient to be near one. However, only 5 of their 10 subjects had significant correlations. Although they concluded that none of the heart rate variability parameters predicted muscle sympathetic nerve activity, under conditions of sympathetic neural stimulation (nitroprusside infusion), there was a better correlation. It seems likely that the low-frequency oscillations of the heart rate result at least in part from oscillations in the sympathetic nerve activity at this frequency, particularly since similar changes are not noted with circulating beta-adrenergic stimulation. Based on these data, it is clear that the sinus node does not have an intrinsic oscillation frequency when it undergoes beta-adrenergic stimulation, at least in the frequency range currently investigated (0.04–0.15 Hz). The variability in the heart rate is likely determined by the variability in the input. It therefore becomes very difficult to evaluate sympathetic effects on heart rate variability without some information on the characteristics of the stimulation. As many conditions are associated with both neural and catecholamine stimulation, currently available heart rate variability techniques may be limited in their ability to quantify sympathetic tone (or sympathovagal balance).

Other types of sympathetic stimulation

Mental stress may be induced by a variety of techniques, including stressful interviews, mental arithmetic, and word or color identification tasks. These techniques may increase both sympathetic neural activity and circulating epinephrine and norepinephrine levels, depending on the stimulus and/or the strength of the stress.[33,41,42] Thus, sympathetic stimulation in this setting may be due to neural stimulation and/or circulating beta-adrenergic agonists. A number of studies have shown that mental stress decreases heart rate variability, as measured by a variety of time-domain techniques.[43–46] When examined in the frequency domain, mental stress has been shown to increase the LF power in only some situations.[47–49] In other situations, despite an increase in the heart rate, consistent with sympathetic stimulation, there has been no significant change in the LF power.[48,50,51] In these studies, changes in the normalized LF power and in the LF/HF power ratio have also been inconsistent. These observations are consistent with the idea that the induced changes in heart rate variability may depend on the type and intensity of stimulation.

Exercise is a well-known physiologic maneuver that is associated with an increase in sympathetic tone and withdrawal of parasympathetic tone. With exercise, there is an increase in both sympathetic neural stimulation and circulating epinephrine, resulting in a mixed type of sympathetic stimulation. Further difficulties in characterizing the effects of exercise on heart rate variability arise from the fact that the intensity of exercise (and consequently sympathetic stimulation) may affect the results.[52] Furthermore, the time window for analysis may be important as exercise-induced changes in heart rate variability may be different during exercise and recovery.[52,53] In addition, exercise is usually associated with an increase in respiratory rate which may itself affect the heart rate spectrum. Finally, spectral analysis requires stationarity of the data; typically, exercise increases nonstationarity. Nevertheless, the effects of exercise on heart rate variability have been studied. At low levels of exercise, Pagani *et al.*[37] reported a predominance of the LF component. In another canine study,[54] it was shown that the absolute LF power may decrease, but that the fractional LF power may increase. Other studies[8,52,53] have suggested a decrease in the LF power and/or the fractional LF power. It is likely that these divergent data are due to the factors described above. Because of the difficulties associated with the analysis of exercise-induced heart rate variability changes, it is difficult to compare the results obtained from these studies.

Myocardial ischemia is another stimulus that results in increased sympathetic tone. Transient coronary occlusion in cats has been shown to result in an increase in sympathetic neural discharge.[55] In humans, acute myocardial infarction has been associated with an increase in both epinephrine and norepinephrine plasma levels.[56] It is therefore likely that the response to this stimulus involves both neural stimulation and circulating beta-adrenergic agonists. Coronary occlusion in conscious dogs has been shown to shorten the RR interval and decrease the RR interval variance.[19] In this study, although the absolute LF power did not increase, there was a significant increase in the fractional low frequency from 3 to 47 normalized units. Although heart rate variability has been extensively evaluated in the postmyocardial infarction period, only limited human information is available regarding the effects of acute ischemia on heart rate variability. As this may also be a condition with significant nonstationarity, these data must be evaluated cautiously. Akselrod *et al.*[57] have shown that, in the acute phase of anterior myocardial infarction, there is a decrease in heart rate variability in both the LF and HF bands, though the decrease in the HF band was more prominent. This decrease in heart rate variability was not noted in the patients with inferior myocardial infarction. Transient asymptomatic ischemia has also been shown to be associated with an increase in heart rate, consistent with enhanced sympathetic tone, accompanied by an increase in the standard deviation and LF power and no significant change in the HF power.[58] Interestingly, the increase in LF power preceded the period of ischemia. Given the divergent data, it is difficult to generalize regarding the effects of ischemia on heart rate variability.

Administration of agents that lower the blood pressure also result in sympathetic activation.[20,22] Nitroprusside infusion in gradually increasing doses results in a progressive increase in muscle sympathetic nerve activity and in the plasma norepinephrine level. Saul *et al.*[20] noted that, over the range tested, the RR interval decreased from approximately 1000 ms to 700 ms, but there was no significant change in the standard deviation of the RR intervals, a time-domain measure of heart rate variability. However, Eckberg *et al.*[22] noted a progressive decline in the respiratory peak to valley RR intervals, also a time-domain measure of heart rate variability. Saul *et al.*[20] did find a progressive increase in the absolute LF power, with a less dramatic increase in the fractional LF power. Studies in dogs[19,36] have shown that nitroglycerin infusion decreases the RR interval variance with an increase in the normalized LF power. Following bilateral stellectomy, a similar decrease in the RR interval variance was noted with nitroglycerin infusion, but the increase in the normalized LF power was prevented.[36] However, Rimoldi *et al.*[19] did not find a significant increase in the absolute LF power.

All these findings demonstrate that the heart rate variability response to sympathetic stimulation is diverse. The factors that are likely to affect the response include the type of stimulation (neural versus circulating beta-adrenergic agonists versus mixed), the intensity of stimulation, and the accompanying level of parasympathetic tone. Other factors such as age and heart disease may also play a role in determining the response of the sinus node to sympathetic stimulation. These findings highlight the complexity of heart rate variability analysis and perhaps provide further directions for research endeavors in this area.

Effects of beta-adrenergic blockade

As discussed above, the resting heart rate variability is predominantly due to parasympathetic tone. Administration of atropine in the baseline state almost completely abolishes the heart rate variability. In contrast, divergent effects of acute beta-blockade have been reported. In the resting supine state, intravenous propranolol has been shown in some studies to have no significant effect on heart rate variability.[7,8] In the study of Ahmed *et al.*[8] acute beta-blockade did not significantly alter the RR interval or any of the time- or frequency-domain measures of heart rate variability. However, Coker *et al.*[10] demonstrated a significant slowing of the heart rate, accompanied by an increase in heart rate variability, in normal controls two hours after pretreatment with 100 mg of oral atenolol. In this study, the RR interval increased from 973 to 1141 ms and the standard deviation of the RR intervals increased from 70 to 103 ms. They postulated that this increase was due to a centrally mediated mechanism. Pagani *et al.*[36] also showed an increase in the RR interval (834 to 1076 ms) and heart rate variability after acute beta-blockade with propranolol (0.2 mg/kg intravenously). Although an increase in the RR interval variance was noted following acute beta-blockade, this was not accompanied by a significant specific increase in either the normalized low- or high-frequency components. Bittiner and Smith[9] studied the effects of four different beta-adrenergic blockers and noted a significant increase in heart rate variability only when the heart rate was significantly slowed. In other settings, the correlation between the RR interval and heart rate variability has also been established.[59] Whether the observed increase in heart rate variability when the heart rate slows results from a central vagotonic effect or simply represents withdrawal of sympathetic tone in some situations is unknown. Chronic therapy with beta-adrenergic blockers has also been shown to result in an increase in heart rate variability.[36,60,61] Thus, a variety of factors may determine whether the heart rate variability increases with beta-blockade. These include whether there is a change in the heart rate, the type of beta-blocker used, and the duration of administration. Possible mechanisms for the increase in heart rate variability include withdrawal of sympathetic tone, a central vagotonic effect, or perhaps altered regulation of beta-adrenergic receptors during chronic administration. Importantly, there is no supine measure of heart rate variability that is attenuated by beta-adrenergic blockade.

In contrast, under conditions of sympathetic stimulation, beta-adrenergic blockade has been shown to have some consistent effects on heart rate variability. As previously discussed, beta-adrenergic blockade significantly decreases the LF power during upright tilt. A similar effect has been demonstrated for the increase in LF power noted with baroreceptor unloading with nitroglycerin. Bilateral stellectomy in dogs prevented the increase in LF power.[36]

Summary

For an index of heart rate variability to be reflective of either sympathetic or parasympathetic tone, it should increase when autonomic tone increases and decrease when it decreases in a monotonic fashion. The time-domain parameters of heart rate variability have been shown to decrease with parasympathetic blockade, parasympathetic stimulation, and sympathetic stimulation. Thus, these parameters are not specific for either parasympathetic or sympathetic tone. Similarly, the HF power has been shown to decrease with parasympathetic stimulation, parasympathetic blockade, and sympathetic stimulation in various situations. The LF power has also been shown to have diverse responses to these kinds of stimuli.

Thus, it seems that although the observed heart rate variability is mediated by the activity of the autonomic nervous system, similar changes in the currently identified parameters may be observed with a variety of different autonomic stimuli. Furthermore, the interaction between parasympathetic and sympathetic tone is complex. It is clear that the effects of parasympathetic and sympathetic tone on the heart rate are not simply additive;[4,18] thus, it is unlikely that their effects on heart rate variability will be simply additive. These findings limit the usefulness of the current heart rate variability indices as determinants of specific levels of autonomic tone in all situations.

However, as has been demonstrated, there are settings in which heart rate variability analysis can provide some information about autonomic tone. The challenge is to identify those situations in which it does provide this kind of information and to adjust the techniques so that they might be applicable to other situations. Nevertheless, as currently performed, heart rate variability analysis has demonstrated clinical utility, as discussed in Chapter 13.

References

1. Chang M, Zipes D. Differential sensitivity of sinus node, atrioventricular node, atrium, and ventricle to propranolol. *Am Heart J* 1988; **116**: 371–8.
2. Higgins C, Vatner S, Braunwald E. Parasympathetic control of the heart. *Pharmacol Rev* 1973; **25**: 119–51.
3. Anrep GV, Pascual W, Rossler R. Respiratory variations of the heart rate. I: The reflex mechanism of respiratory arrhythmia. *Proc Roy Soc London* 1973; **119B**: 191–217.
4. Samaan A. The antagonistic cardiac nerves and heart rate. *J Physiol* 1935; **83**: 332–40.
5. Katona PG, Jih F. Respiratory sinus arrhythmia: noninvasive measure of parasympathetic cardiac control. *J Appl Physiol* 1975; **39**: 801–5.
6. Goldberger J, Ahmed M, Parker M, Kadish A. Dissociation of heart rate variability from parasympathetic tone. *Am J Physiol* 1994; **266**: H2152–7.
7. Pomeranz B, Macaulay RJB, Caudill MA, *et al.* Assessment of autonomic function in humans by heart rate spectral analysis. *Am J Physiol* 1985; **248**: H151–3.
8. Ahmed M, Kadish A, Parker M, Goldberger J. Effect of physiologic and pharmacologic adrenergic stimulation on heart rate variability. *J Am Coll Cardiol* 1994; **24**: 1082–90.
9. Bittiner S, Smith S. Beta-adrenoceptor antagonists increases sinus arrhythmia: a vagotonic effect. *Br J Clin Pharmacol* 1986; **22**: 691–5.
10. Coker R, Koziell A, Oliver C, Smith SE. Does the sympathetic nervous system influence sinus arrhythmia in man? Evidence from combined autonomic blockade. *J Physiol* 1984; **356**: 459–64.

11. Katona PG, Poitras JW, Barnett GO, Terry BS. Cardiac vagal efferent activity and heart period in the carotid sinus reflex. *Am J Physiol* 1970; **218**: 1030–7.
12. Eckberg DL. Human sinus arrhythmia as an index of vagal cardiac outflow. *J Appl Physiol* 1983; **54**: 961–6.
13. Angelone A, Coulter N. Respiratory sinus arrhythmia: a frequency dependent phenomenon. *J Appl Physiol* 1964; **19**: 479–82.
14. Davies C, Neilson J. Sinus arrhythmia in man at rest. *J Appl Physiol* 1967; **22**: 947–55.
15. Hirsch JA, Bishop B. Respiratory sinus arrhythmia in humans: how breathing pattern modulates heart rate. *Am J Physiol* 1981; **241**: H620–9.
16. Randall D, Brown D, Raisch R, Yingling J. Randall W. SA nodal parasympathectomy delineates autonomic control of heart rate power spectrum. *Am J Physiol* 1991; **29**: H985–8.
17. Kunze DL. Reflex discharge patterns of cardiac vagal efferent fibers. *J Physiol* 1972; **222**: 1–15.
18. Pickering T, Gribbin B, Stage-Peterson E, Cunningham D, Sleight P. Effects of autonomic blockade on the baroflex in man at rest and during exercise. *Cir Res* 1972; **30**: 177–85.
19. Rimoldi O, Perini S, Ferrari A, Cerruti S, Pagani M, Malliani A. Analysis of short-term oscillations of RR and arterial pressure in conscious dogs. *Am J Physiol* 1990; **258**: H967–76.
20. Saul JP, Rea RF, Eckberg DL, Berger RD, Cohen RJ. Heart rate and muscle sympathetic nerve variability during reflex changes of autonomic activity. *Am J Physiol* 1990; **258**: H713–21.
21. Goldberger J, Kim YH, Ahmed M, Kadish A. Effects of graded increases in parasympathetic tone on heart rate variability (abstract). *Circulation* 1994; **90**: I-329.
22. Eckberg DL, Rea RF, Anderson OK, *et al*. Baroreflex modulation of sympathetic activity and sympathetic neurotransmitters in humans. *Acta Physiol Scand* 1988; **133**: 221–31.
23. Kollai M, Mizsei G. Respiratory sinus arrhythmia is a limited measure of cardiac parasympathetic control in man. *J Physiol* 1990; **424**: 329–42.
24. Jewett DL. Activity of single efferent fibres in the cervical vagus nerve of the dog, with special reference to possible cardio-inhibitory fibres. *J Physiol* 1964; **175**: 321–57.
25. DiFrancesco D, Ducouret P, Robinson R. Muscarinic modulation of cardiac rate at low acetylcholine concentrations. *Science* 1989; **243**: 669–71.
26. Glitsch H, Pott L. Effects of acetylcholine and parasympathetic nerve stimulation on membrane potential in quiescent guinea-pig atria. *J Physiol* 1978; **279**: 655–68.
27. Sacknoff D, Gleim G, Stachenfeld N, Glace B, Coplan N. Suppression of high-frequency power spectrum of heart rate variability in well-trained endurance athletes (abstract). *Circulation* 1992; **86**: I-658.
28. Talajic M, Villemaire C, Nattel S. Electrophysiologic effects of alpha-adrenergic stimulation. *PACE* 1990; **13**: 578–82.
29. Schuessler RB, Canavan TE, Boineau JP, Cox JL. Baroreflex modulation of heart rate and initiation of atrial activation in dogs. *Am J Physiol* 1988; **255**: H503–13.
30. Warner MR, Loeb JM. Reflex regulation of atrioventricular conduction. *Am J Physiol* 1987; **252**: H1077–85.
31. Robertson D, Johnson G, Robertson R, Nies A, Shand D, Oats J. Comparative assessment of stimuli that release neuronal and adrenomedullary catecholamines in man. *Circulation* 1979; **59**: 637–43.
32. Hortnagl H, Benedict C, Grahame-Smith D. A sensitive radioenzymatic assay for adrenaline and noradrenaline in plasma. *Br J Clin Pharmacol* 1977; **4**: 553–8.
33. Dimsdale J, Ziegler M. What do plasma and urinary measures of catecholamines tell us about human response to stressors? *Circulation* 1991; **183**: 36–42.
34. Binkley P, Nunziata E, Hass G, Nelson S, Cody R. Parasympathetic withdrawal is an integral component of autonomic imbalance in congestive heart failure: demonstration in human subjects and verification in a paced canine model of ventricular failure. *J Am Coll Cardiol* 1991; **18**: 464–72.
35. Vybiral T, Bryg RJ, Maddens ME, Boden WE. Effect of passive tilt on sympathetic and parasympathetic components of heart rate variability in normal subjects. *Am J Cardiol* 1989; **63**: 1117–20.
36. Pagani M, Lombardi F, Guzzetti S, *et al*. Power spectral analysis of heart rate and arterial pressure variabilities as a marker of sympatho-vagal interaction in man and conscious dog. *Cir Res* 1986; **59**: 178–93.
37. Pagani M, Malfatto G, Pierini S, *et al*. Spectral analysis of heart rate variability in the assessment of autonomic diabetic neuropathy. *J Auton Nerv Syst* 1988; **23**: 143–53.
38. Kim YH, Ahmed M, Kadish A, Goldberger J. Response of heart rate variability to sympathetic stimulation (abstract). *Circulation* 1994; **90**: I-331.
39. Lombardi F, Sandrone G, Pernpruner S, *et al*. Heart rate variability as an index of sympathovagal interaction after acute myocardial infarction. *Am J Cardiol* 1987; **60**: 1239–45.
40. Arnold JMO, McDevitt DG. Vagal activity is increased during intravenous isoprenaline infusion in man. *Br J Clin Pharmacol* 1985; **18**: 311–16.
41. Freyschuss U, Faguis J, Wallin B, Bohlin G, Perski A, Hjemdahl P. Cardiovascular and sympathoadrenal responses to mental stress: a study of sensory intake and rejection reactions. *Acta Physiol Scand* 1990; **193**: 173–83.
42. Hjemdahl P, Fagius J, Freyschuss U, *et al*. Muscle sympathetic activity and norepinephrine release during mental challenge in humans. *Am J Physiol* 1989; **257**: E654–64.
43. Ettema J, Zielhuis R. Physiological parameters of mental load. *Ergonomics* 1971; **14**: 137–44.
44. Kalsbeek J, Ettema J. Continuous recording of heart rate and the measurement of perceptual load. *Ergonomics* 1963; **6**: 306–7.
45. Blitz P, Hoogstraten J. Mulder G. Mental load, heart rate and heart rate variability. *Psychol Forsch* 1970; **33**: 277–88.

46. Mulder G, Mulder-Hajonides Van Der Meulen WREH. Mental load and the measurement of heart rate variability. *Ergonomics* 1973; **16**: 69–83.

47. Nandagopal D, Fallen E, Ghista D, Connally S. Reproducibility of resting HRV spectrum and its changes following physiological perturbations. *Automedica* 1985; **6**: 235–47.

48. Pagani M, Mazzuro G, Ferrari A, *et al*. Sympathovagal interaction during mental stress: a study using spectral analysis of heart rate variability in healthy control subjects and patients with a prior myocardial infarction. *Circulation* 1991; **83**: II43–51.

49. Pagani M, Furlan R, Pizzinelli P, Crivellaro W, Cerutti S, Malliani A. Spectral analysis of RR and arterial pressure variabilities to assess sympatho-vagal interaction during mental stress in humans. *J Hypertens* 1989; **7**: S14–15.

50. Langewitz W, Ruddel H. Spectral analysis of heart rate variability under mental stress. *J Hypertens* 1989; **7**: S32–3.

51. Kamada T, Sato N, Miyake S, Kumashiro M, Monou H. Power spectral analysis of heart rate variability in type A's during solo and competitive mental arithmetic task. *J Psychom Res* 1992; **36**: 543–51.

52. Perini R, Orizio C, Baselli G, Cerutti S, Veicsteinas A. The influence of exercise intensity on the power spectrum of heart rate variability. *J Appl Physiol* 1990; **61**: 143–8.

53. Arai Y, Saul JP, Albrecht P, *et al*. Modulation of cardiac autonomic activity during and immediately after exercise. *Am J Physiol* 1989; **256**: H132–41.

54. Rimoldi O, Pagani M, Pagani MR, Baselli G, Malliani A. Sympathetic activation during treadmill exercise in the conscious dog: assessment with spectral analysis of heart period and systolic pressure variabilities. *J Auton Nerv Syst* 1990; **30**: S129–32.

55. Malliani A, Schwartz P, Zanchetti A. Sympathetic reflex elicited by experimental coronary occlusion. *Am J Physiol* 1969; **217**: 703–9.

56. Christensen NJ, Videbaek J. Plasma catecholamines and carbohydrate metabolism in patients with acute myocardial infarction. *J Clin Invest* 1974; **54**: 278–86.

57. Akselrod S, Arbel J, Oz O, Benary V, David D. Spectral analysis of heart rate fluctuations in the evaluation of autonomous control during acute myocardial infarction. *Comput Cardiol* 1985; 315–18.

58. Bernardi L, Lumina C, Ferrai M, *et al*. Relationship between fluctuations in heart rate and asymptomatic nocturnal ischemia. *Int J Cardiol* 1988; **20**: 39–51.

59. Van Hoogenhuyze D, Weinstein N, Martin G, *et al*. Reproducibility and relation to mean heart rate of heart rate variability in normal subjects and in patients with congestive heart failure secondary to coronary artery disease. *Am J Cardiol* 1991; **68**: 1668–76.

60. Cook J, Bigger J, Kleiger R, Fleiss J, Steinman R, Rolnitzky L. Effect of atenolol and diltiazem on heart period variability in normal persons. *J Am Coll Cardiol* 1991; **17**: 480–4.

61. Ewing DJ, Neilson JMM, Travis P. New method for assessing cardiac parasympathetic activity using 24-hour electrocardiograms. *Br Heart J* 1984; **52**: 396–402.

13

Clinical Significance of Heart Rate Variability

A. John Camm and Lü Fei

Introduction

The clinical implications of beat-to-beat heart period variability (usually but inaccurately referred to as heart rate variability, HRV) were not fully appreciated until recently, although respiratory sinus arrhythmia has been recognized for many years. Proper studies on respiratory sinus arrhythmia could not be performed until sometime after the intervention of Einthoven's string galvanometer. In the 1970s, conventional autonomic testing was used to assess diabetic autonomic neuropathy. The physiological basis of beat-to-beat fluctuations was studied in more detail in the early 1980s. Interest in HRV analysis in the field of clinical cardiology stems from the important observation of the Multicentre Post-Infarction Programme (MPIP) that depressed HRV is a powerful and independent risk factor following acute myocardial infarction.[1] The predictive value of HRV following myocardial infarction has since been extensively investigated. Depressed HRV, singly or in combination with other established risk factors, has been shown to significantly improve the prediction of mortality and arrhythmic events after myocardial infarction. Several important investigations listed in Table 13.1 represent the history of this field prior to the MPIP report in 1987.

The prevalence and importance of autonomic dysfunction in cardiovascular disease have been increasingly recognized during the last decade. Recent attention to the role of the autonomic nervous system in clinical cardiology has further stimulated interest in HRV analysis. It is well known that the autonomic nervous system plays an important part in the normal and abnormal mechanical and electrical activities of the heart, but until recently there was no good clinical method for the evaluation of autonomic nervous system function. During the last decade, HRV has been studied in many areas of clinical cardiology (Table 13.2) and considerable knowledge has been assembled.

Analysis of HRV (defined as beat-to-beat fluctuations of sinus RR intervals) has been undoubtedly accepted as a noninvasive method for assessment of autonomic influence on the heart. Although HRV measures autonomic influence at the level of sinus node, it is generally assumed to reflect the global autonomic control of cardiovascular activities. HRV is usually calculated in the time- and frequency-domains. Fractal, chaos and other nonlinear dynamic methods of analysis are being explored as research techniques for the calculation of HRV. The main underlying physiological basis of HRV is generally thought to be vagally-mediated. Spectral analysis of HRV can partially distinguish sympathetic from parasympathetic influence on the heart. The low-frequency component of spectral

Table 13.1 Several important studies on respiratory sinus arrhythmia and heart rate variability

Initial studies on respiratory sinus arrhythmia
Samaan (1935): Section of vagus abolishes respiratory sinus arrhythmia
Clynes (1960): Respiration is the most important stimulus responsible for normal beat-to-beat RR variation

Studies on diabetic autonomic neuropathy
Nathanielsz *et al.* (1967): Abnormal response of heart rate to Valsalva maneuver in diabetic patients with autonomic neuropathy
Wheeler and Watkins (1973): Description of cardiac denervation in diabetes
Ewing *et al.* (1984): Using HRV for diagnosis of autonomic neuropathy in diabetics

Studies on physiological basis of heart rate variability
Akselrod *et al.* (1981): Autonomic blockade on spectral HRV in dogs (physiological basis)
Pomeranz *et al.* (1985): Effects of postures on spectral analysis of HRV in humans

Studies on prognostic value of heart rate variability
Schneider and Costiloe (1965): Sinus arrhythmia decreases with age and is associated with poor prognosis in ischemic heart disease
Hinkle *et al.* (1972): 'Slow heart rate' and increased risk of cardiac death in middle-aged men
Wolf *et al.* (1978): A brief report on prognostic significance of HRV following acute myocardial infarction
Kleiger *et al.* (1987): Powerful independent value of HRV for postinfarction risk stratification

HRV gives a predominant measure of sympathetic activity with some influence from the parasympathetic system. While the high-frequency component is almost exlusively mediated by vagal activity, the low-to-high ratio has been used as an index of the sympathovagal balance to the heart. An increased low-to-high ratio suggests increased sympathetic and/or decreased parasympathetic drive to the heart. Accurate assessment of 'pure' sympathetic activity without the influence of vagal activity using HRV analysis will need further investigations. Obviously, sympathovagal interaction may play a more important role in the modulation of cardiac activity. The physiological basis and methodology of HRV are discussed in detail in other chapters of this book.

HRV in Patients with Chronic Coronary Artery Disease

Animal experiments and clinical observations have shown that transient myocardial ischemia induces significant changes in autonomic activity in patients with myocardial ischemia. Abnormal heart rate responses to autonomic manipulations, such as postural change, Valsalva maneuver and carotid sinus massage are well recognized. For example, a lower heart rate response to deep breathing can be found in 32% of patients with stable coronary artery disease. Changes of HRV induced by transient occlusion of a coronary artery during coronary artery angioplasty have recently been demonstrated. An increased heart rate and low-to-high ratio, and a decreased HF component, have been demonstrated before the onset of transient ischemic episodes. Vagal activity has been shown to be increased 10 minutes preceding the attack of nocturnal variant angina. The fact that not all increased vagal activity is consistently followed by an attack of variant angina suggests that mechanisms other than autonomic changes are also involved in the development of variant angina. Increased sympathetic and/or decreased vagal activity as assessed by spectral HRV analysis also exits in silent ischemia and in syndrome X.

It has been reported that decreased HRV may correlate with the angiographic severity of coronary artery disease,[2] but this observation has not been confirmed so far by other investigators.[3] Depressed HRV in patients with one-vessel coronary artery disease may increase after successful coronary angioplasty. The increase of HRV seems to result from an improvement of segmental left ventricular function since similar changes do not occur

Table 13.2 Clinical assessment of heart rate variability

Cardiovascular system
Acute myocardial infarction
Sudden cardiac death
Ventricular tachyarrhythmias
Congestive heart failure
Chronic coronary artery disease (including variant angina)
Cardiac transplantation (reinnervation and rejection)
Essential hypertension
Long QT syndrome
Hypertrophic and dilated cardiomyopathy
Congenital heart disease (e.g. after surgery)
Patients after catheter ablation of arrhythmias
Syndrome X
Valvular heart disease
Sudden infant death syndrome

Other clinical settings
Diabetes mellitus
Perinatal fetal monitoring
Syncope (e.g. during tilt)
Psychological assessment
Thyrotoxicosis
Chagas' disease
Alcoholism
Chronic renal failure
Obesity
Diagnosis of brain death
Myotonic dystrophy
Familial amyloidotic polyneuropathy
Acquired immunodeficiency syndrome (AIDS)
Aerobic fitness and physical training
Hypoglycemia
Hyperlipidemia
Hypothyroidism
Systemic lupus erythematosus (SLE)
Postprandial hypotension
Central nervous system damage

Evaluation of drug effects
Antiarrhythmic drugs
Angiotensin converting enzyme inhibitors
Autonomic agents (including scopolamine)
Other drugs such as digoxin, magnesium and anesthetics

in patients without abnormal regional wall motion. Reduced HRV in patients with chronic coronary artery disease has prognostic implications. Patients with depressed HRV during conventional antianginal therapy (beta-blockers, heparin and aspirin) are more likely to have an adverse outcome (death, acute myocardial infarction and urgent revascularization). Patients with unstable angina have a more profound decrease in HRV, similar to that in patients who recovered from an acute myocardial infarction. Depressed HRV has been reported to be a potent independent predictor of mortality in the 12 months following elective coronary artery angiography in patients without recent myocardial infarction.

HRV in Patients after Myocardial Infarction

Effects of myocardial infarction on HRV

'Autonomic disturbance' within the early phase of myocardial infarction may cause vagal predominance leading to bradycardia with or without hypotension. Enhanced sympathetic activity, on the other hand, occurs especially in patients with anterior myocardial infarction and results in tachycardia with transient hypertension. These early changes in autonomic activity are thought to be due to either autonomic reflexes elicited by direct effects on the chemoreceptors and mechanoreceptors in the infarcted area, or by adrenaline secretion from the adrenal medulla. Correction of autonomic disturbances may improve survival in patients following myocardial infarction. This hypothesis is supported by the observations of a significant reduction in postinfarction mortality by treatment with beta-blockers.

Animal experiments suggest that myocardial infarction causes a significant decrease in HRV. HRV has been shown to be lower in patients early after myocardial infarction (from a few hours to 2–3 weeks after acute MI) compared with normal controls and begins to return towards normal levels within a few weeks following myocardial infarction. HRV is maximally recovered by 6–12 months after myocardial infarction, but remains lower than in normals.

Mechanisms of HRV changes in myocardial ischemia and infarction

A greater density of receptors on vagal afferents in the inferoposterior wall of the left ventricle may be responsible for the enhanced vasodepressor and cardiopulmonary reflexes in response to ischemia in this area. Myocardial ischemia or infarction not only triggers but also inhibits reflex activation. Prostaglandins released during myocardial ischemia or reperfusion which stimulate chemosensitive vagal endings may contribute to the reflex inhibition of sympathetic nerve activity. Chronic myocardial infarction impairs reflexes that originate in the heart in response to changes in cardiac filling pressure. Afferent and efferent denervation and activation of mechanosensitive sensory nerve endings are likely to be responsible for the lasting autonomic impairment after the acute phase of myocardial infarction. Denervation supersensitivity and reinnervation further complicate the presentation of autonomic dysfunction following myocardial infarction.

HRV for postinfarction risk stratification

The assessment of HRV has become an important clinical technique for risk stratification after myocardial infarction. The predictive value of HRV in patients following myocardial infarction was first suggested by Wolf et al.[4] in 1978, who demonstrated that patients who lacked sinus arrhythmia (defined as the variance of the RR interval on a short electrocardiographic rhythm strip) at the time of admission with acute myocardial infarction had a significantly higher risk of in-hospital mortality. However, the power of HRV prediction was not well recognized until 1987, when Kleiger et al.[1] reported that decreased HRV was associated with an increased mortality in 808 survivors of acute myocardial infarction (relative risk or mortality was 5.3 times higher in the group with a standard deviation of all normal RR intervals in 24-hour recordings <50 ms than in the group with preserved HRV) (Figure 13.1). These findings were later confirmed by several other groups.[5,6] The data of Farrell et al.[5] further suggested that depressed HRV is not only capable of predicting total cardiac mortality after infarction, but also identifies patients at risk of

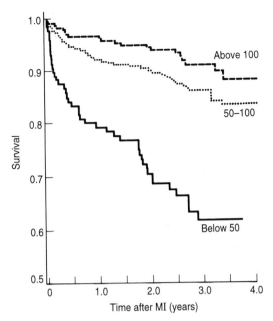

Figure 13.1 Kaplan-Meier survival curves of heart rate variability for all-cause mortality in patients following acute myocardial infarction. (Reproduced with permission from reference 1)

arrhythmic events including sudden cardiac death and sustained symptomatic ventricular tachycardia. Both the short-term (in-hospital) and long-term predictive value of HRV in patients following acute myocardial infarction has now been well established.

It has been shown that exercise elicits a greater reduction in the high-frequency component of HRV in animals susceptible to ventricular fibrillation.[7] This may be of clinical importance, since exercise-induced autonomic and metabolic changes may contribute to the pathogenesis of ventricular arrhythmias and sudden cardiac death. However, this observation has not yet been evaluated in patients following acute myocardial infarction.

The effects of pharmacological (particularly of autonomic agents)[8] and nonpharmacological interventions (such as exercise)[7] on HRV and their value for postinfarction risk stratification remain to be fully defined. It is also uncertain whether the decreased HRV is involved in the mechanism of increased postinfarction mortality or is merely a marker of poor prognosis.

Animal experiments have shown that the change in cardiac autonomic tone with a sympathetic predominance may render the hearts of some animals more susceptible to ventricular fibrillation. Hull et al.[9] investigated HRV in dogs before and one month after experimental myocardial infarction. High- and low-risk animals susceptible to sudden cardiac death after infarction were defined by the development of ventricular fibrillation during an exercise and myocardial ischemia test on a motor-driven treadmill. Prior to infarction there was no significant difference in heart rate or HRV between the high- and low-risk preinfarction animals either at rest or during exercise. However, HRV measured 30 days after myocardial infarction showed a high sensitivity (up to 88%) and specificity (up to 80%) in predicting the susceptibility to ventricular fibrillation (Figure 13.2). Preinfarction HRV did not discriminate between the susceptible and the resistant animals.

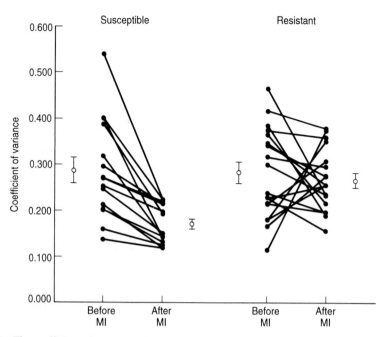

Figure 13.2 The coefficient of variance of RR intervals in 15 susceptible dogs (left) and 18 resistant dogs (right) before and one month after myocardial infarction (MI). Data are expressed as mean ± SE. The difference in HRV after myocardial infarction is highly significant ($p < 0.001$). (Reproduced with permission from reference 9)

It is currently held that increased sympathetic tone and/or decreased vagal tone predispose to ventricular fibrillation and vice versa. Beta-adrenergic blockers increase HRV and reduce the likelihood of ventricular fibrillation following myocardial ischemia or infarction. Suppression of sympathetic activity has been assumed to explain this beneficial effect of beta-blocker therapy. Currently available data suggest that decreased HRV not only reflects the severity of underlying myocardial damage but is also associated with the susceptibility to ventricular tachycardia/fibrillation in patients following acute myocardial infarction.

Comparison of HRV with other risk factors

The predictive value of depressed HRV is independent of other established prognostic predictors, including other Holter features, signal-averaged electrocardiograms (ECGs) and left ventricular ejection fraction. In a study of 416 consecutive survivors of acute myocardial infarction, predischarge HRV, ambulatory ECG and the signal-averaged ECG were assessed.[5] Impaired HRV, late potentials, frequent and repetitive ventricular ectopic beats, decreased left ventricular ejection fraction and Killip class were identified as significant univariate predictors of arrhythmic events. Stepwise Cox regression analysis showed that impaired HRV was the most powerful independent predictor of arrhythmic events (sudden cardiac death and ventricular tachycardia). For prediction of all-cause mortality, the value of HRV was similar to that of left ventricular ejection fraction. HRV, however, was better than left ventricular ejection fraction in predicting arrhythmic events (Figure 13.3).[10] A reduced left ventricular ejection fraction was more likely to reflect situations prone to cardiac failure and was therefore powerfully associated with all-cause mortality.

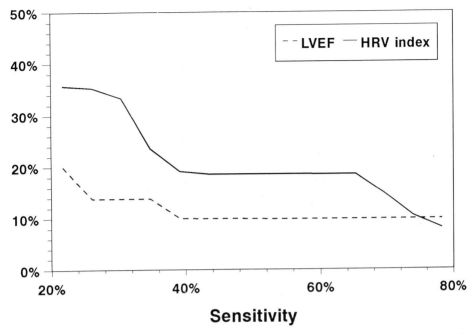

Figure 13.3 Positive predictive accuracy of heart rate variability (HRV) compared with left ventricular ejection fraction (LVEF) for arrhythmic events during the year after acute myocardial infarction, based on the data of the Post Infarct Survey Programme of St George's Hospital Medical School.

The data on the relationship between HRV and inducibility during programmed electrical stimulation in patients following acute myocardial infarction are scarce. A recent study[11] demonstrated that in patients following acute myocardial infarction the low-frequency components (particularly the VLF component) of HRV is significantly reduced in high-risk patients with a history of sustained ventricular tachycardia or cardiac arrest and with inducible ventricular tachycardia compared with low-risk noninducible patients without a history of arrhythmic events.

Combination of HRV with other predictors

The predictive value of HRV alone assessed during the acute phase of myocardial infarction is only modest, although better than any other single variable. Combination of HRV with other risk factors yields better positive predictive accuracy. Combined with left ventricular ejection fraction and/or ventricular ectopic beats, HRV has a positive predicative accuracy of more than 50%. Unfortunately, in these circumstances, the 95% confidence intervals around the point estimates for positive predictive accuracy is wide. Data from our Postinfarction Survey Program showed that, at 50% sensitivity, left ventricular ejection fraction or ventricular ectopic beats gives 10–20% positive predictive accuracy for arrhythmic events within one year after myocardial infarction. HRV alone or combined with left ventricular ejection fraction or ventricular ectopic beats provides 20–30% positive predictive accuracy. More recently, Bigger *et al.*[12] have reported that short-term (2 to 15 minutes) HRV has a predictive accuracy of 24–31%. All the short-term measures of HRV are added to previously established risk factors. The positive predictive accuracy of other established risk predictors (left ventricular ejection fraction, NYHA

Table 13.3 Clinical application of Holter monitoring in postinfarction risk stratification

---

Assessment of cardiac arrhythmias (including bradycardias)
Assessment of heart rate variability (HRV)
Assessment of ST segment alterations
Assessment of QT intervals and its relationship to RR intervals
Assessment of late potentials

---

functional class III and IV, and rales > bibasilar in the coronary care unit) is 26–33%.[12] When combined with the short-term HRV measures, the positive predictive accuracy is significantly improved to between 23% and 47%.

Pedretti et al.[13] reported the combined use of invasive and noninvasive methods for postinfarction risk stratification in 303 patients, 19 of whom died during a 15-month follow-up period. Left ventricular dysfunction, late potentials (and a prolonged filtered QRS duration), frequent (>6 beats/hour) and complex (paired or ⩾2 runs) ventricular ectopic beats, mean heart rate and HRV were univariate predictors of late arrhythmic events. Multivariate analysis showed that only low left ventricular ejection fraction, prolonged QRS duration, reduced HRV and the presence of at least two runs of nonsustained ventricular tachycardia remained as independent risk predictors. The authors also demonstrated that noninvasive risk factors could be used for selecting a sufficiently high-risk group of patients for invasive electrophysiological evaluation. A positive electrophysiological study was found to be the strongest independent predictor, with 81% sensitivity for arrhythmic events in the patients preselected by noninvasive methods. Unfortunately, HRV was not included in the preselection criteria for this study.

As it looks now, combined analysis of several variables from the ambulatory ECGs (Table 13.3) may be the most cost-effective noninvasive technique for risk stratification. Certainly the assessment of HRV, singly or in combination with other established risk factors, has provided a new powerful method for stratifying patients following myocardial infarction into low- and high-risk groups. The high-risk patients identified in this way may then undergo further invasive evaluation and/or aggressive management.

Baroreflex sensitivity and HRV

The baroreceptor reflex plays an important role in the modulation of heart rate. It has been reported that there is a weak ($\gamma = 0.57$–0.63) correlation between baroreflex sensitivity and HRV.[14] A more close relationship between baroreflex sensitivity and cardiac vagal tone (the change in RR interval after complete cholinergic blockade by atropine) has recently been demonstrated. However, little significant relationship between baroreflex sensitivity and HRV was found in the study by Farrell et al.[15] These observations suggest that HRV and baroreflex sensitivity may reflect different aspects of autonomic activity (described by others as 'tonic' and 'phasic', respectively), although baroreceptor reflexes certainly contribute to HRV. Baroreflex sensitivity is decreased in patients following myocardial infarction and a severely depressed baroreflex sensitivity identifies a subgroup at higher risk of arrhythmic events.[16] In animal experiments, baroreflex sensitivity before and after acute myocardial infarction has been shown to predict susceptibility to the development of ventricular fibrillation during an induced ischemic episode following acute myocardial infarction.

Baroreflex sensitivity testing can be safely performed 7–10 days after acute myocardial infarction. Baroreflex sensitivity (expressed as the slope of the regression line relating the beat-to-beat increase in the RR interval to the increase in the preceding systolic arterial pressure induced by phenylephrine) is significantly reduced in patients in whom sustained monomorphic ventricular tachycardia was induced by programmed electrical stimulation. Therefore, programmed electrical stimulation may be appropriately limited to patients with depressed baroreflex sensitivity without much loss of sensitivity and with an overall increase of predictive accuracy. During a one-year follow-up in 122 patients with acute myocardial infarction,[17] depressed baroreflex sensitivity has been shown to be a strong predictor of arrhythmic events (relative risk 23.1).

The relationship between HRV and baroreflex sensitivity in the prediction of postinfarction risk is now being investigated by the ATRAMI (Autonomic Tone and Reflexes in Acute Myocardial Infarction) study, which is being conducted in Europe, Asia and North America. This study will also collect data on the signal-averaged ECG and left ventricular ejection fraction. ATRAMI will recruit 1200 patients and will report shortly.

HRV in Patients Predisposing to Ventricular Tachyarrhythmias and Sudden Cardiac Death

As early as 1972, in a 7-year prospective study of 301 patients, Hinkle *et al.*[18] found that patients with a sustained slow heart rate experienced more sudden cardiac death than expected. In this study, 'slow heart rate' was defined as (1) no expected rise in mean heart rate during daily activities, (2) a low peak heart rate response to standard exercise, (3) little evidence of phasic variation in heart rate with respiration, (4) no evidence of the random abrupt sinus slowing that occurs with sighing, coughing, or straining. This definition of slow heart rate parallels the current concept of a depressed HRV. The observations suggest that patients with depressed HRV are at increased risk of sudden cardiac death. More convincingly, HRV was shown to be significantly reduced in victims of sudden cardiac deaths which were recorded during ambulatory ECG monitoring. Several investigators[19,20] have confirmed that HRV is depressed in survivors of cardiac arrest whether related or not to coronary artery disease. Survivors of out-of-hospital cardiac arrest are believed to be at high risk of recurrence of sudden cardiac death. The one-year mortality in survivors of cardiac arrest is inversely related to the low-frequency component and the standard deviation of all normal RR intervals.[19] Therefore, decreased HRV has a definite prognostic implication in this high-risk patient population. It has been reported[21] that patients with depressed HRV (the standard deviation of normal RR intervals) had a 4-fold higher risk of sudden cardiac death, independent of other risk factors in 6693 consecutive patients who underwent Holter monitoring for screening purposes. Based on the first two hours of ambulatory ECG recordings in the Framingham Heart Study, Tsuji *et al.*[22] demonstrate that HRV is better than other conventional risk factors in predicting all-cause mortality.

Assessment of HRV in patients with ventricular tachyarrhythmias has concentrated on the changes occurring immediately preceding the onset of episodes of ventricular tachycardia/fibrillation. The modification of heart rate prior to the onset of various types of cardiac arrhythmias has been previously documented and discussed. Assessment of HRV prior to the onset of ventricular tachyarrhythmias may further improve our understanding of the contribution of autonomic changes to arrhythmogenesis. In a study of 71 episodes of idiopathic ventricular tachycardia in 23 patients,[23] we demonstrated that there was a significant change in autonomic influence on the heart during the few minutes immediately before the onset of ventricular tachycardia (Figure 13.4). This change of HRV before ventricular tachycardia results mainly from vagal withdrawal rather than enhanced sympathetic input to the heart. A significant change in HRV before sustained ventricular tachycardia has also been demonstrated in patients with coronary artery disease. However, similar autonomic changes are not always followed by ventricular tachycardia/fibrillation. Therefore, changes in autonomic tone are more likely to

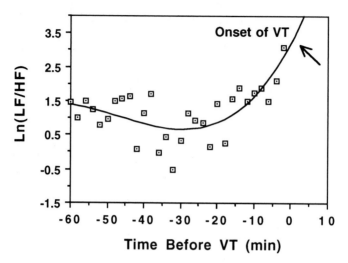

Figure 13.4 There is a significant change in LF/HF ratio immediately before the onset of idiopathic ventricular tachycardia (VT), suggesting there is abnormal autonomic influence on the heart with a sympathetic predominance. This may contribute to the pathogenesis of ventricular tachycardia. (Reproduced with permission from reference 23)

be initiating factors than an intrinsic electrophysiological substrate for ventricular arrhythmias.

HRV in Patients with Congestive Heart Failure

There is substantial evidence that the development of congestive heart failure is associated with significant autonomic dysfunction. Congestive heart failure has been described as a condition of generalized neurohumoral excitation characterized by activation of the sympathetic nervous system (and parasympathetic withdrawal) and activation of the renin–angiotensin–aldosterone systems, with accompanying increased release of vasopressin and endothelin. The increased neuroendocrine activity in such patients maintains blood pressure at the expense of reduced cardiac performance and salt and water retention. Spectral analysis shows that all frequency components of HRV are decreased and that the normal high- and low-frequency peaks of HRV spectra disappear in patients with congestive heart failure. The normal circadian rhythm of heart rate and its variability is lost in patients with congestive heart failure. The overall decrease in HRV simulates the HRV spectra of the denervated heart such as in diabetic patients with cardiac neuropathy and in transplanted patients. Of interest, it has been reported[24] that depressed HRV (measured as the mean difference in the length of consecutive RR intervals in relation to the mean length of RR intervals from 10 minutes of ECG recording in the supine position and expressed in percentage terms) may be an independent risk factor in the development of congestive heart failure. There may be a relative increase in the low-frequency component at the early stage of heart failure, while the low-frequency predominance can no longer be detected owing to the overall decreased response of the heart to sympathetic stimuli. The overall markedly depressed HRV in severe congestive heart failure which resembles that seen in denervated hearts may not merely reflect the autonomic modulation of sinus heart rate as in the normal condition.

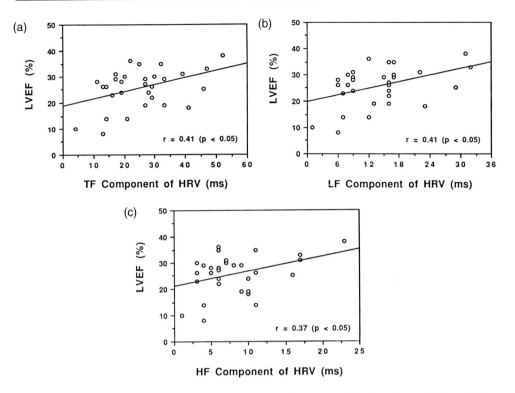

Figure 13.5 All frequency components of heart rate variability are significantly related to left ventricular ejection fraction (LVEF) in patients with congestive heart failure. TF = total frequency; LF = low frequency; HF = high frequency. (Reproduced with permission from reference 26)

Clinical correlates of HRV in patients with congestive heart failure

HRV has mainly been investigated in patients with congestive heart failure secondary to either ischemic heart disease or idiopathic dilated cardiomyopathy. There is no significant difference in any of the frequency components of spectral HRV between these two categories. Several studies have demonstrated that, in patients with congestive heart failure, the decreased HRV is significantly related to left ventricular dysfunction (Figure 13.5) and corresponds to different functional classes. Decompensation may be associated with a further reduction in HRV and, in turn, depressed HRV can be restored towards normal after clinical improvement of congestive heart failure with drug therapy or physical training.

HRV is almost completely abolished following transplantation and progressively increases thereafter. In normal subjects, HRV is significantly related to mean heart rate and age. HRV is also related to mean heart rate in patients with congestive heart failure, but a significant relationship between HRV and age can no longer be demonstrated. This may be due to the overwhelming influence of left ventricular dysfunction and subsequent neurohumoral disturbance. Whether there is a significant relationship between HRV and the severity and frequency of ventricular ectopy is uncertain.[26]

The predictive value of HRV in patients with congestive heart failure

Attention has been paid to the role of the sympathetic nervous system in the pathophysiology of heart failure. Few data are available regarding risk stratification using HRV

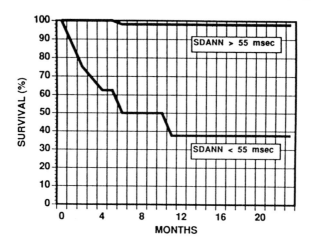

Figure 13.6 Kaplan–Meier survival curves for patients with high and low heart rate variability and congestive heart failure. Total cardiac mortality is the endpoint. *SDANN* = standard deviation of 5-minute mean RR intervals. (Reproduced with permission from reference 25)

analysis in patients with congestive heart failure. Binder *et al.*[25] reported that HRV may be useful in predicting *total* cardiac mortality in congestive heart failure patients waiting for heart transplantation (with a sensitivity of 90% and specificity of 91%). Among the spectal and nonspectral HRV parameters, the standard deviation of a 5-minute mean RR interval (*SDANN*) was the best predictor and an *SDANN* > 55 ms had a 20-fold increased risk of death compared with those with *SDANN* more than 50 ms (Figure 13.6).

Binder *et al.* also demonstrated that HRV parameters were better than other prognostic variables, including left ventricular ejection fraction, in discriminating between groups with high and low risk of death. Patients with congestive heart failure have an abnormal neurohumoral response to vasodilator drugs and to changes of physical posture. An abnormal autonomic response of the heart to such stimuli may be more useful for risk stratification in patients with congestive heart failure. However, our data suggest that HRV analysis, like other techniques such as the signal-averaged ECG and electrophysiology study, may not be useful in predicting patients at risk of *sudden* cardiac death in patients with congestive heart failure.[26]

HRV after heart transplantation

Orthotopic cardiac transplantation has become a standard procedure in the treatment of irreversible congestive heart failure, and the one-year survival rate is now 80% after heart transplantation. HRV after heart transplantation has been shown to be markedly reduced and to lack the distinct frequency components seen in the normal HRV spectrum.[27] A very small fluctuation of heart periods at the respiratory frequency may result from local sinoatrial node stretch reflexes. A non-neurogenic mechanism intrinsic to the heart muscle may contribute to HRV changes during exercise in transplant recipients.

A 'random' (in contrast to the low- and high-frequency component peaks) increase in HRV may indicate the development of allograft rejection in heart transplant recipients. The value of HRV for prediction of allograft rejection has not been fully established. Signs of functional reinnervation can be found in most heart transplantation recipients 20 months following transplantation. However, reinnervation does not occur before 2 months after transplantation. Reinnervation of different parts of the heart may occur together or separately. Therefore, sympathetic reinnervation after cardiac transplantation can be regionally heterogeneous.

HRV in Patients with Essential Hypertension

Blood pressure is influenced by the autonomic nervous system, and enhanced sympathetic activity may play an important role in the pathogenesis of hypertension. However, little is known about vagal activity in hypertensive patients. Insight has been gained into the autonomic status in this patient population using HRV analysis.

Guzzetti *et al.*[28] reported an increased low-frequency component and a decreased high-frequency component of HRV in hypertensive patients compared with normotensive controls. This suggests that there is an increased sympathetic and/or decreased vagal drive to the heart in these patients. The low-frequency components at rest and during tilt are significantly correlated with the level of the hypertension. Passive tilt produces smaller changes in high- and low-frequency components of HRV in hypertensive patients than in controls. The abnormalities of HRV in hypertensive patients have recently been confirmed by other investigators.

In addition to the abnormalities in HRV value, the circadian rhythm of heart rate and HRV is significantly altered in hypertensive patients. There is evidence that both sympathetic and parasympathetic activity and, more importantly, the sympathovagal interaction, may significantly contribute to the impairment of the circadian rhythm of HRV in hypertensive patients. An increase in sympathetic activity during the early morning may contribute to the ominously increased rate of cardiovascular events in the morning hours. However, no correlation between HRV parameters and cardiac arrhythmias has been noted in hypertensive patients without congestive heart failure. Beta-blockade (atenolol) can partially normalize the abnormal spectrum of HRV in hypertensive patients.[28]

HRV in Patients with Other Conditions

Diabetes mellitus

Autonomic neuropathy is a common and severe complication of diabetes mellitus and leads to vagal denervation and sensorimotor and reflex dysfunction of cardiovascular, urogenital and gastrointestinal systems. The diagnosis of neuropathy is usually made by conventional cardiovascular autonomic function tests such as the Valsalva maneuver, the deep-breathing test, and the isometric handgrip test. Autonomic neuropathy has prognostic implications as it is related to retinal ischemia, renal abnormalities, sudden death and other outcomes in diabetic patients. Therefore early diagnosis of autonomic neuropathy is of clinical importance.

The reduced beat-to-beat variation during deep breathing was initially reported by Wheeler and Watkins in 1973.[29] Application of HRV to the diagnosis of diabetic autonomic neuropathy was first reported by Ewing *et al.*[30] in 1984 and was later confirmed by several other investigators. In addition to the global decrease in HRV, the response of HRV to tilt and the circadian variation of HRV are also markedly attenuated. Spectral analysis of HRV has provided a sensitive method for early diagnosis of autonomic neuropathy in diabetes. Vagal impairment is more common than sympathetic damage in diabetic patients. Evaluation of the response of HRV to physiologic stimulation such as active standing or passive tilt and exercise may be helpful in the early diagnosis of autonomic neuropathy, even in patients without significant decrease in HRV at rest.

Hypertrophic cardiomyopathy

Patients with hypertrophic cardiomyopathy are at increased risk of sudden cardiac death (2–4% in adults and 4–6% in children and adolescents). It is generally assumed that sudden cardiac death occurs as a result of ventricular arrhythmias. However, hemodynamic abnormalities may be important contributing factors in the pathogenesis of sudden cardiac death in these patients.

Proposed risk factors include syncope, a positive family history of sudden cardiac death, nonsustained ventricular tachycardia on Holter monitoring, young age at presentation, inducible ventricular tachycardia by programmed electrical stimulation, and increased fractionation of paced right ventricular electrograms. However, the positive predictive accuracy of these risk factors is low and questionable. HRV assessment does not help for identification of those who are at risk of sudden cardiac death in these patients.[31] Ajiki et al.[32] reported that there was an abnormal autonomic activity with sympathetic predominance, as assessed using spectral analysis of HRV, in patients with hypertrophic cardiomyopathy. However, we have not been able to confirm a sympathetic dominance in these patients. HRV is related to the presence of cardiac arrhythmias, exertional chest pain and an adverse family history. The exact underlying mechanisms are unclear.

Chronic valvular heart disease

It has been reported[33] that HRV measured as *SDANN* (the standard deviation of the 5-minute mean RR intervals) is associated with impaired right and left ventricular function and carries important prognostic information in patients with chronic severe mitral regurgitation. HRV predicts development of atrial fibrillation, mortality and progression to valve surgery in this patient population. Reduced HRV in aortic valve disease has recently been reported by Mandawat et al.[34] In contrast, these authors failed to demonstrate any significant association of HRV with left ventricular function (fractional shortening) or the presence of ventricular arrhythmias. However, HRV was significantly related to left ventricular mass index ($r = -0.48$, $p < 0.001$). Similar observations were made in hypertensive patients with left ventricular hypertrophy.

Syncope

Tilt testing has provided a useful clinical method for identification of patients with neurally mediated syncope and is now accepted as a valuable diagnostic maneuver in patients with syncope of unknown origin. As in normal subjects, tilt elicits a significant autonomic alteration in patients with syncope. Patients with vasovagal syndrome show an increased low-frequency component during tilt compared with controls, and this abnormal autonomic response can be prevented after propranolol therapy. Recently, Sneddon et al.[35] reported that there was no significant difference in HRV calculated from 24-hour Holter recordings in 17 patients with neurally mediated syncope compared with 17 control patients with unexplained syncope and a negative tilt test. However, these authors noted that these patients had augmented cardiopulmonary baroreceptor responses to orthostatic stress, which may play an important role in tilt-induced syncope. Furthermore, spectral analysis of HRV suggests impairment of the postprandial autonomic modulation of heart rate in healthy elderly patients, which may contribute to postprandial hypotension and syncope in dysautonomic subjects.

Chagas' disease

Chagas' disease (trypanosomiasis), which is caused by the protozoa *Trypanosoma cruzi*, is the commonest cause of chronic heart disease in Central and South America. It is characterized by a progressive chronic fibrotic myocarditis and degeneration of tissue that is innervated by the autonomic nervous system. Ventricular arrhythmias are a prominent feature of chronic Chagas' disease, and syncope and sudden cardiac death is not infrequent. Both an impaired vagal modulation of heart rate and a reduced sympathetic response have been reported in this clinical setting.

Preliminary observations[36] suggest that a significant alteration of HRV is detectable in patients with Chagas' disease in latent and intermittent phases. The usual responses of HRV to postural changes are attenuated in patients with positive serology without significant changes in HRV at rest. Spectral analysis of HRV has provided an assessment of autonomic function and has proven useful for evaluation of the clinical progression of the disease.

Long QT syndrome

The autonomic nervous system is believed to play an important role in the pathophysiology of this congenital syndrome. Data on the analysis of HRV in patients with long QT syndrome are scarce. Eggeling *et al.*[37] reported that both the low- and high-frequency components of HRV were significantly increased in patients with long QT syndrome compared with normal controls. This increased HRV could be decreased by beta-blocker therapy. Although these observations are partially in line with our knowledge about the long QT syndrome, the behavior of HRV in this setting requires further investigation before any definite conclusions can be drawn.

Catheter ablation of arrhythmias

Recently transcatheter radiofrequency ablation has provided an alternative nonpharmacological method for the management of cardiac arrhythmias. Using spectral analysis of HRV, Kocovic *et al.*[38] reported that radiofrequency ablation of supraventricular tachycardia in the anterior, mid and posterior region of the low interatrial septum may disrupt parasympathetic fibers located in these regions that are destined to innervate the sinus node. Parasympathetic denervation may be one mechanism for persistent inappropriate sinus tachycardia seen after radiofrequency ablation.

Life behavior

Several studies have been conducted to investigate the effects of *mental stress* on HRV. HRV is significantly reduced during mental stress in normal subjects and in patients with coronary artery disease with and without prior myocardial infarction. Recently, Pagani *et al.*[39] observed that psychological stress induced marked changes in sympathovagal balance, mainly characterized by sympathetic predominance. A significant difference in the change of HRV induced by stress has been observed between groups of highly anxious and less anxious women. These observations suggest that influence of emotion should be taken into account when interpreting the results of animal experiments or comparing HRV between different groups of patients.

The effect of acute *alcohol* ingestion on short-term heart rate fluctuations was reported by Gonzalez-Gonzalez *et al.*[40] They demonstrated that acute ingestion of a low dose of alcohol (0.3 g/kg) in 18 normal volunteers did not alter mean heart rate but spectral HRV was significantly changed: the low-frequency oscillations (0.02–0.06 Hz) increased, while middle (0.08–0.15 Hz) and high (0.20–0.35 Hz) frequency oscillations decreased. Acute alcohol intoxication (0.7 g/kg) also reduces HRV. Moderate drinking habits may not much influence HRV. HRV has been shown to be significantly lower in alcohol-dependent patients than in normal subjects. HRV was also depressed in chronic alcoholic neuropathy.

Cigarette smoking caused a transient and significant decrease in the high-frequency component and an increase in the low-frequency component of HRV. Long-term heavy smoking causes a decrease in the high-frequency component of HRV.

Caffeine has been shown to increase HRV in women.

Assessment of the Autonomic Effects of Drugs

Since autonomic activity plays an important role in both the electrical and the mechanical activities of the heart, pharmacological modulation of autonomic activity has been of great interest. However, little was known about drug effects on autonomic activity as there was no simple clinical method available for the assessment of autonomic function during normal daily activities until the recent emergence of HRV analysis. The influence of autonomic agents on HRV has greatly improved our understanding of the physiological basis underlying HRV and, in turn, analysis of HRV can be used to assess the autonomic effects of various drugs.

Reproducibility of HRV

Reproducibility of HRV measures is a prerequisite for the evaluation of drug effects on HRV. HRV is essentially stable over a short period in normal subjects and in patients with decreased cardiac function or ventricular arrhythmias despite significant interindividual HRV variations. This is also true in patients on drug therapy. There is no significant effect of placebo on HRV in normal subjects and in patients with and without cardiac failure. These observations suggest that analysis of HRV can be used for the assessment of pharmacological interventions on cardiac autonomic activity.

Effects of autonomic agents on HRV in normal subjects

Initially the physiological basis of HRV was mainly studied using autonomic blocking and stimulating agents. For example, Akselrod et al.[41] observed that, in the power spectrum of HRV obtained from a 5-minute recording in adult conscious dogs, three distinct components could be distinguished: a high-frequency peak at approximately 0.4 Hz, a mid-frequency peak at approximately 0.15 Hz, had a low-frequency peak at approximately 0.05 Hz. The high- and mid-frequency peaks were abolished and the power of the low-frequency peak was reduced by selective parasympathetic blockade, while combined beta-sympathetic and parasympathetic blockade abolished all frequency components of HRV.

The effect of *atropine* on HRV has been comprehensively studied. Several studies have documented that atropine decreases HRV in animals and in humans. A typical S-shaped dose–response curve has been demonstrated for atropine-induced changes in heart rate. Since vagal modulation of heart rate contributes to both the low-frequency and high-frequency components of HRV, atropine reduces overall HRV including the low- and high-frequency components. Since central anticholinergic agents also decrease HRV, central cholinergic receptors may also be involved in the modulation of heart rate. Ali Melkkila et al.[42] reported that high-dose atropine decreases HRV, while low-dose atropine may increase HRV. *Glycopyrrolate* and *hyoscine butylbromide* also reduce HRV.

Table 13.4 Potential reasons for variable effects of beta-blockers on heart rate variability

Influence of basal autonomic tone?
Influence of sympathovagal interaction?
Influence of pathophysiology of underlying heart disease (myocardial infarction, congestive heart failure)?
Influence of pharmacodynamics ($beta_1$ and $beta_2$ selectivity and intrinsic sympathetic activity)?
Influence of different technique?

Vagal activity is not only attenuated by atropine, but is also modulated by vagomimetic agents. In contrast to the peripheral vagolytic action of high-dose *scopolamine*, low-dose scopolamine exerts a vagomimetic effect. Low-dose transdermal scopolamine has been shown to increase HRV in normal subjects.

Beta-adrenergic stimulation by *isoproterenol* increases the low-frequency component of HRV in normal subjects. However, *beta-blockade* has variable effects on HRV. It may increase, decrease or not affect HRV. Basal autonomic tone may account for the different responses of HRV to beta-blockade. This variable effect of beta-blockade on HRV is consistent with observations of the uncertain significance of the contribution of sympathetic activity to HRV. It has been reported[43] that increased HRV accompanies beta-blockade only in the absence of intrinsic sympathetic activity when bradycardia ensues. Therefore, increase in HRV may reflect augmented vagal tone induced by beta-blockade. Basal state of cardiac vagal tone in various study conditions may be important to the effects of beta-blockers on HRV. The potential explanations for variable effects of beta-blockers on HRV are listed in Table 13.4. Although beta-blockade has significant influence on HRV (principally increases HRV), the effects of *alpha-blockade* on HRV have not been studied. Propranolol suppresses the increase in all frequency components of HRV during tilt in patients with vasovagal syncope. It is interesting to note that HRV is usually decreased in clinical settings associated with increased sympathetic activity. This depressed HRV associated with increased sympathetic activity may be partially explained by subsequent sympathovagal interaction in addition to an increased heart rate.

Effects of antiarrhythmic drugs on HRV

Since the autonomic nervous system plays an important role in the pathogenesis of ventricular tachyarrhythmias, the effects of antiarrhythmic drugs on HRV is of special clinical interest.

Autonomic nervous system function may influence the efficacy of antiarrhythmic drugs under some circumstances. Currently available data suggest that most antiarrhythmic agents decrease HRV. This may be due to their vagolytic or beta-blocking properties.

In a study of 15 patients with ventricular arrhythmias, for example, Lombardi *et al.*[44] showed that *propafenone* significantly decreased the low-frequency component but increased the high-frequency component of HRV, resulting in a significant decrease in the low-to-high ratio (Figure 13.7). Zuanetti *et al.*[45] also reported a significant decrease in HRV (number of times in which the change in successive RR interval was greater than 50 ms, $\approx$ *pNN50*) in patients with ventricular arrhythmias treated with *flecainide* or *propafenone*. This decrease in HRV was reversible with discontinuation of treatment and was not related to arrhythmia suppression, since 24-hour HRV was similar during treatment irrespective of the presence or absence of frequent arrhythmias. This study, using *pNN50* as a measure of HRV, does not preclude a possible relationship between the effects of antiarrhythmic drugs on arrhythmias and those on spectral HRV.

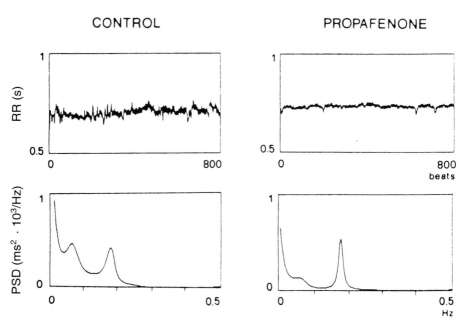

Figure 13.7 Effects of propafenone on spectral heart rate variability in patients with ventricular arrhythmias. The top shows tachograms and the bottom shows autospectra. Note the decreased LF component and an increased HF component of heart rate variability after propafenone. PSD = power spectrum density. (Reproduced with permission from reference 44)

A significant relationship between an increase in *pNN50* and suppression of ventricular ectopic beats has recently been demonstrated. In the study of Zuanetti *et al.*, *amiodarone* was found to have no significant influence on *pNN50* in patients with ventricular arrhythmias. We have noted that low-dose amiodarone (200 mg daily) did not significantly influence spectral HRV in patients with hypertrophic cardiomyopathy, although it significantly reduced heart rate and prolonged QT in a use-independent manner. Hohnloser *et al.*[46] have reported that *sotalol* produced a significant increase in the high-frequency component of HRV but caused no change in the low-frequency component in patients with chronic ventricular arrhythmias.

Several studies have demonstrated that drug effects on HRV are independent of their effects on heart rate. There is evidence that chronic beta-adrenergic blockade leads to a reduction in sympathetic efferent activity and a change in myocardial electrophysiological properties, whereas acute blockade may not have the same effects. However, both acute and chronic administration of *propranolol* has been shown to significantly alter HRV. Although the value of beta-blockers in the prevention of sudden cardiac death has been relatively well established, data on the effects of propranolol on HRV in patients with ventricular arrhythmias are inconclusive. Further studies are needed to define the effect of propranolol on HRV in high-risk patients with and without myocardial infarction. The effects of antiarrhythmic drugs on HRV are summarized in Table 13.5.

Data on the relationship between antiarrhythmic drug-induced alterations of HRV and the drugs' antiarrhythmic and proarrhythmic actions are scarce, although this relationship is obviously important for our understanding of the mechanisms underlying the electrophysiological effects of antiarrhythmic drugs. Bigger *et al.*[47] recently reported that antiarrhythmic drug-induced changes in HRV were not a significant predictor of all-cause mortality during a one-year follow-up after myocardial infarction. However, this

Table 13.5   Effects of antiarrhythmic drugs on HRV

Drug class	Drug	Change of HRV
Class I		
a	Procainamide	Decreases HRV
b	Mexiletine	Decreases RR variance but not normalized LF and HF
c	Propranolol	Decreases HRV but increases normalized LF
	Flecainide	Decreases *pNN50* but does not affect normalized LF and HF
Class II		
	Metoprolol	Increases *SDNN* and *pNN50*
	Propanolol	Increases *SDNN*, *pNN50* and HF
Class III		
	Amiodarone	Does not affect HRV
	Sotalol	Increases *SDNN*, *pNN50* and HF but does not affect LF
Class IV		
	Diltiazem	Decreases *SDNN*
	Nifedipine	No consistent change

HF = high-frequency component of heart rate variability; HRV = heart rate variability; LF = low-frequency component of heart rate variability; *pNN50* = proportion of adjacent intervals more than 50 ms different; *SDNN* = standard deviation of all normal RR intervals.

study does not preclude a possible relationship between antiarrhythmic drug-induced changes in autonomic function and vulnerability to ventricular tachyarrhythmias, although drug-induced changes in ventricular repolarization may be more relevant.

Effects of drugs on HRV in patients following myocardial infarction

Although the predictive value of HRV has been well studied in patients following acute myocardial infarction, few studies address the effect of drugs on HRV in this clinical setting. As in normal subjects, beta-blockers can either decrease (propranolol) or increase (metoprolol) HRV in patients following acute myocardial infarction. Bekheit *et al.*[48] reported that *metoprolol* reduces the low-frequency component of HRV during tilt in patients following myocardial infarction. Since propranolol is a nonselective beta-blocker whereas metoprolol is a beta$_1$-blocker, the differential effects of beta$_1$ and beta$_2$ blockade on HRV is unclear. More recently, Niemelä *et al.*[49] reported that atenolol and metoprolol significantly increased the high-frequency component of HRV to a similar extent (64% versus 62%). These authors also demonstrated that beta-blockade did not significantly influence the circadian rhythm of HRV, but both atenolol and metoprolol blunted the abrupt decrease of the high-frequency component of HRV after arousal.

Scopolamine increases HRV in patients following acute myocardial infarction,[50] as in normal subjects. In a randomized, placebo-controlled study of 61 patients (mean age 58 ± 10 years, left ventricular ejection fraction 44.7 ± 15.5%), 6 days (median) following acute myocardial infarction, Vybiral *et al.*[50] demonstrated that time-domain HRV increases 26–35% in patients given low-dose scopolamine (*n* = 30) compared with patients given placebo (*n* = 31). These authors suggest that this effect of scopolamine on autonomic tone may provide an alternative approach to autonomic modulation for the prevention of sudden cardiac death, particularly in patients in whom beta-blockers are contraindicated.

Bekheit *et al.*[48] have reported that *diltiazem* reduces the low-frequency component of HRV but *nifedipine* does not have consistent effects on HRV in patients following myocardial infarction. Whether drug-induced autonomic alteration in HRV is also associated with a change in prognosis following acute myocardial infarction has yet to be determined. The fact of the spontaneous recovery of HRV following acute myocardial infarction should be taken into account when studying the effects of drugs on HRV in such patients.

Effects of drugs on HRV in patients with congestive heart failure

Angiotensin converting enzyme inhibition may not significantly affect HRV in subjects without cardiac dysfunction. However, *angiotensin converting enzyme inhibitors* consistently improve the depressed HRV in patients with congestive heart failure.[51] Augmentation of parasympathetic tone by angiotensin converting enzyme inhibitors may contribute to their beneficial effect in the treatment of patients with congestive heart failure.

It has been noted that angiotensin II produces a decrease in vagal tone and an increase in sympathetic activity and that blockade of the renin–angiotensin system is involved in the modulation of HRV (the low-frequency component). The removal of central suppression of vagal tone by angiotensin II may be involved in the mechanism underlying the effect of angiotensin converting enzyme inhibition on autonomic tone. In patients with heart failure, there is an abnormal autonomic response to changes in arterial and/or intracardiac pressure and baroreflex sensitivity is also significantly altered. There is evidence that angiotensin II inhibits the baroreceptor reflex and that angiotensin converting enzyme inhibitor therapy improves baroreflex sensitivity in animals and in humans. This improvement in baroreflex sensitivity may contribute to the augmentation of HRV in patients with congestive heart failure. Benedict *et al.*[52] have recently reported that decreased left ventricular ejection fraction plays an important role in the activation of neurohormones in patients with heart failure. Since HRV is also significantly related to left ventricular function, drug-induced alteration of autonomic tone may be partially secondary to the improvement of pathophysiology of this disease caused by drug therapy (including cardiac function and peripheral hemodynamic changes).

Owing to the failure of *encainide* and *flecainide* to reduce mortality after myocardial infarction, and the uncertain role of low-dose *amiodarone* in the prevention of sudden cardiac death and/or reduction of overall mortality in patients with decreased left ventricular function, attention has shifted towards other treatment strategies. Beta-adrenergic blockers may constitute one such approach for the prevention of sudden cardiac death in patients with left ventricular dysfunction, since trials have shown that beta-blockers lead to a consistent reduction in mortality in patients following myocardial infarction, with and without depressed left ventricular function. Correction of autonomic dysfunction may explain the contribution of beta-blockers to improve survival in these patients. At present, little is known about the effects of beta-blockade on HRV in patients with congestive heart failure.

Digoxin has been demonstrated to increase HRV in both time and frequency domains and to decrease the low-to-high frequency ratio in normal subjects.[53] These changes are independent of the effect of digoxin on mean heart rate, since there is no significant change in mean heart rate in patients treated with digoxin compared with those receiving placebo. There is also evidence that digoxin may also affect HRV in patients with congestive heart failure. *Flosequinan* increases the HF and decreases the LF components of HRV despite increasing the heart rate.

Effects on HRV in hypertensive subjects

Several studies have demonstrated that *clonidine* reduces HRV, but *angiotensin converting enzyme inhibitors* either increase or do not affect HRV. Beta-blockade (*atenolol*) has been shown to partially normalize the abnormal spectrum of HRV in hypertensive patients.

Effects of anesthetics on HRV

Several studies have demonstrated that HRV is significantly decreased by anesthesia. It seems that *diazepam* decreases HRV in a dose-dependent manner. A central nervous system mechanism is likely to be involved in the negative influence of sedatives, analgesics and anesthetics on HRV. Since mental activity may also significantly influence HRV in normal subjects and in patients following myocardial infarction, elimination of emotional influences might therefore contribute to the changes in HRV observed during anesthesia.

Effects of other agents on HRV

The fact that HRV decreases after treatment in patients with thyrotoxicosis suggests that *thyroid hormones* may increase HRV. Lethal doses of *cocaine* have been shown to cause a marked decrease in HRV prior to sudden death in conscious ferrets.

Effects of nonpharmacologic interventions on HRV

Exercise training has been shown to increase vagal activity in normal subjects, in patients following myocardial infarction and in patients with congestive heart failure. Exercise training seems to reduce the risk of death in patients following myocardial infarction. There is evidence that biofeedback or self-management training increases vagal tone in sudden cardiac death survivors.

In summary, many drugs have a significant influence on HRV, either directly or indirectly (e.g. through drug-induced hemodynamic changes). The majority of these findings may be explained by their parasympathetic and/or sympathetic blocking or stimulating effects. However, the results of different studies do not always agree, especially on the effects of beta-blockers on HRV. This discrepancy may be due to a different basal state of cardiac vagal tone in a variety of study conditions. In addition, other factors influencing drug effects, such as underlying heart disease and left ventricular dysfunction, may also contribute to inconsistent drug effects on HRV. Nonetheless, analysis of HRV has provided a useful noninvasive method for the assessment of pharmacologic modulation of cardiac autonomic function. From the viewpoint of the clinician, drugs which influence HRV other than ordinary muscarinic and adrenergic agonists and antagonists (such as antiarrhythmic drugs) should be included in the category of autonomic pharmacology. Assessment of drug effects on HRV will further improve our understanding of their pharmacologic mechanisms and suggest strategies of treatment aimed at modification of autonomic nervous system function.

Summary

During the last decade, HRV has been studied in almost all aspects of clinical cardiology and our knowledge about autonomic nervous system function in these clinical settings has been greatly improved. Analysis of HRV has been generally accepted as a noninvasive method for the assessment of autonomic influence on the heart.

HRV for risk stratification. Depressed HRV is a new and powerful risk factor following myocardial infarction. The predictive value of HRV is independent of other parameters established for postinfarction risk stratification, such as left ventricular ejection fraction, ventricular ectopic activity and late potentials. For prediction of all-cause mortality, the value of HRV is similar to that of left ventricular ejection fraction, while HRV is superior to left ventricular ejection fraction in predicting arrhythmic events. HRV, singly or in combination with other risk factors, significantly improves the positive predictive accuracy for death. HRV has also been studied as a stratification technique in survivors of cardiac arrest, congestive heart failure and hypertrophic cardiomyopathy. The data on stratification value of HRV in these patients are few.

HRV for assessment of autonomic influence on the heart. Assessment of HRV and thereby autonomic activity is of great clinical significance, particularly in certain clinical settings such as cardiac arrhythmias, cardiac failure and diabetic autonomic neuropathy. HRV is markedly reduced in patients with congestive heart failure. This decreased HRV is related to the severity of left ventricular dysfunction and can be improved after successful treatments. Changes in HRV (autonomic influence) prior to the onset of ventricular tachyarrhythmias may contribute to arrhythmogenesis. HRV analysis has provided an insight into the autonomic aspects of essential hypertension, chronic ischemic heart disease and other local and systemic disorders. Assessment of HRV is a useful clinical method for monitoring autonomic nervous system function and can be used for evaluation of the effects of pharmacological and nonpharmacological interventions. Of particular interest is the autonomic modulation induced by antiarrhythmic drugs.

References

1. Kleiger RE, Miller JP, Bigger JT, Moss AJ, and the Multicenter Post-Infarction Research Group. Decreased heart rate variability and its association with increased mortality after acute myocardial infarction. *Am J Cardiol* 1987; **59**: 256–62.
2. Hayano J, Sakakibara Y, Yamada M, Ohte N, Fujinami T, Yokoyama K, Watanabe Y, Takata K. Decreased magnitude of heart rate spectral components in coronary artery disease: its relation to angiographic severity. *Circulation* 1990; **81**: 1217–24.
3. Nolan J, Flapan AD, Reid J, Neilson JM, Bloomfield P, Ewing DJ. Cardiac parasympathetic activity in severe uncomplicated coronary artery disease. *Br Heart J* 1994; **71**: 515–20.
4. Wolf MM, Varigos GA, Hunt D, Sloman JG. Sinus arrhythmia in acure myocardial infarction. *Med J Aust* 1978; **2**: 52–3.
5. Farrell TG, Bashir Y, Cripps T, Malik M, Poloniecki J, Bennett ED, Ward DE, Camm AJ. Risk stratification for arrhythmic events in postinfarction patients based on heart rate variability, ambulatory electrocardiographic variables and the signal-averaged electrocardiogram. *J Am Coll Cardiol* 1991; **18**: 687–97.
6. Bigger JT, Fleiss JL, Steinman RC, Rolnitzky LM, Kleiger RE, Rottman JN. Frequency domain measures of heart rate variability and mortality after myocardial infarction. *Circulation* 1992; **85**: 164–71.
7. Billman GE, Hoskins RS. Time-series analysis of heart rate variability during submaximal exercise: evidence for reduced cardiac vagal tone in animals susceptible to ventricular fibrillation. *Circulation* 1989; **80**: 146–57.
8. Adamson PB, Huang MH, Vanoli E, Foreman RD, Schwartz PJ, Hull SS. Unexpected interaction between beta-adrenergic blockade and heart rate variability before and after myocardial infarction: a longitudinal study in dogs at high and low risk of sudden death. *Circulation* 1994; **90**: 976–82.
9. Hull SS, Evans AR, Vanoli E, Adamson PB, Stramba-Badiale M, Albert DE, Foreman RD, Schwartz PJ. Heart rate variability before and after myocardial infarction in conscious dogs at high and low risk of sudden death. *J Am Coll Cardiol* 1990; **16**: 978–85.
10. Odemuyiwa O, Malik M, Farrell T, Bashir, Y, Poloniecki J, Camm AJ. Comparison of the predictive characteristics of heart rate variability index and left ventricular ejection fraction for all-cause mortality, arrhythmic events and sudden death after acute myocardial infarction. *Am J Cardiol* 1991; **68**: 434–9.
11. Huikuri H, Koistinen MJ, Yli-Mäyry S, Airaksinen KE, Ikäheimo MJ, Myerburg RJ. Impaired very low frequency oscillation of heart rate in patients with life threatening arrhythmias (abstract). *J Am Coll Cardiol* 1994; **23**: 38A.
12. Bigger JT, Fleiss JL, Rolnitzky LM, Steinman RC. The ability of several short-term measures of RR variability to predict mortality after myocardial infarction. *Circulation* 1993; **88**: 927–34.
13. Pedretti R, Etro MD, Laporta A, Braga SS, Carù B. Prediction of late arrhythmic events after acute myocardial infarction from combined use of noninvasive prognostic variables and inducibility of sustained monomorphic ventricular tachycardia. *Am J Cardiol* 1993; **71**: 1131–41.
14. Bigger JT, La Rovere MT, Steinman RC, Fleiss JL, Rottman JN, Rolnitzky LM, Schwartz PJ. Comparison of baroreflex sensitivity and heart period variability after myocardial infarction. *J Am Coll Cardiol* 1989; **14**: 1511–18.
15. Farrell TG, Paul V, Cripps TR, Malik M, Bennett ED, Ward DE, Camm AJ. Baroreflex sensitivity and electrophysiological correlates in patients after acute myocardial infarction. *Circulation* 1991; **83**: 945–52.
16. La Rovere MT, Specchia G, Mortara A, Schwartz PJ. Baroreflex sensitivity, clinical correlates, and cardiovascular mortality among patients with a first myocardial infarction: a prospective study. *Circulation* 1988; **78**: 816–24.

17. Farrell TG, Odemuyiwa O, Bashir Y, Cripps TR, Malik M, Ward DE, Camm AJ. Prognostic value of baroreflex sensitivity testing after acute myocardial infarction. *Br Heart J* 1992; **67**: 129–37.

18. Hinkle LE, Carver ST, Plakun A. Slow heart rates and increased risk of cardiac death in middle-aged men. *Arch Intern Med* 1972; **129**: 732–48.

19. Dougherty CM, Burr RL. Comparisons of heart rate variability in survivors and nonsurvivors of sudden cardiac arrest. *Am J Cardiol* 1992; **70**: 441–8.

20. Lü Fei, Anderson MH, Katritsis D, Sneddon J, Statters DJ, Malik M, Camm AJ. Decreased heart rate variability in sudden cardiac death survivors not associated with coronary artery disease. *Br Heart J* 1994; **71**: 16–21.

21. Algra A, Tijssen JG, Roelandt JR, Pool J, Lubsen J. Heart rate variability from 24-hour electrocardiography and the two-year risk for sudden death. *Circulation* 1993; **88**: 180–5.

22. Tsuji H, Venditti FJ, Manders ES, Evans JC, Larson MG, Feldman CL, Levy DL. Reduced heart rate variability and mortality risk in an elderly cohort: the Framingham Heart Study. *Circulation* 1994; **90**: 878–83.

23. Lü Fei, Statters DJ, Hnatkova K, Poloniecki J, Malik M, Camm AJ. Change of the autonomic influence on the heart immediately before the onset of spontaneous idiopathic ventricular tachycardia. *J Am Coll Cardiol* 1994; **24**: 1515–22.

24. Eriksson H, Svärdsudd K, Larsson B, Ohlson LO, Tibblin G, Welin L, Wilhelmsen L. Risk factors for heart failure in the general population: the study of men born in 1913. *Eur Heart J* 1989; **10**: 647–56.

25. Binder T, Frey B, Porenta G, Heinz G, Wutte M, Kreiner G, Gössinger H, Schmidinger H, Pacher R, Weber H. Prognostic value of heart rate variability in patients awaiting cardiac transplantation. *PACE* 1992; **15**: 2215–20.

26. Lü Fei, Keeling PJ, Gill JS, Bashir Y, Statters DJ, Poloniecki J, McKenna WJ, Camm AJ. Heart rate variability and its relation to ventricular arrhythmias in congestive heart failure. *Br Heart J* 1994; **71**: 322–8.

27. Sands KE, Appel ML, Lilly LS, Schoen FJ, Mudge GH, Cohen RJ. Power spectrum analysis of heart rate variability in human cardiac transplant recipients. *Circulation* 1989; **79**: 76–82.

28. Guzzetti S, Piccaluga E, Casati R, Cerutti S, Lombardi F, Pagani M, Malliani A. Sympathetic predominance in essential hypertension: a study employing spectral analysis of heart rate variability. *J Hypertens* 1988; **6**: 711–17.

29. Wheeler T, Watkins PJ. Cardiac denervation in diabetes. *Br Med J* 1973; **4**: 584–6.

30. Ewing DJ, Neilson JM, Travis P. New method for assessing cardiac parasympathetic activity using 24-hour electrocardiograms. *Br Heart J* 1984; **52**: 396–402.

31. Counihan PJ, Lü Fei, Bashir Y, Farrell TG, Haywood GA, McKenna WJ. Assessment of heart rate variability in hypertrophic cardiomyopathy: association with clinical and prognostic features. *Circulation* 1993; **88**: 1682–90.

32. Ajiki K, Murakawa Y, Yanagisawa-Miwa A, Usui M, Yamashita T, Oikawa N, Inoue H. Autonomic nervous system activity in idiopathic dilated cardiomyopathy and in hypertrophic cardiomyopathy. *Am J Cardiol* 1993; **71**: 1316–20.

33. Stein KM, Borer JS, Hochreiter C, Okin PM, Herrold E, Devereux RB, Kligfield P. Prognostic value and physiological correlates of heart rate variability in chronic severe mitral regurgitation. *Circulation* 1993; **88**: 127–35.

34. Mandawat MK, Wallbridge DR, Pringle SD, Riyami AA, Latif S, Macfarlane PW, Lorimer AR, Cobbe SM. Heart rate variability in left ventricular hypertrophy. *Br Heart J* 1995; **73**: 139–44.

35. Sneddon JF, Counihan PJ, Bashir Y, Haywood GA, Ward DE, Camm AJ. Assessment of autonomic function in patients with neurally mediated syncope: augmented cardiopulmonary baroreceptor responses to graded orthostatic stress. *J Am Coll Cardiol* 1993; **21**: 1193–8.

36. Loyo LG, Puigbó JJ, Pérez DV, Moleiro F, Barroyeta R, Braun I, Ruggiero A. Autonomic dysfunction evidenced by heart rate variability abnormalities in latent or indeterminate phase of Chagas' disease (abstract). *J Am Coll Cardiol* 1994; **23**: 151A.

37. Eggeling T, Osterhues H, Höher M, Kochs M. Influence of beta-blocker therapy on heart rate variability in patients with long QT syndrome (abstract). *Circulation* 1993; **88**: I-116.

38. Kocovic DZ, Harada T, Shea JB, Soroff D, Friedman PL. Alterations of heart rate and of heart rate variability after radio frequency catheter ablation of supraventricular tachycardia: delineation of parasympathetic pathways in the human heart. *Circulation* 1993; **88**: 1671–81.

39. Pagani M, Mazzuero G, Ferrari A, Liberati D, Cerutti S, Vaitl D, Tavazzi L, Malliani A. Sympathovagal interaction during mental stress: a study using spectral analysis of heart rate variability in healthy control subjects and patients with a prior myocardial infarction. *Circulation* 1991; **83**: II-43–51.

40. Gonzalez-Gonzalez J, Mendez-Llorens A, Mendez-Novoa A, Cordero-Valeriano JJ. Effect of alcohol ingestion on short term heart rate fluctuations. *J Stud Alcohol* 1992; **53**: 86–90.

41. Akselrod S, Gordon D, Ubel FA, Shannon DC, Barger AC. Power spectrum analysis of heart rate fluctuation: a quantitative probe of beat-to-beat cardiovascular control. *Science* 1981; **213**(4504): 220–22.

42. Ali Melkkila T, Kaila T, Antila K, Halkola L, Iisalo E. Effects of glycopyrrolate and atropine on heart rate variability. *Acta Anaesthesiol Scand* 1991; **35**: 436–41.

43. Bittiner SB, Smith SE. Beta-adrenoceptor antagonists increase sinus arrhythmia, a vagotonic effect. *Br J Clin Pharmacol* 1986; **22**: 691–5.

44. Lombardi F, Torzillo D, Sandrone G, Dalla-Vecchia L, Finocchiaro ML, Bernasconi R, Cappiello E. Beta-blocking effect of propafenone based on spectral analysis of heart rate variability. *Am J Cardiol* 1992; **70**: 1028–34.

45. Zuanetti G, Latini R, Neilson JM, Schwartz PJ, Ewing DJ. Heart rate variability in patients with ventricular arrhythmias: effects of antiarrhythmic drugs. *J Am Coll Cardiol* 1991; **17**: 604–12.

46. Hohnloser SH, Klingenheben T, Zabel M, Just H. Effect of sotalol on heart rate variability assessed by Holter monitoring in patients with ventricular arrhythmias. *Am J Cardiol* 1993; **72**: 67A–71A.

47. Bigger JT, Rolnitzky LM, Steinman RC, Fleiss JL. Predicting mortality after myocardial infarction from the response of RR variability to antiarrhythmic drug therapy. *J Am Coll Cardiol* 1994; **23**: 733–40.

48. Bekheit S, Tangella M, El-Sakr A, Rasheed Q, Craelius W, El-Sherif N. Use of heart rate spectral analysis to study the effects of calcium channel blockers on sympathetic activity after myocardial infarction. *Am Heart J* 1990; **119**: 79–85.
49. Niemelä MJ, Airaksinen KE, Huikuri HV. Effect of beta-blockade on heart rate variability in patients with coronary artery disease. *J Am Coll Cardiol* 1994; **23**: 1370–77.
50. Vybiral T, Glaeser DH, Morris G, Hess KR, Yang K, Francis M, Pratt CM. Effects of low-dose transdermal scopolamine on heart rate variability in acute myocardial infarction. *J Am Coll Cardiol* 1993; **22**: 1320–26.
51. Flapan AD, Nolan J, Neilson JM, Ewing DJ. Effect of captopril on parasympathetic activity in congestive cardiac failure secondary to coronary artery disease. *Am J Cardiol* 1992; **69**: 532–5.
52. Benedict CR, Johnstone DE, Weiner DH, Bourassa MG, Bittner V, Kay R, Kirlin P, Greenberg B, Kohn RM, Nicklas JM, McIntyre K, Quinones MA, Yusuf S, and the SOLVD Investigators. Relation of neurohumoral activation to clinical variables and degree of ventricular dysfunction: a report from the Registry of Studies of Left Ventricular Dysfunction. *J Am Coll Cardiol* 1994; **23**: 1410–20.
53. Kaufman ES, Bosner MS, Bigger JT, Stein PK, Kleiger RE, Rolnitzky LM, Steinman RC, Fleiss JL. Effects of digoxin and enalapril on heart period variability and response to head-up tilt in normal subjects. *Am J Cardiol* 1993; **72**: 95–9.

SECTION IV

High-Resolution Electrocardiography

Introduction by Nabil El-Sherif

There are several low-level electrocardiographic (ECG) potentials whose manifestations on the body surface are too small to be detected by routine measurement techniques. These include the potentials produced by the His–Purkinje system and by slow, nonhomogeneous conduction in depressed ventricular myocardium (usually called 'late potentials'). These potentials are small because the activation front is slow and fractionated or the mass of tissue undergoing depolarization is small, or both. However, measurement of the bioelectric potentials produced by these tissues is important for diagnostic purposes. Identification of the His–Purkinje potential can localize the site of atrioventricular conduction disorders, and detection of late potentials may identify patients at high risk for malignant ventricular tachyarrhythmias. The problem in identifying these potentials is that the signal is smaller than the electrical noise produced by various sources. Two different techniques have been adopted to improve the signal-to-noise ratio (SNR):

1. *Ensemble or temporal averaging* (usually referred to as 'signal averaging'). This technique is applicable only to repetitive electrocardiographic signals and cannot detect moment-by-moment dynamic changes in the signals.
2. *Spatial averaging.* This technique can record the His–Purkinje signal and late potentials on a beat-to-beat basis.

The signal-averaged (SA) technique has been utilized more often in the last few years, and the averaged signal can be analyzed in either time domain, frequency domain, or a combination of both time and frequency display in the form of spectrotemporal maps. The term 'high-resolution ECG' should be considered to encompass any technique that results in improvement of the signal-to-noise ratio. This includes both temporal and spatial averaging techniques.

Time-Domain Signal-Averaged ECGs

Time-domain analysis of the SAECG derives data from the QRS vector magnitude (the root-mean-square of averaged X, Y and Z leads) that has been subjected to bandpass digital filters. The analysis usually includes determination of three typical parameters: (1) the filtered QRS duration (*QRSD*), (2) the root-mean-square voltage of the terminal 40 ms of the QRS (*RMS 40*), and (3) the duration of the low-amplitude signal; i.e. the time that the filtered QRS complex remains below 40 μV (*LAS 40*).

According to the Task Force Committee of the European Society of Cardiology, as well as the American Heart Association and the American College of Cardiology,[1] the definition of a late potential and the scoring of an SAECG as normal or abnormal have not yet been standardized. Representative criteria include that a late potential exists (using 40 Hz highpass bidirectional filtering) when (1) the filtered QRS complex is greater than 114 ms; (2) there is less than 20 μV of signal in the last 40 ms of the vector magnitude complex; and (3) the terminal vector magnitude complex remains below 40 μV for more than 38 ms. Other criteria have been used, and the predictive value varies with the specific criterion applied and the prevalence of disease in the population studied; for example, a vector magnitude complex of less than 25 μV at 25 Hz and less than 16 μV at 40 Hz highpass filtering.[2] At present it is suggested that each laboratory should define its own normal values.

The most common clinical application of time-domain SAECG is risk stratification of postinfarction patients for vulnerability to malignant ventricular tachyarrhythmias.[3] Risk stratification of patients with remote infarction and nonsustained ventricular tachycardia (VT) constitutes another application. Studies have demonstrated that patients with abnormal SAECG are more prone to inducible sustained monomorphic VT. The SAECG could be used for both risk stratification and management of those patients.[4] The SAECG could also be applied to investigate unexplained syncope, for the evaluation of the results of thrombolytic therapy and antiarrhythmic surgery, and for the recognition of acute rejection in patients with cardiac transplant. Other applications are risk stratification for serious arrhythmic events in patients with organic heart disease other than coronary artery disease, like hypertrophic cardiomyopathy, idiopathic dilated cardiomyopathy, right ventricular dysplasia, etc. Signal-averaging of the P wave has also been used to detect patients susceptible to paroxysmal atrial fibrillation.

The Need for Different Criteria of Time-Domain SAECGs

Two general approaches have been used to derive criteria for an abnormal time-domain SAECG. The first approach investigated 'normal' study groups to obtain 'upper limits' for the normal SAECG. This approach has been criticized because 'normal' study groups are not representative of the population with coronary artery disease. The second approach evaluated the predictive value of the SAECG criteria for patients with spontaneous and/or inducible sustained VT. In this group of patients, the time-domain SAECG criteria reflecting the presence of late potentials (i.e. *RMS 40* and/or *LAS 40*) were usually the most predictive. The electrophysiologic rationale for the predictive value of these criteria was that late potentials represent the slowed and disorganized conduction of localized myocardial zones that could provide the anatomic–electrophysiologic substrate for re-entrant VT. It does not necessarily follow that these criteria would also be predictive in the postmyocardial infarction (MI) period where the majority of serious arrhythmic events are fatal ventricular tachyarrhythmias rather than nonfatal sustained VT.[5]

The above concept is justified by the results of a recent multicenter NIH-sponsored study that was conducted to define the best predictive criteria of time-domain SAECG in the post-MI period.[5] A cohort of 1160 patients was followed for an average of 10.3 $\pm$ 3.2 months. Forty-five patients (4.3%) suffered serious arrhythmic events (42 sudden cardiac deaths judged to be due to arrhythmias, and 3 nonfatal sustained VT). Using the Cox proportional hazards regression model, and controlling for clinical variables that showed a significant difference, the SAECG parameters were found to be independently predictive of arrhythmic events. A filtered *QRSD* of at least 120 provided the best predictive criterion. The addition of other dichotomized SAECG parameters did not improve the predictive value of the test. Thus in this study, the signal-averaged *QRSD* at a 40 Hz highpass filter was found to be the single best predictive criterion for subsequent serious arrhythmic events. The electrophysiologic rationale as to why this parameter best predicts fatal arrhythmic events in the first year post-MI is not clear. However, it is possible that this may reflect the slowed and nonhomogeneous conduction of a larger mass of ventricular myocardium. Such hearts may be more vulnerable to fast VT/VF.

Frequency-Domain Signal-Averaged ECGs

Current techniques for time-domain late potential analysis have several limitations. As mentioned earlier, there is a lack of agreement at present as to the optimal filter characteristics, as well as to the best numerical criteria of abnormality. The numerical measurements are sensitive to the specific algorithm used for determining QRS termination. In the presence of intraventricular conduction defect and/or bundle branch block, which many patients at potential risk have, interpretation of late potentials may be difficult. Several authors have reported promising results employing frequency analysis techniques for VT risk assessment. Cain and associates performed a fast Fourier transform (FFT), after Blackman Harris windowing, upon a variable length of SAECG from each orthogonal lead X, Y and Z comprising the terminal 40 ms of the QRS complex in addition to the whole of the ST segment.[6] Abnormality was indicated by the presence of increased signal components in the 20–50 Hz range as measured by a variety of indices (area ratio or magnitude ratio) whose numerical definitions have been somewhat modified over the course of subsequent publications. However, several authors have shown that this technique is sensitive to the position and duration of the signal. Because of the limitations of the traditional FFT technique, several investigators utilized a spectrotemporal technique. The rationale for this technique is the observation that the QRS, late potentials, and ST segment waveforms in the SAECG have different spectral characteristics; or, in other words, that the ECG signal has a time-varying spectrum. However, some techniques that utilize a 'normality factor' analysis were shown to be nonreproducible, primarily because of sensitivity of the measurement to QRS offset localization.

A novel frequency-domain analysis technique, which may overcome some of the disadvantages of both time-domain late potential analysis and previously advocated methods of frequency analysis, is called 'spectral turbulence analysis'.[7] In this technique, the hallmark of arrhythmogenic abnormality is postulated to be frequent and abrupt changes in the frequency signature of QRS wavefront velocity as it propagates throughout the ventricle around and across areas of abnormal conduction, resulting in a high degree of spectral turbulence. This technique was initially shown to provide a more accurate marker for the anatomic–electrophysiologic substrate of re-entrant tachyarrhythmias. However, recent studies suggest that the spectral turbulence criteria for prediction of inducible sustained VT may not apply for risk stratification of post-MI patients and that a different set of criteria in these patients is required.[8]

Combined Time- and Frequency-Domain Analysis of SAECGs

One of the limitations of time-domain late potentials analysis of the SAECG is that partial obscuring of late potentials may occur if the abnormal myocardial region is activated relatively early during the QRS complex. This occurs more often with anterior wall (AW)

MI than inferior wall (IW) MI and may partially explain the higher incidence of false-positive abnormal recordings in patients with IWMI. On the other hand there is a higher incidence of abnormal spectral turbulence in AWMI compared with IWMI leading to a high incidence of false-positive abnormal test results in patients with AWMI. A recent study investigated the hypothesis that combined time-domain (TD) and spectrotemporal (ST) analysis of the SAECG could improve its predictive accuracy in post-MI patients.[8] Combined TD/ST was found to significantly improve the positive predictive accuracy of the test to 35% in the total group and to 40% in patients with first AWMI or IWMI. The best results were obtained in patients with first AWMI where the positive predictive accuracy of combined analysis was 50%.

Conclusions

Time-domain SAECG has been established as a useful test for risk stratification of malignant ventricular tachyarrhythmias in the post-MI period. It has a very high negative predictive accuracy but a relatively low positive predictive power. That is why it is suggested that the test be utilized as part of an algorithm in conjunction with several other risk stratifiers like ejection fraction, ambulatory arrhythmias, heart rate variability, etc. Holter monitoring with high-frequency capability (1000 Hz) would permit the simultaneous analysis of the SAECG in the time and frequency domains with arrhythmia and heart rate variability parameters.

The most urgent technical requirement is to standardize the algorithm for detection of QRS offset among different commercial machines so that clinical data can be exchanged. There is evidence that somewhat different criteria for an abnormal recording may be required in different clinical situations. Frequency-domain analysis of the SAECG is under active clinical investigation, with the technique of spectral turbulence analysis showing promising results. The recent approach of combined time- and frequency-domain analysis of the SAECG may improve further the predictive accuracy of this test. In this regard, the chapters by Breithardt and Rubel and their associates in this section are especially instructive.

Time-domain SAECG is now being applied to the analysis of atrial activity, and recent studies indicate that the P-wave SAECG is useful for identifying patients at risk for atrial fibrillation. The following chapter by Steinberg and Ehlert provides a summary of the current work in the field and is particularly enlightening in view of the rapid advances being made.

References

1. Breithardt G, Cain ME, El-Sherif N, Flowers NC, Hombach V, Janse M, Simson MB, Steinbeck G. Standards for analysis of ventricular late potentials using high-resolution or signal-averaged electrocardiography: a statement by a Task Force Committee of the European Society of Cardiology, the American Heart Association, and the American College of Cardiology. *J Am Coll Cardiol* 1991; **17**: 999–1006.
2. Caref EB, Turitto G, Ibrahim BB, Henkin R, El-Sherif. Role of bandpass filters in optimizing the value of the signal averaged electrocardiogram as a predictor of the results of programmed stimulation. *Am J Cardiol* 1989; **64**: 16–26.
3. Kuchar D, Thorburn C, Sammuel N. Prediction of serious arrhythmic events after myocardial infarction: signal-averaged electrocardiogram, Holter monitoring and radionuclide ventriculography. *J Am Coll Cardiol* 1987; **9**: 531–8.
4. Turitto G, Fontaine JM, Ursell SM, Caref EB, Bekheit S, El-Sherif N. Risk stratification and management of patients with organic heart disease and nonsustained ventricular tachycardia: role of programmed stimulation, left ventricular ejection fraction, and the signal-averaged electrocardiogram. *Am J Med* 1990; **88**: 1-35N–41N.
5. El-Sherif N, Denes P, Katz R, Capone R, Mitchell LB, Carlson M, Reynolds-Haertle R. Definition of the best prediction criteria of the time-domain signal-averaged electrocardiogram for serious arrhythmic events in the post-infarction period. *J Am Coll Cardiol* 1995; **25**: 908–14.
6. Cain ME, Ambos HD, Witkowski FX, Sobel BE. Fast Fourier transform analysis of signal averaged ECGs for identification of patients prone to sustained ventricular tachycardia. *Circulation* 1984; **69**: 711–20.

7. Kelen GJ, Henkin R, Starr A-M, Caref EB, Bloomfield D, El-Sherif N. Spectral turbulence analysis of the signal-averaged electrocardiogram and its predictive accuracy for inducible sustained monomorphic ventricular tachycardia. *Am J Cardiol* 1991; **67**: 965–75.
8. Ahuja RK, Turitto G, Ibrahim B, Caref EB, El-Sherif N. Combined time-domain and spectral turbulence analysis of the signal-averaged electrocardiogram improve its predictive accuracy in post-infarction patients. *J Electrocardiol* 1994; **27**(Suppl): 206–9.

14

P Wave Signal-Averaging

Jonathan S. Steinberg and Frederick A. Ehlert

Introduction

The P wave signal-averaged electrocardiogram (SAECG) has been designed to predict the development of atrial fibrillation (AF). This chapter will summarize the relevant characteristics of AF, and discuss in detail the methodology and published experience with the P wave SAECG.

Epidemiology of Atrial Fibrillation

AF is the most common sustained arrhythmia seen in clinical practice and is responsible for more hospital admissions than any other arrhythmia. AF causes significant morbidity and is associated with decreased survival. Complications of AF include the symptoms and hemodynamic consequences associated with rapid ventricular rates, the loss of AV synchrony and shortened diastole. The most important complication of AF is the creation of atrial thrombus which can dislodge and cause systemic emboli, especially stroke.

The prevalence of AF increases with age. It is uncommon below the age of 40, being present in about 0.2% of this segment of the population. For patients above the age of 60, the prevalence may be higher than 5%. As many as 1–1.5 million Americans have nonvalvular AF. With its first appearance in a patient, AF is often a transient and short-lived arrhythmia that has a variable frequency and duration but usually reverts to sinus rhythm spontaneously. As time passes, AF often becomes more persistent as it advances to a chronic phase. Most typically, AF occurs in the setting of established heart disease. Although previously a consequence of rheumatic heart disease, it is now primarily a complication of hypertension and coronary artery disease. Many other chronic and acute disorders can provoke AF, such as cardiomyopathy, mitral valve prolapse, cardiac surgery and hyperthyroidism. In a substantial proportion of AF patients, there is no demonstrable heart disease, a condition termed idiopathic or lone AF. The subset of AF patients who fall into this category has varied in published data, ranging between as low as 2% and as high as 30%.

AF is generally not innocuous. Death from cardiovascular causes doubles in the presence of AF. AF increases the risk of stroke almost five-fold and is directly responsible for approximately 15% of all strokes, the most common consequence of systemic embolism. Patients with lone AF may be spared the higher risk of complications of AF.

The cerebral infarction resulting from AF is often large and results in significant physical disability. Clearly prevention is desirable, and recent randomized trials have strongly endorsed the prophylactic use of anticoagulation with either coumadin or aspirin.

Many other symptoms can result from AF, including angina, congestive heart failure, syncope, fatigue and palpitations. The degree of symptomatology is highly variable and depends at least in part on the presence and severity of underlying cardiac disease, especially LV function and coronary artery disease.

Noninvasive Risk Prediction

Risk modification depends upon the accurate prediction of which patients will develop the clinical condition in question. Because the prevention of AF may be accompanied by a reduction in likelihood of stroke or hemodynamic embarrassment, risk assessment may lead to effective treatment strategies targeted to those most likely to develop AF and its complications. Furthermore, estimating the risk of recurrence of AF after its initial presentation may also facilitate appropriate interventions. Targeting treatment strategies at those at highest risk may avoid indiscriminant treatment or unnecessary investigation, which should translate into more cost-effective and safer approaches to disease prevention.

Prophylactic treatment of AF is evolving. Greater recognition of the risks of antiarrhythmic therapy has tempered enthusiasm for the widespread use of class I antiarrhythmic drugs. Beta-blockers have a proven role in the prevention of AF after cardiac surgery, but the failure to use this approach aggressively has left the incidence of AF distressingly high. Beta-blockers have unproven benefit in other patient groups. Enormous progress has been made regarding the use of anticoagulation, a treatment aimed at preventing the complications of AF rather than the arrhythmia itself.

Because new pharmacologic and nonpharmacologic antiarrhythmic therapeutic approaches are being actively investigated, it is logical and prudent that clinical trials will attempt to enroll patients in appropriate risk categories. Noninvasive methods have long been used to identify those at lowest risk and to pinpoint subjects at greatest risk. For example, the SAECG, Holter monitoring and LV ejection fraction have all been used successfully to select patients for diagnostic or therapeutic procedures in studies of post-MI patients. We expect similar efforts to be made with regard to AF, especially as the era of clinical trials is entered.

In general, noninvasive methods have distinct advantages over invasive strategies. The equipment is usually less expensive to purchase, use and maintain. They have, by definition, a lower risk even though many invasive tests are safe and commonly employed. Noninvasive methods are often portable and are typically available in a variety of settings, from the primary physician's office to the tertiary hospital laboratory. For these reasons, noninvasive screening is often easily obtainable, inexpensive and safe. Of course, the specific screening process must be of proven value and must lead to sound and effective intervention.

Mechanism of Atrial Fibrillation

Previously, speculation had focused on several possible mechanisms as responsible for AF, such as abnormal automaticity and various forms of re-entry. With the advent of high-density computerized mapping systems, it has become possible to map the initiation, activation and termination patterns during AF so that detailed and serial snapshots can reveal insights into the mechanism. Much of this data has been generated from animal models, with some confirmatory data from clinical investigations.

It has become generally accepted that Moe's multiple wavelet hypothesis was correct, as elegantly shown by the work of Alessie et al.[1] According to this concept, there are several independent re-entrant circuits operating simultaneously in the atrial myocardium. These circuits, or wavelets, are constantly changing size, velocity, and direction according to the state of tissue excitability. A minimum number of wavelets must persist for the maintenance of AF.

Fundamental to the mechanism of re-entry is the presence of specific tissue electrophysiologic characteristics needed for the circuit to start and persist. It is convenient to use the concept of wavelength[2] to estimate whether tissue conditions are ripe for the development of AF. Wavelength is defined as the product of conduction velocity and refractory period. When the wavelength is short, re-entry is more readily inducible and sustainable. Conversely, when the wavelength is long, re-entry is more difficult to initiate and maintain. Conditions that reduce conduction velocity or refractory period will promote AF. On the other hand, interventions designed to accelerate conduction velocity – or more likely prolong refractory period – may be therapeutic.

Mapping studies have supported the notion that conduction delay shortens the wavelength and facilitates the formation of wavelets of AF. Clinical studies have provided confirmatory data regarding the importance of slowed conduction. Invasive recordings have shown intra-atrial conduction delay[3] as well as fragmentation of atrial electograms[4] as important determinants of AF.

The central importance of the relationship between conduction velocity and the development of AF directly influenced the conceptual and technical framework that led to the P wave SAECG.

Development of the P Wave Signal-Averaged Electrocardiogram

Signal-averaging of the QRS complex of the surface electrocardiogram has become a widely used tool in the noninvasive evaluation of patients with known or suspected ventricular arrhythmias. This high-resolution electrocardiographic technique averages multiple QRS complexes, thus minimizing the signal contamination by noise and exposing microvolt level signals called 'late potentials'. In ventricular tissue, these late potentials were shown to arise from areas of delayed or fractionated conduction, the substrate of re-entrant arrhythmias. Over a decade ago, late potentials were first associated with clinical ventricular arrhythmias in humans; since that time the SAECG has become a useful tool in risk stratification of patients with myocardial infarction[5] and the evaluation of patients with syncope.[6]

As discussed above, the re-entrant nature of AF requires areas of conduction delay to initiate and sustain the arrhythmia. It would seem that, just as the presence of QRS late potentials indicates slowed conduction and the anatomic substrate for re-entrant arrhythmias, atrial conduction delay would create high-frequency low-amplitude signals and prolong the duration of the P wave on the surface electrocardiogram. However, this technology was neither completely nor directly transferable from the QRS complex to the P wave. The earliest attempts at applying high-resolution electrocardiography to atrial activity correlated poorly with atrial arrhythmias.[7] More recent attempts at signal-averaging of the P wave have modified existing technology in important ways and as a result have achieved significantly better correlation with atrial arrhythmias.[8–10] Clinically, abnormalities in the P wave SAECG have been associated with AF.[11,12] In a manner analogous to the SAECG of the QRS complex, abnormalities of the P wave SAECG have been used to predict the occurrence of AF in certain populations.[8,9,13,14]

As high-resolution electrocardiography has achieved wider clinical usage, the number of commercially available systems have proliferated. However, acquisition and filtering technologies differ considerably among these systems; efforts are under way to standardize several aspects of QRS signal-averaging and analysis. In the newly emerging field of P wave signal-averaging, a thorough understanding of the acquisition and analysis technology being employed is even more essential for accurate interpretation and clinical application.

Methods for P Wave Signal Acquisition

The lead system

Signal-averaging of P waves from the surface electrocardiogram is performed in a manner similar to standard signal-averaging of the QRS complex. As with QRS SAECG acquisition, the skin at the site of lead attachment is abraded to decrease impedance, which generates noise. Silver/silver-chloride electrodes are typically used because the low half-cell potential also reduces noise.

Most studies in the time domain have used an orthogonal lead arrangement to record surface electrograms in three dimensions. The X lead is positioned at the 4th intercostal space from the left (positive) to right midaxillary line (negative). The Y lead is positioned from the superior aspect of the manubrium (positive) to either the proximal left leg or left abdomen (negative). The Z lead is positioned from the 4th intercostal space and the left of the sternum (positive) to a position directly posterior to the left of the spine (negative).

In our laboratory, P waves are recorded until a noise endpoint of 0.3 μV is achieved in the TP segment. Approximately 200–500 beats are typically necessary to complete the signal-averaging, and data acquisition usually requires approximately 20 minutes. As with QRS signal-averaging, signals from each lead are amplified and digitized at sampling frequencies of 1000–2000 times per second. Analog-to-digital convertors have at least 12-bit precision.

Signal alignment and beat rejection

Commercially available signal-averaging systems use the largest deviation from baseline (QRS complex) as the 'trigger' for alignment of the 'window' used for template correlation and signal acquisition. Selection of the 'trigger', or fiducial point, is often a nonprogrammable function of the signal-averaging system and cannot be altered, whether attempting to analyze the QRS complex or the P wave. However, selection of the 'window' used for P wave signal-acquisition obviously differs significantly from the window for the QRS complex. In order to analyze P wave segments, the software must allow alteration in the relation of the analysis window to the QRS trigger. For the QRS SAECG, the fiducial point typically lies on the left side of the analysis window. However, the P wave SAECG requires that the fiducial point by located on the extreme right side of the analysis window, thereby exposing the P wave and PR segment for analysis. Some commercially available systems, like the 'Predictor' system (Corazonix Corporation, Oklahoma City) used in our laboratory, allow software reprogramming, permitting this critical alteration in the acquisition process.

A second necessary condition for the use of commercially available systems for the P wave SAECG is that software modification must permit the P wave to serve as a template. For P wave signal-averaging, the window width or duration is typically set between 100 and 150 ms. Within that window, each point (one per millisecond with sampling frequencies of 1000/s) of the acquired digitized signal is compared with an operator-selected sinus P wave template. P waves that do not match the template with a high degree of correlation are excluded from averaging; typical correlation coefficients range from 0.95 to 0.99. P waves which fail to correlate with the template P wave are beats of ectopic origin, P waves with excessive noise, or misaligned P waves due to PR interval variations related to fluctuations in autonomic tone.

Because the potential abnormalities in atrial signals being studied are of high frequency and low amplitude, the importance of precise waveform alignment cannot be overemphasized. Misalignment, or 'jitter', makes detection and interpretation of these high-frequency signals unreliable. Quantitative assessment of template fit is essential to guarantee that only identical beats are averaged. Earliest attempts at P wave signal-averaging used only QRS templates.[7] As a result, misalignment of P waves created artificially prolonged P wave durations and resulted in little correlation between atrial arrhythmias and P wave SAECG abnormalities. Some investigators have attempted to use a 'visual assessment of fit'.[10] These qualitative comparisons may also result in small but significant misalignments. In order to resolve these high-frequency differences sufficiently, an alignment variation <1.0 ms is required. To achieve this level of template fit, our laboratory and others[8,9] have utilized quantitative fitting of the digitized signal for each sampling interval and thus have demonstrated improved correlation.

Other investigators have developed custom-made software to allow P wave triggering. Fukunami *et al.*[9] have developed their own computer software which is able to use the P wave signal as a secondary 'trigger' following primary triggering off the QRS complex. Preliminary results from this group appear promising, but the system software is not yet commercially available.

Analysis of the P Wave SAECG

Signal filtering

Before analysis can be performed, the electrocardiographic signal must be 'processed' using a variety of filters. Signals from the surface electrocardiogram are filtered prior to additional processing in order to eliminate contamination by low-frequency artifact, to ensure isolated detection of depolarization (without contamination by repolarization), and to enhance detection of onset and offset of the low-amplitude signals. The latter is especially important when analyzing low-amplitude P waves. For time-domain analysis, filter characteristics and frequencies are crucial.

Significant controversy remains regarding the optimal filtering methodology for the QRS SAECG. Each method of processing produces unique results and has its own set of values defined as normal. As a result, while acquisition and analysis guidelines have been developed for the QRS SAECG, the optimal filtering methodology has yet to be determined. For the less well-established technique of P wave signal-averaging, filtering methodology is also still being investigated.

A wide variety of filtering types have been used for P wave SAECG analysis; the type of filter used is frequently determined by the default settings of equipment and software at the individual institution. Some investigators[13,15] have used uni- and bidirectional filters. These filters are of a fourth-order Butterworth design and the digital equivalent of the standard analog filtering. Bidirectional filtering is commonly employed in QRS signal-averaging. Chang *et al.*[12] have used the finite impulse response filter, which is a linear phase response filter. Our laboratory uses the least-squares-fit filter, which is also a linear phase response filter (see discussion below). With this filter, the width of the filter window controls the duration of the parabola fitted to the signal of interest and thereby controls the bandpass. Paylos *et al.*[16] have used a fast Fourier transform filter. This form of spectral filtering is performed in the frequency domain and requires subsequent conversion back to the time domain.

While several comparisons between filter types have been made for the QRS SAECG, only one such evaluation has been made for the P wave SAECG.[17] These results have suggested that least-squares-fit filtering may offer advantages over other methods. P wave SAECG data obtained from 30 subjects (15 patients with documented previous AF

Table 14.1 Signal-averaged P wave duration by filter type and patient group

Filter type	Group 1 (AF) ($n = 15$) (ms)	Group 2 (Controls) ($n = 15$) (ms)	P	Odds ratio
Unidirectional	150 ± 17	136 ± 16	0.04	2.3
Bidirectional	150 ± 17	136 ± 16	0.04	2.3
Finite impulse response	122 ± 25	110 ± 16	NS	1.0
Least-squares-fit	159 ± 14	137 ± 12	0.005	26
Spectral	143 ± 19	122 ± 23	0.02	5.5

AF = atrial fibrillation; NS = not significant; P wave values are in milliseconds.

and 15 age-, sex- and disease-matched controls) were analyzed. Five filtering techniques were evaluated; unidirectional, bidirectional, finite impulse response, fast Fourier transform (spectral) and least-squares-fit filtering. Differences between AF patients and controls as demonstrated by odds ratios were statistically significant for all filtering methods except the finite impulse response filter. Among the P wave filtering methods, the least-squares-fit filter demonstrated the strongest association with AF with an odds ratio of 26 (95% confidence intervals, 7–45). These results are presented in Table 14.1.

These data from our laboratory also demonstrated that unidirectional and bidirectional filtering methods produced identical results for the P wave SAECG. This finding makes sense when the methodology of bidirectional filtering is reviewed. In bidirectional filtering, initial components of the QRS are filtered antegrade and terminal components are filtered retrograde; filtering in both directions terminates in the center of the QRS. This termination is determined by the window 'trigger' point and is a nonprogrammable feature of the system software. P waves, which fall far to the left of the QRS, will be filtered normally by unidirectional antegrade (left-to-right) filters. However, retrograde (right-to-left) filtering will terminate in the QRS and never reach the P wave window. This finding provides an excellent example of the types of limitations of which users must be cognizant when applying commercial systems to P wave signal-averaging.

Filtering frequency

Filtering of surface electrocardiographic signals is designed to eliminate unwanted, contaminant signals which would obscure the low-amplitude 'late potentials' of tissue depolarization. Highpass filters, typically set at frequencies of 10 to 100 Hz, remove low-frequency contamination. These low-frequency contaminants arise from two major sources: repolarization and respiratory motion artifact. Filters in this frequency range are effective because these contaminant signals are slowly-changing (low frequency) relative to signals arising from normal and delayed depolarization. For the QRS SAECG, increases in the highpass filter frequency have been shown to result in significant decreases in the filtered QRS duration and may alter other late potential parameters.

Few studies have attempted to characterize the effects of highpass frequency filter on the P wave SAECG. Fukunami et al.,[9] using P wave triggered signal-averaging, applied highpass filters of 20, 30, 40, 60 and 80 Hz to P wave SAECGs from 9 patients. All demonstrated decreases in vector P wave duration with increasing filter frequency. These results are presented in Figure. 14.1. Work from our laboratory[17] evaluated various bandpass filtering frequencies applied to the least-squares-fit filter. With this filter, the width of the filter window controls bandpass frequency: a window width of 200 ms yields an equivalent highpass cutoff of 14 Hz, a window width of 100 ms yields a highpass cutoff of 29 Hz, and a window width of 50 ms yields a highpass cutoff of 60 Hz.

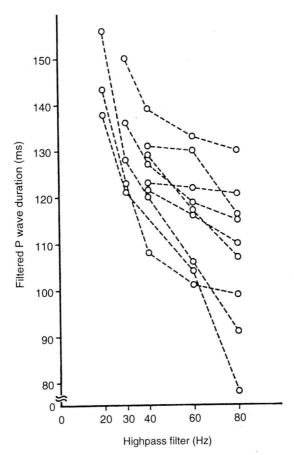

Figure 14.1 The effect of a highpass filter on the duration of the P wave. Dotted lines show data from the same patient. As the frequency of highpass filtering increases (horizontal axis), the filtered P wave duration (vertical axis) progressively decreases. (Reproduced with permission from reference 9: © American Heart Association)

Table 14.2 Signal-averaged P wave duration by patient group and filtering frequency using the least-squares-fit filter type

Filter frequency	Group 1 (AF) (n = 15) (ms)	Group 2 (Controls) (n = 15) (ms)	P	Odds ratio
14–250 Hz (window width = 200 ms)	132 ± 24	108 ± 15	0.01	3
29–250 Hz (window width = 100 ms)	159 ± 14	137 ± 12	0.005	26
60–250 Hz (window width = 50 ms)	138 ± 14	128 ± 15	NS	4

The signal-averaged P wave durations resulting from these three highpass filtering frequencies were evaluated for the strength of their association to atrial fibrillation. Results are presented in Table 14.2. A bandpass filtering frequency of 29–250 Hz produced the strongest association with AF with a calculated odds ratio of 26 (95% confidence intervals, 7–45).

Lowpass filters, typically set at frequencies of 250 or 300 Hz, remove contamination with high-frequency noise. The selection of low-bandpass filters in this range has relatively little effect on the final signal (unless in the range of 100 Hz or less) and, as a result, the selection of filter frequency is less controversial. Very little cardiac depolarization energy resides in these very high frequency ranges.

Total P Wave Duration and the Role of Individual Leads

P wave signal-averaged data are typically analyzed in the form of a composite vector. This vector P wave is calculated from the three bipolar leads combined by the formula $(X^2 + Y^2 + Z^2)^{1/2}$. Onset and offset of the vector P wave may be determined manually or automatically and are defined as the first deflection from baseline noise and the return of the atrial signal to baseline, respectively. A representative vector magnitude signal is presented in Figure 14.2.

The criteria for an abnormal composite vector signal-averaged P wave have not been established. Fukunami et al.,[9] comparing patients with paroxysmal AF to controls, noted significantly longer P wave SAECG durations (137 ± 14 versus 119 ± 11 ms, $p < 0.0001$). From their data, they defined a vector P wave signal duration above 120 ms as abnormal. Guidera and Steinberg[8] also demonstrated a significantly lower P wave SAECG in patients with AF compared with age-, sex- and disease-matched controls (162 ± 15 versus 140 ± 12 ms, $p < 0.01$). Based on their data, these authors defined a filtered vector P wave signal duration above 155 ms as abnormal. More recent work from the same group[11] has suggested that a filtered vector P wave duration above 140 ms may be a better definition of abnormal. Further work will be required to establish the range of normal and abnormal values for this P wave SAECG parameter.

It is possible that a composite vector signal-averaged P wave may miss information available from each of the individual orthogonal leads. Work at our laboratory[17] has evaluated the potential contribution of individual orthogonal leads in P wave signal-averaging. P wave duration measurements for each of the individual X, Y and Z leads as

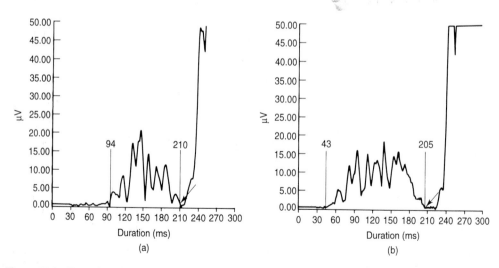

Figure 14.2 Examples of measured P waves from the vector combination of filtered orthogonal leads. (a) SAECG from a control subject with a measured P wave duration of 116 ms. (b) Recording from a patient with atrial fibrillation who had a P wave duration of 162 ms. (Reproduced from reference 8 with permission of the American College of Cardiology)

well as a 'total atrial activation', defined as the time from the earliest onset of atrial activation in any one of the individual leads to the latest offset of atrial activation in any one of the individual leads, were evaluated. These data demonstrated a strong correlation among the individual leads; however, neither the individual leads nor the 'total atrial activation' derived from them significantly improved upon the ability of the composite vector P wave to predict AF.

Terminal P Wave Measurements

Another method used to identify conduction delay in the atrium is measurement of the RMS voltage of the terminal segment of the signal-averaged P wave; low voltage in this segment suggests low-amplitude 'late potentials'. Fukunami *et al.*[9] noted that AF patients had significantly lower RMS voltages in the terminal 10 ms and 20 ms segments of the vector P wave signal. Based on these data, they suggested that a root-mean-squared voltage below $3.5\,\mu V$ in the terminal 20 ms of the P wave be defined as abnormal.

Conflicting data exist regarding the value of terminal P wave RMS voltages. Recently published data from our laboratory[17] have shown that RMS voltage of terminal 10, 20, 30 and 40 ms of the composite vector P wave and the entire P wave did not differ between patients with and without AF.

Other authors have defined additional parameters to identify abnormal signal-averaged P waves. Stafford *et al.*[10] measured the RMS voltage of each quarter of the signal-averaged P wave; they found a significant increase in RMS voltage in the third quartile in patients with AF. Paylos *et al.*[16] found significantly lower terminal RMS voltages in P wave signals recorded from orthogonal leads facing the posterior and posterolateral atrium. These leads correlate to regions of the atrium where slow conduction and conduction block have been described. Further work is needed to resolve issues arising from these conflicting reports. It is apparent, however, that total P wave duration provides consistently useful data.

Reproducibility of Signal-Averaged P Wave Measurements

While the reproducibility of QRS SAECG has been studied in detail, no previous work has evaluated the reproducibility of the P wave SAECG. Recent data from our laboratory[18] have confirmed the reproducibility of duration measurements for the P wave SAECG both when repeat testing was performed immediately and at 24–48 hours. Correlation coefficients in excess of 0.90 were noted in control subjects, in patients with underlying heart disease and in patients with a documented history of AF. These results are presented in Figure 14.3. In addition, the P wave SAECG also remained highly reproducible in patients with signal-averaged P wave durations defined as abnormal (>155 ms).

Clinical Value of the P Wave SAECG

Association with atrial fibrillation

Because AF is an arrhythmia based on a re-entrant process which depends on slow conduction, it was hypothesized that the body surface detection of the atrial conduction substrate would correlate with risk of AF. The SAECG procedure attenuates electrical noise from a variety of sources and would thus facilitate the measurement of the entire atrial activation sequence, even from tissue generating small electrical signals on the

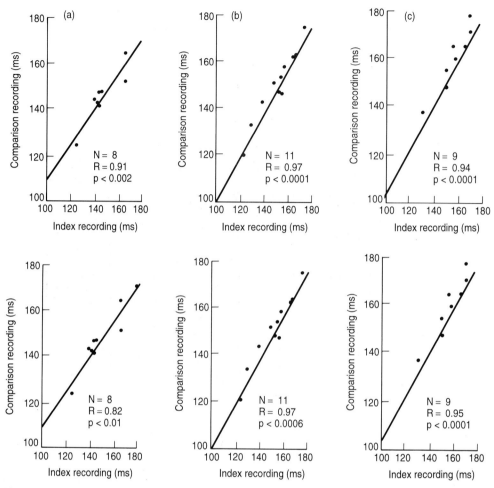

Figure 14.3 Linear regression plots comparing initial signal-averaged P wave duration with immediate (above) and short-term reacquisition (below) measurements for (a) control subjects, (b) cardiac patients, and (c) patients with known AF. Correlation coefficients for each of the curves are presented next to that line. P wave duration obtained at initial SAECG acquisition are represented on the x axis; P wave durations obtained at immediate (O) and short-term (X) reacquisition are represented on the y axis.

body surface. We proposed that the P wave SAECG would provide a rapid and noninvasive means for identifying atrial conduction delay.

In our initial study,[8] we enrolled 15 patients who had previously experienced AF. Of these 15, ten had paroxysmal AF and five had recently been converted to normal sinus rhythm with DC countershock. The second group in this investigation comprised 15 control subjects selected to match the age and disease distribution in the AF group. The control group had never experienced AF. Clinical characteristics were similar between the two groups and represented the typical spectrum of cardiovascular diseases associated with AF. Only two patients in the AF group were receiving antiarrhythmic drugs at the time of the SAECG recording; both patients were on sotalol, a drug known to have no effect on myocardial conduction. No patient was being treated with class I antiarrhythmia drugs or amiodarone.

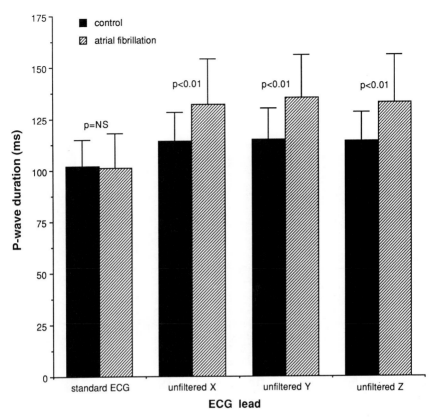

Figure 14.4 P wave duration as measured by standard and unfiltered signal-averaged electrocardiogram (ECG). The mean ($\pm$SD) P wave duration for 15 patients with atrial fibrillation (hatched bars) and 15 control subjects (black bars) are shown. The difference in P wave durations between the two groups is not statistically significant as measured by standard ECG, but P wave duration as measured by signal-averaged ECG is significantly prolonged in the X, Y and Z leads in patients with atrial fibrillation relative to that in control subjects. (Reproduced from reference 8 with permission of the American College of Cardiology)

The P wave duration was measured on the standard ECG (Figure 14.4) and was nearly identical in the two groups. Three patients in each group had a P wave duration above 110 ms on the standard ECG, a value commonly used to indicate prolonged atrial conduction. Thus the standard ECG was incapable of discriminating between patients with and without AF.

In contrast to the standard ECG, the SAECG has undergone noise reduction and signal amplification. The P wave duration on the unfiltered orthogonal leads all increased after signal-averaging, but the increment was much greater in the patients with AF. In the patients with AF, P wave duration increased from 101 $\pm$ 17 ms to 132 $\pm$ 22 ms ($p < 0.01$), 135 $\pm$ 21 ms ($p < 0.01$) and 133 $\pm$ 23 ms ($p < 0.01$) in the X, Y and Z leads, respectively. In the control group, the P wave increased from 102 $\pm$ 13 ms to 114 $\pm$ 14 ms ($p < 0.01$), 115 $\pm$ 15 ms ($p < 0.01$) and 114 $\pm$ 14 ms ($p < 0.01$) in the X, Y and Z leads, respectively.

The next step in the post-averaging process is filtering. After filtering with a least-squares-fit filter (100 ms window), the P wave duration increased further. Presumably, this increase was related to amplification and enhanced detection of low-amplitude signal, but the filter itself may have caused some prolongation of the atrial signal. In the

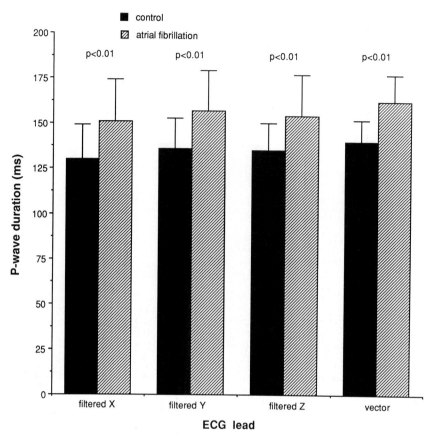

Figure 14.5   P wave duration (mean ± SD) measured by SAECG in each of three orthogonal leads, and their vector combination after filtering. There is significant P wave prolongation in the 15 patients with atrial fibrillation (hatched bars) relative to that in the 15 control subjects (black bars) in each individual lead and in the vector composite. (Reproduced from reference 8 with permission of the American College of Cardiology)

AF group, the P wave duration increased from 132 ± 22 ms to 151 ± 23 ms ($p < 0.01$), from 135 ± 21 ms to 157 ± 22 ms ($p < 0.01$), and from 133 ± 23 ms to 154 ± 23 ms ($p < 0.01$) in the X, Y and Z leads, respectively. In the control patients, the P wave duration increased after filtering from 114 ± 14 ms to 130 ± 19 ms ($p < 0.01$), from 115 ± 15 ms to 136 ± 17 ms ($p < 0.01$), and from 114 ± 14 ms to 135 ± 15 ms ($p < 0.01$) in the X, Y and Z leads, respectively.

Comparison of P wave durations from SAECG revealed striking differences between the AF patients and their matched controls (Figure 14.4.). Each unfiltered orthogonal lead was longer in the patients with a history of AF than in the control subjects. The difference was in the range of 20 ms. Within each patient group, there was no difference between each of the three orthogonal leads.

Filtered P wave durations were also longer in patients with AF than in the control patients (Figure 14.5). Again the differential was approximately 20 ms. There was no difference in filtered P wave duration among the individual leads within each group.

The three filtered leads were combined into a vector composite lead and compared between the two patient groups. Patients with a history of AF had P wave duration that

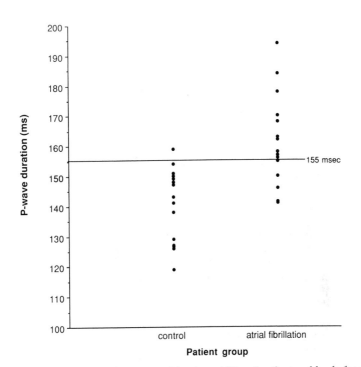

Figure 14.6   The P wave duration of vector combination of filtered orthogonal leads for all 15 patients with atrial fibrillation and the 15 control subjects. A P wave duration ⩾155 ms identified patients with a history of atrial fibrillation with a sensitivity of 80% and a specificity of 93%. (Reproduced from reference 8 with permission of the American College of Cardiology)

was 16% longer than the control subjects: 162 ± 15 ms versus 140 ± 12 ms ($p < 0.01$) (Figure 14.5). The clinical value of the P wave SAECG was estimated using the filtered vector combination leads (Figure 14.6) which maximized the differences between patient groups. Using a P wave duration ⩾155 ms yielded a sensitivity of 80%, specificity of 93% and positive predictive value of 92% for identifying risk of AF.

These results clearly demonstrated that the SAECG was superior to the standard ECG for detecting atrial conduction delay, and that the prolonged activation times of SAECG were associated with a history of AF. The results were simple and readily obtainable from commercially available SAECG equipment (with appropriate software modification).

In a report from Fukunami et al.,[9] the SAECG was also used to identify patients with AF. The SAECG system used by these investigators was custom designed and was P wave triggered. Patients were selected because of a history of paroxysmal AF ($n = 42$) and were compared with matched controls ($n = 50$). Several SAECG variables distinguished AF patients, including the total filtered P wave duration, but AF patients also had lower voltage in terminal segments of the P wave. Importantly, left atrial dimension measured on the echocardiogram did not differ between the patients with paroxysmal AF and the controls. Accounting for the presence of underlying structural heart disease did not alter the SAECG results. Stafford et al.[10] reported similar results in a smaller study of patients with paroxysmal AF.

In another preliminary report, hypertrophic cardiomyopathy patients with AF could be distinguished by the left atrial dimension on echocardiogram but also by the P wave SAECG.[12]

Relationship to severity of atrial fibrillation

AF often appears first as a paroxysmal arrhythmia. The severity of symptoms and the risk of complications, especially thromboembolic, are intimately related to the anatomic size of the atria and the frequency and duration of recurrences. In addition, paroxysmal AF often progresses to chronic AF which may require a different strategy for effective management.

The ability to predict the progression, if any, of AF after initial presentation would have definite clinical advantages. The P wave SAECG has been explored to this end, but only limited data are available. Iwakura *et al.*[14] examined the frequency and duration of paroxysmal attacks of AF as they related to findings on the P wave SAECG in 46 patients. They subdivided their patients into those with frequent attacks, one or more times per month, and those with infrequent attacks, less than one per month. They also classified their patients into those with prolonged episodes, at least 2 hours, and those with shorter episodes.

These authors found that the frequency of AF episodes was related to the duration of the P wave, but not to any of the amplitude calculations they performed. The duration of episodes, however, had no relationship to any P wave variable. Thus it appears that prolonged conduction may contribute to the spontaneous frequency of paroxysmal AF.

The clinical application of these data is potentially very useful. However, further investigation in larger clinical series is clearly needed.

Predicting development of atrial fibrillation

The P wave SAECG was designed to screen populations of patients at risk of atrial tachyarrhythmias in order to identify the subset at greatest risk. This goal is best accomplished in a prospective clinical study. To date there has been only one such investigation,[11] a study involving patients following cardiac surgery.

AF is a predictable complication of cardiac surgery. It is common, affecting roughly one-quarter of all patients. AF typically begins within the first few days of surgery and can be associated with stroke, hemodynamic embarrassment and a prolonged hospitalization. Many prophylactic measures have been tested, but beta-blockers are the only clearly effective intervention to reduce the incidence of AF in this setting. The response to beta-blockers implicates catecholamine excess or perhaps heightened catecholamine sensitivity following beta-blocker withdrawal for surgery. Although beta-blockers are effective, they are often withheld to avoid the perceived risk of hemodynamic compromise in the early postoperative state.

Steinberg *et al.*[11] enrolled 130 patients undergoing elective surgery, primarily coronary artery bypass graft surgery. Patients were excluded if there was a previous history of AF or if the patient was treated with class I or III antiarrhythmic therapy. AF developed in 25% of this cohort, usually 2 or 3 days following surgery. The average duration of AF was 2.3 days before self-termination, or chemical or electrical cardioversion.

A variety of clinical characteristics typically available to the clinician were analyzed. Only two were found to be predictive: left ventricular hypertrophy on preoperative ECG and the LV ejection fraction. This observation suggests that the risk of AF was dependent on the presence of underlying heart disease, not simply the postoperative state. Previous studies of AF in this setting have had conflicting results regarding clinical predictors, but have often identified older age or absence of beta-blocker therapy.

The P wave duration on the SAECG emerged as the most potent predictor of postoperative AF. It was far superior to the significant clinical variables, reduced EF and LV hypertrophy on ECG. The P wave duration was almost 10% longer in the AF patients than in those patients who did not develop AF: 152 ± 18 ms versus 139 ± 17 ms ($p < 0.001$).

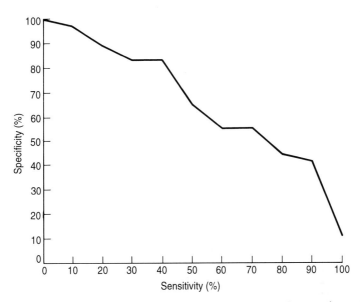

Figure 14.7 Receiver–operator characteristic curve of the SAECG P wave duration for predicting atrial fibrillation after cardiac surgery. (Reproduced with permission from reference 11: © American Heart Association)

Sensitivity and specificity were strongly related to the results of the P wave SAECG (Figure 14.7). AF occurrence was optimally predicted by a P wave duration above 140 ms with a sensitivity of 77%, specificity of 55%, positive predictive accuracy of 37% and negative predictive accuracy of 87%. With a P wave duration above 150 ms, maximal specificity (70%) with adequate sensitivity (50%) was obtained. Results remained the same if the analysis was restricted to patients who underwent coronary artery bypass surgery rather than valve replacement.

A multivariate analysis was performed with logistic regression. Only one variable was identified as predictive of AF: P wave duration above 140 ms on the SAECG. The likelihood of developing AF was increased almost four-fold if the P wave duration was prolonged. Addition of clinical variables to the logistic regression model failed to improve prediction.

Interestingly, separate analysis failed to identify clinical variables, such as EF or left ventricular hypertrophy, that were predictive of the P wave duration. This and the previous findings suggest that the SAECG is detecting a unique atrial characteristic that is not closely related to other known risk factors of AF or atrial disease.

As discussed in preceding sections, the finding of a prolonged P wave duration implies slowed atrial conduction resulting in lengthened atrial activation time. Thus the relationship of slowed conduction and re-entrant AF was confirmed in a clinical setting, specifically AF after cardiac surgery. It is particularly noteworthy that the P wave SAECG was recorded preoperatively. Thus the atrial conduction delay was present prior to surgical intervention and prior to the changes or complications that may follow surgery. We concluded that these patients had a preoperative predisposition to AF due to a primary electrical abnormality. Because these patients had never experienced AF, we must assume that one or more of the many stresses present in the postoperative state triggered AF when the substrate (prolonged atrial conduction) was present. This supposition is consistent with the observed clustering of AF in the first few days following surgery.

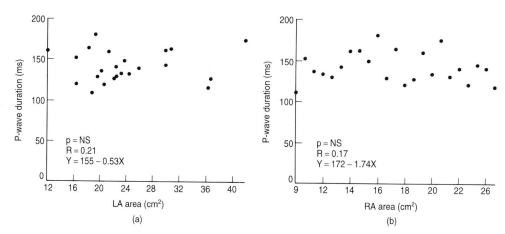

Figure 14.8   (a) Relationship of P wave duration on the SAECG to left atrial area measured on the 2-D electrocardiogram. (b) Relationship of the P wave duration on the SAECG to right atrial area measured on the 2-D electrocardiogram. LA = left atrial; RA = right atrial.

The factors responsible for prolonged atrial conduction in these patients are unknown. Postoperative anatomic or dynamic conditions resulting from surgery were clearly excluded. Experimental data would suggest that atrial enlargement and hypertrophy create the electrophysiologic milieu that promotes AF.[19] Definitive data are not yet available in clinical contexts to answer these questions, but our initial analyses suggest that the electrical abnormality is independent of atrial chamber enlargement.

In a subset of the larger study population, M-mode and 2-D echocardiographic data were carefully examined to determine if the P wave duration was correlated with atrial dimensions.[20] Of the entire cohort, 23 patients had echocardiography performed during their hospital stay. In this subset, 12 patients had a prolonged P wave duration on SAECG above 140 ms and 11 patients did not. These two groups were well matched for all clinical and surgical characteristics. We then compared these two groups with respect to left atrial dimension and area and right atrial dimension. There were no differences in any atrial echocardiographic parameter in the two study groups. Furthermore, in the 23 patients we examined whether there was any relationship between these atrial echocardiographic measurements and the P wave duration. By linear regression, P wave duration was not correlated to any of these values (Figure 14.8). Interestingly, in this subset of 23 patients, the atrial size was not related to the development of postoperative AF, yet the P wave duration was. These findings lead us to believe that prolongation of atrial conduction in this population of patients is not due to atrial enlargement. Instead, it may represent a specific atrial conduction abnormality that is a determinant of postoperative AF risk.

The clinical usefulness of the P wave SAECG will need to be confirmed in other populations before the results described in the postoperative patient can be extrapolated. Suitable candidates include other high-risk populations such as patients with valvular heart disease, hypertension or coronary artery disease.

Advances in Defining the Mechanism and Management of Atrial Fibrillation

The availability of a noninvasive procedure that provides reliable and informative data about atrial conduction can have important applications as a research tool. For example, it has already been uncovered that the development of AF after cardiac surgery depends at least in part on the presence of a fixed underlying atrial conduction abnormality rather than solely on postoperative developments. Other data[9,11] have suggested that the development of paroxysmal AF or AF after cardiac surgery is not related to underlying abnormalities of atrial structure, but is an independent electrical abnormality.

Further work will be needed to determine if other anatomic or functional determinants are responsible for the prolonged conduction detected on the P wave SAECG. For example, more data regarding the effects of increased atrial pressure, rather than simply size, would be informative. In addition, abnormalities of structure and function of the right atrium should not be ignored and will need to be studied in conjunction with the left atrium. This type of thorough investigation will answer the question of whether the atrial late potential is indeed a primary electrical abnormality.

As clinical investigation proceeds, other patient groups will receive scrutiny using the P wave SAECG. Many patient groups are known to have increased risk for the development of AF, and the P wave SAECG may help risk stratification efforts. Some patient groups present both a mechanistic and clinical quandary. In particular, lone AF develops in substantial numbers of patients, yet in most we have no clear understanding why it has occurred nor the likelihood for recurrence. One may speculate that pockets of fibrosis in atrial myocardium which escapes clinical detection may predispose to disorders of atrial conduction and AF in at least some of these patients. The P wave SAECG could help address hypotheses such as this.

The P wave SAECG represents an important contribution to the field of noninvasive electrocardiology. It will undoubtedly see increasing use as an investigative tool for screening populations at risk of AF, especially as advances are made in prevention of AF or its complications. The P wave SAECG may also serve as a noninvasive probe into the mechanism of AF and thus provide the means to better understand the development of AF in specific patient groups and clinical settings.

References

1. Allessie MA, Lammers WJ, Bonke FI, Hollin J. Experimental evaluation of Moe's multiple wavelet hypothesis of atrial fibrillation. In: Zipes D, Jalife J (eds), *Cardiac Electrophysiology Arrhythmias*. New York: Grune & Stratton, 1985: 265–75.
2. Janse MJ, Allessie MA. Experimental observations in atrial fibrillation. In: *Atrial Fibrillation: Mechanism and Management*. New York: Raven Press, 1992: 41–57.
3. Simpson RJ, Foster JR, Gettes LS. Atrial excitability and conduction in patients with intraatrial conduction defects. *Am J Cardiol* 1982; **50**: 1331–7.
4. Ohe T, Matsuhisa M, Kamakura S, Yamada J, Sato I, Nakajima K, Shimomura K. Relation between the widening of the fragmented atrial activity zone and atrial fibrillation. *Am J Cardiol* 1983; **53**: 1219–22.
5. Steinberg JS, Regen A, Sciacca RR, Bigger JT, Fleiss JL. Predicting arrhythmic events after acute myocardial infarction using the signal-averaged electrocardiogram. *Am J Cardiol* 1992; **69**: 13–21.
6. Steinberg JS, Prystowsky E, Freedman RA, Moreno F, Katz R, Kron J, Regen A, Sciacca RR. Use of the signal-averaged electrocardiogram for predicting inducible ventricular tachycardia in patients with unexplained syncope: relationship to clinical variables in a multivariate analysis. *J Am Coll Cardiol* 1994; **23**: 99–106.
7. Engel TR, Vallone N, Windle J. Signal-averaged electrocardiograms in patients with atrial fibrillation or flutter. *Am Heart J* 1988; **115**: 592–7.
8. Guidera SA, Steinberg JS. The signal-averaged P wave duration: a rapid and non-invasive marker of atrial fibrillation. *J Am Coll Cardiol* 1993; **21**: 1645–51.
9. Fukunami M, Yamada T, Ohmori M, Kumagai K, Umemeto K, Sakai A, Kondoh N, Minamoto T, Hoki N. Detection of patients at risk for paroxysmal atrial fibrillation during sinus rhythm by P wave triggered signal-averaging electrocardiogram. *Circulation* 1991; **83**: 162–9.
10. Stafford PJ, Turner I, Vincent R. Quantitative analysis of signal-averaged P waves in idiopathic paroxysmal atrial fibrillation. *Am J Cardiol* 1991; **68**: 751–5.
11. Steinberg JS, Zelenkofske S, Wong SC, Gelernt M, Sciacca R, Menchavez E. The value of the P-wave signal-averaged electrocardiogram for predicting atrial fibrillation after cardiac surgery. *Circulation* 1993; **88**: 2618–22.
12. Chang AC, Winkler JB, Fananapazir L. P wave signal averaging identifies hypertrophic cardiomyopathy patients with paroxysmal atrial fibrillation (abstract). *J Am Coll Cardiol* 1990; **15**: 191A.

13. Klein MS, Evans SJL, Cataldo L, Bodenheimer MM. Prediction of atrial fibrillation following coronary artery bypass grafting by the use of P-wave-triggered P-wave signal-averaging (abstract). *Circulation* 1992; **86**: I-131.
14. Iwakura K, Abe Y, Ohmori M, Yamada T, Kondoh N, Minamino T, Tsujimara I, Fukunari M. Relationship between frequency and duration of paroxysmal atrial fibrillation attacks and atrial late potential (abstract). *Circulation* 1992; **86**: I-131.
15. Ozin MB, Oto MA, Saki MC, Muderrisaglu H, Korkmaz M, Ider YZ. Analysis of signal averaged P wave identifies patients at risk for paroxysmal atrial fibrillation (abstract). *Circulation* 1992; **86**: I-131.
16. Paylos JM, Cordero B, Lopez-de-Sa E, Calzado CS. Spatial temporal mapping of P waves in subjects with and without paroxysmal atrial fibrillation (abstract). *J Am Coll Cardiol* 1993; **21**: 181A.
17. Steinberg JS, Korenstein D. Comparison of techniques for analysis of the P-wave signal-averaged ECG (abstract). *Circulation* 1993; **88**: I-311.
18. Steinberg JS, Ehlert FA, Menchavez-Tam E. Immediate and short-term reproducibility of the P-wave signal-averaged electrocardiogram (abstract). *J Am Coll Cardiol* 1994; **23**: 252A.
19. Boyden PA, Hoffman BF. The effects on atrial physiology and structure of surgically induced right atrial enlargement in dogs. *Circulation* 1981; **49**: 1319–31.
20. Zelenkofske S, Brown E, Mogtader A, Menchavez E, Steinberg JS. Prolonged SAECG P-wave duration is not due to atrial enlargement (abstract). *Circulation* 1993; **88**: I-311.

15

Ventricular Late Potentials: Time Domain

Markku Mäkijärvi, Thomas Fetsch, Lutz Reinhardt, Antoni Martinez-Rubio, Martin Borggrefe and Günter Breithardt

High-resolution electrocardiography using the signal-averaging technique has been developed to detect cardiac electrical activation in the microvolt range from the body surface.[1] These low-amplitude signals may stem from the bundle of His or from areas of myocardial infarction and are termed 'ventricular late potentials'. They have been regarded as a marker of an arrhythmogenic substrate, and are considered to herald an increased risk of sustained ventricular tachyarrhythmias.[2] A combination of ambulatory ECG and signal-averaging has been proposed for assessment of spontaneous ventricular ectopy and detection of ventricular late potentials.

This chapter will review the subject of ventricular late potentials, by addressing the pathophysiology of re-entrant ventricular tachyarrhythmias, describing the methodology of high-resolution ECG, and demonstrating its current clinical applications.

Anatomic and Electrophysiologic Bases of Ventricular Late Potentials

Re-entrant excitation occurs when the propagating activation wavefront persists after complete activation of the atria and/or ventricle and re-excites either of them after the end of the refractory period. The most frequently applied model of re-entrant excitation is circus movement.[3] In this type of re-entry, the activation wavefront encounters a site of unidirectional conduction block, and slowly propagates in a circuitous pathway before retrogradely re-exciting the tissue proximal to the site of block after the refractory period has ended. Circus movement means the kind of impulse propagation which traverses a re-entrant loop. A major prerequisite for re-entry to occur is the presence of inhomogeneities of conduction. This may be due to intrinsic anisotropy of conduction parallel or perpendicular to fiber orientation, or to structural abnormalities as a result of myocardial scarring.[4–8]

After myocardial infarction, delayed myocardial activation is caused by depolarization of surviving myocardium around the islands of fibrosis at the border zone of or within an area of infarction. Extracellular electrograms recorded from the endocardial surface of such bundles of myocardial tissue usually have small amplitudes and demonstrate fractionation because of the interposed layers of fibrous tissue and small diameter of the surviving muscle bundles. When individual bundles are separated by connective tissue, heterogeneous patterns of activation may occur, resulting in fragmentation of local extracellular electrograms. Signals that can be recorded from these areas by using bipolar electrodes may appear at the time of normal ventricular activation (i.e. during the QRS complex) or after completion of normal activation.[7] In the latter case, these signals have been termed 'late potentials'.[10] They can also be recorded from the body surface using appropriate recording techniques.[11,2,8]

Noninvasive Recording of Late Potentials

Real-Time Recording

Late ventricular activity

Late ventricular electrical activity detected from the body surface is caused by delayed activation of myocardium. This late activity was first recorded in dogs with experimental infarction and corresponded in time with fragmented and delayed electrograms recorded from the epicardium.[1] In humans, late ventricular activity in the body surface electrocardiogram has been accompanied by late, fragmented electrograms recorded directly from the heart.[4,8,9] Fragmented electrograms can be recorded from many patients after Q wave myocardial infarction.[2] However, in patients with ventricular tachycardia after infarction, the abnormal delayed activation is more profound and detectable at multiple cardiac sites.

The finding of fragmented local electrograms during direct catheter mapping, or late ventricular activity in the body surface electrocardiogram, may indicate that the substrate for re-entry is present.[8] Although late ventricular activity seems to represent a fixed substrate for re-entrant excitation, additional triggering mechanisms – such as one or more premature beats, modulating factors such as imbalance of the autonomous nervous system or ischemia – may also be required for the manifestation of re-entry and clinical arrhythmia. In addition, a recent intracardiac mapping study has shown that late potentials detected from the body surface may also lie at sites distant from the site of origin of ventricular tachycardia.[9]

Electrodes and ECG leads

Silver/silver-chloride electrodes are most commonly used for high-resolution electrocardiographic recordings. The skin is cleansed and abraded in order to decrease impedance. Most studies have used bipolar X, Y and Z leads. According to the standards for high-resolution electrocardiography, the X lead is positioned at the 4th intercostal space in both midaxillary lines (V6R and V6 positions), the Y lead is positioned on the superior aspect of the manubrium and on either the upper left leg or left iliac crest, and the Z lead is at the 4th intercostal space (V2 position) with the second electrode directly posterior on the left side of the vertebral column.[10] Positive electrodes are left (X lead), inferior (Y lead) and anterior (Z lead). The original Frank vector-cardiographic lead system has also been used (Figure 15.1).

Noise reduction

Noise in SAECG measurements arises by three mechanisms: patient noise, instrument noise and power-line interference. Adequate noise reduction is essential for analysis of SAECG recordings. To decrease the patient noise, the skin must be prepared carefully by

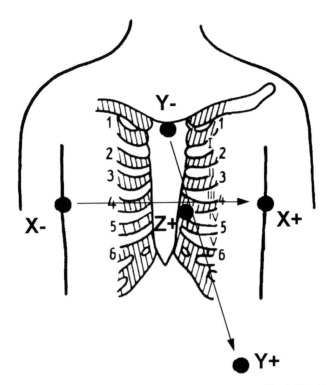

Figure 15.1   Electrode positioning in SAECG measurements. Horizontal lead (X−, X+): 4th intercostal space at the midaxillary lines. Vertical lead (Y−, Y+): suprasternal notch and the anterior–superior iliac crest. Anteroposterior lead (Z+, Z−): parasternal 4th intercostal space (V2) and directly posterior.

cleansing it with alcohol and abrading it with very fine sandpaper. The patient should be relaxed, and a few minutes waiting time before starting the measurement can lower the noise level significantly. Also, cessation of breathing after a long expiration has been used for decreasing the noise generated by thoracic muscles and the diaphragm. Warm and peaceful surroundings are helpful in patient relaxation.

Instrument noise in electronic amplifiers was a problem in the early 1980s, but low-noise equipment is now available. Nowadays, low-noise silver/silver-chloride electrodes are also commercially available but only a few types are suitable for high-resolution recordings.

Noise in the surroundings is a problem of varying significance. Especially in older electrical installations, it may be very disturbing, and may not always be removed by adequate grounding. It is mainly due to power-line noise causing 50 Hz (or 60 Hz) interference, usually combined with its harmonics. The disturbing effect of the power-line interference can be reduced by using notch filters which, however, tend to distort the true signal. The other possibility is to record in a shielded environment. The extent of noise also depends on the type of filter used.

Amplification and analog-to-digital conversion

The ECG signals are recorded with low-noise analog amplifiers at bandpass filter settings of 0.5 to 250 Hz. Analog/digital conversion is usually performed with 12-bit resolution at a sampling rate of 1 kHz or more. All ECG leads are recorded and converted simultaneously.

Signal-averaging

The signal-averaging technique requires that a reference beat or a template is extracted before starting the averaging process. Ectopic beats or extremely noisy beats are excluded by the computer algorithm. Each input beat is aligned by matching it against the template. High-frequency signals are attenuated during the signal-averaging process if the alignment of incoming beats is not exact (trigger jitter). Therefore, the trigger jitter, measured with an artificial QRS complex, should be less than 1 ms, and ideally less than 0.5 ms. A cross-correlation technique can also be used for alignment. After averaging, the waveforms are usually stored on a computer disk.

Filtering

Usually, analog bandpass filtering (e.g. 0.5–250 Hz) is applied before analog-to-digital conversion in order to stabilize the baseline in the ECG and to prevent aliasing of higher frequencies during the digitization process. In order to further increase the signal of interest (the late potential) in relation to the background signal (normal depolarization), different types of highpass filters have been used, mostly at 25 Hz or 40 Hz cutoff frequencies. Analog and digital filters have both been used for this purpose.

The various late potential parameters depend on the digital filter used for enhancement of the recorded signal. The most widely used filter is the fourth-order Butterworth infinite impulse response highpass filter. The optimal highpass filter cutoff frequency for detecting late ventricular activity after myocardial infarction was first proposed to be 25 Hz. Later, a cutoff frequency of 40 Hz was found to be more suitable for identifying patients with sustained ventricular tachycardia. It has been reported that a higher cutoff frequency has better sensitivity but lower specificity for identifying ventricular tachycardia.[11] Other cutoff frequencies (from 50 to 100 Hz) have also been used.

Analysis of the signal-averaged electrocardiogram

The modern type of quantitative analysis of the SAECG for late potential detection in the time domain was first proposed by Simson.[7] His method is based on analysis of the time–voltage relation in the terminal 40 ms of the vector magnitude of the filtered leads: $(X^2 + Y^2 + Z^2)^{1/2}$ (filtered QRS complex).

The most important step in analysis is the identification of the transition between the filtered QRS complex and the ST segment. This transition is searched for retrogradely until the root-mean-square voltage in a searching window exceeds a predefined limit. The end of the filtered QRS complex has been defined as the midpoint of a 5 ms segment in which the mean voltage first exceeds the mean noise level plus three times the standard deviation of the noise sample. The same principle is applied to the onset of the filtered QRS complex. The automatically determined endpoints are verified visually.

The initial late potential analysis presented by Simson included determination of the filtered QRS duration and the root-mean-square voltage of the terminal 40 ms of the filtered QRS. The duration of the low-amplitude signal below 40 μV has also been used in separating ventricular tachycardia patients[12] (Figure 15.2).

Reproducibility of signal-averaged electrocardiograms

In several studies, the immediate reproducibility has been shown to be excellent. As a rule, the filtered QRS duration has the highest reproducibility ($r^2 = 0.95$–0.97), followed by the root-mean-square voltage ($r^2 = 0.92$–0.94) of the terminal 40 ms of the QRS complex and the duration of the low-amplitude signal under 40 μV in the terminal portion of the QRS complex ($r^2 = 0.90$–0.92). The reproducibility of an initially normal SAECG has been reported to be 92%, compared with a reproducibility of 96% of an initially abnormal SAECG. SAECG data with 40 Hz highpass filtering have been demonstrated to be more reproducible than data with 25 Hz highpass filtering.[12] Also, the short-term (3 days) reproducibility has been shown to be good.

Spatial-Averaging

In the spatial-averaging technique, potentials recorded simultaneously from multiple pairs of electrodes are averaged. The averaging reinforces the coherent signals and attenuates the uncorrelated signals such as electromyographic noise. For example, four pairs of electrodes will approximately halve the noise. Increasing the distance between the electrode pairs (i.e. between the two composite electrodes) improves the signal-to-noise ratio. An electrode pair separation of 2–4 inches (5–10 cm) has been found desirable. With the spatial-averaging technique, both His–Purkinje signals and late potentials have been detected. The ensemble in spatial averaging is limited by the size of the subject's torso, perimeters of the positive and negative fields on the chest, and the size of the electrodes. In practice, the noise reduction achieved with this technique alone is insufficient and other noise-reduction measures must also be applied.

Beat-to-Beat Recordings

Dynamic changes in the microsignals can be detected only by continuous beat-to-beat recordings. The detection of microsignals during complex cardiac arrhythmias requires beat-to-beat techniques as well. The temporal or morphological changes in micropotentials may be clinically relevant. In experimental and clinical studies, it has been suggested that spontaneous arrhythmias may be associated with a Wenckebach-like conduction pattern in a potentially re-entrant pathway.[3] Thus, recording of late potentials on a beat-to-beat basis has the potential for directly identifying dynamic changes in the electrophysiologic milieu. However, this technique has not yet been demonstrated to be clinically useful even though it has been available for some time.

Several different systems for recording beat-to-beat have been proposed.[13] Bipolar electrodes have been utilized with or without spatial averaging. Electrode positioning depends on the microsignals to be detected. Uncorrected orthogonal XYZ leads along the heart axis are the most commonly used. Highpass filtering varies from 0 to 100 Hz and lowpass filtering from 70 to 300 Hz. Many systems also use notch filters: 50/100 Hz or 60/120 Hz. Most groups have recorded in shielded environments.

Several problems are associated with the analysis of beat-to-beat recordings. Both quantitative and qualitative approaches have been used, but the reported methods are all user-dependent, and the definitions of pathological findings either vary or have not been stated. The reported noise levels have varied between 0.8 and $4\,\mu V$, but are hardly comparable because of different noise-reduction methods (filtering, spatial averaging, etc.) and different ways of calculating the noise. In at least two systems, frequency analysis has been used instead of temporal analysis.

Figure 15.2 (*over page*)   Schematic of the principles of calculating high-resolution parameters in the time domain. The total duration of the filtered vector magnitude QRS complex is measured (QRS duration). In (a) and (b) the shaded areas represent the root-mean-square voltages at the terminal 40 ms time interval of the filtered QRS complex (*RMS 40*). In (c) and (d) the shaded areas represent the duration of the low-amplitude signal below the threshold value of $40\,\mu V$ at the terminal part of the filtered QRS complex (*LAS 40*). (a) and (c) characterize normal *RMS 40* and *LAS 40*: (b) and (d) represent a ventricular late potential finding, reduced terminal RMS voltage and lengthened terminal LAS duration.

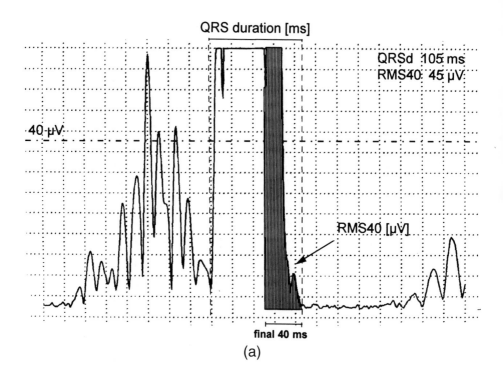

(a)

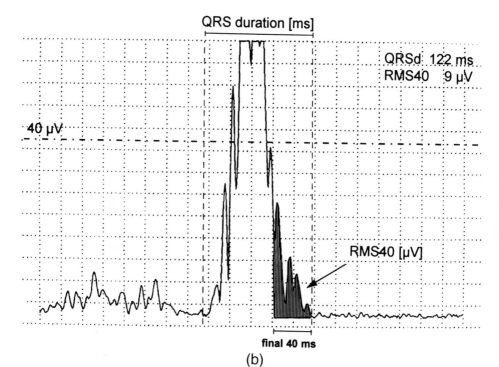

(b)

Figure 15.2

QRS duration [ms]

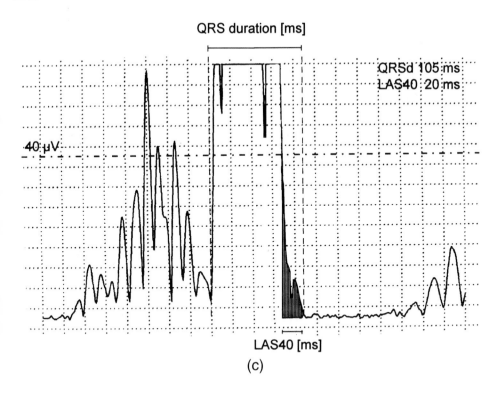

QRSd 105 ms
LAS40 20 ms

40 µV

LAS40 [ms]

(c)

QRS duration [ms]

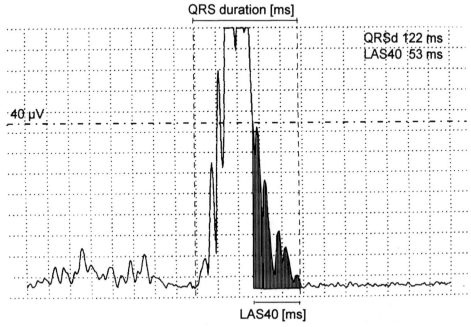

QRSd 122 ms
LAS40 53 ms

40 µV

LAS40 [ms]

(d)

Figure 15.2 continued

The reported recovery rate of microsignals has varied greatly. His bundle potentials have been detected with a sensitivity of 31–64% and ventricular late potentials with 52–90%. All studies state that complementary information can be gained from high-resolution ECG beat-to-beat recordings when compared with conventional signal-averaging.[13] Other problems of beat-to-beat recordings include electromyotonic noise, power-line interference and instrument noise. The lack of standardization and quantification of the results makes it difficult to compare the results of different groups.

Only one study has evaluated the diagnostic performance of real-time, nonaveraged high-resolution ECG. A sensitivity of 93% and a specificity of 65% for identifying ventricular tachycardia patients was reported.[13] Visual analysis of the high-resolution ECG parameters was used, which could in part explain the rather low specificity obtained.

Holter-Based Analysis of Late Potentials

In 1989, data acquisition from Holter tapes for detection of ventricular late potentials was introduced.[14] The ability to record and analyze signal-averaged high-resolution electrocardiograms from Holter tapes offers clear advantages: easy handling of the recordings and the option of several analysis periods during 24 hours of registration, as well as the chance to assess arrhythmias, ST segment changes, heart rate variability and late potentials from one data source. However, this technique also leads to significant technical problems, such as speed stability of the recording and playback processes, a possible increase in background noise due to the patient's activities or inadequate electrode contact, and a restricted frequency bandwidth of the tape-recorder.

A three-channel Holter system providing this technique is available commercially (Del Mar Avionics, Irvine, CA). It stores the analog ECG raw data on a conventional 60-minute audio tape without any preselection. The frequency response of the recorder is limited (0.1–100 Hz, ±3 dB) compared with the wider frequency band of real-time systems (0.5–300 Hz, ±3 dB). At the beginning of each recording, 6 minutes' of calibration pulses are obtained to adjust the amplitudes and facilitate channel alignment in the scanning mode. Resting periods within the 24-hour recording without conspicuous disturbances in the ECG have to be selected. Segments of 800 s are then digitized from the tape at a scanning speed of 120 times the recording speed, with 1.000 Hz real-time conversion rate per channel. Signal-averaging is subsequently performed using a manually selected QRS complex as a template. The resulting averaged QRS complex of each lead is then stored on hard disk for further analysis.

Kelen et al.[14] found a close morphologic similarity and a high concordance of parameters between real-time and Holter-recorded signal-averaged high-resolution ECGs. They obtained SAECGs using both techniques in 18 patients with known positive late potential findings and a previous myocardial infarction as well as a history of spontaneous or induced sustained ventricular tachycardia, and in 14 healthy volunteers. The analysis was performed using identical software for all recordings. The linear correlations for QRSD, LAS 40 and RMS 40 were $r = 0.99, 0.93$ and 0.95, respectively. The patient categorization into normal and abnormal SAECGs did not change in any case between real-time and Holter-based recordings using similar criteria.

We performed a comparative study to determine whether the new method is feasible in a daily routine and whether the previously described limitations result in a significantly reduced reliability in detection of late potentials, comparing the Holter-based system to conventional real-time equipment (1200 EPX, ART, Houston). 110 subjects were studied, of whom 21 were healthy people and 89 consecutive patients with coronary artery disease suffering from myocardial infarction. Previous episodes of ventricular tachycardia were documented in 40 patients. Each subject served as his own control, with the Holter recording performed directly before or after real-time acquisition in a randomized order using the same skin electrodes. The linear correlations comparing the individual late potential parameters calculated with both techniques ranged from 0.48 to 0.70. A major interesting result was that the mean noise levels of the ECG recordings were identical for both recording techniques. The clinical value of both equipments was similar, showing no significant differences in sensitivity and specificity in detecting patients with previous episodes of ventricular tachycardia.

However, the feasibility of a diagnostic tool in clinical practice is particularly dependent on the reproducibility of its results. The signal-averaging process of the Holter-based equipment is different from most of the real-time systems, in so far as a manual template setting for the averaging process has to be performed which may influence the results. We therefore averaged and analyzed 30 tapes four times using different template settings. The high linear correlation found for the late potential parameters confirmed the fair reproducibility of time-domain analysis from Holter-recorded signal-averaged ECG.

In conclusion, the use of Holter-recorded ECGs for detection of ventricular late potentials in the time domain is feasible and yields results which are comparable to those of real-time systems. Holter recording provides the ability to perform several noninvasive analytical procedures of risk stratification from one medium. However, some technical limitations still have to be overcome. Future Holter systems using solid-state memory without tape-recordings will enhance the quality of signal-averaged ECGs and even allow frequency analysis methods without the current frequency restrictions.

Technical Standards of Commercial Late Potential Systems

Various equipment has been introduced offering signal-averaging ECG acquisition and analysis with different levels of technology. Some early systems were simply modified digital ECG devices, whereas others were specifically created for late potential analysis. Equipment ranges from simple bedside recording units presenting a fixed time-domain analysis, up to high-end systems with online or post-processing signal-averaging, individual template settings, single lead analysis, and a variety of time- and frequency-domain analysis programs such as spectrotemporal mapping, spectral turbulence analysis or adaptive frequency analysis. Other options include selectable filter cutoff frequencies for time-domain analysis, several filter types or flexible definitions of late potential parameters (i.e. *RMS 30*, the root-mean-square voltage of the last 30 ms of QRS, instead of *RMS 40* which is more generally used). Batch-processing options allow full automatic analysis of hundreds of raw data files, producing numerical results stored in a database or in ASCII files which can subsequently be used with statistical software for further investigation.

A variety of studies have demonstrated significant differences in late potential findings depending on the equipment used.[15] While the hardware settings (lead systems, amplifiers, A/D converters) of the majority of commercial systems meet comparable standards, the signal-processing software differs markedly and will continue to do so with the development of new algorithms. Furthermore, the filter design most commonly used for time-domain analysis, namely the 4-pole bidirectional Butterworth bandpass filter, is partly protected by an international patent. Many equipment manufacturers attempt to circumvent this patent by creating their own filter algorithms.

The clinical usefulness of this noninvasive method has been evaluated in fairly large prospective trials. It is desirable to use identical, or at least comparable, signal-processing techniques and similar definitions for late potential parameters in clinical routine or in research. This obviously has not been the case. Therefore, in 1991 a statement by a joint Task Force Committee of the European Society of Cardiology, the American Heart Association and the American College of Cardiology provided standards for analysis of ventricular late potentials using high-resolution electrocardiography.[16] It recognized a variety of technical considerations as standards, starting with electrodes and the lead systems, leading to the signal-averaging and data-analysis process. Measurement of noise level and definition of the endpoint of the QRS complex in the time domain were described following the method of Simson.[7]

However, it should be noted that several years after publication of the Task Force Committee statement, obvious differences remain in time-domain signal processing in commercial late potential devices. Even for basic items like noise measurement or the QRS endpoint definition, no consensus has been achieved. We tested the results of signal processing of six commercial devices using an artificial signal as common analog input. The six late potential systems showed a wide range of differences. The noise levels differed from 0.25 to $0.6\,\mu V$ owing to different methods of measurement. Hence differences in parameter calculations occur depending on the equipment used, which may lead to misinterpretations of late potential findings in individual patients. For this reason, either individual abnormality cutoffs for each commercial system have to be established in large prospective trials, or a consensus on standards has to be accepted.

Effects of Pharmacologic and Nonpharmacologic Interventions

Pharmacologic interventions

All drugs prolonging the duration of the QRS complex and slowing the conduction velocity also affect the SAECG recording. In patients taking an antiarrhythmia drug, abnormalities of the SAECG may be more pronounced than before drug therapy. Separating patients who will benefit from antiarrhythmia drugs from those in whom these drugs are ineffective, or even proarrhythmia, is a desirable goal that has not yet been achieved. Further studies are necessary before the technique can be used to generate useful information.

Antitachycardia surgery

Another indication for the SAECG is to study patients before and after surgery for drug-refractory ventricular tachycardia. Normalization of an abnormal preoperative SAECG predicts surgical success for removal of the tachycardia structures. The change in SAECG is not related to other factors such as left ventricular function, aneurysmectomy, the site of endocardial resection or the site of origin of ventricular tachycardia. If a preoperatively abnormal SAECG is postoperatively normal, there is a high chance of remaining free of subsequent tachyarrhythmias.

Lack of normalization does not exclude surgical success, because in about half of patients with late potentials persistently present, ventricular tachycardia is no longer inducible after surgery – suggesting that a critical amount of the re-entrant pathway has been removed despite the remaining abnormal electrical activity.

Catheter ablation

Very few studies have evaluated the effects of catheter ablation on the SAECG. In small-scale studies, no significant changes in SAECG parameters have been found although the ablation procedure itself was successful. These 'negative' findings could be explained by the fact that the amount of scar tissue producing the delayed fragmented electrical activity is much greater than the amount of tissue critical for arrhythmia induction and continuation which can be ablated.

Few studies have investigated the effects of catheter ablation on the SAECG in patients with supraventricular arrhythmias. No pathological changes could be demonstrated.

Effects of autonomic function on the SAECG

The effects of increased or decreased sympathetic and parasympathetic activity on the SAECG have received very little attention. In a recent study,[17] sympathetic activation induced by the head-up tilt test did not modify the incidence of late potentials or of individual SAECG parameters. Moreover, physical exertion, like marathon running, has been shown to have no influence on SAECG parameters.

Clinical Studies of Ventricular Late Potentials

Coronary artery disease and documented ventricular tachyarrhythmias

The most important application of SAECG is the prediction of subsequent sustained ventricular arrhythmias such as ventricular tachycardia, ventricular fibrillation and sudden cardiac death, especially in patients following myocardial infarction.[7,10] At least as important is its ability to identify those patients who will not have these events (high specificity). In general, ventricular tachycardia is predicted better than ventricular fibrillation or sudden cardiac death, which may have arrhythmogenic mechanisms other than re-entry[5,7,20] (Figure 15.3).

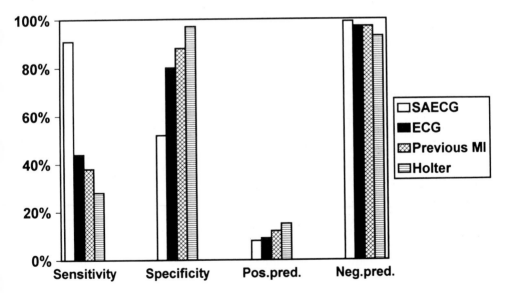

Figure 15.3 Sensitivity, specificity, positive and negative predictive values of the signal-averaged ECG (SAECG), occurrence of nonsustained ventricular tachycardia in ambulatory 24-hour ECG (Holter), Selvester score >10 (ECG), and history of previous infarction (previous MI), for prediction of arrhythmic events after acute myocardial infarction. The highest sensitivity of 91% and negative predictive accuracy of 99% for identifying patients with and without arrhythmic events was achieved by SAECG, and the highest specificity of 97% and positive predictive accuracy of 15% by nonsustained ventricular tachycardia in 24-hour ambulatory ECG. All parameters had very high negative predictive values (93% to 99%).

Several retrospective studies have demonstrated abnormal late ventricular activity to differentiate postmyocardial infarction patients with and without a history of sustained ventricular tachycardia. In addition, risk stratification of patients with remote infarction having nonsustained ventricular tachycardia appears promising using the high-resolution ECG technique. Studies have demonstrated that patients with abnormal high-resolution ECGs are more prone to inducible sustained monomorphic ventricular tachycardia.[11] Prospective studies suggest that the high-resolution ECG could be utilized for risk stratification and management of patients with old myocardial infarction and nonsustained ventricular tachycardia.

Sensitivity and specificity of the different parameters have been reported to depend on the corner frequency of the highpass filter. Specificity is higher with the lower cutoff frequencies, whereas sensitivity is higher with the higher cutoff frequencies. The widely used 40 Hz highpass cutoff seems to be a good compromise.

Detection of late potentials appears likely to be most useful as a noninvasive predictor of inducibility of ventricular tachycardia, especially in patients with previous myocardial infarction. Particularly, an abnormal SAECG may indicate ventricular tachycardia inducibility in patients with nonsustained ventricular tachycardia, in contrast to patients who have a normal SAECG and are more likely to be noninducible. In combination with normal left ventricular function, a high negative predictive value has been associated with a normal SAECG.

Patients with acute myocardial infarction

Natural history. Late potentials may show time-dependent changes in patients with acute myocardial infarction (MI). They can be detected as early as 3 hours after the onset of acute MI. The first 24–48 hours after onset of MI are electrophysiologically unstable. They show an increasing incidence of late potentials. Late potentials have been found to be most prevalent in the period 6–30 days after MI. Most positive SAECGs (93%) are recorded in the period 6–14 days after MI.[18] The later appearance of a new late potential is rare without a new myocardial infarction. Transient late potentials are uncommon. In a recent study,[19] the loss of late potentials during the first months after MI did not decrease the risk of subsequent arrhythmic events.

Abnormalities in the SAECG occur in 20–52% of cases after MI. Especially patients with Q wave infarction, high total creatinine phosphokinase (CPK) values, and inferior infarct location have been demonstrated to present more abnormal findings in SAECG than those with non-Q-wave infarction, low CPK values and anterior infarction. In post-MI patients developing sustained ventricular tachycardia, the SAECG is abnormal in 73–100% of cases, compared with 7–15% of post-MI patients without sustained VT.

Prediction of arrhythmic events. Prospective studies in post-MI patients have confirmed the increased likelihood of spontaneous sustained ventricular tachycardia and sudden cardiac death in patients having an abnormal high-resolution ECG defined by the investigators.[2,5,6,20] Thus, results of multivariate analysis show that risk stratification based on the high-resolution ECG is independent of more traditional determinants of risk that include left ventricular ejection fraction and the presence and complexity of ventricular ectopy. According to the literature, 14–29% of patients recovering from MI with abnormal high-resolution ECGs will experience sustained VT within the first year, but only 0.8–4.5% of those in whom the high-resolution ECG is normal.[5,6,20] Another 3.6–40% of patients with late ventricular activity are going to die suddenly, compared with 0–4.3% of patients without late ventricular activity.

The predictive accuracy of the high-resolution ECG can be increased by combining its results with measures of left ventricular function, mainly left ventricular ejection fraction.[20] Overall, the high-resolution ECG is a sensitive, noninvasive method for risk stratification of patients recovering from MI. The optimal time after MI for recording the high-resolution ECG has not been clearly defined. Recordings obtained during the second week after MI have been proposed to have the highest predictive accuracy for future arrhythmic events. However, follow-up of post-MI patients has shown that a normal SAECG could identify patients with a patent infarct-related vessel with 86% positive predictive accuracy and 56% negative predictive accuracy. Vessel patency is an important factor improving prognosis after MI, independently from left ventricular function.

Thrombolytic therapy and late potentials. Several large-scale studies have confirmed the reduced risk and improved survival after successful thrombolytic therapy following acute MI. Many studies have shown that patients with patent infarct-related vessel after thrombolysis have a reduced incidence of late potentials. However, this seems to be true only in cases with early (within 4–6 hours) revascularization either by thrombolytic agents or angioplasty. This effect has been demonstrated to be independent of other measures of successful reperfusion therapy, such as preserved left ventricular function.

Several studies have demonstrated that successful reperfusion therapy is related to decreased incidence of late potentials in the SAECG, especially in inferior infarctions. Reperfusion also seems to cause preservation of the initial RMS voltage in the anteroseptal infarcts and terminal RMS voltage in patients treated during the first two hours after infarction.

Comparison with clinical variables. The use of the SAECG and of left ventricular ejection fraction together have been reported to result in an improved risk stratification after first myocardial infarction.[5,20] In our study,[21] a prospective series of 733 males below 66 years of age surviving the acute phase of MI underwent routine clinical evaluation, standard 12-lead ECG, exercise testing, signal-averaged ECG, and 24-hour ambulatory ECG before hospital discharge. In Cox regression analysis of the variables that were significant in univariate analyses, an abnormal signal-averaged electrocardiogram, nonsustained ventricular tachycardia on ambulatory ECG, Selvester ECG score >10 (an ECG surrogate for the extent of left ventricular involvement), and a history of previous myocardial infarction, were the only independent predictors of the 32 arrhythmic events (12 sustained ventricular tachycardia, 8 ventricular fibrillation, 12 sudden cardiac deaths) during the 6-month follow-up (Figure 15.3). Based on the regression coefficients of these variables in the model, a new risk score for arrhythmic events after acute MI was created. An abnormal signal-averaged electrocardiogram gave 4 points, nonsustained ventricular tachycardia on ambulatory ECG 3 points, and a Selvester ECG score >10 or history of previous MI gave 2 points each. Patients without risk factors got 0 points. Patients with higher risk scores had clearly a worse outcome (Figure 15.4). The high-risk patients with scores from 8 to 11 (26 patients, 4% of all patients) had a relative risk of 9.1 (95% confidence limit, 4.5–18.6) for subsequent arrhythmic events compared with low-risk patients with scores 0 or 6. Only 69% of patients with risk scores from 8 to 11 were event-free, compared with 97% of patients with risk scores 0–7. The positive predictive value of this classification was 31%.

This study shows that the high risk of arrhythmic events after acute MI is identified by the following four parameters: an abnormal signal-averaged ECG; the occurrence of nonsustained ventricular tachycardia on 24-hour ambulatory ECG; a Selvester ECG score >10; and a history of previous myocardial infarction. Using this type of screening, patients can be divided into groups with different prognoses. Patients with high risk (scores from 8 to 11) should be directed to further diagnostic work-up and intensified follow-up. Whether there is a role for invasive electrophysiologic studies followed by prophylactic antiarrhythmic drug therapy or implantation of an automatic defibrillator in this special patient group remains to be studied.

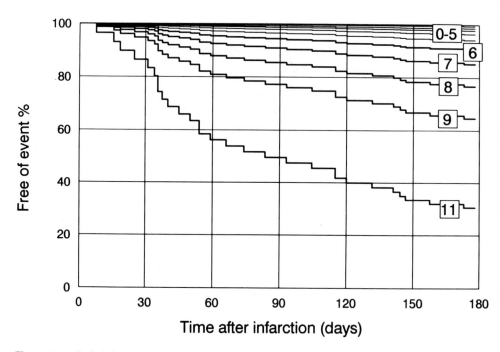

Figure 15.4 Probabilities of remaining free of arrhythmic events after acute myocardial infarction for patients cross-classified by signal-averaged ECG, occurrence of nonsustained ventricular tachycardia in ambulatory 24-hour ECG, Selvester score >10, and history of previous infarction. The groups from 0 to 11 were formed according to points given by different positive risk factors. Especially, patients with scores from 8 to 11 have clearly higher risk arrhythmic events than other patients. Only 69% of patients with risk scores from 8 to 11 were event-free, compared with 97% of patients with risk scores 0–7.

Patients with syncope

The SAECG has a limited role in assessment of the patient presenting with unexplained syncope, depending on the type of underlying cardiac disorder.[22] In 25–40% of cases with organic heart disease, sustained ventricular tachycardia has been reported as the most probable cause of syncope. In such patients, a negative SAECG excludes ventricular tachycardia or ventricular fibrillation as the cause of syncope, with a high predictive value. In mixed cohorts of patients presenting with syncope, about half of those with late potentials have ventricular tachycardia as an underlying mechanism, amounting to about 80% in those with CAD.

A normal SAECG does not preclude ventricular tachycardia as a mechanism, since not even all patients with re-entrant ventricular tachycardia have late potentials, and ventricular tachycardia may also be due to other mechanisms such as abnormal automaticity. Thus, the indication for invasive electrophysiologic studies is based more on the history and type of underlying heart disease and less on the presence of late potentials. If present, they strengthen the indication, but when absent the need for an electrophysiologic study is governed by the history of the patient.

Patients with cardiomyopathy and heart failure

An abnormal SAECG can also predict the occurrence of sustained ventricular tachyarrhythmias and sudden death in patients with dilated cardiomyopathy.

A positive SAECG is usually seen only in patients with dilated hearts. However, an abnormal SAECG does not correlate with increased risk of either spontaneous or induced sustained ventricular tachycardia. Patients with dilated cardiomyopathy have a high incidence of serious arrhythmic events. An abnormal SAECG was found in 83% of patients with nonischemic congestive cardiomyopathy presenting with sustained ventricular arrhythmia, compared with 14% of patients without these arrhythmias. Life-table analysis showed that the probability of remaining free from sudden death was lower in patients with an abnormal SAECG than in patients with a normal SAECG (68% versus 100%, $p < 0.01$).

The SAECG seems to be predictive of sudden cardiac death in younger patients with hypertrophic cardiomyopathy. The prevalence of late potentials in this disease ranges between 12.5% and 20%. Late potentials have been found to have a 50% sensitivity and a 93% specificity for predicting independently a history of spontaneous nonsustained ventricular tachycardia or cardiac arrest.[23] In addition, among patients with hypertrophic cardiomyopathy undergoing programmed electrical stimulation, 74% with inducible ventricular tachycardia had late potentials – yielding a sensitivity of 74% and a specificity of 86%. On the other hand, attempts that have been made to use the signal-averaged ECG as a predictor of spontaneous or inducible arrhythmias have had poor results. In one study, a weak association was demonstrated between sudden cardiac death and late potentials in young hypertrophic cardiomyopathy patients.

Some reports have shown possible clinical applications of the SAECG for predicting sustained ventricular tachycardia in patients with arrhythmogenic right ventricular cardiomyopathy. It should be noted that the criteria for an abnormal finding in this group of patients differ from those used in ischemic heart disease.

In 123 patients the presence of late potentials correctly identified those with inducible ventricular tachycardia (sensitivity 78%, specificity 74%), extensive right ventricular disease (96% and 63%, respectively), and abnormal fibrolipomatous infiltration (35% and 77%, respectively).[24] The predictive value of SAECG was further improved by additional analysis of the clinical arrhythmia (sustained or nonsustained ventricular tachycardia).

Patients with ventricular tachycardia without heart disease

The incidence of late potentials in patients with sustained ventricular tachycardia and structurally normal heart has been reported to be 37%, compared with 5% in patients with nonsustained ventricular tachycardia and a normal heart. The presence of late potentials was specific but not sensitive as a correlate of abnormal endomyocardial biopsy results. Late potentials have been reported to be particularly rare in patients with ventricular tachycardia originating in the right ventricular outflow tract. These findings may be explained by early activation of this area during sinus rhythm, by the small size of the arrhythmogenic substrate, and the fact that most of these arrhythmias probably originate from abnormal automaticity and not re-entry.

Patients after heart transplantation

Early studies have suggested the use of the SAECG for monitoring cardiac transplant rejections.[25] The SAECG recorded at the time of the first normal endomyocardial biopsy is compared with subsequent recordings. According to limited studies, an abnormal SAECG predicted rejection earlier than scheduled biopsies. The SAECG has also been found to be much more sensitive than the standard ECG or clinical parameters. Especially, cyclosporin-treated transplant patients having rejection experience gradual changes in these parameters, rendering them less sensitive. The abnormal values for a positive SAECG finding differ from those used in arrhythmia prediction.

Late potentials and ischemia

The SAECG has only rarely been reported to detect ischemia induced by dipyridamole or exercise.

Limitations of the SAECG

The SAECG has several limitations in the time domain, and these should be kept in mind when applying the method in clinical settings. Patients with bundle branch block or implanted pacemakers have to be excluded, as do those with atrial fibrillation and flutter which have been reported to produce false-positive late potentials. The algorithms for detecting QRS onset and offset are all based on measuring noise before or after the QRS. This means that QRS endpoint detection can fail in cases with noise levels that are too high or too low.

Although most commercial and custom-made recording systems use a similar approach, real standardization of the method and the criteria are still needed. Highpass filtering is a very important part of SAECG data processing. Very few studies have investigated the effects of different highpass filter settings on SAECG signals. All types of filtering affect the signals. For example, the commonly used bidirectional filters distort the middle portion of the QRS complex, and finite impulse response filters tend to spread the signal. A study to evaluate the effects of different filter types on SAECG signals in the clinical setting is yet to be performed.

Although the reproducibility of the method has been demonstrated to be excellent, it is known that even a slight change of the electrode positions may have a great influence on SAECG signals and their classification.

The criteria for a normal or an abnormal SAECG have been studied only to a limited degree, although gender, stature and the underlying heart disease may have effects on the high-resolution parameters. Recently, the effects of age and infarct location have been proposed. Criteria for abnormality of a high-resolution ECG depend on many factors: technical details, data processing, and the patient material studied. Therefore, it is necessary for each research group to determine their own criteria for abnormality, especially when custom-made systems are used.

Evaluation of the diagnostic performance of a screening method is difficult. In many studies, sensitivity and specificity have been chosen instead of predictive value, for three main reasons:

1. Only a few studies have been performed prospectively.
2. Predictive accuracy depends a great deal on the prevalence of endpoints in the study (arrhythmic events, induced arrhythmias etc.).
3. Studies have mainly used sensitivity and specificity for optimizing the diagnostic performance of the SAECG method, which enables direct comparison of the results.

However, one should be careful when comparing studies that specify definite clinical endpoints (e.g. documented sustained ventricular tachyarrhythmias or sudden death) with studies that have nonclinical or other endpoints (induced arrhythmias, nonsustained arrhythmias). In addition, results obtained using arbitrarily dichotomized parameters and their combinations should not be compared directly with results obtained using continuous data.

Many SAECG studies reported in the literature have included heterogeneous patient populations. Patients with sustained or nonsustained ventricular tachycardia with different types of underlying organic heart disease have been compared with patients without arrhythmias, or even with normals. Some studies have used the inducibility of sustained ventricular arrhythmias as an endpoint.

Application of the SAECG in Clinical Settings

Use of the SAECG as one of the methods for stratifying risk after acute myocardial infarction seems well-founded. The efficacy of the method increases when it is combined with other risk indicators, especially left ventricular ejection fraction. The SAECG method is still open to refinement. Different features and parameters can be of different value when the clinical setup is changed. It seems highly probable that the SAECG can provide useful information both in therapy and in pathophysiological studies of cardiac diseases and arrhythmias.

Several studies have shown that post-MI patients with unexplained syncope and abnormal high-resolution ECG are more prone to sustained ventricular tachycardia during programmed ventricular stimulation. However, since in some patients ventricular tachycardia may be inducible when SAECG is normal, an abnormal SAECG is not required prior to electrophysiological study.

Patients with a previously positive high-resolution ECG, who have been operated on for recurrent ventricular tachycardia and in whom the high-resolution ECG reverts to normal after surgery, have been reported to have a high likelihood (about 90%) of no recurrence of these arrhythmias. Successful catheter ablation of any arrhythmia has not been shown to have any effect on the SAECG.

In patients with arrhythmogenic right ventricular cardiomyopathy, the SAECG can identify those with more extensive right ventricular involvement, a history of sustained ventricular tachycardia, and of inducible ventricular tachycardia during programmed ventricular stimulation. In patients with dilated cardiomyopathy, the SAECG might prove to be helpful for detecting propensity to spontaneous ventricular tachycardia. A significant correlation has been found between young patients with hypertrophic cardiomyopathy and the risk of sudden cardiac death. Data on the assessment of risk in patients with mitral valve prolapse or antiarrhythmic drug efficacy are too limited to allow any definite conclusions. Another application concerns the follow-up of patients after heart transplantation, to detect rejection; changes in SAECG seem to correlate with signs of rejection.

In conclusion, the high-resolution ECG has a definite independent role in improving the predictive accuracy of conventional risk-evaluation techniques. Risk stratification is an important clinical task because of improved therapeutic possibilities. Directed nonpharmacologic treatment has been shown to improve the prognosis of patients with documented life-threatening arrhythmias. Recognizing the patients at risk before the arrhythmic event is the first step towards advanced diagnostic and preventive treatment. Noninvasive techniques are desirable as screening methods compared with invasive techniques. Although it is not yet known how these patients at risk should be handled, the detection of risk is important for follow-up and essential for any prospective study evaluating the alternative management strategies.

Future Perspectives

Real-time SAECG has already established its value in clinical decision-making. In the near future, new hardware and software may enable us to study beat-to-beat recordings and achieve ambulatory high-resolution monitoring. It may be possible to study arrhythmia mechanisms other than re-entry. Developments may also improve the detection of arrhythmic components of cardiac electrical activation in patients without coronary heart disease. Combining SAECG and related methods with other forms of analysis (frequency-domain, etc.) and other parameters related to arrhythmia is a way to optimize the use of this sophisticated technique in clinical practice.

References

1. Berbari EJ, Scherlag BJ, Hope RR, Lazzara R. Recording from the body surface of arrhythmogenic ventricular activity during the ST-segment. *Am J Cardiol* 1978; **41**: 697–702.
2. Breithardt G, Becker R, Seipel L, Abendroth RR, Ostermeyer J. Noninvasive detection of late potentials in man – a new marker for ventricular tachycardia. *Eur Heart J* 1981; **2**: 1–11.
3. El-Sherif N, Scherlag BJ, Lazzara R, Hope RR. Re-entrant ventricular arrhythmias in the late myocardial infarction period. I: Conduction characteristics in the infarction zone. *Circulation* 1977; **55**: 686–702.
4. Gardner PI, Ursell PC, Fenoglio JJ, Wit AL. Electrophysiologic and anatomic basis for fractionated electrograms recorded from healed myocardial infarcts. *Circulation* 1985; **72**: 596–611.
5. Kuchar DL, Thorburn CW, Sammel NL. Prediction of serious arrhythmic events after myocardial infarction: signal-averaged electrocardiogram, Holter monitoring and radionuclide ventriculography. *J Am Coll Cardiol* 1987; **9**: 531–8.
6. Malik M, Odemuyiwa O, Poloniecki J, Kulakowski P, Farrell T, Staunton A, Camm AJ. Late potentials after acute myocardial infarction: performance of different criteria for the prediction of arrhythmic complications. *Eur Heart J* 1992; **13**: 599–607.
7. Simson MB. Identification of patients with ventricular tachycardia after myocardial infarction from signals in the terminal QRS complex. *Circulation* 1981; **64**: 235–42.
8. Simson MB, Untereker WJ, Spielman SR, Horowitz LN, Marcus NH, Falcone RA, Harken AH, Josephson ME. Relation between late potentials on the body surface and directly recorded fragmented electrocardiograms in patients with ventricular tachycardia. *Am J Cardiol* 1983; **51**: 105–12.
9. Hood MA, Pogwizd SM, Peirick J, Cain ME. Contribution of myocardium responsible for ventricular tachycardia to abnormalities detected by analysis of signal-averaged ECGs. *Circulation* 1992; **86**: 1888–901.
10. Breithardt G, Cain ME, El-Sherif N, Flowers NC, Hombach V, Janse M, Simson MB, Steinbeck G. Standard for analysis of ventricular late potentials using high-resolution or signal-averaged electrocardiography. *Circulation* 1991; **83**: 1481–7.
11. Caref EB, Turitto G, Ibrahim BB, Henkin R, El-Sherif N. Role of bandpass filters in optimizing the value of the signal-averaged electrocardiogram as a predictor of the results of programmed stimulation. *Am J Cardiol* 1989; **64**: 16–26.
12. Denes P, Santarelli P, Hauser RG, Uretz EF. Quantitative analysis of the high-frequency components of the terminal portion of the body surface QRS in normal subjects and in patients with ventricular tachycardia. *Circulation* 1983; **67**: 1129–38.
13. Zimmermann M, Adamec R, Simonin P, Richez J. Beat-to-beat detection of ventricular late potentials with high-resolution electrocardiography. *Am Heart J* 1991; **121**: 576–85.
14. Kelen G, Henkin R, Lannon M, Bloomfield D, El-Sherif N. Correlation between the signal averaged electrocardiogram from Holter tapes and from real-time recordings. *Am J Cardiol* 1989; **63**: 1321–5.
15. Zimmermann M, Adamec R, Simonin P, Fromer M, Richez J. Noninvasive detection of ventricular late potentials: direct comparison of 7 different high-gain recording systems. *Am J Noninvas Cardiol* 1992; **6**: 154–67.
16. Breithardt G (chairman), Cain M, El-Sherif N, Flowers N, Hombach V, Janse M, Simson MB, Steinbeck G. Standards for analysis of ventricular late potentials using high-resolution electrocardiography – a statement of a Task Force Committee between the European Society of Cardiology, the American Heart Association and the American College of Cardiology. *Eur Heart J* 1991; **12**: 473–80. Also *J Am Coll Cardiol* 1991; **17**: 999–1006. Also *Circulation* 1991; **83**: 1481–8.
17. Lombardi F, Finocchiaro ML, Dalla Vecchia L, Sala R, Garimoldi M, Baselli G, Cerutti S, Malliani A. Effects of tilt and exercise on signal-averaged electrocardiogram after acute myocardial infarction. *Eur Heart J* 1990; **11**: 421–8.
18. El Sherif N, Ursell SN, Bekheit S, Fontaine J, Turitto G, Henkin R, Caref EB. Prognostic significance of the signal-averaged ECG depends on the time of recording in the postinfarction period. *Am Heart J* 1989; **118**: 256–64.
19. Kuchar DL, Thorburn CW, Sammel NL. Prognostic implications of loss of late potentials following acute myocardial infarction. *PACE* 1993; **16**: 2104–11.
20. Farrell TG, Bashir Y, Cripps T, Malik M, Poloniecki J, Bennett D, Ward DE, Camm AJ. Risk stratification for arrhythmic events in postinfarction patients based on heart rate variability, ambulatory electrocardiographic variables and the signal-averaged electrocardiogram. *Am J Coll Cardiol* 1991; **18**: 687–97.
21. Maekijaervi M, Fetsch T, Reinhardt L, Martinez-Rubio A, Borggrefe M, Breithardt G. A new diagnostic algorithm for noninvasive risk stratification after acute myocardial infarction using ECG techniques. *Circulation* 1994; **90**: 501.
22. Winters SL, Stewart D, Gomes JA. Signal averaging of the surface QRS complex predicts inducibility of ventricular tachycardia in patients with syncopy of unknown origin: a prospective study. *J Am Coll Cardiol* 1987; **10**: 775.
23. Cripps TR, Counihan PJ, Frenneaux MP, Ward DE, Camm AJ, McKenna WJ. Signal-averaged electrocardiography in hypertrophic cardiomyopathy. *J Am Coll Cardiol* 1990; **15**: 956–61.
24. Wichter T, Fetsch T. Time domain analysis and spectral turbulence analysis of the signal-averaged ECG identify high-risk subgroups in arrhythmogenic right ventricular cardiomyopathy. *Circulation* 1994; **90**: 229.
25. Haberl R, Weber M, Reichenspurner H. Frequency analysis of the surface electrocardiogram for recognition of acute rejection after orthotopic cardiac transplantation. *Circulation* 1987; **76**: 101–8.

16

Spectral Analysis of High-Resolution ECGs

P. Rubel, J. Ph. Couderc, D. Morlet, J. Fayn, F. Peyrin and P. Touboul

Introduction

Accurate noninvasive detection of patients at risk of developing sustained ventricular tachycardia (VT) and sudden cardiac death is one of the most challenging issues in cardiology.

In the prediction of ventricular tachyarrhythmia, one consideration is to detect the small areas of diseased myocardium that could be at the origin of malignant re-entries after myocardial infarction. Around these diseased areas, the depolarization wavefront is delayed and disorganized. This results in late, fractionated potentials in the electrocardiogram. Early studies showed that an altered depolarization can also be manifested as an increased number of notches and slurs within the QRS complex.[1] In contrast, spectral analysis has revealed reduction of high-frequency energy in patients after myocardial infarction.[2]

Nowadays, a widely used prognostic investigative tool is high-resolution electrocardiography (HRECG). One basic hypothesis in HRECG is that the low-amplitude fractioned potentials manifested after altered depolarizations can be taken from the body surface by signal-averaging techniques. The goal in HRECG signal acquisition is to improve the signal-to-noise ratio of the ECG; resolution of signals to the order of $0.5\,\mu V$ is required to detect late potentials accurately.[3]

The first method proposed for analysis of the signal-averaged HRECG was in the time domain. Today this is by far the most widely used technique. Standard time-domain analysis is based on the concept of late ventricular potentials defined as high-frequency (usually above 25 Hz), low-amplitude potentials in the terminal 40 ms of the QRS complex. However, time-domain analysis remains very dependent on accurate determination of the end of the QRS and on prior filtering.[4]

Since time-domain analysis is limited to the terminal QRS complex, fractionated potentials appearing within the QRS are not detected and myocardial regions activated too early in the QRS complex may not be detected at all. Furthermore, patients with bundle branch blocks are generally excluded from this analysis or modified criteria must be used.

Several other methods have been proposed in the literature to highlight fractionated potentials in signal-averaged HRECGs. They are based on standard frequency-domain analysis techniques,[5] time–frequency domain techniques, like short-time Fourier analysis,[6,7] autoregressive modeling,[8] the Wigner–Ville distribution,[9,10] and time–scale techniques like the wavelet transforms.[4,11,12]

Most of these studies concentrated on portions of the cardiac cycle that contain late potentials detectable by time-domain analysis, such as the terminal QRS complex and/or the ST segment. Spectral analysis was used to search for specific frequency features that characterize late ventricular potentials and the entire cardiac cycle. However, results of spectral analysis are difficult to reproduce since the basic requirement for signal stationarity is not fulfilled. Advanced multiresolution time-varying spectral analysis techniques should overcome this problem.

In the following, we briefly review the signal processing methods that are currently being used for analysis of HRECGs in the frequency domain, discuss their most salient properties, present novel wavelet analysis methods for the stratification of postinfarction patients, and speculate on their potential.

Frequency-Domain Analysis of High-Resolution ECGs

Time-Invariant Spectral Analysis

Spectral analysis consists in the transformation of a time signal, such as the ECG, into the frequency domain so that power is represented as a function of frequency. The frequency spectrum is computed by means of the Fourier transform:[3]

$$S(\omega) = \int_{-\infty}^{+\infty} s(t) \exp(-j\omega t)\, dt.$$

The relative power of each frequency component is given by the power density spectrum $P(\omega)$ defined by:

$$P(\omega) = |S(\omega)|^2.$$

The Fourier transform of a signal $s(t)$ performs a decomposition of the signal following a series of sine and cosine waves of appropriate phases and amplitudes. Theoretically, the power spectrum of a pure sinusoid of frequency f_0 is a single impulse; i.e. a single spectral line at the frequency f_0 of the sine wave. In practice, however, because the Fourier transform is computed over a limited duration T, and because the signal is usually first multiplied by a window function $w(t)$, the power is spread over a frequency range. The effective spectral resolution Δf (i.e. the effective frequency bandwidth of a pure sinusoid containing 95% of its power) is given by

$$\Delta f = K_w / T,$$

where T is in seconds, Δf in hertz (Hz), and K_w is a constant depending on the characteristics of the window. Typical values for K_w range from 3.6 to 4.0.

Δf defines the frequency difference between two adjacent spectral components that could be accurately distinguished from each other.

Following Lander and Berbari,[3] there are three serious limitations in applying spectral analysis to high-resolution ECGs. These are (1) inadequate spectral resolution, (2) technique-induced artefacts, and (3) significant variability in the spectral estimates owing to nonstationarity of the ECG signals.

Since the spectrum of an ECG is continuously varying over time, the power spectral estimates computed by a standard Fourier analysis represent only the time average of all power spectra existing during the analysis interval. To achieve a time analysis of these changes, we have to consider methods of performing time-varying spectral analysis. The issue is that of representing the ventricular activity in a two-dimensional plane where one axis is time and the second is frequency. The objective of this so-called 'spectrotemporal mapping' of the ECG is to model its time–frequency structure and to extract useful and reproducible features from it.

The measurement of time-varying spectra characteristics is presently an active research topic in digital signal processing. We will review in the following sections three approaches: the fast Fourier transform, the Wigner–Ville distribution, and time–scale methods based on wavelet transforms. A discussion of autoregressive modeling approaches and signal-dependent kernel analysis can be found in reference 3.

Time–Frequency Analysis

The Short-Time Fourier Transform

The short-time Fourier transform is the best known and most widely used time–frequency representation. Spectrotemporal mapping is performed by segmenting the signal into a series of overlapping frames of duration $2T$ with an overlap duration of $(2T - \Delta)$.[3,6] For each time frame, the short-time Fourier transform $SF(t,\omega)$ is computed:

$$SF(t,\omega) = \int_{-T}^{+T} s(\tau)w^*(\tau - t) \exp(-j\omega\tau)\, d\tau$$

where $s(t)$ is the signal, $w(t)$ is the window function and $w^*(t)$ is the complex conjugate of $w(t)$. The signal is assumed to be zero everywhere outside the window interval. Typical are the rectangular window and the Blackman–Harris window.

The squared magnitude of the short-time Fourier transform is called the *spectrogram*. $w(t)$ can be considered as a window that selects a particular portion of signal centered around a given time location, and the Fourier transform of the windowed signal yields the frequency content at that time. The shorter the window, the better the time resolution, but the worse the frequency resolution. The rectangular window has the best resolution, but yields a series of sidelobes. The Blackman–Harris windows have very low sidelobes but relatively poor frequency resolution.

Figure 16.1 shows the 3-dimensional plots of 25 spectrograms of two postinfarction patients with and without ventricular tachycardia (VT). The total duration of the time frame is $2T = 80$ ms. Each time frame has been shifted by a value $\Delta = 3$ ms. The first time frame (segment 1) started 52 ms after the end of the QRS. The subsequent segments started progressively earlier in the ST segment, by steps of 3 ms, up to segment 25 that started within the QRS complex, 20 ms before the end of the QRS. Thus in Figure 16.1 time progresses from back to front, from QRS end minus 20 ms to QRS end plus 52 ms, by steps of 3 ms, and the frequency increases from the left to the right from 0 to 200 Hz. Certain differences can be observed, mainly the high-frequency content at the end of the QRS of the patient with VT, between 120 and 160 ms.

The Wigner–Ville transform

The shortcomings of the short-time Fourier transform has prompted several investigators to search for methods that provide high-resolution estimation, both in time and in frequency, of the bidimensional time–frequency distribution $P(t,f)$ of the ECG signal.

Several time–frequency transforms may be used to represent the distribution of the ECG signal energy in the time–frequency plane.[13] Among these is the class of shift-invariant quadratic time–frequency representations (Cohen's class), in which the Wigner distribution (WD) and its variants, the 'pseudo Wigner distribution' (PWD) and the 'smoothed pseudo Wigner distribution' (SPWD), play major roles. We briefly present

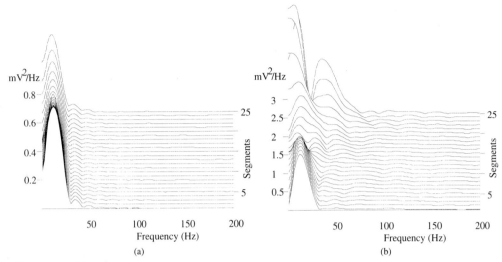

Figure 16.1 Short Fourier spectrotemporal mappings of the HRECG magnitude vector in postinfarction patients, (a) without VT, and (b) with VT. In (b), segments 15–25 show an increase in the high-frequency components and a decrease in the segment-to-segment spectral correlation, typical of delayed ventricular activation.

some basic definitions and the relationships between these representations. A more thorough description can be found in reference 13.

The Wigner distribution of a signal $s(t)$ is defined by:

$$WD_s(t,\omega) = \int_{-\infty}^{+\infty} s\left(t + \frac{\tau}{2}\right) s^*\left(t - \frac{\tau}{2}\right) \exp(-j\omega\tau) \, d\tau$$

where $s^*(t)$ is the complex conjugate of $s(t)$. The WD is always real and has a number of interesting mathematical properties. It satisfies the marginal properties, meaning that its projections on the time and frequency axes, respectively, give the signal's instantaneous power and spectral energy density:

$$\int_{-\infty}^{+\infty} P(t,f) \, df = |s(t)|^2 \quad \text{and} \quad \int_{-\infty}^{+\infty} P(t,f) \, dt = |s(f)|^2.$$

Compared with other distributions, the WD provides an improved, near-optimum time–frequency resolution.[3] Its major drawback, however, is the appearance of interference 'cross-terms'. These spurious interference terms appear between the signal frequencies, and present oscillations whose orientation and frequency depend on the positions of the interfering structures. For example, if there will be frequency components at 5 and 15 Hz respectively, there will be a spurious peak at 10 Hz. This makes it difficult to interpret the representation.

In order to reduce the interference terms, other techniques are necessary. Martin and Flandrin showed that most of the cross-terms feature cosine amplitude dependency, so they can easily be removed by a variety of smoothing techniques.[14] The pseudo-Wigner distribution is obtained by multiplying the temporal signal $s(t)$ by a window $w(t)$:

$$PWD_s(t,\omega) = \int_{-\infty}^{+\infty} \left| w\left(\frac{\tau}{2}\right) \right|^2 s\left(t + \frac{\tau}{2}\right) s^*\left(t - \frac{\tau}{2}\right) \exp(-j\omega\tau) \, d\tau.$$

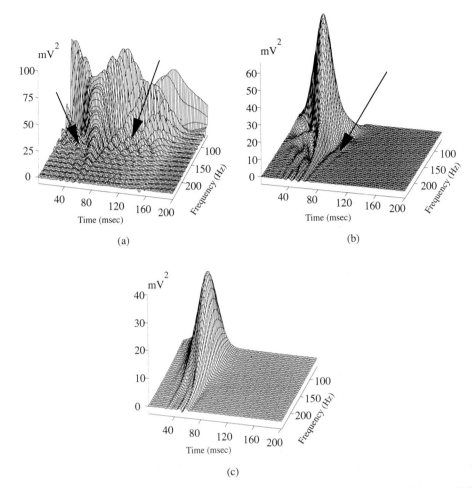

Figure 16.2 Time–frequency representations of (a, b) the Wigner–Ville and (c) the pseudo Wigner–Ville distributions of the HRECG magnitude vector of a healthy subject between QRS onset and QRS onset plus 200 ms. (a) shows the raw ECG signal, (b) the signal after baseline and T wave removal, and (c) the same signal as in (b) after temporal smoothing as performed by the pseudo Wigner–Ville transform. The arrows indicate the presence of cross-terms.

The smoothed pseudo-Wigner distribution is obtained by smoothing the result with an additional temporal window $h(t)$:

$$SPWD_s(t,\omega) = \int_{-\infty}^{+\infty} \left| w\left(\frac{\tau}{2}\right) \right|^2 \left(\int_{-\infty}^{+\infty} h(u-t)\, s\left(u+\frac{\tau}{2}\right) s^*\left(u-\frac{\tau}{2}\right) du \right) \exp(-j\omega\tau)\, d\tau.$$

The SPWD (and as a particular case the PWD) are related to the WD by:

$$SPWD_s(t,\omega) = \int_{-\infty}^{+\infty} \int_{-\infty}^{+\infty} WD_s(t',\omega')\, h(t-t')\, WD_w(0,\omega-\omega')\, dt'\, d\omega'.$$

Figure 16.2 shows the Wigner–Ville distribution of the high-resolution ECG of a young healthy subject. The representation is quite concentrated, but as indicated by the arrows, many oscillatory cross-terms are apparent, some of which are inherited by the interference between the QRS and the T waves. Removing the T wave and compensating for the baseline drift greatly improves the result. The pseudo Wigner–Ville transformation further enhances the time–frequency representation by suppressing the remaining cross-terms. However, this is done at the expense of a significant smoothing that lowers the spectrotemporal resolution.

The Wavelet Transform

Time–scale representations

The wavelet transform $S_g(a,b)$ of a signal $s(t)$ is the decomposition of this signal onto a set of analyzing functions $g_{a,b}(t)$ that are derived from a generic analyzing wavelet $g(t)$ by temporal translations (parameter b) and, according to whether the scale parameter a is greater or less than unity, by dilatation or contraction:

$$g_{a,b}(t) = \frac{1}{\sqrt{|a|}} g\left(\frac{t-b}{a}\right).$$

The continuous wavelet transform of $s(t)$ for wavelet $g(t)$ at scale a and time b is defined as:

$$S_g(a,b) = \int_{-\infty}^{+\infty} s(t)\, g_{a,b}^*(t)\, dt$$

where $g_{a,b}^*(t)$ denotes the complex conjugate of $g_{a,b}(t)$.

In order to be accepted as a basic wavelet, the function $g(t)$ must be integrable and square-integrable, and it must satisfy the following 'admissibility' condition:[15]

$$\int_{-\infty}^{+\infty} \frac{|G(\omega)|^2}{|\omega|}\, d\omega < \infty$$

where $G(\omega)$ denotes the Fourier transform of $g(t)$.

As an additional restriction, $g(t)$ and $G(\omega)$ should satisfy the following conditions:

$$\int_{-\infty}^{+\infty} t^2 |g(t)|^2\, dt < \infty \qquad \text{and} \qquad \int_{-\infty}^{+\infty} \omega^2 |G(\omega)|^2\, d\omega < \infty.$$

Under these additional assumptions, $G(0)=0$ or, equivalently,

$$\int_{-\infty}^{+\infty} g(t)\, dt = 0$$

and $g(t)$ looks like a 'small wave' well localized in time and in frequency.

The analyzing wavelet is chosen *a priori*. The first basic wavelet to be introduced was the modified Gaussian function described in 1984 by Morlet and Grossman:[16]

$$g(t) = \exp(i\omega_0 t)\exp(-t^2/2)$$

Admissibility conditions are satisfied with ω_0 between 5.0 and 6.0.

Figure 16.3 shows the time-domain graph of Morlet's wavelet for $\omega_0 = 5.33$ rad/s, together with the graphs of the orthogonal Meyer wavelet, a cubic B-spline wavelet and the first six derivatives of the Gaussian function $f(t) = \exp(-t^2/2)$.

B-spline wavelets of degree n are polynomial spline functions $g^n(t)$ that can be approximated by the following function:[17]

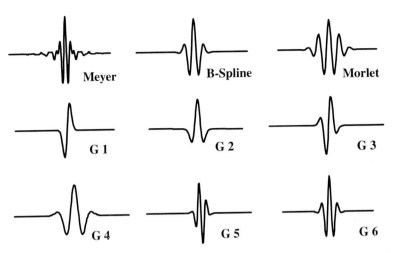

Figure 16.3 Time-domain representation of the nine basic analyzing wavelets considered for the analysis of HRECGs. G1 to G6 refer to the six first-derivatives of a Gaussian function. All wavelets are nonorthogonal except the Meyer.

$$g^n(t) \approx \sqrt{\left(\frac{6}{\pi(n+1)}\right)} \exp[-6t^2/(n+1)].$$

Defining the Meyer wavelets is much less straightforward. First, the generic wavelets are defined in the frequency domain in the following way:[18]

$G(f) = \exp(-j\pi f)\theta(f)$ with $g(t) = TF^{-1}(G(f))$

$\theta(f) = \theta(-f) \quad \forall f$

$\theta(f) \neq 0 \quad \forall |f| \in [\frac{1}{2} - \varepsilon, 1 + 2\varepsilon]$

$\theta(f) = 1 \quad \forall |f| \in [\frac{1}{2} + \varepsilon, 1 - 2\varepsilon]$

$\theta^2(f) + \theta^2(1 - f) = 1 \quad \forall |f| \in [\frac{1}{2} - \varepsilon, \frac{1}{2} + \varepsilon]$

$\theta(2f) = \theta(1 - f) \quad \forall |f| \in [\frac{1}{2} - \varepsilon, \frac{1}{2} + \varepsilon]$

with $0 < \varepsilon \leq 1/6$.

Then, $g(t)$ is computed by taking the inverse Fourier transform of $G(f)$:

$$g(t) = TF^{-1}(G(f)).$$

Finally, the different wavelets $g_{a,b}(t)$ are computed from $g(t)$ for different values of a and b, with the restriction that $a = 2^j$ and that j and b are integers.

Unlike the short-time Fourier transform, the frequency–resolution properties of the wavelet transform are frequency-dependent. To analyze high frequencies the analyzing wavelet is compressed in time (small scales) and thereby expanded in frequency, whereas at low frequencies (large scales) it uses large windows (Figure 16.4). It thus avoids poor frequency-domain resolutions in short segments, which is prevalent in Fourier analysis.

This so-called 'time–scale' technique is especially relevant for analyzing the underlying fractal structure of the signal and for the detection of transient signals.

Figure 16.5 shows the magnitudes of the Morlet wavelet transforms for a set of artificial test signals. Panel (a) simulates a very smooth QRS wave, obtained by computing the first

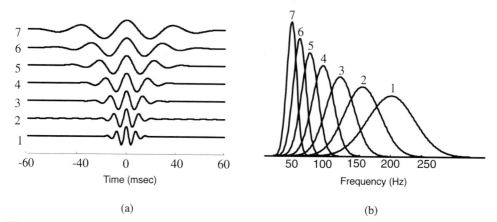

Figure 16.4   (a) Real part and (b) frequency spectrum of the Morlet wavelet, for $b = 0$ and for seven values of the scale parameter $a = 40 \times 2^{-m}$, with m ranging from 1.75 to 3.25 in steps of 0.25.

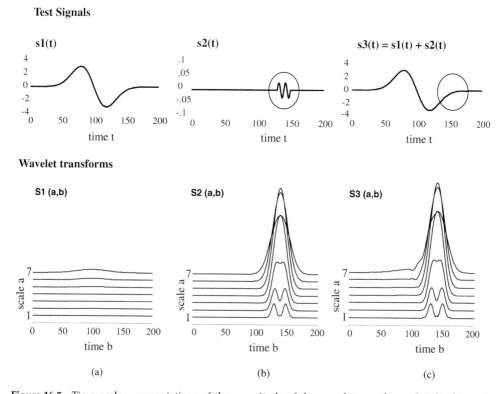

Figure 16.5   Time–scale representations of the magnitude of the wavelet transforms $Sn(a,b)$ obtained from three test signals $s1$–$3(t)$ using the Morlet wavelet at the seven scales defined in Figure 16.4. In (a), $s1(t)$ is the derivative of a Gaussian function. In (b), $s2(t)$ is a truncated sinusoidal function. In (c), $s3(t) = s1(t) + s2(t)$. (Reproduced with permission from reference 4)

derivative of the Gaussian function $f(t) = \exp(-t^2/2)$. The test signal in (b) was a small 100 Hz sinusoidal function, limited in time over two periods. The test signal in (c) was a combination of both. The added signal is clearly highlighted in the time–scale representation, although it is not visible in the time-domain representation. The highest local maximum of the wavelet transform is obtained in scale 5, whose middle frequency is the closest to the frequency of the additional sinusoidal signal. The local maxima in scales 1–3 coincide with the onset and the end of the sinusoid. This illustrates one of the main issues in multiscale analysis; that is, to relate singularities and any other local properties of the signal to the changes of the transform values when the scale varies. It confirms previous findings, where the authors have reported that the evolution of local maxima of the wavelet transform across scales could detect sharper variations of the signal.[4,19]

Time–frequency representations

Every analyzing wavelet $S_g(a,b)$ has a very precise bandpass filtering characteristic that is also precisely located in time. The equivalent time–frequency window of a basic analyzing wavelet $g(t)$ is a rectangle with centre (t^*,ω^*) and width $(2\Delta_g \times 2\Delta_G)$, defined by:

$$t^* = \frac{\displaystyle\int_{-\infty}^{+\infty} t|g(t)|^2 dt}{E_g^2} \quad \text{and} \quad \Delta_g^2 = \frac{\displaystyle\int_{-\infty}^{+\infty} (t - t^*)|g(t)|^2 dt}{E_g^2}$$

$$\omega^* = \frac{\displaystyle\int_{-\infty}^{+\infty} \omega|G(\omega)|^2 d\omega}{E_g^2} \quad \text{and} \quad \Delta_G^2 = \frac{\displaystyle\int_{-\infty}^{+\infty} (\omega - \omega^*)|G(\omega)|^2 d\omega}{E_g^2}$$

where E_g^2 is the energy of wavelet g:

$$E_g^2 = \int_{-\infty}^{+\infty} |g(t)|^2 dt = \int_{-\infty}^{+\infty} |G(\omega)|^2 d\omega.$$

For convenience, we shall consider basic wavelets centered at $t^* = 0$. It follows that the wavelet transform $S_g(a,b)$ of a signal $s(t)$ localizes the signal with a 'time-window' centered at $t = b$: $[b - a\Delta_g, b + a\Delta_g]$; and it also provides localized information of the spectrum of s within a 'frequency-window': $[\omega^*/a - \Delta G/a, \omega^*/a + \Delta G/a]$.

Hence, for a given basic wavelet, every point $(b,\omega^*/a)$ in the time–frequency plane (t,ω) associates with a rectangular 'time–frequency' window centered at $(b,\omega^*/a)$, with time width $2a\Delta_g$ and bandwidth $2\Delta_G/a$. The window area $(4\Delta_g\Delta_G)$, and the ratio of the center frequency to the bandwidth $(\omega^*/2\Delta_G)$ are independent of scaling factor a. However, the window automatically narrows for detecting high-frequency (small-scale) characteristics and it widens for investigating low-frequency (large-scale) behavior.

Figure 16.6 shows the time–frequency characteristics for cubic B-spline, Meyer, Morlet and first-order Gaussian derivative wavelets for a scaling factor a computed as $a = 2^{-m}$, with m varying linearly, which leads to a logarithmic progression of the central frequencies (peak amplitude frequency response). Only the windows of the orthogonal Meyer wavelets are not overlapping (Figure 16.7). This feature makes the Meyer wavelets especially suitable for data-compression.[20] From our experience, however, it appears that having overlapping windows is not necessarily a handicap. This propriety has been largely used to detect redundancies across adjacent scales, a method which has proven to have superior performance for the stratification of the risk of ventricular tachycardia by localizing strings of connected local maxima at the end or after the end of the QRS wave, that are indicative of the presence of singularities and of fractional potentials in the raw signal.

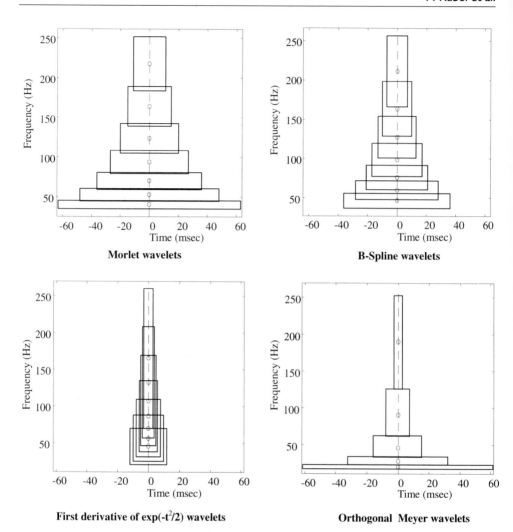

Figure 16.6 Time–frequency representations of the time duration and locations, and of the frequency bandwidth and central frequencies of the Morlet, B-spline, first-derivative Gaussian function, and orthogonal Meyer wavelets. The number of scales for the Meyer wavelets was determined by the process of construction of an orthogonal dyadic wavelet base that corresponds to a set of adjacent, nonoverlapping time–frequency windows, whereas the number of scales for the nonorthogonal wavelets has been fixed arbitrarily to seven. The first-derivative Gaussian function is the most accurate in the time domain, but it lacks in frequency resolution. The Morlet wavelet, on the other hand, has better accuracy in the frequency domain. 0 = central frequency location of each analyzing wavelet.

However, there is no general methodology for the design of an optimal series of analyzing wavelets. In practice, the basic wavelet g, and the set of scales considered, should be chosen in such a way that the bandwidth covered by the time–frequency windows includes the bandwidth of interest in the signal.

Figure 16.8 highlights the differences between the short-time Fourier transform, the pseudo Wigner–Ville transform and the wavelet transform for two postinfarction patients, one without VT (left panels), and the other with VT (right side).

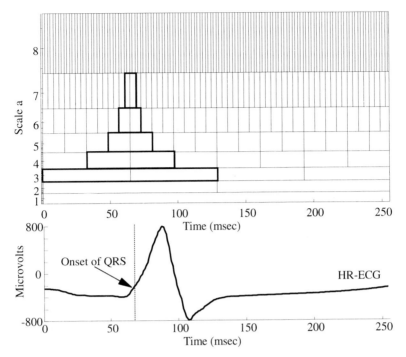

Figure 16.7 Time–scale representation of an eight-scale dyadic orthogonal Meyer wavelet base with $2^8 - 1 = 255$ wavelets and the corresponding 255 nonoverlapping characteristic windows. Decomposition of the HRECGs is performed between QRS onset minus 64 ms and QRS onset plus 192 ms.

Assessment of Wavelet Transform Analysis in Postinfarction Patients

Several authors have used advanced time–frequency methods to map the ECG signal into the time–frequency and the time–scale planes, but only a few have extracted from the corresponding representations quantitative descriptors that would allow automation of the stratification of patients at risk.

To quantify the changes between the spectrograms of each analyzed segment, Haberl et al.[6] computed the correlation coefficient between each spectrum and the reference spectrum corresponding to the first analyzed segment. Some authors have considered the cumulative energy in given frequency bands,[21,22] or have explored the ECG spectrum amplitude.[23,24]

In earlier studies, we investigated the way in which wavelet analysis of signal-averaged HRECGs could be used to detect abnormalities resulting from a possible disorganization of the depolarization wavefront over all the QRS–ST segment, and eventually to discriminate patients at risk. In a first study, we showed that an improved graphic representation of the wavelet transform provides an accurate visual characterization of patients prone to ventricular tachycardia.[25] In a further study, we worked out an original algorithm for the detection and the localization of sharp variations of the signal, based on coherent detection of the local maxima of the wavelet transform, and we derived a risk stratification method based on the detection of at least one such singularity at or after a point defined with reference to the QRS onset.[4,11]

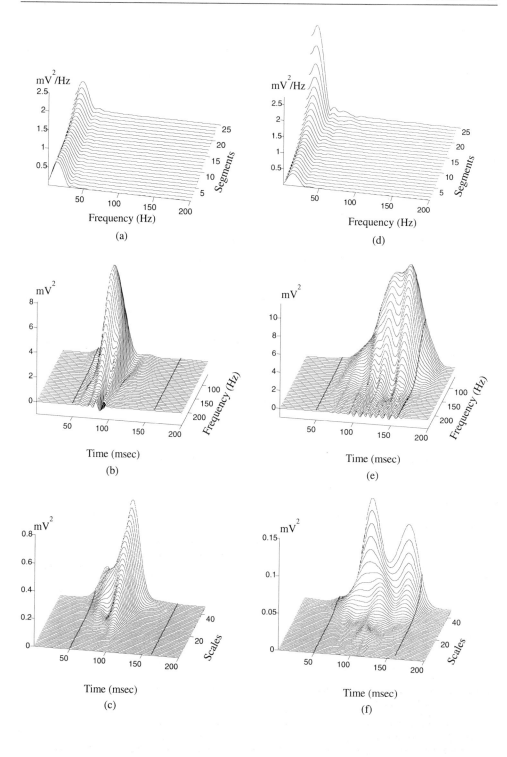

(a)

(d)

(b)

(e)

(c)

(f)

In the most recent study, we assessed the influence of the choice of analyzing wavelet, and determined whether specifically analyzing the wavelet transform of each lead could bring more information than globally analyzing a vector magnitude.[11]

In the following, we report these studies and show how combining advanced signal-processing techniques and pattern recognition methods can improve the stratification of postinfarction patients at risk of ventricular tachycardia.

Materials and Methods

Study populations

Three groups of patients were studied. Two groups of 20 patients following myocardial infarction constituted a 40-patient training set for ventricular tachycardia risk stratification. These patients were free of any complete bundle branch block. One group of 10 young, healthy volunteers served as a control group.

Group 1 (MI with VT) consisted of 20 consecutive postinfarction patients admitted to the coronary care unit of the Lyon cardiology hospital between September 1989 and May 1991 for cardiac arrest or ventricular tachycardia. All the patients were men, with a mean age of 58 ± 9 years. All of them had at least one period of sustained ventricular tachycardia that was not associated with acute myocardial infarction. The high-resolution ECG was recorded within the week following the arrhythmia.

Group 2 (MI without VT) consisted of 20 consecutive patients (18 men and 2 women; mean age 57 ± 8 years) admitted to the same coronary care unit for myocardial infarction between August and November 1988. The high-resolution ECG was recorded 10–21 days after the infarction. These patients were free of arrhythmic events 3 years after their inclusion.

Group 3 (normal patients) consisted of 7 men and 3 women, with a mean age of 27 ± 5 years.

Data acquisition

Bipolar pseudo-orthogonal X, Y, Z leads were acquired using an ART® 1200 EPX (Arrhythmia Research Technology, Austin, TX) high-resolution signal-averaging system. The sampling rate was 1000 per second and the resolution was 16 bits. Signal-averaging was performed from 154 ± 94 beats (range 51–500 beats). The noise level was determined from 40–250 Hz filtered vector magnitude by the ART program. The mean root-mean-square value of the noise was 0.3 ± 0.1 μV for the three groups.

Averaged unfiltered ECG signals were transferred to a personal computer. Conventional time-domain analysis was performed using the ART version 3.00 analysis software. The wavelet analysis program was implemented using PC-MATLAB® (Math-Works, Natik, MA).

Conventional time-domain analysis

The analysis was based on bidirectional bandpass filtering and on study of the vector magnitude of the filtered leads, called the filtered QRS complex, according to Simson's method.[26]

Figure 16.8   Time–frequency and time–scale representations of (a, d) the short-time Fourier transform, (b, e) the pseudo Wigner–Ville transform, and (c, f) the Morlet wavelet transform of the HRECG magnitude vector. (a)–(c) are from a postinfarction patient noninducible for VT, (d)–(f) from a VT-inducible postinfarction patient. (d)–(f) show evidence of an increase of the high-frequency energy in the vicinity of the end of QRS. The heavy lines designate respectively the onset and the end of QRS as determined by the ART program prior to bidirectional filtering. QRS durations are 112 ms (left panels) and 111 ms (right panels).

As recommended by a joint Task Force Committee of the European Society of Cardiology, the American Heart Association, and the American College of Cardiology,[27] the filter setting was 40–250 Hz and three parameters were considered for detection of late potentials: (1) the filtered QRS duration, (2) the root-mean-square voltage of the terminal 40 ms of the filtered QRS (*RMS 40*), and (3) the amount of time that the filtered QRS complex remained below 40 μV (*LAS 40*).

We specifically considered the following recommended cutoff points: (1) QRS duration should be greater than 114 ms; (2) *RMS 40* should be less than 20 μV; (3) *LAS 40* should be more than 38 ms. We also computed global results that were obtained for one, two and three criteria satisfied.

The predictive power of these parameters was further assessed in terms of receiver operating characteristics computed from the 40 postinfarction patients. The receiver characteristic curve is a diagrammatic representation of the interdependence of the sensitivity and specificity of a test when the cutoff point of the test varies.

Wavelet transform of the ECG signal

Let us call $s(n)$ one of the three sampled, averaged, unfiltered ECG leads. There are two possible approaches to computing the sampled wavelet transform $S_g(a,n)$. The first, and the most direct, way consists in computing the inner product of $s(n)$ by the sampled wavelet at scale a. The second consists in first computing the spectrum $\bar{S}_{g,a}(\omega)$ of $S_g(a,n)$, then in computing the complex wavelet transform $S_g(a,n)$ by taking the inverse Fourier transform of $\bar{S}_{g,a}(\omega)$. The first step reduces to the product of the digital Fourier transform $S(\omega)$ of signal $s(n)$ by the digital Fourier transform $G_a(\omega)$ of the analyzing wavelet $g_a(n)$:

$$\bar{S}_{g,a}(\omega) = S(\omega) \cdot G_a^*(\omega)$$

where $G_a(\omega) = \sqrt{a} \cdot G(a\omega)$ and $G_a^*(\omega)$ is the complex conjugate of $G_a(\omega)$. In our study, we used the complex analytic form of the basic wavelet.

For each of the three ECG leads we then computed the magnitude of the resulting complex wavelet transforms, which we called, depending on the basic wavelet used, $WTX_g(a,n)$, $WTY_g(a,n)$ and $WTZ_g(a,n)$. An example of such time–scale representations is given in Figure 16.8. In addition, we computed the so-called 'vector magnitude' of the wavelet transform (see Figure 16.9):

$$WTM_g(a,n) = \sqrt{WTX_g^2(a,n) + WTY_g^2(a,n) + WTZ_g^2(a,n)}$$

Thus, for each high-resolution signal-averaged ECG recording, and for each of the studied wavelets, we obtained three time–scale representations, corresponding to the three individual leads, and one additional time–scale representation synthesizing the information contained within the three leads.

The number of scales for each basic wavelet was uniformly fixed to eleven. The scaling factor a was determined as $a = 2^{-m}$ with m varying linearly, which as already stated leads to a logarithmic progression of the central frequencies. The extreme values of m were determined so that the largest scale shows a frequency window going not below 25 Hz, and the smallest scale displays a frequency window stretching up to 250 Hz. This complies with the common understanding that fractionated potentials are detected somewhere between these two frequencies.

Singularity detection

It has been reported that frequency-direction ridges in the time–scale representation detect sharper variations of the signal.[19] We have developed a new method for the detection of irregular structures, or singularities, in the raw signal. This consists in

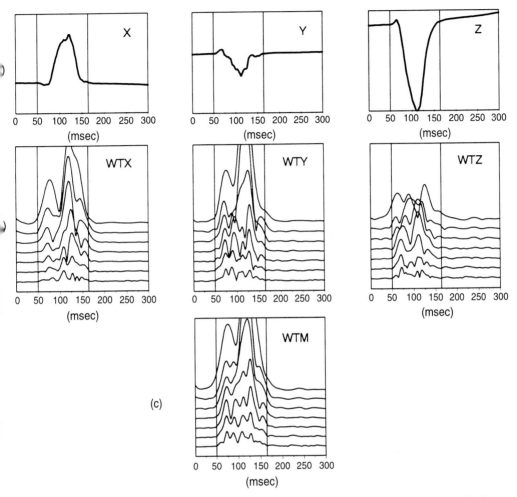

Figure 16.9 Wavelet transforms computed for a postinfarction patient with ventricular tachycardia. In each graph, the two vertical lines denote, respectively, the onset and the end of the QRS as determined by the ART program prior to bidirectional filtering. (a) Unfiltered averaged X, Y, Z leads. (b) Magnitude of the complex wavelet transform: *WTX* for lead X, *WTY* for lead Y, and *WTZ* for lead Z. (c) vector magnitude *WTM*. (Reproduced with permission from reference 4)

tracking the evolution of so-called 'local maxima' of the wavelet transform across scales.[4,11] It develops in three steps: (1) detection of local maxima, (2) localization of connected local maxima, and (3) acknowledgement of connected local maxima as signal singularities. Figure 16.10 illustrates the method.

1. On a given scale, a local maximum is detected at the point where the wavelet transform magnitude is greater than the amplitude of the two nearest neighbors, or where the transform shows a small plateau within a raising or a falling front. A more formal definition can be found elsewhere.[11] In order to discard small local maxima due to noise, only maxima with a magnitude greater than a given adaptive amplitude threshold (AMPLTHR) are considered. The threshold is defined as a fixed percentage of the maximal amplitude of the wavelet transform in the smallest scale.

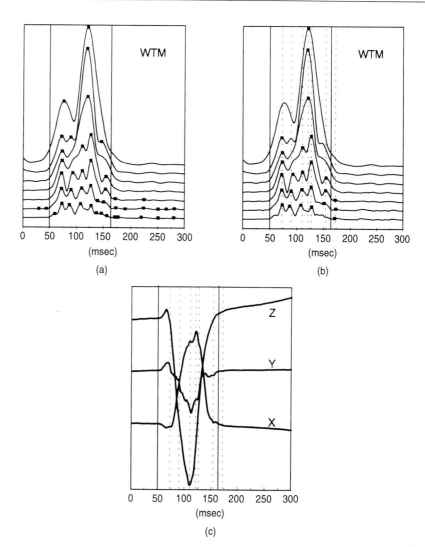

Figure 16.10 Algorithm for the detection and localization of signal singularities for the same patient as in Figure 16.9. (a) Detection of *WTM* local maxima. (b) Location of strings of connected local maxima (dotted lines). (c) Location of the detected singularities in the raw signal (dotted lines). The vertical solid lines denote the onset and the end of the QRS. (Reproduced with permission from reference 4)

2. A local maximum in any scale, and a local maximum in the smallest scale, are said to be connected if the deviation between their respective time locations is not greater than a given scatter threshold (SCATTHR).
3. A signal singularity is detected when the number of local maxima found to be connected to one same local maximum in the smallest scale is greater than a given number, called RIDGLEN (meaning the minimum length for a ridge). The time location of the singularity is assigned the time location of the local maximum in the smallest scale.

Assigning a value to the three parameters AMPLTHR, SCATTHR and RIDGLEN defines one algorithm for singularity detection, and leads to a specific location of signal singularities for each time–scale representation of each recording. We considered the segment [QRS onset, QRS onset + 250 ms], where the onset of QRS is determined by the ART program prior to bidirectional filtering.

Results

Conventional time-domain analysis

Figure 16.11 shows the receiver operating characteristic curves of the three standard parameters, with an identification of the points corresponding to the standard criteria.

The receiver operating characteristic curves of *RMS 40* and *LAS 40* demonstrate a poor predictive value of these parameters. The recommended criteria based on *RMS 40* and *LAS 40* provide balanced, but poor, sensitivity and specificity figures. The predictive value of parameter *QRS dur* is better. The recommended criterion based on *QRS dur* gave alone a sensitivity of 80% and a specificity of 90%.

For postinfarction patients, considering at least one, two or three standard time-domain criteria satisfied gave, respectively, points *a, b* and *c* of the graph in Figure 16.11.

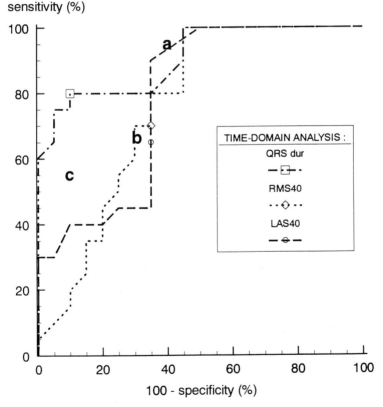

Figure 16.11 Receiver operating characteristics of the three standard time-domain parameters computed from 40 postinfarction patients, with an identification of the points corresponding to the standard criteria (QRS duration > 114 ms, RMS 40 $< 20\,\mu V$, LAS 40 ≥ 38 ms). Points (a), (b) and (c) illustrate the performance data obtained when considering, respectively, at least one, two or three of these standard criteria to be satisfied. (Reproduced with permission from reference 4)

Considering at least one criterion satisfied provided the highest sensitivity (95%), but a low specificity (60%). Considering two or more criteria satisfied provided a poor sensitivity (65%) and a poor specificity (70%). Considering the three criteria satisfied gave a good specificity (90%), but a very low sensitivity (55%). Because of the weakness of *RMS 40* and *LAS 40* results, these combined results are poorer than the performance data of *QRS dur* considered alone.

Wavelet analysis

In a first study, we arbitrarily fixed the amplitude threshold AMPLTHR = 4%, the scatter threshold SCATTHR = 3 ms and the minimum length of a ridge RIDGLEN = 3.

The mean number of irregularities detected between QRS onset and QRS onset + 250 ms was 5.3 ± 2.2 for the MI-with-VT patients, 3.5 ± 1.6 for the MI-without-VT patients, and 3.2 ± 1.5 for the healthy subjects.

In MI-with-VT patients, singularities spread out in the whole analyzed interval. In the MI-without-VT patients, only one singularity was detected after the point QRS onset + 100 ms. None of the healthy subjects showed a singularity 100 ms after the point QRS onset + 96 ms.

These results led to the definition of a ventricular tachycardia risk stratification criterion which is based on the detection of singularities at or after a limit defined as 'QRS onset plus T milliseconds'. In order to select an optimum value of this threshold T, the rates of well-classified patients in the two infarction groups (i.e. the sensitivity and the specificity of the criterion) have been plotted as a function of T varying from 30 to 250 ms.[4] The two curves intersect at a level where sensitivity and specificity equal 85%, for T ranging from 95 to 97 ms. For T equal to 98 and 99 ms, sensitivity was still 85%, and specificity reached 90%.

The receiver operating characteristic curve of this criterion showed consistently an improvement of almost 5% in sensitivity over the results obtained by standard time-domain parameters. The optimum cutoff point was $T = 98$ ms.

In a second study, we searched for a pertinent setting of the parameter quadruplets [AMPLTHR, SCATTHR, RIDGLEN, NBRIDG] and [AMPLTHR, SCATTHR, RIDGLEN, SEGBEG], where NBRIDG yields the number of ridges in the [QRS onset, QRS onset + 250 ms] segment, and SEGBEG involves a shorter search segment starting at QRS onset + SEGBEG and ending at QRS onset + 250 ms, giving optimal diagnostic efficacy and leading to optimal algorithms for risk stratification.[11] On the whole, more than 30 000 combinations of four parameters were tested.

The optimal diagnostic efficacy, (sensitivity + specificity)/2, was never less than 77.5%. In some instances it reached 95%. Wavelets G2 to G6 and the Morlet wavelet as a whole showed very similar performance. Wavelet G1 globally gave poorer results than the other basic wavelets. We further noticed that the three individual leads did not systematically show enhanced results, when compared with the vector magnitude. A combination of two leads among three led to the best results, mainly for wavelets G3 to G6, with both risk stratification methods. One of the best results (sensitivity = 90%, specificity = 100%) was given by the variable segment length method (SEGBEG = 95–105 ms) applied to the vector magnitude of the Morlet wavelet, which was the basis for our previous study.

To design an optimal risk stratification algorithm in each time–frequency representation, we considered the diagnostic efficacy as a function defined in the 4-D space made up by the parameter quadruplets. We observed that this 'efficacy function' passes through a set of maxima for connected domains of the parameters. Among the parameter values leading to optimal classification, the adaptive amplitude threshold for maxima detection (AMPLTHR), the variable segment length begin (SEGBEG) and, to a lesser extent, the minimal number of singularities to be detected (NBRIDG], were found to be the less scattered ones. In contrast, once these parameters had been fixed, both parameters allowing singularity detection (SCATTHR and RIDGLEN) seemed to be almost unaffected.

Filtering the 'efficacy function' led to more precisely localized maxima of this function, and the corresponding values of the parameters were taken as optimal quadruplets. Optimal parameter quadruplets for risk stratification based on the Morlet wavelet and on the vector magnitude are: AMPLTHR = 7%, SCATTHR = 2–5 ms, RIDGLEN = 3, and SEGBEG = 95–105 ms.

Discussion

In this section we refer to a series of studies that support the idea that time–frequency and time-scale analysis could improve the discrimination of patients prone to ventricular tachycardia. The methods consist of detecting a possible disorganization of the depolarization wavefront in the patients at risk in the years following a myocardial infarction. This fragmentation of the front of activation is expected to result in irregularities, appearing in and shortly after the QRS complex of the high-resolution signal-averaged ECG. However, the problem is not so much to have nice 3-D time–frequency or time–scale representations that are very difficult to interpret, but also to set up quantitative data-analysis and pattern-recognition methods that could highlight distinguishing features between the transformed signals.

In a first study, using a training set of 40 postinfarction patient records, we implemented an automated risk stratification algorithm based on the location of sharper variations of the signal. We used the wavelet transform, a technique that is of particular interest for the detection of transient signals. In contrast to the classical short-time Fourier transform, which uses a single analysis window, the wavelet transform uses short windows at high frequencies (small scales), and long windows at low frequencies (large scales). It thus avoids the problem of poor frequency resolution in short segments, which occurs in Fourier analysis.

Analysing the relative locations of the local maxima of the wavelet transform across the scales makes it possible to detect singularities. We implemented a method based on this property, using the vector magnitude computed from the wavelet transforms of three bipolar pseudo-orthogonal unfiltered leads.

All analysed recordings showed irregularities in the QRS complex. Although this effect was lower in postinfarction patients without ventricular tachycardia and in normals, the total number of detected irregularities did not appear as a significant criterion to discriminate patients with ventricular tachycardia. However, an essential difference was the systematic presence of singularities roughly more than 100 ms after the beginning of the ventricular depolarization in postinfarction patients with ventricular tachycardia, in a region where, as a general rule, no irregular activity was detected in the recordings of the other patients.

The main conclusion was that the detection of strings of connected local maxima of the vector magnitude of the wavelet transform at or after the point QRS onset plus 98 ms was a reasonable criterion for VT risk stratification in postinfarction patients, with a sensitivity of 85% and a specificity of 90%.

As a reference point, we assessed the results of the conventional time-domain analysis methods on the same training set of 40 postinfarction patients. Among the time-domain parameters, the duration of the filtered QRS showed the best predictive values. This standard criterion gives, after optimization, a sensitivity of 80% and a specificity of 90%.

Nevertheless, the QRS-duration receiver operating characteristic curve consistently lies under the wavelet-analysis receiver operating characteristic curve, which implies a slightly lower predictive power of the time-domain parameter. One could have expected similar results from these two criteria because the time-domain criterion is based on the measure of the filtered QRS duration, and the wavelet-analysis criterion implies the detection of singularities at or after a point near the normal expected end of QRS. The longer the filtered QRS complex, the greater the probability of finding singularities more than 98 ms after the onset of QRS. One fundamental difference is that our approach does not require any prior knowledge of the end of QRS. This point is noteworthy, because one of the major weaknesses of time-domain analysis is the difficulty in accurately determining the end of QRS.

In a more recent study, we checked the validity of *a priori* choices such as applying the Morlet wavelet, and computing a vector magnitude.[11] At the same time, we searched for optimal values of the parameters of the algorithms. The final goal was to improve the diagnostic efficacy of the risk stratification process. Our method consisted in assessing the risk stratification results in terms of sensitivity and specificity in the same 40-patient learning group, for several basic wavelets, for several configurations of the signal-singularities detection algorithm, and for individual leads as well as for lead combinations.

We studied seven basic wavelets, namely the six first-derivatives of a Gaussian function, and the Morlet wavelet. These nonorthogonal, easy-to-implement analytic wavelets are known to be quite suitable for signal detection.

Using a logarithmic progression of the central frequencies, we fixed the eleven scaling parameters for a precise coverage of the 25–250 Hz frequency band, which leads to noninteger values of the exponent m of the scaling parameter a. With this definition of the scaling parameter, the central frequencies and the bandwidths of the various basic wavelets at matching scales (numbers 1 to 11) obviously do not coincide. However, when considering the eleven scales as a whole, comparable frequency information is globally restored in the transformed signal, whatever the basic wavelet applied. Another method would have consisted of aligning the central frequencies of corresponding scales; we discarded this method because it would have defined frequency zones of the signal that would have been different according to the basic wavelet.

The time–frequency windows of the first derivative of a Gaussian function have a narrow time-width (10 ms for the largest scale) and large frequency overlap of the scales (see Figure 16.6). These properties materialize in the ECG wavelet transform as numerous well-located maxima, with an obvious information redundancy in the eleven scales. They could explain the poor results obtained by G1 with our stratification method, since it is based on the presence of complementary frequency information in the scales.

The ECG wavelet transform based on the sixth-order derivative (G6) obviously reveals more frequency information. Indeed, this wavelet shows much narrower frequency width, and a smaller overlap of the frequency bands. It therefore provides much better results in risk stratification, even if it shows poorer time location properties.

The Morlet wavelet shows balanced time and frequency widths, and reduced frequency overlap. The good results obtained by this basic wavelet method could thus be explained by the significance of the presence of synchronous relative maxima in the wavelet transform, due to the relatively smaller information redundancy of the scales.

With regard to relative maxima, two types are detected. The first are real maxima, i.e. points where the derivative of the function is zero. The second type are points of inflection of the curves, corresponding to some ridges that a filtering effect distorts because of the presence of another high-amplitude ridge in close proximity.

However, obviously not all the singular points detected in the time signal by this method correspond to fractionated late potentials. We started with the hypothesis that singularities in general denote some change in the orientation or in the velocity of the activation wavefront. They may be observed all over the QRS, even in normal subjects. In a recent study we assessed two methods for ventricular tachycardia risk stratification.[11] Method 1 was based on the hypothesis that a patient at risk will globally show more singularities inside the QRS complex and in the ST segment than a patient without ventricular tachycardia. Method 2, in a more customary way, looked for fractionated potentials in the terminal portion of the QRS, and in the ST segment. It could be observed that the optimal starting point of the analyzing segment actually lies between 90 and 110 ms; that is, surrounding the end of QRS. An additional study showed that the results are in practice independent of the terminal end of the segment under investigation, when this point lies in a zone surrounding the point 250 ms after the onset of QRS. We thus set to QRS onset plus 250 ms the terminal end of the segment to be investigated in method 1 and in method 2. In both methods, no preliminary detection of the end of QRS is required. This point removes a possible source of erroneous results, because of the specific difficulty in determining accurately the offset of QRS.[28]

Assessment of the sensitivity and specificity results clearly shows that none of the individual leads is relevant for risk stratification, whatever the method.[11] An opposite result would have worked in favor of the hypothesis of a privileged direction of the potentials of interest. On the other hand, an acceptable diagnostic efficacy is obtained in searching for singularities in at least two leads among three. Equivalent results are obtained in analyzing a vector magnitude of the three wavelet transforms, which makes it possible to say that computing a vector magnitude does not drastically decrease the signal-to-noise ratio. Moreover, when compared with the methods based on the detection of singularities in at least two leads among three, the vector-magnitude-based methods save time because they require the analysis of only one time-scale representation, instead of three. For all these reasons, we would recommend the use of a method based on the vector magnitude.

Normal subjects were analyzed using the algorithms that led to optimal results in the pathological population. The whole normal population was well classified with risk stratification method 2, and using the vector magnitude, whatever the basic wavelet, G1 being excluded. The relative superiority of method 2 in classifying this population as a population without risk could be explained by the large number of singularities detected inside the QRS complexes of this young healthy population.

Optimizing the values of the four parameters of the algorithms using our learning set might be considered as a rather hazardous task, because of the small number of patients. However, because parameter settings leading to optimal diagnostic efficacy belong to large connected domains,[11] we may suggest that the results of the risk stratification algorithms are not very dependent on the values of the parameters but more on what they represent.

In order to further check the robustness of the results, the method for optimal determination of the parameter setting was applied to two subsets of 20 patients, which were chosen at random among the 40 patients population. For this, Group 1 was split into two groups of 10 patients at risk (G_1^1 and G_1^2) and Group 2 was split into two groups of 10 patients without ventricular tachycardia (G_2^1 and G_2^2). The 20 patients in G_1^1 and G_2^1 made up a subset called P1, and subgroups G_1^2 and G_2^2 a subset called P2. Risk stratification method 2 was applied to the vector magnitude of the wavelet transform based on the Morlet basic wavelet. The diagnostic efficacy function was computed and filtered in both subsets, and an optimal parameter setting was inferred for the discrimination of patients at risk, respectively in P1 and in P2. Optimal parameters obtained from P1 were then applied to the patients in P2, and conversely optimal parameters obtained from P2 were applied to the patients in P1.

The parameter set obtained from P1 correctly classified all patients in G_2^1 and in G_2^2, 9 patients in G_2^1, and 8 patients in G_1^2. The two parameter sets obtained from P2 correctly classified all patients in G_1^2 and in G_2^2, 8 patients in G_1^1, and respectively 8 and 7 patients in G_2^1.

Parameter values AMPLTHR = 7% and SCATTHR = 5 ms were obtained in both populations, and they corresponded to the optimal values determined from the whole learning set. The parameter RIDGLEN could reasonably be fixed to 3, which is the minimum number required for aligned maxima to make up a string. Concerning SEGBEG, optimal values were different from one learning set to another. For a more precise definition of this parameter, however, a larger learning set and an independent test set are required.

Although they show promise, most of the methods recently developed for the prediction of ventricular tachycardia are still based on the detection of late fractionated potentials in the terminal portion of the QRS complex and in the ST segment. We recently developed a new technique based on orthogonal decomposition of the whole HRECG following a dyadic Meyer wavelets network with central frequencies at 28, 47, 97, and 195 HZ.[29] This supports the hypothesis that there should be a relationship between the position of the malignant re-entry site and the temporal location of the fractionated potentials. As the infarction site has different locations in the myocardium, we tried to detect abnormal potentials in the ST segment and also in the whole QRS complex.

The time-scale transforms were computed from QRS onset to QRS onset plus 256 ms on the same set of 40 patients as reported before. The results of the wavelet decomposition were further stratified by means of an optimal stepwise-linear discriminant analysis. The reproducibility was tested with an additional set of 10 MI patients recorded twice at 10-minute intervals.

Among the 120 decomposition coefficients tested, the four most relevant were at QRS onset + 48 ms and QRS onset + 64 ms, at the end of the QRS at QRS onset + 128 ms, and in the ST segment at QRS onset + 224 ms. The latter was mainly used to discriminate normals from postinfarction patients. All four wavelets corresponded to the highest frequency scale, which corresponded to a 125–250 Hz bandpass filter.

In comparison with patients without VT, the high-frequency content for the patients with VT was lowered at QRS onset + 48 ms, but increased at QRS onset + 64 ms and at QRS onset + 128 ms. The figures for the overall population ($N = 50$) were 95% in sensitivity and 95% in specificity.

Conclusions

Spectral analysis of high-resolution ECGs is a promising approach for detecting patients at risk of sudden cardiac death or of sustained ventricular tachycardia after acute myocardial infarction.

Time-invariant spectral analysis offers several advantages for the identification and characterization of ECG signals. It gives a complete description of the ECG and may disclose information that could be difficult to distinguish in the raw or in the filtered signal. It is very relevant for studying the variability of the heart rate and of the repolarization phase and their relationship to the neuro-vegetative system. However, this approach has severe shortcomings for the study of fractionated potentials, mainly because of the nonstationarity of the ECG signals.

The central issue in time-varying spectral analysis is to precisely model the time–frequency structure of the ECG by mapping its spectrotemporal components in the time–frequency plane. The best known and most widely used time–frequency analysis method is the short-time Fourier transform. This technique, however, suffers from a poor spectrotemporal resolution. The greater the length of each analyzing time window, the better the spectral resolution but the worse the temporal resolution.

The Wigner–Ville distribution in theory offers a near-optimal spectrotemporal resolution (about twice that of the short-time Fourier transform), without the need for an analyzing window. But in practice it suffers heavily from the introduction of interference terms that affect the terminal part of the QRS, and this renders interpretation very difficult. These cross-terms can only be removed by signal-dependent smoothing, which in turn lowers the spectrotemporal resolution. Further research is necessary to assess its validity.

The recently introduced wavelet transform provides a fruitful alternative. Unlike the short-time Fourier transform, the frequency resolution properties of the wavelet transform are frequency-dependent. The time resolution increases at high frequencies at the expense of frequency resolution, and vice versa. From our earlier studies, one can expect it to prove beneficial for the detection of high-frequency components both within and after the QRS complex. Preliminary results show a 10–15% performance improvement over conventional time-domain analysis methods for the stratification of the HRECG after myocardial infarction. The best results are obtained when considering a vector magnitude computed from the wavelet transforms of three pseudo-orthogonal leads. Analyzing the individual leads gave poor results. From the studied wavelets, the most stable results were obtained with the very commonly used J Morlet wavelet. Improvements might still be obtained by optimizing the analyzing wavelet; i.e. by determining a wavelet specifically adapted to the detection of cardiac micropotentials.

Having developed sound mathematical techniques that allow precise mapping of cardiac signals in the time–frequency and time–scale planes, the next important issue is to extract from these representations information that best reflects the electrophysiologic and anatomic derangements unique to patients at risk of life-threatening arrythmias and other cardiac diseases. Observation of the various time–frequency representations suggested the computation of some distinguishing features. Spectral slice-to-slice correlation has been used together with median or 95% energy frequency tracking for the analysis of time–frequency maps. In former studies, we worked out an original algorithm for the detection and the location of sharp variations of the signal, based on coherent detection of the local maxima of the wavelet transform, and we derived risk stratification methods based on the detection of at least one such singularity at or after a point defined with reference to the QRS onset. We have also developed a unique risk stratification method based on the orthogonal decomposition of the HRECG signals following a dyadic wavelets network combined with optimal stepwise linear discriminant analysis.

However, alternative features might offer even more promise. Further studies are required to develop and implement procedures to maximally extract and quantitate these features, and to test them on much larger groups than has been done before. Numerical Holter recorders have an enormous potential for collecting such large datasets in real-life situations, and could give a new dimension to the research in the field of high-resolution ECG monitoring.

References

1. Flowers NC, Horan LG, Thomas JR, Tollesson WJ. The anatomic basis for high-frequency components in the electrocardiogram. *Circulation* 1969; **39**: 531.
2. Goldberger AL, Bhargava V, Froelicher V, *et al.* Effect of myocardium infarction in high-frequency QRS potentials. *Circulation* 1981; **64**: 34.
3. Lander P, Berbari EJ. Principles and signal processing techniques of the high-resolution electrocardiogram. *Prog Cardiovasc Dis* 1992; **35**: 169–88.
4. Morlet D, Peyrin F, Desseigne P, Touboul P, Rubel P. Wavelet analysis of high-resolution signal-averaged ECGs in postinfarction patients. *J. Electrocardiol* 1993; **26**: 311–19.
5. Cain ME, Ambos HD, Witkowski FX, Sobel BE. Fast-Fourier transform analysis of signal-averaged electrocardiograms for identification of patients prone to sustained ventricular tachycardia. *Circulation* 1984; **69**: 711–20.
6. Haberl R, Jilge G, Pulter R, Steinbeck G. Spectral mapping of the electrocardiogram with Fourier transform for identification of patients with sustained ventricular tachycardia and coronary artery disease. *Eur Heart J* 1989; **10**: 316–22.
7. Lander P, Jones D L, Berbari J, Lazzara R. Time–frequency structure of the high-resolution ECG. *J Electrocardiol* 1992; **27**(Suppl): 207–12.
8. Haberl R, Schels HF, Steinbigler P, Jilge G, Steinbeck G. Top-resolution frequency analysis of the electrocardiogram with adaptive frequency determination: identification of late potentials in patients with coronary artery disease. *Circulation* 1990; **82**: 1183–92.
9. Hessen SF, Kidwell GA, Waldo D, Prabhakara Rao C, Greenspon AJ. Joint time–frequency analysis of the signal-averaged electrocardiogram using the Wigner–Ville distribution. *Circulation* 1988; **78**(Suppl II): 138.

10 Peyrin F, Karoubi B, Morlet D, Dupont F, Rubel P, Desseigne P, Touboul P. Application of the Wigner distribution to the detection of the late potentials in ECG. In: Luk (ed.), *Advanced Signal Processing Algorithms, Architectures and Implementations III*. SPIE, 1992: 418–28.

11. Morlet D, Couderc JP, Touboul P, Rubel P. Wavelet analysis of high-resolution ECGs in postinfarction patients: role of the basic wavelet and of the analyzed lead. *Int J Biomed Comp* 1995; **39**: 311–25.

12. Jones DL, Touvannas JS, Lander P, Albert DE. Advanced time–frequency methods for signal-averaged ECG analysis. *J Electrocardiol* 1992; **25**:(Suppl): 188–94.

13. Hlawatsch F, Boudreaux-Bartels GF. Linear and quadratic time–frequency signal representations. *IEEE Signal Processing Magazine* 1992; 21–67.

14. Martin W, Flandrin P. Wigner–Ville spectral analysis of nonstationary processes. *IEEE ASSP* 1985; **33**: 1461.

15. Chui C K. *An Introduction to Wavelets*. San Diego: Academic Press, 1992.

16. Grossmann A, Morlet J. Decomposition of hardy functions into square integrable wavelets of constant shape. *Siam Math Anal* 1984; **15**: 723–36.

17. Unser M, Aldroubi A. Polynomial splines and wavelets: a signal processing perspective. In: Chui CK (ed.), *Wavelets: A Tutorial in Theory and Applications*. San Diego: Academic Press, 1992: 91–122.

18. Bertrand O, Bohorquez J, Pernier J. A reversible discrete wavelet transform. Application to the filtering of transient electrical brain signals. In: Meyer (ed.), *Wavelets and Applications*. Paris: Masson, 1992; 105–9.

19. Mallat S, Zhong S. Wavelet maxima representation. In: Meyer (ed.), *Wavelets and Applications*. Paris: Masson, 1992: 207–84.

20. Antonini M, Barlaud M, Mathieu P. Digital image compression using vector quantization and the wavelet transform. In: Meyer (ed.), *Wavelets and Applications*. Paris: Masson, 1992: 160–94.

21. Diego J, Ruben M, Hugo C. Spectral analysis of the surface electrocardiogram in patients with Chagas' disease. In: Morruci R, Coatrieux JL, Laxminarian S (eds), *Proceedings of the 14th Annual International Conference of the IEEE Engineering in Medicine and Biology Society*. New York: IEEE, 1992: 514–15.

22. Shinnar M, Simson MB. Wavelets and the multifractal substrate of ventricular tachycardia (abstract). *Circulation* 1992; **86**:(Suppl I): I–319.

23. Kavesh NG, Cain ME, Ambos HD, Arthur RM. Enhanced detection of distinguishing features in signal-averaged electrocardiograms from patients with ventricular tachycardia by combined spatial and spectral analyses of the entire cardiac cycle. *Circulation* 1994; **90**: 254–63.

24. Cain ME, Ambos HD, Markham J, Lindsay BD, Arthur RM. Diagnostic implications of spectral and temporal analysis of the entire cardiac cycle in patients with ventricular tachycardia. *Circulation* 1991; **83**: 1637–48.

25. Morlet D, Peyrin F, Desseigne P, Touboul P, Rubel P. Time-scale analysis of high-resolution signal-averaged surface ECG using wavelet transformation. In: Murray and Arzbaecher (eds), *Computers in Cardiology 1991*. Los Alamitos, CA: IEEE Computer Society, 1991: 393–6.

26. Simson MB. Use of signals in the terminal QRS complex to identify patients with ventricular tachycardia after myocardial infarction. *Circulation* 1981; **64**: 235–42.

27. Breithardt G, Cain ME, El-Sherif N, Flowers NC, Hombach V, Janse M, Simson MB, Steinbeck G. Standards for analysis of ventricular late potentials using high-resolution or signal-averaged electrocardiography: a statement by a Task Force Committee of the European Society of Cardiology, the American Heart Association, and the American College of Cardiology. *JACC* 1991; **17**: 999–1006.

28. Morlet D, Rubel P, Amaud P, Willems JL. An improved method to evaluate the precision of computer ECG measurement programs. *Int J Biomed Comput* 1988; **22**: 199–216.

29. Couderc JP, Morlet D, Fayn J, Kirkorian G, Rubel P, Touboul P. A new efficient method to detect patients prone to ventricular tachycardia using orthogonal wavelet transform of high-resolution ECG (abstract). *Circulation* 1994; **90**(Part 2): I–230.

30. Oeff M, von Leitner ER, Sthapit R, Breithardt G, Borggrefe M, Karbenn U, Meinertz T, Zotz R, Clas W, Hombach V. Höpp HW. Methods for noninvasive detection of ventricular late potentials: a comparative multicenter study. *Eur Heart J* 1986; **7**:25–33.

17

Clinical Utility of High-Resolution Monitoring

Vinzenz Hombach, Martin Höher,
Hans-Heinrich Osterhues and Matthias Kochs

Introduction

In the conventional ECG, only the activation and recovery processes of the atria and ventricles can be detected, because the depolarization amplitudes of the sinus node and the His–Purkinje system are at the microvolt level and are thus usually buried within the baseline noise. A prolonged intraventricular conduction of larger areas of ventricular myocardium may be demonstrated by the typical hemiblock or complete bundle branch block patterns of the conventional ECG. A delayed activation of smaller areas of ventricular myocardium (e.g. in the periphery of an infarction zone or in right ventricular dysplasia) will, however, be lost, owing to the small amplitude of the signals of interest. Such low level signals from sinus node depolarization or His-bundle activation, as well as from areas of late ventricular depolarization, can be detected by direct intracardiac catheter recordings or mapping procedures, methods which are invasive, technically demanding and somewhat complicated. High-resolution ECG equipments are therefore very attractive and allow noninvasive low-noise recordings from the body surface in larger patient populations.

The signal-averaging technique was adopted from other research areas to significantly reduce noise and improve the signal-to-noise ratio in the highly amplified surface ECG. In the early years many researchers concentrated on detecting His bundle and sinus node potentials from the body surface. Later on the main interest shifted to the retrieval of ventricular late potentials (VLPs), and this now represents by far the most frequent application of low-noise body-surface ECG recordings.

From a clinician's viewpoint, two areas of high-resolution electrocardiographic monitoring are of major interest:

1. The analysis of pre- and post-atrial to ventricular electrical activity to detect sinus node and His bundle depolarization. This should help to better define the functional role of sinus node pacemaker activity in normal and abnormal clinical situations, and to locate the area of impaired or blocked conduction in patients with second-degree AV-block, which in turn would provide a more precise separation of patients at risk of severe bradycardia and/or asystole.
2. The analysis of a localized conduction delay within the ventricular myocardium, which may constitute the slow conduction area of a re-entrant circuit to initiate life-

threatening ventricular tachyarrhythmias. This analysis could principally separate patients at risk of ventricular tachycardia (VT) or fibrillation (VF) from those without increased electrical instability of ventricular myocardium.

In this chapter, these two main areas will be discussed with respect to risk stratification and treatment in patients prone to bradycardia or asystole, as well as to those who are prone to ventricular tachyarrhythmias, which may deteriorate to VF with subsequent sudden cardiac death (SCD).

High-Resolution Monitoring of Atrial Depolarization and Atrioventricular Conduction

When averaging the pre- and post-P-wave intervals, using the initial slope of the P wave as the trigger point, it is possible in principle to retrieve regularly occurring physiological preatrial signals (possible sinus node potentials), as well as atrial repolarization, from baseline noise. From animal studies and direct endocardial catheter recordings from the sinus node area in man, it became clear that the depolarization process of the pacemaker cells resembles a slow up- or downsloping wave with an interval from its beginning to the abrupt transition into the atrial depolarization signal of 40–80 ms in humans.[1–3] In individuals with sinus node disease, sinoatrial conduction times of more than 100 ms have been reported. In principle, preatrial signals from the body surface may be detected by both the signal-averaging (SASE) and the real-time beat-by-beat high-resolution surface electrocardiogram (RT-HRSE) technique, and the following formal character-istics of supposed sinus node potentials should be present:

1. Only DC or 0.05 Hz highpass filtering should be used in order to avoid cutoff of the lower frequencies.
2. The signals of interest should show a ramp or slope-like depolarizing wave with abrupt merging into the P wave.
3. The interval to the beginning of the P wave should be in the range of 40–80 ms.

Using these techniques and criteria, preatrial signals have been reported by Wajszczuk *et al.* in 32 out of 36 noise-free recordings,[2] and with bandpass filtering of 30–300 Hz, preatrial intervals of 20–40 ms were measured. The longest intervals were recorded with the transthoracic Z lead. All recordings were made in patients during regular sinus rhythm, and none of them suffered from sinus node dysfunction, and no comparison was made with simultaneous endocardial electrograms recorded directly from the region of the sinus node.

We have seen preatrial potentials in the SASE in 23 out of 37 individuals (85%) with two different shapes depending on the low-frequency cutoff used. Only those signals that disappeared with 50 Hz highpass filtering showed intervals of 50–165 ms and were considered as true sinus node potentials.[1] In a second small cohort of 13 individuals, we found preatrial signals in none of the 8 normals, but in 2 out of 5 with coronary artery disease using the RT-HRSE; in 7 out of 13 of these individuals, reproducible preatrial potentials were seen within the SASE. Simultaneous intracardiac recordings from the sinus node region to validate the surface signals as true sinus node potentials were not performed.

The clinical significance of these pilot studies is limited by at least two facts:

1. Since only individuals with normal sinus rhythm were studied with the SASE and the RT-HRSE techniques, no information is available as to the behavior of preatrial signals in sinus node arrest or sinoatrial block and the correlation with patients' symptoms.

2. Only the RT-HRSE would reveal dynamic changes of sinus node function in sinus node disease, but the recovery rates of sinus node potentials were very poor with the RT-HRSE technique.

Therefore the high-resolution surface ECG seems to play no role at all for diagnosing symptomatic sinus node dysfunction, and decision-making for pacemaker implantation is primarily based on patients' symptoms and the results of one or several conventional 24-hour ambulatory ECG recordings rather than high-resolution ECG (Figure 17.1).

A similar situation may be found as far as the clinical significance of surface His bundle recordings in the SASE or RT-HRSE is concerned. His bundle recordings represented the first applications of the signal-averaging technique,[1,3] and when using the initial 'crude' technology with less accurate trigger stability His bundle spikes were seen in the SASE in about 30–50% of cases. Later on the retrieval rates were found in up to 66% of cases. In a recent study of a large group of 434 consecutive patients, we found a clear-cut isoelectric line between the end of the P wave and the beginning of the QRS complex in 395 patients, and in only 41 out of 395 individuals (10%) reproducible and stable signals were recorded within the PR segment,[3] which resembled His bundle deflections, despite the fact that the most recent and highly sophisticated signal-averaging equipment (Predictor, Corazonix, USA) was used. Simultaneous intracardiac catheter recordings to confirm that these signals were true His bundle deflections were not performed. An even more sophisticated method of signal analysis was used by our group (Höher *et al.*, unpublished data), but the results were not strikingly better: with both special precordial 'adapted leads' and post-processing averaging of the high-resolution ECG of 16 beats with bidirectional Bessel 80 Hz highpass filtering, a signal probability factor was calculated for

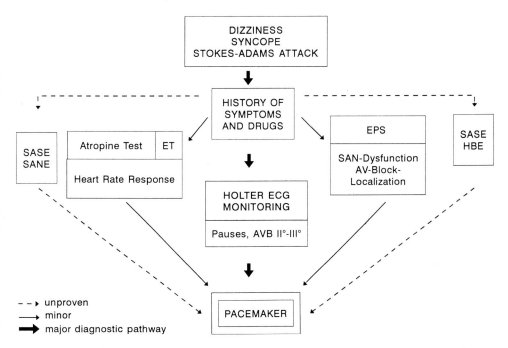

Figure 17.1 Flow chart of major and minor diagnostic pathways in patients with dizziness, syncope or Stokes–Adams attacks, to assess the need for implanting a cardiac pacemaker. Note that signal-averaged ECG parameters to detect sinus mode dysfunction or abnormal AV conduction are of practically no value for clinical decision-making. SASE = signal-averaged surface ECG; SANE = sinoatrial node electrogram; ET = exercise test; AVB = AV block; SAN = sinoatrial node; HBE = His bundle electrogram.

each signal point within the PR segment. Signals exceeding the noise level outside a 95% confidence interval were given the number +1 or −1 depending on their polarity, and those within the noise level the number 0. Thereafter, the number of 'confident' points occurring along the time sector of the His bundle electrogram, as given by a simultaneous intracardiac recording from the His bundle area, were counted. A total of 15 patients had a peak of 'confident' points at the time of the His bundle potential, but in only 7 out of 15 were these points correlated exactly with the timing of the true intracardiac His bundle signal.[3] Again, none of the patients had a disturbed AV conduction like an AV block of second or third degree.

In a few pilot studies using the RT-HRSE technique, the recovery rates of His bundle potentials were similar to or lower than those known for the averaging technique.[3] In none of these reports were patients with higher-degree AV blocks studied, in order to locate the site of block noninvasively – which would be of some help in assessing the risk of a given patient suffering severe bradycardia or long pauses of cardiac arrest. Just one report in the literature describes a so-called 'automated discrimination circuit' to locate the site of block (supra-His versus infra-His) within the averaged surface electrocardiogram.[4] After eliminating superimposed P and R wave segments, post-P-wave triggering was performed which showed either a P wave without His bundle spike (supra-His block) or with subsequent His spike (infra-His block). In a total of 10 patients with complete AV block, 6 had supra-His block and 4 infra-His block within the intracardiac His bundle recording. Five patients did not show a His bundle spike in the post-P interval of the selectively averaged ECG (supra-His block), whereas 4 patients had a His deflection following the P wave of the averaged ECG (infra-His block). Thus, in 9 out of 10 patients the site of AV block was correctly classified by the intelligent surface ECG averaging algorithm. However, this procedure was not completely 'noninvasive', since atrial electrograms from esophageal electrodes were used to record larger atrial deflections for reasons of safer triggering. Since many patients may complain about swallowing an esophageal electrode, they may refuse screening sessions for follow-up studies of normal or impaired AV conduction in order to assess the future risk of higher degrees of AV block.

In summary, then, body surface recordings of His bundle potentials are not reliable for verifying that a given patient's symptoms like dizziness or Stokes–Adams attacks are caused by second- or third-degree AV block, or for assessing the risk of relevant future bradycardic events.

Since recordings of preatrial potentials are not helpful in defining the type and severity of sinus node dysfunction, the decision to implant a pacemaker in a symptomatic patient with bradycardia has to be based on other clinical variables. The main criteria are the history of the patient's syncopal or Stokes–Adams attacks or dizziness, drug intake, clinical examination, and the result of single or repeat 24-hour ambulatory ECG recordings, by which ideally bradycardic or asystolic episodes can be correlated with the patient's symptoms (Figure 17.1). Heart rate response to exercise or IV atropine (the so-called 'atropine test') are of minor importance in uncovering sinus node dysfunction, and intracardiac ECG recordings and stimulation protocols to assess sinus node function and AV conduction are only indicated in a few cases in whom the abovementioned major clinical criteria have failed to provide clear results.

Another interesting new application of P wave averaging relates to atrial delayed depolarization and its role in characterizing patients prone to atrial fibrillation. Steinberg *et al.*[5] have published a prospective study on 130 consecutive patients after cardiac surgery, 33 of whom developed atrial fibrillation (AF) 2.6 days after surgery. P wave duration of the SASE was significantly longer (152 ± 18 ms) in patients with subsequent AF than in those without future AF (139 ± 17 ms). An SASE P wave duration of above 140 ms predicted AF with sensitivity of 77%, specificity of 55%, positive predictive accuracy of 37% and negative predictive accuracy of 87%. The P wave SASE results were independent of other clinical variables by multivariate analysis.

In this report, a comparison of SASE P wave duration was performed with only lead II of the standard 12-lead ECG. From recent large studies it is well known that AF may occur after CABG in 19–28% of cases.[6] Although postoperative AF is often benign and self-limiting, severe sequelae like postoperative stroke may occur. Therefore it seems reasonable and important to predict the risk of an individual patient developing AF after cardiac surgery. However, it should be mentioned that P wave duration obtained from standard 12-lead ECG recordings may provide a similar prognostic power as from SASE. Buxton and Josephson,[7] in a cohort of 99 patients undergoing cardiac surgery, identified total P wave duration of >110 ms from leads I, II and III as a significant predictor of AF or atrial flutter. The P wave duration in lead II alone did not separate patients without and with AF, but total P wave duration in all three leads did. Because of considerable overlap, an isoelectric interval (IEI; subtraction of the longest P wave duration in lead II from total P wave duration in the three limb leads) was used and considered prolonged if above 10 ms. This criterion had a 72% sensitivity, 82% specificity, and a 39% positive predictive accuracy to identify patients prone to AF. The corresponding values of a combination of a prolonged P wave and IEI > 10 ms were: sensitivity 66%, specificity 82%, and positive predictive accuracy 48%. If these results are confirmed by further prospective studies, the question arises whether SASE P wave analysis should be used at all for predicting the risk of postoperative AF, if the conventional ECG provides a similar predictive power, whereas its registration is simpler, easier, less time-consuming and less expensive than signal averaging.

In another study, SASE P wave recordings from surface and esophageal leads were used and analyzed in 45 patients with idiopathic AF and 33 normal controls, to characterize individuals at risk of AF attacks.[8] Both techniques revealed a prolonged P wave duration in patients compared with controls, but only the esophageal lead identified the presence of atrial late potentials as defined by the RMS criterion of the averaged ECG. The predictive power of P wave duration >110 ms alone and in combination with RMS voltage of the last 10 ms < 6.5 μV was: sensitivity 85% and 80%, specificity 100% and 100%, and positive predictive accuracy 100% and 100%, respectively. The authors concluded from their study that the signal-averaged transesophageal lead produces a higher amplitude signal, which detects fractionation of atrial activation in AF and allows identification of individuals predisposed to this arrhythmia.

This study requires several comments. Placing an esophageal electrode in patients is not an entirely 'noninvasive' procedure, and many patients may refuse to swallow such an electrode. The atrial signal from the esophageal electrode represents a more local electrical event as compared with the surface ECG, and therefore some information on the electrical behavior of both atria may be lost. It is not surprising that the predictive power of the signal-averaged esophageal ECG was found to be very high, because patients with idiopathic AF were compared with normal volunteers. Moreover, further clinical criteria like atrial dimensions within the echocardiogram have not been reported. It would be interesting to see what the predictive power of the signal-averaged ECG would be when comparing the patients with idiopathic AF with a matched group with respect to atrial dimensions, age, and risk factors of microvascular disease such as diabetes. And lastly, it would be very important to know whether the analysis of the P wave duration in the routine 12-lead ECG would have had the same predictive power as the signal-averaged ECG, which – as stated above – is more complicated, expensive and time-consuming.

Therefore, the role of P wave analysis from the signal-averaged ECG to predict AF remains to be further clarified and warrants larger and prognostic studies which include all major clinical and anatomical variables.

High-Resolution Monitoring of Ventricular Depolarization

A widespread clinical application of the signal-averaging technique relates to the recovery of VLP. The pathophysiological background for the functional role of VLPs has been shown by the fact that re-entrant pathways play a major role in the initiation and maintenance of ventricular tachycardias. Prerequisites of re-entry are unidirectional block, slow conduction within a partially damaged zone of myocardium, and recovery of excitability of the tissue ahead of the excitation wavefront. Since delayed and fractionated electrical activity during diastole after the QRS complex has been shown to be the correlate of slow conduction, one may principally be able to recover one functional substrate of a re-entrant circuit noninvasively by detecting VLPs from the body surface. Sudden cardiac death (SCD) is most frequently encountered in CDH patients, in whom VT/VF is considered the lethal arrhythmic event, and VLPs seem to be an attractive and promising sign of ventricular electrical instability, which may potentially help to identify individuals at risk of SCD.

The larger studies on the prognostic value of VLPs have been performed almost exclusively with the signal-averaging technique in CHD patients with acute ischemic syndromes, with subacute and chronic stable syndromes, and in patients with cardiomyopathies (dilated, hypertrophic). Only a small number of studies have been devoted to the clinical and prognostic value of RT-HRSE or to the improvement of signal analysis to overcome the limitations of the ECG criteria in the time and frequency domains presently used in high-resolution surface electrocardiography.

Although arrhythmias during transient episodes of myocardial ischemia with ST elevation or ST depression may be observed in a significant number of cases, their electrophysiological mechanism has not been clarified as yet. It is estimated that approximately one-third of SCD episodes are due to VT-fibrillation precipitated by myocardial ischemia. Therefore, there is great interest in knowing whether acute myocardial ischemia may alter the regional electrical conduction and thus may precipitate ventricular arrhythmias. A small number of studies have been devoted to the effect of acute myocardial ischemia as induced by IV administration of dipyridamole or by exercise testing on the incidence of VLPs. In none of these studies were significant differences in the time domain parameters of VLPs observed during myocardial ischemia as compared with baseline values, and in one study with VBP counting no correlation was found between exercise-induced ischemia, VLPs and the number and severity of VPBs.[3] The reason for these negative results may be that myocardial ischemia induced either by dipyridamole or by exercise was not severe enough to produce a conduction delay of a significant amount of myocardium, or that dynamic changes like Wenckebach patterns of conduction delay may have been induced but lost by the averaging process. Therefore, at present the SASE seems to have no real clinical value in the study of patients with acutely provoked myocardial ischemia.

It is well known that systemic or intracoronary thrombolysis may significantly decrease infarct size, preserve left ventricular function and improve prognosis in patients with acute myocardial infarction. The question arises, whether this improvement of prognosis goes parallel with a reduction of myocardial electrical instability, which could be documented by the detection of VLPs. A limited number of studies has been devoted to this problem, with in part conflicting results.[3] The incidence of VLPs in patients with thrombolysis was 5–17%, compared with 23–34% without thrombolysis and 9% with an open versus 39–50% with an occluded infarct related coronary artery. No clear-cut and significant correlation could be found between the incidence of VLPs and VPBs during the acute phase and late arrhythmic events during follow-up. From these studies it was concluded that thrombolysis and patency of an infarct-related coronary artery significantly reduce the rate of VLPs independently of global left ventricular function. This was interpreted as an improved ventricular electrical stability, despite the lack of differences in the incidence of late arrhythmic events in both patient groups.[3]

These discrepancies may be explained in the following way. VLPs in post-MI patients may arise from viable myocardium interspersed in the infarct zone with delayed conduction or from slow activation in the infarct border zone. Any intervention aimed at reducing the extent of infarcted myocardium may not necessarily modify the anatomic substrate for VLPs, and thrombolysis may not provide an antiarrhythmic effect. This fact is not surprising because the result of reperfusion may not be uniform, since the extent of myocardial ischemia may be reduced, but heterogeneity of de- and repolarization may be enhanced. Thus, it may be concluded that in post-MI patients VLPs in the SASE and complex ventricular arrhythmias represent two different electrophysiological substrates.

In the past the incidence and prognostic significance of VLPs in the immediate post-MI period and the first year thereafter has been studied extensively. Patients were investigated routinely 3–4 weeks post-MI before hospital discharge and followed for one to three or more years.[3,9] The incidence of VLPs before discharge was different and ranged between 10% and 55%, depending on the equipment and methodology used. The rate of SCD was 0–4.1% in patients without and 3.6–40% with VLPs during follow-up. The most important message of these studies was that the predictive value of a negative test was very high, between 95% and 99%, whereas the predictive value of a positive test was very low, in the range of 4% to 30%. It should be mentioned that the predictive value of a positive test (VLP present) can be considerably enhanced up to 50%, when further clinical parameters like EF and repetitive VPBs are added, but this goes parallel with a decrease of sensitivity, whereas the negative predictive value may approach 100%.[3,9–11]

From these results it can be concluded that patients without demonstrable VLPs in the third to fourth week post-MI have an excellent prognosis in the first year of follow-up. The problem arises if VLPs are present, because two out of three of those patients do not develop serious arrhythmias as the precursor of SCD. These patients may be screened with further noninvasive methods like echocardiography or RNV to assess LV function, ambulatory monitoring to detect repetitive VPBs and/or to assess heart rate variability, and the test results combined in order to increase the predictive value. However, because of the tendency of subsequent decrease of sensitivity and/or specificity in patients with two or three positive test results, further evaluation has to be considered (e.g. EPS with programmed ventricular stimulation, PVS).

This stepwise approach has recently been described and tested by Pedretti et al.[12] in 303 consecutive patients surviving an AMI. Patients with more than two abnormal noninvasive parameters (EF < 40%, repetitive VPBs, and VLPs) were considered eligible for EPS. Nineteen of 303 patients had an arrhythmic event during follow-up. During multivariate analysis, LV-EF <40%, prolonged filtered QRS complex (VLPs), reduced HRV index and more than two runs of unsustained VT had an independent relation to the arrhythmic event. In 47 out of 67 eligible patients, PVS was performed and a positive EPS result was found to be the strongest predictor of events among patients preselected by noninvasive techniques (sensitivity 81%, specificity 97%, predictive value of a positive test 65%, and predictive value of a negative test 99%).

In conclusion, SCD is a multifactorial syndrome, which is electrophysiologically based on regional conduction delays within certain zones of damaged myocardium (e.g. border zone of an infarct), and which may serve as the electrophysiologic substrate of a re-entrant circuit. However, delayed conduction during sinus rhythm, as seen by VLPs in the averaged ECG, may represent depolarizations of myocardial zones that may not necessarily be an integral part of the re-entrant circuit (so-called 'bystander area'). On the other hand, the most likely initiating mechanism of a re-entrant circuit may be a successive Wenckebach-type conduction delay due to external or internal stimuli (increased sympathetic activity, ischemia, wall stress, etc.), which would be lost by the averaging process. This may explain the high number of false positive results with the

SASE technique to predict SCD. It seems also conceivable that only a certain type of VPBs may act as the trigger event to initiate the intraventricular re-entrant circuit, and according to experimental results the Wenckebach conduction delay type seems to be the best candidate for 'malignant' VPBs, whereas the focal type of VPB, which may not be able to initiate re-entrant excitations, would be 'benign'. Therefore, it would be extremely valuable to have RT-HRSE equipments to detect these dynamic Wenckebach conduction events for VPB- and subsequent VT induction and to allow the identification and differentiation of malignant versus benign types of VPBs. At present, only the above-mentioned two-step approach can be recommended for an effective risk stratification of patients following AMI; that is, *first step*: non-invasive screening for VLPs, repetitive VPBs, and EF <40% or HRV; *second step*: EPS in patients with two or more pathological noninvasive criteria. Patients with inducible sustained VT should then be treated very aggressively by antiarrhythmia drugs (serial EPS testing), catheter ablation or by implantation of an ICD.

In patients with chronic stable CHD remote from MI, the prognostic significance of VLPs within the SASE seems to be limited (sensitivity to predict SCD within two years of follow-up 94%, specificity 50%, positive predictive value 16%, negative predictive value 99%).[3] In a recent larger study at our institution (Höher *et al.*, unpublished data) on 1426 patients with chronic CHD, studied by modern sophisticated SASE techniques, only 31% of patients had two of three VLP criteria positive (filtered QRS duration, RMS value, LAS duration). For a mean follow-up period of 18 months, the predictive value of VLPs to identify SCD candidates was: sensitivity 47%, specificity 70%, positive predictive value 6%, and negative predictive value 97%.[3] From this it can be concluded that, again, a negative test (no VLP) in patients with chronic stable CHD heralds an excellent outcome, but a positive test is of no real value and should not initiate further extensive examinations of these patients unless further criteria of instability are evident (e.g. severe LV dysfunction, spontaneous VTs).

The prognostic power of VLPs has also been studied in patients with nonischemic dilated cardiomyopathy (DCM). The prevalence of VLPs was relatively low in the range 10–20%, the predictive power to either predict the risk of spontaneous VT (sensitivity 83–93%, specificity 68–88%, positive predictive value 53–71%, and negative predictive value 93–96%) or of SCD (sensitivity 0–71%, specificity 66–96%, positive predictive value 0–24%, and negative predictive value 93–94%) was moderate to limited.[13] The message from these results is that a given patient with DCM without demonstrable VLPs will have a good prognosis with regard to the risk of arrhythmic SCD, whereas a positive test result again requires additional noninvasive parameters. In a recent larger prognostic study on 114 patients with nonischemic DCM, multivariate analysis revealed that both the SASE and NYHA functional class were independent predictors of survival.[14] Further extended prognostic studies have to be conducted to show the reproducibility of these results.

The limitations of the SASE as a predictive tool in patients with DCM may also be explained by the following experiences and considerations:[13]

1. The increased rate of bundle branch block in DCM patients, which limits the ability of the SASE to identify local slow conduction.
2. Serious ventricular arrhythmias may account for SCD in only 40–59% of cases, whereas electromechanical dissociation or bradycardia or asystole may account for more than 50% of SCD.
3. The high rate of bundle branch re-entry as the cause of VTs, which cannot be predicted by VLPs.
4. Hemodynamic changes or further pathophysiological influences (electrolyte imbalance, hypoxia, catecholamines, etc.) may not significantly alter the 'fixed' electrophysiologic substrate, but may significantly contribute to the increased risk of fatal ventricular tachyarrhythmias.

According to our own experiences and the literature, the SASE seems to have virtually no value in predicting SCD in patients with hypertrophic cardiomyopathy.[15] Since no signs of initial or terminal slow conduction can be found, which correlate with sustained VTs or SCD,[15] these findings may indicate that fixed re-entrant circuits may not prevail and other electrical or mechanical mechanisms may be responsible for the patients' SCD.

The significance of the SASE in patients with unexplained syncope seems to be limited as well.[3] Beside the fact that more than 50% of those patients may suffer from hemodynamic rather than electrophysiological disturbances, only in individuals with structural heart disease and ventricular arrhythmias may VLP be detected. In a recent larger prognostic multicenter study on 189 consecutive patients with syncope,[16] in all of whom SASE and EPS were performed, multivariate analysis disclosed two variables independently predictive of inducible VTs: previous myocardial infarction and an abnormal SASE. When fitting a logistic regression model using clinical history (age, gender, previous MI), two groups could be identified, a low-risk group and a moderate-risk group. The SASE was able to stratify the risk, so that the post-test probability of inducible VT exceeded 50% (7/11 = 64% of patients with inducible VT had a post-test probability >50%, compared with 6/19 = 32% without inducible VT and a post-test probability >50%). Of the three noninvasive tests (LV ejection fraction, repetitive VPBs, and VLPs), the detection of VLPs seemed to be superior to clarify the likelihood of spontaneous or induced VTs. For practical purposes in patients with unexplained syncope, only those with structural heart disease, particularly with CHD and previous MI, should be studied with SASE, and individuals with moderate risk should then be subjected to PVS to uncover the propensity to VT as the cause of syncope.

Dynamic Behavior of Ventricular Late Potentials

As pointed out earlier, VTs may be initiated by a progressive conduction delay like a Wenckebach pattern within zones of damaged myocardium, which may result in single (one VPB) or repetitive re-entrant circles (nonsustained to sustained VT). One can expect that dynamic alterations of VLPs, like timing relative to the preceding QRS complex or their amplitudes or base width, may indicate a higher degree of electrical instability than stable VLPs. However, only RT-HRSE would be able to detect such unstable and changing VLP patterns. Our own preliminary studies in CHD patients and patients with the long QT-syndrome have shown that dynamic late ventricular activation may be present and may better indicate the risk of SCD than SASE with stable VLPs.[3] However, in trying to significantly enhance the prognostic power of unstable VLPs, one should be able to retrieve the abovementioned Wenckebach progressive conduction delay pattern with one or repetitive ventricular re-entrant excitations, that would represent the malignant type of VPBs, and to differentiate these VPBs from the focal type (no fractionated electrical activity prior to onset of VPB, benign type of VPBs). Thus, a further goal of long-term monitoring is the retrieval of a possibly limited number of malignant VPBs in a 24-hour ambulatory ECG and the separation from a potentially huge number of benign VPBs. Unfortunately, owing to present limitations of technology, the desired low ECG noise levels cannot be achieved in ambulatory recordings; but research capabilities should be directed to this important field to design and commercialize digital ambulatory RT-HRSE equipments.

One approximate solution to uncover a dynamic behavior of VLP may be the recovery of VLPs from conventional Holter tapes, particularly at time periods which precede attacks of unsustained or sustained VTs. Although several reports have described the feasibility and reliability of VLP retrieval from Holter tapes,[17] studies on the relative distribution of VLPs during day and night and possible changes of VLP patterns one hour or minutes prior to the onset of malignant ventricular tachyarrhythmias have not been reported up to now. One might argue that significantly more precise information on ventricular electrical instability prior to the onset of ventricular tachyarrhythmias may not be obtained by analyzing the specific VLP pattern during this period, since preliminary observations on HRV by power spectral analysis as an indicator of sympathetic/parasympathetic imbalance one hour before the onset of SCD did not show consistent changes of the power spectra of the sort one would expect to trigger ventricular fibrillation.[18]

This problem may be approached in another way by recording the RT-HRSE over longer periods to include VPBs, which may potentially trigger re-entrant VT episodes. A preliminary study by Höher et al.[19] disclosed that VLP variability, as measured by QRS and LAS duration, was significantly greater in patients with VLPs in the SASE as compared with those without VLPs, and was also significantly greater in patients with inducible VT versus those without inducible VT. Three different class I drugs increased QRS and LAS duration, and one of these class I drugs, propafenone, increased the variability of QRS and LAS duration. On the other hand, the class III drug sotalol decreased significantly the LAS variability. In this study the effect of variable QRS and LAS duration on the initiation of complex VPBs was not tested. The latter problem is now under study in a much larger cohort of CHD patients with and without spontaneous or induced VTs.

Future Developments

Because of the limited value of static VLPs within the SASE to identify patients at risk of sudden cardiac death, alternative methods are mandatory to increase the predictive power of specific HRSE criteria. One solution has been developed by Höher and coworkers by introducing neural network analysis techniques. A back propagation network[3,20] was fed with common SASE parameters obtained from 147 patients undergoing PVS and trained according to the result of EPS (inducibility or noninducibility of VT). The result of this analysis was compared with the common Simson criteria of VLP, and the following differences were found with regard to predicting the inducibility of VTs:

1. *Simson criteria*: sensitivity 64%, specificity 67%, predictive value of a positive test 50%, predictive value of a negative test 78%.
2. *Neural network analysis*: sensitivity 72%, specificity 96%, predictive value of a positive test 90%, predictive value of a negative test 87%.

Thus, trained network analysis of averaged ECG criteria proved to be superior to the standard time-domain criteria to identify CHD patients prone to spontaneous or inducible sustained VT. This method is currently under continuous improvement and will soon be applied to beat-to-beat RT-HRSE parameters.

Another way to further improve the chance to detect episodes of incremental conduction delays resulting in re-entrant excitations may be the development of digital ambulatory RT-HRSE equipments. In the future, modern electrode design and amplifier technology together with a 'localized shielding' of the recording electrode plus amplifier should enable recordings of selected periods and later on of a full 24-hour RT-HRSE, which would contain the most interesting and important episodes of normal to ectopic single or repetitive ventricular depolarizations.

Moreover, the type and number of so-called 'malignant VPBs' could be assessed, counted and differentiated from the benign types of VPB. Thus, a much more specific approach to risk assessment and therapy may be possible by trying to suppress specifically most or all of the malignant VPBs by antiarrhythmia drugs or by catheter ablation. In principle such technology is in part already available and we have to wait for the first prototypes of such revolutionary equipment modules.

As stated above, SCD due to VT and VF is a complex and multifactorial process. In most SCD victims an arrhythmogenic substrate is present at the site of ventricular myocardium, in which a re-entrant excitation pathway can be initiated by a number of specific triggers like LV wall stress (diastolic, systolic), VPBs, ischemia or an increased sympathetic drive of the heart (Figure 17.2). It is very likely that none of the methods to detect one of these triggers will be specific enough to differentiate a candidate at high-risk of life-threatening ventricular tachyarrhythmias from one with a low risk; but rather a multiple trigger-factor recording approach should be developed and introduced into clinical evaluation, as outlined in Figure 17.2. Such ambulatory monitoring equipment should include invasive pulmonary and arterial blood pressure measurements (diastolic and systolic LV wall stress), detection of VPBs, of ST-segment changes (ischemia) and heart rate and QT variability, eventually in combination with skin impedance or sweat behavior analysis (sympathetic drive), and last but not least a RT-HRSE mini-recorder module (documentation of Wenckebach conduction patterns prior to malignant VPBs). Simultaneous recordings and evaluations of these biologic parameters would help to characterize the whole biologic chain, along which disturbances of the cardiorespiratory and central nervous system will result in the catastrophic event of ventricular fibrillation. Most components of such a complex system are available and used separately, but have not been integrated and matched together in a technically feasible and appropriate way.

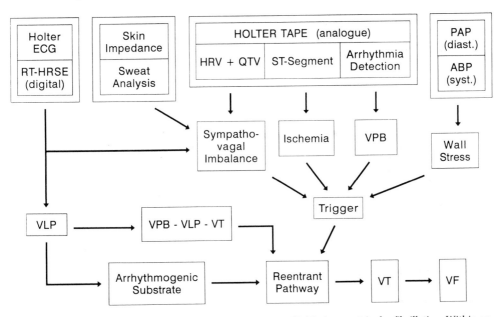

Figure 17.2 The arrhythmogenic substrate trigger concept of initiating ventricular fibrillation. Within an arrhythmogenic myocardial area, re-entrant pathways may be initiated by triggers like LV wall stress, ventricular premature beats, ischemia and/or increased sympathetic drive. A 'multiarrhythmia risk factor ambulatory monitoring' device (MARFAM device) should be able to uncover trigger parameters by simultaneous recordings of pulmonary arterial and arterial blood pressure (diastolic and systolic wall stress), ventricular arrhythmias (VPBs), heart rate and QT interval variability together with skin impedance or sweat analysis (sympathetic drive) and RT-HRSE (Wenckebach conduction type of VLPs to induce one or repetitive re-entrant excitations). By this means the whole 'biological chain' could be assessed, which leads to the catastrophic event of ventricular fibrillation. PAP = pulmonary artery pressure; ABP = arterial blood pressure; HRV = heart rate variability; QTV = QT interval variability; RT-HRSE = real-time (beat-to-beat) high-resolution surface ECG; VPB = ventricular premature beat; VLP = ventricular late potential; VT = sustained ventricular tachycardia; VF = ventricular fibrillation.

It is hoped that a research team will design and make available such a sophisticated 'multi-arrhythmia risk factor ambulatory monitoring' (MARFAM) device.

References

1. Hombach V, Braun V, Höpp HW, *et al*. The applicability of the signal averaging technique in clinical cardiology. *Clin Cardiol* 1982; **5**: 107–24.
2. Wajszczuk WJ, Palko T, Przybylski J *et al*. External recording of sinus node region activity in animals and in man. In: Hombach V, Hilger HH (eds), *Signal Averaging Techniques in Clinical Cardiology*. New York: Schattauer Publishers, 1981: 65–79.
3. Hombach V, Höher M, Kochs M, *et al*. Clinical significance of high resolution electrocardiography – sinus node, His bundle and ventricular late potentials. In: Gomes JA (ed.), *Signal Averaged Electrocardiography: Concepts, Methods and Applications*. Boston: Kluwer Academic, 1993: 267–95.
4. Takeda H, Kitamura K, Takanashi T, *et al*. Noninvasive recording of His–Purkinje activity in patients with complete atrioventricular block. *Circulation* 1979; **60**: 421–6.
5. Steinberg JS, Zelenkofske S, Wong SC, *et al*. Value of the P-wave signal averaged ECG for predicting atrial fibrillation after cardiac surgery. *Circulation* 1993; **88**: 2618–22.
6. Seifert M, Josephson ME. Editorial: P-wave signal averaging – Hightech or an expansive alternative to the standard ECG? *Circulation* 1993; **88**: 2980–82.
7. Buxton AE, Josephson ME. The role of P-wave duration as a predictor of postoperative atrial arrhythmia. *Chest* 1981; **80**: 68–73.
8. Villani GQ, Piepoli M, Cripps T, *et al*. Atrial late potentials in patients with paroxysmal atrial fibrillation detected using a high gain signal averaged esophageal lead. *PACE* 1994; **17**: 1118–23.
9. Breithardt G, Borggrefe M, Martinez-Rubio A. Late potentials in the post-infarction period: prognostic significance. In: El-Sherif N, Turitto G (eds), *High-Resolution Electrocardiography*. Mount Kiski, NY: Futura, 1992; 405–25.
10. Hombach V, Eggeling T, Weismüller P, *et al*. High resolution ECG, Holter ECG monitoring and electrophysiologic studies for risk stratification and evaluation of antiarrhythmic therapy. *J Ambul Monit* 1989; **2**: 33–45.
11. Ip JH, Winters SL, Gomes JA. Risk stratification of post myocardial infarction identification of patients at risk of sudden cardiac death. In: Gomes JA (ed.), *Signal Averaged Electrocardiography: Concepts, Methods and Applications*. Boston: Kluwer Academic, 1993; 459–68.
12. Pedretti R, Etro MD, Laporta A, *et al*. Prediction of late arrhythmic events after acute myocardial infarction from combined use of noninvasive prognostic variables and inducibility of sustained monomorphic ventricular tachycardias. *Am J Cardiol* 1993; **71**: 1131–41.
13. Finkle JK, Marchlinski FE. The signal averaged ECG in patients with cardiomyopathy. In: Gomes JA (ed.), *Signal Averaged Electrocardiography: Concepts, Methods and Applications*. Boston: Kluwer Academic, 1993: 327–43.
14. Mancini DM, Wong KL, Simson MB. Prognostic value of an abnormal signal-averaged electrocardiogram in patients with nonischemic congestive cardiomyopathy. *Circulation* 1993; **87**: 1083–92.
15. Kulakowski P, Counihan PJ, Camm AJ, *et al*. The value of time and frequency domain, and spectrotemporal mapping analysis of the signal-averaged electrocardiogram in identification of patients with hypertrophic cardiomyopathy at increased risk of sudden death. *Eur Heart J* 1993; **14**: 941–50.
16. Steinberg JS, Prystowsky E, Freedman RA, *et al*. Use of the signal averaged electrocardiogram for predicting inducible ventricular tachycardia in patients with unexplained syncope: relation to clinical variables in a multivariate analysis. *J Am Coll Cardiol* 1994, **23**: 99–106.
17. Kennedy HL, Bavishi NS, Buckingham TA. Ambulatory (Holter) electrocardiography signal-averaging: a current perspective. *Am Heart J* 1992; **124**: 1339–46.
18. Öri Z, Monir G, Weiss J, *et al*. Heart rate variability-frequency domain analysis. In: Kennedy HL (ed.), *Ambulatory Electrocardiography*. Philadelphia: Cardiology Clinics, 1992: 499–533.
19. Höher M, Axmann J, Eggeling T, *et al*. Beat-to-beat variability of ventricular late potentials in the unaveraged high resolution electrocardiogram: effects of antiarrhythmic drugs. *Eur Heart J* 1993; **14**(Suppl E): 33–9.
20. Höher M, Kestler HA, Palm G, *et al*. Neural network based QRS classification of the signal averaged electrocardiogram (abstract). *Eur Heart J* 1994; **15**(Suppl): 734.

SECTION V

The ST Segment

Introduction by Peter Cohn

The use of a Holter monitor for documenting ST segment changes is not new and, in fact, Holter's first article dealt with both ST changes and arrhythmias. Fortunately, the issue of whether or not ST segment changes recorded on Holter monitors are reliable indicators of myocardial ischemia is no longer as controversial as it once was when continuous ambulatory monitoring was introduced as a clinical tool in the 1960s. There are still problem areas, however. Whatever the ECG recording procedure employed – Holter, exercise tests, etc. – it is well known that ST segments are labile and notoriously susceptible to hyperventilation, electrolyte abnormalities, drugs, and so on. In addition, since most of the equipment currently in use at hospitals and diagnostic laboratories is an amplitude-modulated (AM) tape system, it is important that physicians also have assurances that the report they receive is accurate. Lambert et al.[1] have provided assurances for the reliability of such devices in their study of low-frequency requirements for recording ischemic ST segment abnormalities. Their conclusion – that current AM models are as reliable as the 'gold standard' frequency-modulated (FM) systems – has been confirmed by Shook et al.[2] in a separate study protocol.

Ironically, as the issue appears to be resolved, another has emerged. A new type of Holter monitor using real-time analysis has been developed. This has presented a new set of problems. In the final analysis, the use of these real-time devices depends on validation studies comparing the devices with conventional AM and FM monitors, as has been done with several systems.

These technical problems notwithstanding, ST segment changes have been used to document ischemia clinically for over 20 years. Stern and Tzivoni[3] were the first to demonstrate ST segment abnormalities on Holter monitoring in a series of 80 patients with chest pain syndromes, normal resting electrocardiograms and normal exercise tests. Thirty-seven of the 80 patients had ischemic ST segment abnormalities (either elevation or depression) on their ambulatory recordings. Many of these episodes were unaccompanied by pain. In the initial 12-month follow-up period, one of these 37 patients developed a myocardial infarction; 23 others developed increasing chest pain or further ECG changes suggestive of coronary artery disease.

In the late 1970s, other groups also attempted to correlate ambulatory ECGs with the results of coronary arteriograms. Crawford and colleagues[4] studied 70 patients (39 with and 31 without coronary artery disease) with 24-hour ambulatory monitors, exercise stress tests, as well as coronary arteriography. Twenty-four of the 39 patients (62%) with coronary artery disease had ischemic ST segment abnormalities on the 24-hour monitors. This compared with 26 patients (or 67%) who had positive stress tests. By contrast, in the 31 patients free of coronary artery disease, 19 (61%) had no ischemic abnormalities on 24-hour monitoring. The exercise stress test was negative in 23 of the 31 subjects (75%).

Most of the studies cited above dealt peripherally with the issue of silent myocardial ischemia. The first Holter study to specifically evaluate the significance of asymptomatic episodes was that of Schang and Pepine.[5] Twenty patients with angiographically confirmed coronary artery disease and positive exercise tests were each monitored for several 10-hour periods over the course of 16 months. In the total of 2826 hours of technically adequate recordings, 411 episodes of transient ST segment abnormalities were documented. Of the 411 episodes, 308 (or 75%) were asymptomatic. Most of these occurred during sleep, sitting or periods of slow walking and at heart rates very much less than those at which patients complained of angina during their stress tests. Schang and Pepine indirectly 'proved' that the silent ST segment episodes were truly ischemic by markedly reducing their occurrence with the frequent, prophylactic use of nitrate preparations. This was an important feature of their study since, as noted previously, considerable criticism had been directed toward the use of the ST segment as a marker of ischemia.

However, it was not until the study by Deanfield and coworkers appeared that this criticism abated.[6] This study and its successor succeeded in refuting much of the skepticism concerning the occurrence and significance of symptomatic versus asymptomatic episodes. In 30 patients with stable angina and positive exercise tests, ambulatory ST segment monitoring was used to record episodes of transient ischemia during daily life. All patients had four consecutive days of monitoring, and in 20 patients long-term variability was evaluated by repeated 48-hour monitoring and exercise testing over an 18-month period. Of the 1934 episodes of horizontal or downsloping ST segment depression, only 470 (or 24%) were accompanied by angina – a figure almost identical to that of Schang and Pepine in their study published six years earlier. Physiologic validation of the ST segment change was an especially important part of their second study, which included 34 patients. That ischemia could occur without angina was documented by positron tomography with the occurrence of ST segment depression being consistently underestimated by symptoms.

As more and more studies using the Holter monitor have been published, it is apparent that episodes involving ST elevation often have similar characteristics to episodes involving ST depression in regard to heart rate, duration of ischemia, etc.; that there is a circadian variation in these episodes, with most coming after arousal in the morning or waking and rising at night, perhaps related to enhanced platelet aggregation or variations in vascular tone; that silent events are also common in patients with unstable angina and are more common in patients with positive rather than negative exercise tests; and that Holter monitoring is useful in assessing success of coronary angioplasty. The day-to-day variability in these events must be considered, however.

The use of Holter monitoring to document silent myocardial ischemia in patients with known symptomatic coronary disease seems well established. Still uncertain, however, is whether ST changes seen in otherwise healthy individuals (who have not undergone coronary arteriography) and in patients with stable coronary disease, have the same connotation and prognostic implications as that found in patients with high-risk coronary disease. The role of routine Holter monitoring in detecting coronary artery disease in a totally asymptomatic population remains unclear. The four chapters that make up this section explore these questions and, in addition, explore new approaches to the detection and clinical significance of Holter-recorded ST segment shifts.

References

1. Lambert CR, Imperi GA, Pepine CJ. Low-frequency requirements for recording ischemic ST-segment abnormalities in coronary artery disease. *Am J Cardiol* 1986; **58**: 225.
2. Shook TL, Balke W, Kotilainen PW, Hudelbank M, Selwyn AP, Stone PH. Comparison of amplitude-modulated (direct) and frequency-modulated ambulatory techniques for recording ischemic electrocardiographic changes. *Am J Cardiol* 1987; **60**: 895.
3. Stern S, Tzivoni D. Early detection of silent ischaemic heart disease by 24-hour ECG monitoring during normal daily activity. *Br Heart J* 1974; **36**: 481.
4. Crawford MH, Mendoza CA, O'Rourke RA, White DH, Boucher CA, Gorwit J. Limitations of continuous ambulatory electrocardiogram monitoring for detecting coronary artery disease. *Ann Intern Med* 1978; **89**: 1.
5. Schang SJ, Pepine CJ. Transient asymptomatic ST segment depression during daily activity. *Am J Cardiol* 1977; **39**: 396.
6. Deanfield JE, Shea M, Ribiero P, deLandsheere CM, Wilson RA, Horlock P, Selwyn AP. Myocardial ischemia during daily life in patients with stable angina: its relation to symptoms and heart rate changes. *Lancet* 1983; **2**: 753.

18

Ischemia Detected by Holter Monitoring in Coronary Artery Disease

Prakash C. Deedwania

Introduction

Although, traditionally, ambulatory ECG monitoring (AEM) has been used largely for the evaluation of patients with cardiac arrhythmias, during the past decade there has been a growing interest in using AEM for evaluation of myocardial ischemia detected by ST segment changes on ECG. The first report regarding the technical feasibility and use of Holter monitoring for detection of myocardial ischemia by recording ST segment changes was described in 1961 by Normal Holter, the inventor of the technique.[1] However, it was not until the pioneering work of Stern and Tzivoni in 1973 that the medical community started believing in the diagnostic accuracy of ST segment depression recorded on Holter monitoring in identifying periods of myocardial ischemia.[2] Subsequent work by Schang and Pepine,[3] as well as by Deanfield and coworkers,[4] emphasized the clinical importance of AEM in detecting asymptomatic ST segment depression on ECGs recorded during ambulatory monitoring for identification of silent ischemic episodes. A large number of studies have now shown that transient ischemic episodes, which are largely asymptomatic (silent), occur frequently in patients with a variety of acute as well as chronic ischemic syndromes.[5–7] The results of several recent studies have also demonstrated that, despite the absence of anginal symptoms, episodes of silent myocardial ischemia detected by AEM in patients with coronary artery disease (CAD) have a poor prognosis.[5,6] Some of these studies have emphasized the clinical importance of performing AEM in patients with stable and unstable angina by showing that silent ischemia may persist despite medical therapy that is effective in controlling anginal symptoms. Furthermore, considerable new evidence that has emerged in recent years clearly emphasizes that it is the presence of myocardial ischemia, regardless of its association with anginal symptoms, that determines the prognosis in patients with CAD.

In this chapter, the available data regarding the clinical utility and significance of AEM in detecting asymptomatic ST segment depression will be reviewed, followed by a brief discussion on important technical aspects.

Definition of Silent Ischemia

Silent ischemia is defined as the objective evidence of myocardial ischemia in the absence of chest pain or other anginal equivalent symptoms.[5,6] The presence of myocardial ischemia can be inferred from transient ST segment changes on ECG, reversible myocardial perfusion defect, or regional wall motion abnormalities. A number of techniques, including exercise testing, ambulatory ECG (Holter) monitoring, radio-nuclide imaging, and stress echocardiography can be utilized for detection of silent myocardial ischemia. Of the available diagnostic tools, AEM has been the most widely used method because of the distinct advantage due to its ability to record ischemic episodes in the ambulatory setting while the patient is engaged in usual daily activities.

Although a variety of definitions have been used to describe an episode of myocardial ischemia during AEM, the definition adopted at the National Institute of Health Workshop on Silent Ischemia is the one accepted by most investigators in this area.[6] This definition, which is typically referred to as the $1 \times 1 \times 1$ rule, describes a transient ischemic event during AEM as horizontal or downsloping ST segment depression greater than or equal to 0.1 mV measured 60–80 ms from the J point, lasting for 1 minute, and separated from another episode by at least 1 minute. Although this definition provides specific criteria for the identification of an ischemic episode during AEM, it does not specify the onset and offset points for ST segment depression, which are essential to measure the duration of ischemic events. Because of the lack of specific guidelines, many investigators have measured the duration of ischemic events as the total time from the point when ST segment depression begins to the point when ST segment returns to the baseline. More recently, others have used the onset point when the ST segment depression reaches the 1 mm level and the offset point had been defined as the time when ST depression becomes less than 1 mm. Lack of a standardized technique for measuring duration of ischemic events may explain, in part, the variation in results reported by several investigators.

Reliability of Ischemic Changes Detected by ST Segment Depression

Although, in the past, ST segment depression during AEM was not well accepted as unequivocal evidence of myocardial ischemia, findings from recent studies have demonstrated an excellent correlation between ST depression during AEM and other objective evidence of ischemia, such as simultaneous reversible perfusion defects on thallium-201 scintigraphy, regional wall motion abnormalities on radionuclide angiocardiography, and hemodynamic abnormalities.[5] Investigators comparing the diagnostic value of exercise testing and AEM for detection of myocardial ischemic changes have reported good correlation between the exercise test and AEM findings. Tzivoni and colleagues compared ST segment changes on ambulatory ECG recordings with ST segment changes during submaximal treadmill exercise test in 144 patients. In this study, findings from both tests were found to be in agreement in 96% of subjects.[8]

The specificity of the ST depression during AEM as an indicator of myocardial ischemia has been further evaluated in studies of normal individuals who underwent 24-hour AEM. In a study of 33 normal ambulatory individuals, no flat ST depression was noted during Holter monitoring. In another study of 80 volunteers free of clinical CAD, only two subjects exhibited transient ST depression during the monitoring period.[5,6] Nonspecific ST (e.g. unsloping ST depression) or T wave changes, however, are not specific for myocardial ischemia and have been noted in 30–40% of normal subjects. Therefore, it is important to emphasize that only ST segment changes meeting the diagnostic criteria, as described previously, should be considered.

Several recent studies have demonstrated that if the established diagnostic criteria are used, episodes of ST depression during AEM have a good correlation with the presence of myocardial ischemia in patients with proven CAD.

Clinical Significance of Asymptomatic ST Segment Depression

Traditionally, the evaluation of patients with coronary artery disease (CAD) has been based on the subjective description of angina or anginal equivalent symptoms. Recent findings from studies in various subsets of patients with CAD, however, indicate that symptoms are unreliable markers of disease activity.[5] This problem is further compounded by the fact that most episodes of myocardial ischemia detected during continuous electrocardiographic (ECG) recording by Holter monitoring in the hospital or during routine daily activities, are not associated with any symptom. These findings have led to the growing interest in evaluating CAD patients with AEM for detection of silent myocardial ischemia. In patients with symptomatic CAD, the findings from several recent investigations in various subsets of patients indicate a frequent occurrence of silent ischemic events during Holter monitoring.[9–16] In general, it is estimated that in patients with unstable coronary syndromes and in those with chronic stable CAD, more than 80% of all transient ischemic episodes remain silent (Figure 18.1) and can be detected only by the presence of ST segment changes recorded during ECG monitoring. The largest group of patients at risk of transient silent ischemia consists of patients with stable CAD. Of the 5 million Americans suffering from chronic stable CAD, it is estimated that nearly 2 million might have evidence of silent ischemia which can be detected by AEM.

Several studies in patients admitted with the clinical diagnosis of unstable angina indicate that transient myocardial ischemia can be detected during continuous ECG monitoring in 11–66% of the patients.[5,6] In these patients, most ischemic events were not associated with symptoms (Figure 18.2). In some of these studies, intensive antianginal drug treatment was provided at the outset. However, despite control of symptoms, transient ischemic changes were detected in 34–66% of patients.[5,6,9,10] In one study, even thrombolytic therapy was administered after the initial ECG monitoring demonstrated transient episodes of myocardial ischemia.[13] After thrombolytic therapy, repeat ECG monitoring within 4 days still revealed ischemic changes in 61% of the patients.

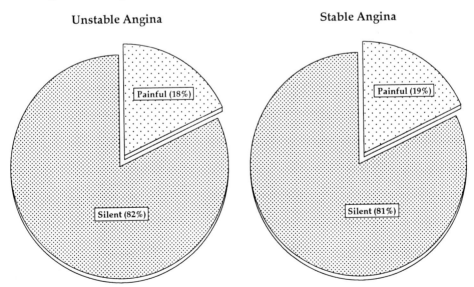

Figure 18.1 Distributions of silent and symptomatic episodes of myocardial ischemia during Holter monitoring in patients with unstable angina and in those with stable coronary artery disease and angina. (Adapted with permission from reference 6)

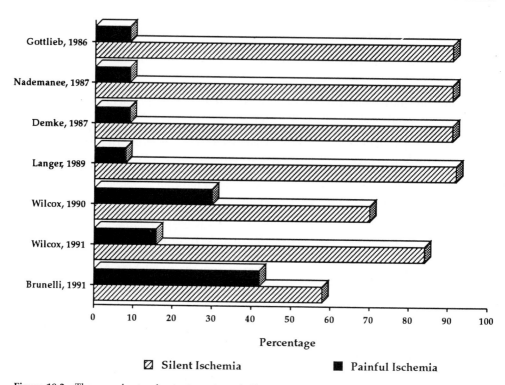

Figure 18.2 The prevalence of symptomatic and silent myocardial ischemia in patients with unstable angina. (Adapted with permission from reference 6)

The prevalence of silent ischemia in the nearly 6 million Americans with chronic stable CAD has been estimated to be between 40% and 50%.[5,6,14–16] This makes transient episodes of silent myocardial ischemia the most common manifestation of CAD. Several studies in patients with known CAD and stable angina evaluated by exercise treadmill testing and ambulatory ECG monitoring have shown that episodes of silent ischemia are more common than symptomatic episodes.[5,6,14,15] In patients with CAD and stable angina undergoing AEM, asymptomatic ST segment depressions (Figure 18.3) have been detected in 41–59% of patients.[5,6,14–16] Based on the data from these observations, it can be estimated that between 2 and 3 million Americans with stable CAD have evidence of silent myocardial ischemia.

Studies in patients with CAD clearly show that conventional or intensive antianginal drug therapy, aimed at symptom control, does not eliminate silent ischemic episodes.[5,6] In a recent study of 105 patients with stable angina and CAD, ambulatory ECG monitoring was performed while patients were receiving treatment with one or more conventional antianginal drugs.[5] In this study, we found that despite adequate control of angina symptoms, 43% of patients showed episodes of silent ischemia during AEM. Most ischemic episodes were associated with minimal or lack of physical activity, and most patients did not have symptoms during the monitoring period.

It is important to emphasize that, without AEM, the residual ischemia present in these patients would have remained unrecognized because both patients and their physicians thought that the therapy was adequate for control of anginal symptoms.

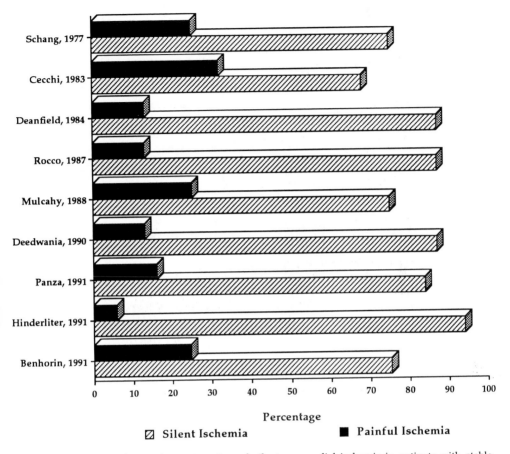

Figure 18.3 The prevalence of symptomatic and silent myocardial ischemia in patients with stable coronary artery disease. (Adapted with permission from reference 6)

Defining the Pathophysiology of Myocardial Ischemia During Daily Life

Recent findings from several studies in patients undergoing AEM have revealed substantial information to help explain the pathophysiologic mechanism(s) responsible in the genesis of transient myocardial ischemia during daily life.

Although the precise mechanism responsible for the development of transient ischemic episodes in the ambulatory setting is not well understood, previous studies suggested that a reduction in coronary blood flow may play a dominant role. This assumption had been based primarily on results showing relatively small increases in the heart rate during the 5–15 minute period preceding the ischemic episodes during AEM.[5,6] This concept was further supported by demonstrating a smaller increase in heart rate preceding ischemic events during daily life when compared with the increase in heart rate observed during exercise-induced ischemia in the same patient.[5,6] Also, since most silent ischemic episodes on AEM occur during minimal or no strenuous activity, it had been postulated that an increase in myocardial oxygen demand was unlikely to play a significant role.

However, several recent studies have shown that an increase in myocardial oxygen demand does play a significant role in the development of ambulatory silent myocardial ischemia.[5,6,17] In a study of 25 patients with documented CAD, stable angina, and a positive exercise treadmill test, simultaneous ambulatory ECG and blood pressure monitoring were performed for 24–48 hours.[17] In this study, we had demonstrated that the majority of transient ischemic events during daily life were preceded by significant increases in heart rate and systolic blood pressure. These circulatory changes, observed prior to the onset of silent ST segment depression during ambulatory ECG monitoring, closely resembled those involved in the pathophysiology of angina pectoris. These data, along with the results of other recent studies showing beneficial effects of beta-blocking agents in the treatment of silent ischemic events,[18,19] confirm the role of increased myocardial oxygen demand in the pathogenesis of most episodes of silent ischemia during daily life.

Circadian Rhythmicity of Silent Ischemic Events

Ambulatory ECG monitoring is a useful tool to evaluate the pattern of ischemic activity during the 24-hour period. Previous data from large epidemiological studies had provided evidence for circadian variation of acute myocardial infarction and sudden cardiac death. Recently, several studies in patients with coronary artery disease have demonstrated that transient myocardial ischemia, as evidenced by silent or symptomatic ST segment depressions during ambulatory ECG monitoring, also show a circadian pattern with increased incidence of ischemic events in the morning hours.[5,6,17–19] In a study of 25 patients evaluated by 24-hour AEM, a morning surge in silent ischemic events was observed and paralleled the morning increases in heart rate and systolic blood pressure.[17] In a large, multicenter, prospective study of 306 patients with CAD and evidence of silent ischemia during 48-hour AEM, we have recently demonstrated that transient ischemic episodes during daily life show a definite morning peak between 9am and 10am and a secondary peak at around 8pm.[19] Numerous studies have shown that treatment with beta-blockers is highly effective in suppressing the circadian rhythm of silent ischemia.[5,18–19] Because this circadian pattern of silent ischemic events is quite similar to that observed for the onset of acute myocardial infarction, as well as sudden death, it would be reasonable to assume that transient ischemic events may indeed be an important substrate for acute MI and sudden death.

Predictors of Silent Ischemia during AEM

Because ambulatory AEM for ischemia monitoring is not readily available, and its routine use in patients with stable angina would increase the cost of health care considerably, it is essential to identify the predictors of ambulatory silent ischemia in patients at risk. Comparison of various clinical features, coronary risk factors, and exercise test findings have revealed that certain exercise parameters can be used to predict reliably the risk of silent ischemia during AEM.[20,21]

In a study of 277 patients with stable angina and CAD undergoing 48-hour AEM, Mulcahy and coworkers found that most patients developing ischemia during AEM (131 of 187, 70%) had evidence of ischemia during exercise testing. Patients with a negative exercise test rarely developed ischemia during AEM (19 of 90, 21%).[20] The results of other recent studies also indicate that the majority (65–95%) of patients at risk of developing myocardial ischemia during ambulatory ECG monitoring can be identified based on an earlier onset (within second stage or <6 minutes of standard Bruce protocol) of ischemia during exercise testing.[6,21] Furthermore, it appears that there is a relationship between the time to onset of exercise-induced ischemia and the duration of myocardial ischemia during AEM.[6,21] It has been shown that the earlier the onset of exercise-induced ischemia and the more severe the degree of ST segment depression during exercise testing, the greater the duration of ambulatory myocardial ischemia detected by AEM.

Prognostic Importance of Silent Myocardial Ischemia

Although silent ischemia detected by AEM does not produce discomfort, its presence has been associated with an adverse clinical outcome and poor prognosis. Patients with unstable angina who demonstrate silent ischemic events during continuous ECG monitoring have been found to have an increased risk of experiencing an acute MI, cardiac death, or need for coronary artery bypass surgery during the follow-up.[9–12]

In a report of 70 patients with unstable angina receiving intensive drug therapy with nitrates, beta-blockers, and calcium-channel blockers, patients (53%) with one or more episodes of silent ischemia during ECG monitoring had a higher risk for MI or need for coronary revascularization during the subsequent 30 day follow-up.[9] In a smaller study of 49 patients with unstable angina who underwent AEM after their condition was stabilized with one or more antianginal agents, 29 patients had silent ischemia.[11] Those with more than 60 minutes of ischemia during AEM had increased risk of acute MI or need for coronary artery bypass surgery, compared with patients with under 60 minutes of ischemia or those without ischemia. Similar findings were reported in another study of 135 patients with unstable angina who underwent AEM during the acute phase.[10] In this study, significantly more patients (48%) with transient ischemia during ECG monitoring had an unfavorable outcome (MI, death, or need for aortocoronary bypass or percutaneous transluminal coronary angioplasty) compared with patients without ST segment changes during AEM (20%, odds ratio 3.79). The patients with more than 60 minutes of ischemia had significantly greater risk of nonfatal MI and death (20% rate) compared with those without ST shift (4%). There was no significant difference compared with those patients with less than 60 minutes of ischemia (11%). In another study of 66 patients with unstable angina evaluated by continuous ECG monitoring, Wilcox and coworkers found that during the 13.3-month follow-up period, all patients (7 of 7, $p <$ 0.005) with transient ischemia during ECG monitoring required coronary revascularization (aortocoronary bypass or coronary angioplasty) compared with 42% of patients without ischemia during ECG monitoring.[12]

In patients with chronic stable angina, silent ischemia during AEM has been found to carry adverse prognostic significance. A study of 86 patients with chronic exertional angina revealed that episodes of silent myocardial ischemia during AEM were associated with an increased risk for unstable angina and coronary revascularization procedures during a 12-month follow-up.[14] In a study of 107 patients with known CAD and exertional angina, those with presence of silent ischemia during AEM had a three-fold risk of sudden cardiac death and fatal MI compared with patients without ischemia (24% versus 8% mortality, $p = 0.02$) during the 2-year follow-up.[16] In a more recent study, Yeung and associates evaluated the long-term prognostic significance of silent ischemia during AEM in 138 patients with stable angina.[22] In this study, those patients with ischemic episodes during AEM had a significantly higher relative risk (>10) of developing death or MI at 2-year follow-up. For all cardiac events, including coronary revascularization, the patients with ischemia during AEM had a higher relative risk (2.82) throughout the 37-month follow-up compared with patients without ischemia recorded during AEM. Based on the above data, it is clear that episodes of silent myocardial ischemia detected by ambulatory ECG monitoring during routine daily activities are associated with an adverse clinical outcome.

Prognostic Significance of Asymptomatic ST Depression

Data from recent studies suggest that the presence of silent ischemic episodes during AEM provide additional prognostic information in high-risk CAD patients, when compared with data available from an exercise tolerance test.[23,24] In a study of 224 patients recovering from acute myocardial infarction who underwent exercise treadmill tests and ambulatory ECG monitoring, Tzivoni and coworkers evaluated the prognostic significance of myocardial ischemia during AEM in patients with exercise-induced ischemia.[23] In this study, the patients with myocardial ischemia during AEM had a significantly higher rate (51% versus 20%, $p < 0.001$) of cardiac events (cardiac death, nonfatal myocardial reinfarction, unstable angina, and coronary revascularization) compared with patients with ischemia during exercise testing but without ischemic events during AEM.

In a recent study, we prospectively examined and compared the prognostic value of silent ischemia during AEM with exercise test parameters in patients with stable angina and documented CAD.[24] In this study of 86 patients, all of whom had exercise-induced ischemia and who were prospectively followed for a mean period of 2 years, those with evidence of silent ischemia during AEM had significantly higher mortality (23% versus 4% mortality, $p < 0.008$) compared with patients without evidence of ischemia during AEM. The presence of ischemia during AEM did indeed provide additional prognostic information to that available from the previously established poor prognostic indicators derived from exercise test findings. It is known that patients with a total exercise duration less than 6 minutes, as well as those with early (within second stage of Bruce protocol) onset of ischemia, have worse prognosis and poor clinical outcome. The findings from our study showed that ischemia recorded by AEM further stratified these patients into high- and low-risk subsets. Patients with evidence of ischemia during AEM within these subsets had significantly higher risk of cardiac death during the follow-up period. Peak exercise heart rate less than 120 bpm has also been shown to predict poor clinical outcome. Our data revealed that in patients with peak exercise heart rate less than 120 bpm, as well as in those with at least 120 bpm, the presence of ischemia during AEM identified the patients who had worse prognosis and increased risk of cardiac death. Evaluation by multivariate regression analysis of several clinical exercise tests and AEM variables, revealed silent ischemia during AEM as the most powerful predictor of cardiac death ($p < 0.001$).

The reason for adverse clinical outcome and increased cardiac mortality in association with silent ischemia detected during Holter monitoring is not clear. Limited data from a few studies could be used to explain, in part, the adverse outcome associated with silent ischemia.[5,6,16] Findings from studies conducted in experimental animals have indicated that repeated brief episodes of myocardial ischemia can produce small but distinct areas of subendocardial necrosis. In a study of patients with CAD undergoing cardiac surgery, intraoperative biopsy specimens revealed abnormalities of nuclei, mitochondria, and a reduction of contractile material in the subendocardium. Although there was no gross histologic evidence of MI, there was a loss of myocytes and an increased amount of fibrosis. These changes were also associated with evidence of localized hypokinesias. The effects of transient ischemia on myocardial structure and ventricular function have also been evaluated. Histopathologic examination of the myocardial biopsy samples obtained from left ventricle in patients with CAD undergoing open heart surgery showed muscle fiber hypertrophy and increased interstitial nonmuscular tissue in the endocardial layers of the transiently ischemic myocardium with normal function at rest. There was, however, evidence of ischemia-induced regional wall motion abnormalities during exercise in these areas of myocardium. Thus, it is conceivable that repeated episodes of transient ischemia over a long period may result in left ventricular dysfunction. It is also possible that silent ischemia may result in lethal ventricular arrhythmias. Although there is no direct evidence of such an association, the results of some recent studies suggest that silent ischemia may indeed be a forerunner of malignant ventricular arrhythmias.

The results of studies in patients with stable angina clearly indicate that silent ischemia is far more prevalent than anginal symptoms. Because it is the presence of ischemia that determines the prognosis, it is imperative that clinicians carefully evaluate their patients for the presence of residual ischemia. In general, the patients at risk of silent ischemia during daily life can be identified by either early onset of ischemia, or ischemia developing at relatively low double product (>20 000 heart rate × systolic blood pressure) during treadmill exercise testing. Although the benefit of eliminating all episodes of silent ischemia is not yet proven, early identification of such patients may help stratify the patients into high- and low-risk subsets.

Technological Requirements for ST Segment Monitoring

In order to perform ambulatory ECG monitoring for detection and evaluation of myocardial ischemia, two pieces of equipment are needed: a recorder and a playback, scanning device. Some of the essential technical considerations for proper electrocardiographic monitoring are listed in Table 18.1 (see also Chapter 1 in this volume).

The recording device

Currently, three types of ECG recorders are available for the evaluation of ST segment changes on AEM: amplitude-modulated (AM), frequency-modulated (FM), and solid-state digital. FM recorders have been considered the 'gold standard' for assessment of myocardial ischemia because they have ideal frequency response (<2 Hz) characteristics and are less prone to phase shifts.[7] However, findings from recent studies in patients with coronary artery disease indicate that the amplitude-response characteristics of electrocardiographic recording equipment do not require an extended low-frequency range (such as that found in FM systems) to reproduce accurately ischemic ST segment

Table 18.1 Technical considerations of ambulatory ECG monitoring for myocardial ischemia

---

Equipment choice
AM versus FM
Continuous versus event recording devices
Digital (solid-state) systems

Hook-up technique
Thorough-skin preparation (dermabrasion)
Stress loop use
Test for impedance
Postural recordings
Calibration signal input

Angina/activity diary: review needed

Scanning of recorded tapes
Playback units and software
Experienced personnel
Speed of review (60–120 times)
Positional changes/artifact

abnormalities in humans. Furthermore, recent studies comparing the currently available AM and FM systems have demonstrated that the newer AM monitoring devices with improved low-frequency recording and playback systems can reliably reproduce the ST segment deviation recorded during FM monitoring. Both AM and FM systems have problems with background electrical activity. However, the signal-to-noise ratio (tape noise) is higher in FM than in AM recording devices.

Continuous versus intermittent recording devices

Although the hardware implementation of the continuous and intermittent recorders is similar, intermittent (event) recorders have a limited capability to store short segments of data, usually when the recording is triggered by the patient with the onset of symptoms or by the characteristic ECG changes previously set to a threshold point. There is no system currently available that has a reliable algorithm for automated detection of diagnostic ST segment changes. Because of this limitation, it has been suggested that continuous ECG monitoring is more useful than intermittent event recording for the evaluation of ambulatory silent ischemia.

Playback and scanning devices

A variety of systems are available for the analysis of AEM tapes. These offer a wide range of data displays, including full disclosure and trending ability as well as statistical summary options.[7] Proper trending of heart rate and ST segment level are essential in analyzing data for transient myocardial ischemic events. Many systems have a spectrum of capabilities for automatic or manual interaction during signal processing. This is necessary because no machine provides perfect discrimination between an 'unusual' but physiologic signal and noise or artifact.

Current ambulatory ECG monitoring techniques for detection and evaluation of transient myocardial ischemia require an interactive, user-dependent analytic system that can modify detection and classification parameters on an ongoing basis in order to customize the processing to specific requirements. Therefore, even when automatic scanners are used, quantitative assessment of ST segment changes should always include a visual editing process (physician over-read) based on uniform morphologic guidelines and established definitions of transient ischemic events.

Patient Selection for ST Segment Monitoring by AEM

At present, ambulatory ECG monitoring should be performed to detect and evaluate transient myocardial ischemia only in patients who are at high risk of developing ischemic episodes and in patients with anginal symptoms at rest, or during emotional or specific physical activities where other tests are not feasible or have been previously negative. Ambulatory ECG monitoring might be considered as an alternative diagnostic modality for evaluation of myocardial ischemia in patients with physical disability as well as in preoperative evaluation of patients referred for vascular surgery.

With the exception of these categories of patients, AEM is not recommended for screening healthy individuals for detection of asymptomatic CAD. It is important to recognize that, because of the high rate of false positive results, AEM is not suitable for ischemia monitoring in patients with pre-existing baseline ST segment changes, LVH, bundle branch blocks, pre-excitation syndrome, and atrial flutter/atrial fibrillation. Also, patients receiving medications such as digoxin, diuretics and phenothiazines may not be suitable candidates for AEM to detect silent myocardial ischemia because of the potential high false positive rate.

Methodological Considerations

For optimal diagnostic accuracy, a great deal of attention should be given to the methodology used, including lead selection, hook-up technique, and careful evaluation of subjective entries in the diaries.[7] A minimum of two leads should be selected for ambulatory ECG monitoring. Each lead should have an individual negative or reference electrode. This should prevent losing data from a single channel malfunction and also allow for a better and thorough analysis of the recorded data covering more than one anatomical location of the heart. Preferably, the selected leads should match the leads with the greatest ST segment depression during exercise testing. Leads which are recommended for general use simulate a V1 and a V5 lead axis. Other lead systems may be more appropriate on a case-by-case basis as dictated by specific clinical situations. Leads showing evidence of previous myocardial infarction on a 12-lead ECG should be avoided. Also, it is essential to select the leads with an R wave voltage of at least 8 mm, since it has been shown that the chances of detecting diagnostic ST segment changes diminish considerably with a lower R wave amplitude. Furthermore, thick areas of adipose tissue, heavy muscle masses, and the abdominal area should not be used. This will minimize movement artifact as well as avoid increased electrical impedance.

Skin preparation and proper electrode application are absolute requirements during the AEM hook-up procedure. A meticulous approach is required to ensure maximal adhesiveness and a clear signal, and to minimize patient discomfort and skin–electrode impedance. A bath or shower with plain soap and water prior to the monitoring session will help reduce the skin–electrode impedance.

After a careful hook-up, it is essential to test for ST segment changes during hyperventilation and various common postures (supine, prone, lateral and sitting positions). Patients with postural changes are not suitable for ST segment monitoring.

An accurate and complete record of the patient's symptoms and activities is crucial in the evaluation of myocardial ischemic activity detected during AEM. Patients should be instructed in keeping a log of symptoms, including the time of occurrence and disappearance of each symptom as well as the associated activity. Also, certain activities, even when not associated with symptoms, should be regularly recorded in the diary (e.g. physical activity, meals, emotional states, driving, wake and sleep cycles). Timing of events is best recorded by referring to a digital clock incorporated in the recorder. Upon return of the patient, a thorough review and confirmation of the diary entries should be performed before the patient leaves the office.

AEM Recording Time and Variability of Ischemic Episodes

For most clinical purposes, a minimum recording period of 24 consecutive hours has been recommended. In a study of 16 patients with chronic angina pectoris undergoing AEM, Khurmi and coworkers found that the number and duration of ST segment depressions during 24-hour AEM at the baseline were reproducible at 6 weeks.[25] Because of the demonstrated variability in the number and duration of ischemic events similar to that described for ventricular arrhythmia, a 24-hour recording period may not be sufficient, particularly when the results of AEM are to be used in the evaluation of therapeutic response.[26] In a report from a study of 42 patients with stable angina and documented CAD, Nabel *et al.* suggested that, as a result of intraindividual variability, at least 48 hours of AEM should be performed when evaluating ischemic activity.[26] These principles should also be taken into consideration when monitoring episodes of ischemic ST depression within groups of patients.

Based on these findings, it seems appropriate to perform ambulatory ECG monitoring for at least 48 hours when evaluating patients at risk of developing myocardial ischemia during daily life, particularly when it is essential to evaluate the response of anti-ischemic therapy.

The Role of AEM in the Management of Patients with CAD

The clinical management of patients with CAD has, traditionally, focused on the assessment and monitoring of anginal symptoms, with the primary goal of relieving symptoms. As discussed earlier, the available evidence suggests clearly that chest pain is an insensitive indicator of transient myocardial ischemia and that the severity of angina has poor correlation with prognosis.

Because silent ischemic events occur frequently in patients with stable and unstable CAD and are associated with an adverse clinical outcome and risk of cardiac death,[5,6] it has been suggested that anti-ischemic therapy should be directed at reducing the total ischemic activity (silent and symptomatic) during daily life. Ambulatory ECG monitoring can be reliably used in the evaluation of anti-ischemic therapy directed towards control of total ischemic burden. Data from several studies in patients with CAD indicate that ambulatory ECG monitoring provides a good index of the frequency and magnitude of recurring myocardial ischemia during daily life before and after anti-ischemic drug therapy. The results of recent studies indicate that anti-ischemic drugs can differ significantly in their effects on transient ischemic events.[18,27] Ambulatory ECG monitoring is also quite useful in evaluating the distribution of ischemic events during the 24–48 hour period before and after drug therapy.

Although treatment of all ischemic episodes, regardless of associated symptoms, has been empirically recommended by many investigators, little convincing evidence is available to show that such therapy is effective in reducing the associated adverse prognosis.[27] More studies are needed to examine this critical and clinically important question.

Clinical Implications of ST Segment Evaluation by AEM

Ambulatory ECG monitoring is a useful diagnostic modality in the assessment of myocardial ischemic events during daily life. Several recent studies have shown that most of the transient ischemic events that occur in the ambulatory setting are not associated with symptoms and may remain undetected unless evaluated by AEM. Based on the results of recent studies it seems reasonable to conclude that, despite control of anginal symptoms, residual ischemia detected by AEM may be present in as many as 50% of patients with CAD. Because it is the presence of ischemia, regardless of associated symptoms, that carries the adverse prognosis in patients with CAD, it seems logical to consider that detection of such residual ischemia by AEM would be useful in identifying the high-risk CAD patients.

Recent advances in AEM techniques (which are discussed in subsequent chapters) should make ambulatory ECG monitoring for myocardial ischemia even more reliable and readily accessible in the evaluation of patients with coronary artery disease.

References

1. Holter N. New method for heart studies: continuous electrocardiography of active subjects over long periods is now practical. *Science* 1961; **134**: 1214–20.
2. Stern S, Tzivoni D. Dynamic changes in the ST–T segment during sleep in ischemic heart disease. *Am J Cardiol* 1973; **32**: 17–20.

3. Schang S, Pepine C. Transient asymptomatic ST segment depression during daily activity. *Am J Cardiol* 1977; **39**: 396–402.

4. Deanfield J, Shea M, Ribiero P, *et al*. Transient ST-segment depression as a marker of myocardial ischemia during daily life. *Am J Cardiol* 1984; **54**: 1195–200.

5. Deedwania P, Carbajal E. Silent myocardial ischemia: a clinical perspective. *Arch Intern Med* 1991; **151**: 2373–82.

6. Deedwania P, Carbajal E. Ambulatory electrocardiographic evaluation of asymptomatic, unstable, and stable coronary artery disease patients for myocardial ischemia. *Cardiol Clin* 1992; **10**: 417.

7. Deedwania P, Carbajal E. Ambulatory ECG monitoring for myocardial ischemia – 'state-of-the-art'. *J Myocardial Isch* 1992; **4**: 52–71.

8. Tzivoni D, Benhorin J, Gavish A, *et al*. Holter recording during treadmill testing in assessing myocardial ischemic changes. *Am J Cardiol* 1985; **55**: 1200–3.

9. Gottlieb SO, Weisfeldt ML, Ouyang P, *et al*. Silent ischemia as a marker for early unfavorable outcomes in patients with unstable angina. *New Engl J Med* 1986; **314**: 1214–19.

10. Langer A, Freeman M, Armstrong P. ST segment shift in unstable angina: pathophysiology and association with coronary anatomy and hospital outcome. *J Am Coll Cardiol* 1989; **13**: 1495–1502.

11. Mody F, Nademanee K, Intarachot V, *et al*. Severity of silent myocardial ischemia on ambulatory electrocardiographic monitoring in patients with stable angina pectoris: relation to prognostic determinants during exercise stress testing and coronary angiography. *J Am Coll Cardiol* 1988; **12**: 1169–76.

12. Wilcox I, Freedman B, Li J, *et al*. Comparison of exercise stress testing with ambulatory electrocardiographic monitoring in the detection of myocardial ischemia after unstable angina pectoris. *Am J Cardiol* 1991; **67**: 89–91.

13. Brunelli C, Spallarossa P, Chigliotti G, *et al*. Thrombolytic therapy in refractory unstable angina: the role of Holter monitoring. *Clin Cardiol* 1991; **14**: 297–304.

14. Rocco M, Nabel E, Campbell S, *et al*. Prognostic importance of myocardial ischemia detected by ambulatory monitoring in patients with stable coronary artery disease. *Circulation* 1988; **78**: 877–84.

15. Deedwania P, Carbajal E. Prevalence and patterns of silent myocardial ischemia during daily life in stable angina patients receiving conventional antianginal drug therapy. *Am J Cardiol* 1990; **65**: 1090–6.

16. Deedwania P, Carbajal E. Silent ischemia during daily life is an independent predictor of mortality in stable angina. *Circulation* 1990; **81**: 748–56.

17. Deedwania P, Nelson J. Pathophysiology of silent myocardial ischemia during daily life: hemodynamic evaluation by simultaneous electrocardiographic and blood pressure monitoring. *Circulation* 1990; **82**: 1296.

18. Deedwania P, Carbajal E. Anti-ischemic effects of atenolol versus nifedipine in patients with coronary artery disease and ambulatory silent ischemia. *J Am Coll Cardiol* 1991; **17**: 963.

19. Deedwania P, Pepine CJ, Cohn P, *et al*., for the ASIST Study Group. The morning increase in myocardial ischemia is effectively suppressed by atenolol. *Circulation* 1993; **88**(4 Pt 2): 1594.

20. Mulcahy D, Keegan J, Crean P, *et al*. Silent myocardial ischemia in chronic stable angina: a study of its frequency and characteristics in 150 patients. *Br Heart J* 1988; **60**: 417–23.

21. Deedwania P, Carbajal E. Exercise-test predictors of ambulatory silent ischemia during daily life in stable angina pectoris. *Am J Cardiol* 1990; **66**: 1151–6.

22. Yeung A, Barry J, Orav J, *et al*. Effect of asymptomatic ischemia on long-term prognosis in chronic stable coronary disease. *Circulation* 1991; **83**: 1598–604.

23. Tzivoni D, Gavish A, Zin D, *et al*. Prognostic significance of ischemic episodes in patients with previous myocardial infarction. *Am J Cardiol* 1988; **62**: 661–4.

24. Deedwania P, Carbajal E. Usefulness of ambulatory silent myocardial ischemia added to the prognostic value of exercise test parameters in predicting risk of cardiac death in patients with stable angina pectoris and exercise induced myocardial ischemia. *Am J Cardiol* 1991; **68**: 1279–86.

25. Khurmi N, Raftery E. Reproducibility and validity of ambulatory ST segment monitoring in patients with chronic stable angina pectoris. *Am Heart J* 1987; **113**: 1091–6.

26. Nabel, *et al*. Variability of transient myocardial ischemia in ambulatory patients with coronary artery disease. *Circulation* 1988; **78**(1): 60.

27. Deedwania P. Is there evidence in support of the ischemia suppression hypothesis? *J Am Coll Cardiol* 1994; **24**(1): 21.

19

New Approach to Detection of Ischemic-Type ST Segment Depression

Jesaia Benhorin, Fabio Badilini, Arthur J. Moss,
W. Jackson Hall, Mario Merri and Wojciech Zareba

Introduction

Episodes of transient myocardial ischemia during daily activities are often associated with transient ST segment displacements on the ECG. These displacements can be detected by 24-hour ambulatory ECG recording and are usually indicative of low-threshold myocardial ischemia that is commonly clinically silent.[1-8] Prior to the advent of digitized ECG, 24-hour analog tapes were visually scanned to identify transient ischemic episodes. Currently, digitized ECG is the data input to most ST segment analytic systems. However, most conventional computer algorithms for ST segment analysis are still heavily dependent on the operator's interactions that are accomplished by visual inspection. These interactions are mainly needed to identify the isoelectric reference baseline and to determine the proper temporal locations for the ST segment amplitude measurements. Furthermore, the output of these algorithms is conventionally categorized by a set of discrete definitions for diagnosing the occurrence of transient 'ischemic-type' ST segment displacements (commonly 1 mm of horizontal or downsloping ST segment depression for 1 minute or more, measured 60–80 msec after the J point). Using such definitions obviously creates a diagnostic grey zone of 'borderline' ischemic cases that are conventionally visually categorized using real-time ECG output. Consequently, currently available methods for ST segment analysis on ambulatory ECG recordings are relatively deficient in terms of their reproducibility.[9]

We will report here a robust, fully automatic algorithm that extracts reliable operator-independent beat-to-beat ST segment amplitude measurements. Rather than identifying discrete sequential short occurrences of ST segment displacement, this approach utilizes frequency distributions of the ST segment amplitude measurements for each 24-hour recording (typically of 50 000) to 100 000 beats) in order to yield a better global perspective of ST segment shifts that have occurred during the whole recording period. Several statistical parameters that describe these frequency distributions are extracted and tested for their diagnostic accuracy in identifying patients with transient myocardial ischemia.

345

Details of the New Approach

The population

The population studied consisted of 63 normal individuals (ages 23–58 years; 6 females) and 37 patients with ischemic heart disease (ages 39–85 years; 6 females). All normals were asymptomatic, medication-free individuals with no history of cardiovascular disorders and with normal physical examination, normal 12-lead ECG and a negative Bruce protocol exercise test. All ischemic patients had typical effort angina, transient ischemic changes on a Bruce protocol exercise test, reversible ischemic defects on stress thallium scintigraphy, and several transient ischemic episodes on 24-hour ambulatory ECG recording (analyzed by conventional methods). All ischemic patients were off digoxin, and did not have prominent ST segment displacements on their resting 12-lead ECG. Twenty-four of them (65%) also had evidence of significant coronary artery disease (>70% stenosis of at least one major coronary artery) by coronary arteriography.

Data acquisition

Ambulatory ECG tracings ($n = 100$, 24-hour each) were acquired with three different recorders (ACS 8300 analog series, Marquette 8500 analog series, and Marquette Digital SEER). Bipolar V1-like and V5-like leads were connected using silver/silver-chloride electrodes. Only the V5-like data were used for the ST-segment analysis. All analog ECGs were played back on a dedicated Marquette Laser Holter System and digitized at a sampling frequency of 128 Hz. The ECGs recorded with the Marquette Digital SEER (which implements 120 Hz sampling frequency) were also downloaded on the Marquette Laser Holter System. Digitized ECGs were stored in a compressed format, each sample quantified with 10-bit resolution. The total digital file size for a 24-hour recording was approximately 44 Mbyte. The digitized ECG data were then transferred to a reel-to-reel 9-track magnetic tape with a streaming tape drive (Digi-Data Corporation Series 2000) hard-connected to the Marquette system. The 9-track tapes were finally read by a Sun Sparcserver 4/470 computer where the analysis was carried out.

Digital processing

A dedicated computer program read one or two channels of raw digital ECG data. The calibration pulse signal was identified first and automatically measured. The reading pointer was then positioned at the first low-noise 30-second segment identified. The input ECG signal and its first and second derivatives were then loaded, 10 seconds at a time, in three parallel circular buffers that served a series of beat-to-beat sequential subroutines that are detailed below.

   QRS complex detection. The QRS detection procedure was activated each time the first derivative of the ECG signal reached a dynamic threshold (initialized at 0.6 the maximum derivative of the first 10 seconds of clean signal). The sample with the highest absolute amplitude in an interval centered around the threshold-crossing location of the first derivative was found, and a parabolic interpolation was then fitted around this sample. The peak of the parabola estimated the peak of the R wave.

   QRS complex classification. In order to verify whether an identified QRS complex was a sinus beat, a single-layer neural network (Perceptron) was applied. A vector containing 500 ms of ECG data (300 ms before and 200 ms after an identified R wave) was fed into a feature selector which reduces the dimension of the vector to 10. This vector was finally fed into the Perceptron which labeled the QRS complex as normal (sinus) or abnormal (noise or any form of premature beat). The training of the network was achieved with two selected libraries, one of sinus beats (of different morphologies), and one of abnormal beats (different shapes of nonsinus beats, including artefactual ECG portions). The classification performance of the Perceptron was compared with that of other commonly used classifiers such as Fisher discriminant and the quadratic Gaussian classifiers and was found to be superior.[10]

Isoelectric point detection. A fiducial isoelectric point was searched for in an 80 ms interval prior to the R wave peak by minimizing the first derivative and the absolute product of the first derivative and the signal itself. Commonly, the locations of the two minima coincided; however, when they did not, the one with an amplitude more similar to that of the fiducial point that corresponded to the previous sinus beat was labeled as the current fiducial point. This double minimization technique avoids common errors like labeling a prominent Q wave as a fiducial point while using the 'derivative only' technique.[11]

Beat-to-beat isoelectric baseline estimation. A beat-specific estimated isoelectric baseline was constructed by fitting third-order polynomes (cubic splines) to six consecutive fiducial points (5 splines), three preceding (and including) the index beat and three following it. The 20 spline parameters (4 per each spline) were estimated by matching the inner first and second derivatives. The resulting estimated baseline was a smoother curve that adjusted for the commonly seen 'baseline sway' in ambulatory ECG. The application of a cubic spline interpolation technique as a baseline estimator has been proposed in the past in opposition to the use of linear filters.[12,13] Indeed, the cubic spline, not being a filter, avoids ST segment phase distortions which can be quite prominent.[14]

Beat-specific noise setting. A beat-to-beat 3-level noise code was set and used further on in defining a set of exclusion criteria. Each level in the code took into account different noise tests that were run for the beat under analysis.

The first level was based on the measured RR and RTm (R wave peak to T wave peak) intervals and its code was set to an exclusion value when either the RR interval, the RTm interval or their ratio were out of prespecified physiologic ranges.[15] In addition, a particular value at this level was set when the QRS was labeled as a nonsinus beat (premature beat or noise).

The second level involved the estimated beat-specific baseline: high maximum amplitude shifts (>10 mm) of the fiducial points used for the cubic spline interpolation, a low correlation coefficient (<0.5) of the regression line fitting the fiducial points, or certain combinations of the above set the code to exclusion values.

At the third level, the stability of the ECG signal within the ST segment was quantified by counting the number of 'strokes' in a fixed-length window. A stroke was defined as a single change in the derivative sign combined with changes in the signal amplitude above predefined thresholds. In order to select the set of stroke counts that would best classify an ST segment as too noisy or unacceptable for analysis, 24-hour ambulatory recordings of 10 normal individuals and 10 certified ischemic patients were analyzed. Forty segments of ECG data (2 segments of daytime and nighttime per individual, 3 minutes/segment) were randomly extracted from each recording and visually analyzed by two experienced cardiologists. Beat-specific visual calls (analyzable versus non-analyzable ST segment) on this subset of approximately 10 000 beats were finally used to set the threshold values for the stroke count procedure.

ST segment analysis. The algorithm calculates the magnitude of ST displacement (relative to the estimated beat-specific isoelectric baseline) at two heart-rate dependent

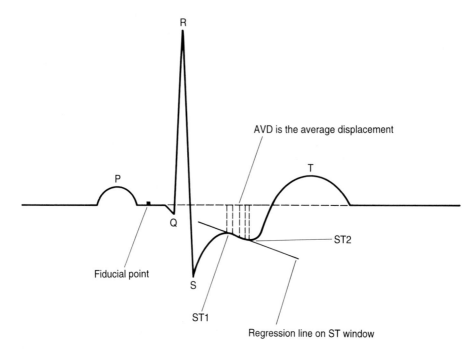

Figure 19.1 Beat-to-beat ST segment measurements.

intervals (R–ST1 and R–ST2) that are measured starting from the R wave peak, and the average ST displacement (AVD) over the time-window between R–ST1 and R–ST2 (Figure 19.1).

The heart-rate dependent R–ST1 and R–ST2 intervals are defined according to the following empirical formulas: R–ST1 = 40 + K1 (SQRT(R–R)); R–ST2 = 40 + K2 (SQRT(R–R)), where K1 and K2 are two *a priori* determined constants, and R–ST1, R–ST2 and RR are expressed in milliseconds. The constant of 40 ms in both equations corresponds to the estimated average interval from the R wave peak to the J point in a normal QRS complex. We empirically selected K1 = 0.948 and K2 = 2.21 to get R–ST1 = 70 ms and R–ST2 = 110 ms for a heart rate of 60 bpm (RR = 1000 ms). The reliability of the ST displacement measurements at R–ST1 and R–ST2 versus a variety of white noise levels has been validated. A linear fit of the samples available within the R–ST1 to R–ST2 time-window was used in calculating the AVD, and in estimating the ST segment slope (mV/ms) on a beat-to-beat basis.

Ischemia variables

The frequency distribution (histogram) of the AVD time series (over 24 hours) served as the basis for extracting several parameters that might be indicative of transient myocardial ischemia. Ischemic episodes of ST segment deviation on ambulatory ECG monitoring are transient and typically last only for several minutes. Therefore, an ischemic frequency distribution is expected to be skewed to the left and to be asymmetrically spread around an average deviation of less than 0 mm. In contrast, a nonischemic frequency distribution is expected to be narrow and symmetric and to have an average deviation close to 0 mm.

Several statistical parameters of the AVD frequency distribution were examined as potential indicators of transient ischemic episodes. All parameters were defined as percentile functions to allow for the fact that ST displacement is not expected to be normally distributed in cases with evident transient ischemic episodes. Ischemic parameters were grouped according to six categories as follows.

Percentiles. Percentile (Pxx) values (mm) in the AVD distribution function of P01, P05, P10, P25, P50, and of the mean AVD.

Spread measures. Percentile-dependent spread parameters (SPx) were defined as differences between specific percentiles according to the following formulas: SP1 = P75 − P25; SP2 = P90 − P10; SP3 = P95 − P5; SP4 = P50 − P25; SP5 = P50 − P10; SP6 = P50 − P5; SP7 = P50 − P1. Note that SP1, SP2 and SP3 are symmetrical spread measures, whereas SP4, SP5, SP6 and SP7 are asymmetrical spread measures.

Skewness measures. Three percentile-dependent skewness parameters (SKx, all with normalized units) were considered:

$$SK1 = (2{*}P50 - P25 - P75)/(P75 - P25);$$

$$SK2 = (2{*}P50 - P10 - P90)/(P90 - P10);$$

$$SK3 = (2{*}P50 - P5 - P95)/(P95 - P5).$$

ST segment slope measures. An additional ischemic feature that is not directly related to the frequency distribution of ST displacement, but rather to the morphology of the ST segment itself, was included as well. Since ST segment depression of the ischemic type depicts horizontal or downsloping morphology (as opposed to the upsloping morphology that is commonly observed among normals), two percentile-dependent ST segment slope variables (MS1 and MS5) were defined as the average ST slope measured in the beats contained in the lower 1%, and the lower 5% tails of the AVD frequency distribution, respectively.

Correlations of ST displacement with heart rate. Transient ischemic episodes are commonly accompanied by a significant transient heart rate increase. To account for this phenomenon, AVD was linearly regressed and correlated with the cycle length (RR) for beats contained in the lower 1% and 5% tails of the AVD frequency distribution. The slopes of the corresponding linear regressions (S1 and S5, respectively) and the corresponding correlations between AVD and RR (C1 and C5, respectively) were selected as potential ischemia variables.

Temporal sequencing of ST displacement. One of the limitations of the statistical approach that extracts ischemia parameters from AVD frequency distributions is the loss of information regarding the temporal sequencing of ischemic beats. In order to partially compensate for this loss, a 'clustering' subroutine was applied. This subroutine checked the temporal sequences of all beats contained in the lower 5% tail (P5) of the AVD frequency distribution. If some of the beats contained in P5 were part of an ischemic episode they should cluster in time, rather than be randomly related in time to each other. Since P5 varied across subjects, the clustering process was independent of an absolute ST segment displacement cutoff. A cluster was defined as a 20-second ECG portion that included less than 50% nonanalyzable beats, and within which two-thirds or more of all analyzable beats had an AVD less than P5. All clusters that were no more than 2 minutes apart from each other were lumped and labeled as 'potential super-clusters'. Potential super-clusters were labeled as 'true super-clusters' if they contained 50 beats or more that had an AVD less than P5. The number of true super-clusters (NC), and the total number of beats within all true super-clusters that had an ADV less than P5 (NB), were selected as potential ischemia variables. NC and NB are surrogates for two commonly used conventional ischemia parameters in ambulatory monitoring: the number of ischemic episodes, and the total duration of ischemia, respectively.

Statistical analysis

Univariate analysis. Mean values of all selected ischemia variables ($n = 24$) were compared between normal individuals and ischemic patients by employing the non-pooled Student's t-test (that allows unequal variances), and the Mann–Whitney test (that allows the comparison of variables that are not normally distributed). A p value under 0.002 (according to a Bonfferoni correction) was considered statistically significant.

Multivariate analysis. In order to determine which ischemia variables independently contribute to the discrimination of ischemic patients from normal individuals after adjustment to other covariates, a logistic regression model was used. All variables that came out as significant discriminators in the univariate analysis at the 0.05 significance level (and their interactions) were initially submitted to the model. Variables selection by the model was carried out twice using the forward and the backward selection procedures, respectively. The final output of the model included individual p values that correspond to the final set of independent predictors of ischemia, and an estimated probability of ischemia for each 24-hour recording that was analyzed. Estimated probabilities of ischemia were set to range between 0 and 1, where 0 corresponds to the lowest probability and 1 corresponds to the highest probability. The capability of the model to classify normals versus ischemic patients was quantified by a simple count of false negative and false positive cells, using an estimated probability of 0.45 as an arbitrary probability cutoff. Corresponding sensitivity and specificity were computed.

Results

Representative AVD frequency distributions of a normal control and of an ischemic patient are presented in Figures 19.2 and 19.3. Typical frequency distributions were based on more than 50 000 heart beats. Of note are the different shapes of the two distributions in terms of width and symmetry. The lower left tail of the distribution function of the ischemic patient is especially prominent.

Univariate comparison between normals and ischemic patients

Tables 19.1 and 19.2 summarize the comparison between 63 normal controls and 37 ischemic patients. Normal controls had significantly higher percentile values, significantly lower AVD heart-rate relation parameters (C1, C5, S1 and S5), and significantly lower clustering parameters (NC and NB) than ischemic patients. None of the spread or skewness measures were significantly different in the two subsets.

Multivariate analysis

Table 19.3 summarizes the results of the multivariate analysis. The final set of ischemia variables that were selected by the logistic regression model as independent predictors of ischemia were: P10 (the tenth percentile value), MS5 (the mean ST segment slope of beats contained in the lower 5% tail of the AVD distribution), C5 (the correlation between AVD and heart rate of beats contained in the lower 5% tail of the AVD distribution), and NB

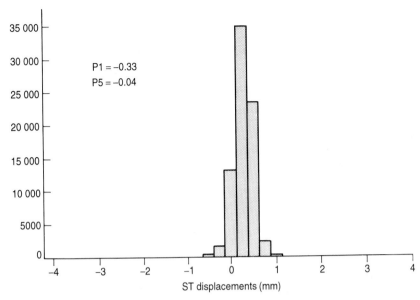

Figure 19.2 Frequency distribution of the average ST segment displacement in a normal individual. The number of beats is shown on the vertical axis. P1 and P5 are the AVD values of the first and fifth percentiles, respectively.

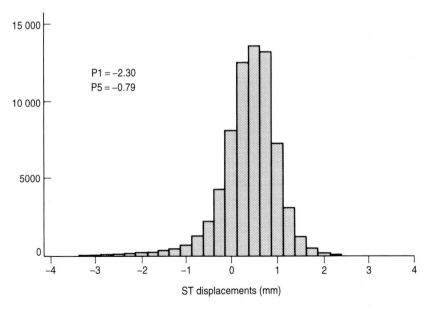

Figure 19.3 Frequency distribution of the average ST segment displacement in an ischemic patient.

Table 19.1 Percentile values and spread measures of AVD frequency distributions

	Normals (n = 63)		Ischemics (n = 37)		
	Mean	SD	Mean	SD	p value
Percentile					
P01	−1.106	0.686	−2.316	0.869	<0.001
P05	−0.347	0.564	−1.462	0.606	<0.001
P10	−0.070	0.502	−1.188	0.565	<0.001
P25	0.250	0.515	−0.835	0.523	<0.001
P50	0.537	0.559	−0.523	0.519	<0.001
Mean	0.504	0.580	−0.567	0.518	<0.001
Spread measures					
SP1	0.547	0.268	0.576	0.193	0.53
SP2	0.133	0.545	1.205	0.422	0.46
SP3	1.314	0.667	1.409	0.532	0.43
SP4	0.286	0.133	0.313	0.120	0.31
SP5	0.607	0.259	0.665	0.255	0.28
SP6	0.884	0.368	0.940	0.356	0.46
SP7	1.602	0.563	1.793	0.787	0.20

Table 19.2 Skewness, ST segment slope, heart rate relation and clustering parameters of AVD frequency distributions

	Normals (n = 63)		Ischemics (n = 37)		
	Mean	SD	Mean	SD	p value
Skewness					
SK1	0.060	0.110	0.076	0.104	0.46
SK2	0.099	0.141	0.110	0.174	0.76
SK3	0.139	0.174	0.127	0.194	0.77
ST segment slope					
MS1	0.01294	0.0093	−0.00107	0.0093	<0.001
MS5	0.01257	0.0120	−0.00098	0.0069	<0.001
Heart rate relations					
C1	0.016	0.029	0.044	0.067	0.02
C5	0.054	0.063	0.132	0.107	<0.001
S1	0.00039	0.00061	0.00083	0.00079	0.005
S5	0.0011	0.00109	0.00178	0.00148	0.17
Clustering					
NC	2.286	2.217	4.054	2.403	<0.001
NB	445	502	1106	808	<0.001

MS1 and MS5 are the mean ST segment slopes of beats contained in the lower 1% and 5% tails of the AVD frequency distribution, respectively. C1 and C5 are correlations between AVD and heart rate for beats contained in the lower 1% and 5% tails of the AVD frequency distribution, respectively. S1 and S5 are slopes of the linear regression of AVD on heart rate for beats contained in the lower 1% and 5% tails of the AVD frequency distribution. NC and NB are the number of ischemic 'super-clusters' and the number of beats within them, respectively.

Table 19.3 Independent predictors of ischemia in 24-hour ambulatory ECG analysis based on AVD frequency distributions

	Parameter estimate	Standard error	p value	Odds ratio	95%–CI
Intercept	−3.5212	1.244	0.0046	—	—
P10	−3.6149	1.078	<0.001	0.0269	0.00325–0.222
MS5	−2.6885	1.1236	<0.001	0.680	0.00751–0.614
C5	1.26011	0.6549	0.041	3.526	0.9768–12.727
NB	1.5136	0.8118	0.039	4.543	0.9254–22.303

In order to make the magnitude of the parameter estimates comparable, MS5 (mm/s) was multiplied by 100, C5 was multiplied by 10 and NB was divided by 1000. CI are confidence intervals for the odds ratio.

(the number of beats contained in all 'true super-clusters'). These results were consistent with both backward and forward variables selection procedures. Similar results were obtained using ischemia variables that were derived from frequency distributions of the ST segment displacement at R–ST1 or R–ST2. The overall fit of the model was highly significant ($p < 0.001$), and was not significantly improved by any interaction term. In order to make the magnitude of the parameter estimates comparable, MS5 (mm/s) was multiplied by 100, C5 was multiplied by 10 and NB was divided by 1000. The odds ratio was defined as the relative probability of ischemia per unit increase of an ischemia variable, while keeping all other ischemia variables constant. According to these definitions, the odds for ischemia are increased: 37.17-fold (1/0.0269) when P10 decreases by 1 mm, by 6.8% when MS5 decreases by 1 mm/s, 3.5-fold when C5 increases by 0.1, and 4.5-fold when NB increases by 1000 beats.

Classification of ischemic patients and normal controls

The estimated probability of ischemia in the two patient subsets is presented graphically in Figure 19.4. The different spreads of the estimated probabilities among the two subsets highlight the prominent discriminating power of the multivariate model. A probability cutoff of 0.45 correctly classified the two subsets with two false negatives and three false positives (95% sensitivity and 95% specificity, respectively).

Comments

The new ST segment analytic system was able to correctly classify 95% of the study population while being fully automatic and totally independent of any operator inter-actions (and thus must yield 100% reproducible results on a reread situation). More accurate beat-to-beat measurement schemes of both the ST segment amplitude and the isoelectric baseline, which are key figures in creating the final diagnostic output of such an analysis, played a major role in achieving the abovementioned diagnostic perform-ance. These mainly include the double minimization technique in the identification of the isoelectric fiducial points; application of the cubic-spline method for estimating the beat-to-beat isoelectric baseline; and application of a heart-rate dependent interval (R–ST1 to R–ST2) that depicts more accurately where, over the ST segment, the ST amplitude should be measured. Relating the ST measurement points to the R wave excluded the need to identify the J point, which is quite inaccurate in many cases.

In addition to these 'technical' improvements, a new concept of focusing on ST-segment-displacement frequency distributions rather than on discrete sequential occur-rences of ST displacements over time has been introduced. By fitting a multivariate

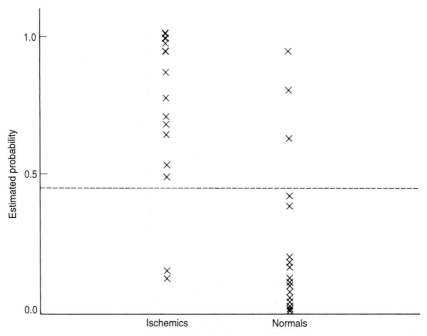

Figure 19.4 Estimated probabilities of ischemia on ambulatory monitoring, by patient subset, according to a multivariate analysis based on AVD frequency distribution parameters. The broken line corresponds to an estimated probability of 0.45.

model based on a variety of statistical variables related to the ST frequency distribution, we were able to identify independent predictors of ischemia, and to assign a probability score to each studied case. Such a probability score is actually a quantitative diagnostic call that might serve the clinician better than the conventional discrete diagnostic call. The probability cutoff of 0.45 that was used in this study is obviously the one that yielded the best classification of the study population. Different probability cutoffs might perform better among other patient populations.

Further studies are needed in order to test this new approach among large patient populations with proven coronary disease in whom the probability of ischemia should be correlated with prognostic indices.

References

1. Stern S, Tzivoni D. Early detection of silent ischemic heart disease by 24-hour electrocardiographic monitoring of active subjects. *Br Heart J* 1974; **36**: 481–6.
2. Stern S, Tzivoni D, Stern Z. Diagnostic accuracy of ambulatory ECG monitoring in ischemic heart disease. *Circulation* 1975; **52**: 1045–9.
3. Schang SJ, Pepine CJ. Transient asymptomatic ST segment depression during daily activity. *Am J Cardiol* 1977; **39**: 396–402.
4. Deanfield JE, Maseri A, Selwyn AP, *et al.* Myocardial ischemia during daily life in patients with stable angina: its relation to heart rate changes. *Lancet* 1983; **2**: 753–8.
5. Deanfield JE, Ribiero P, Oaklay K, *et al.* Analysis of the ST-segment changes in normal subjects: implications for ambulatory monitoring in angina pectoris. *Am J Cardiol* 1984; **54**: 1321–5.
6. Tzivoni D, Benhorin J, Gavish A, *et al.* Holter recordings during treadmill testing in assessing myocardial ischemic changes. *Am J Cardiol* 1985; **55**: 1200–3.
7. Akselrod S, Norymberg M, Peled I, *et al.* Computerized analysis of ST segment changes in ambulatory electrocardiograms. *Med Biol Eng Comput* 1987; **25**: 513–19.

8. Benhorin J, Tzivoni D, Banai S, *et al*. Circadian variations in ischemic threshold and their relation to the occurrence of ischemic episodes. *Circulation* 1993; **87**: 808–14.
9. Moss AJ, Goldstein RE, Hall WJ, *et al*. Detection and significance of myocardial ischemia in stable patients after recovery from an acute coronary event. *JAMA* 1993; **269**: 2379–85.
10. Badilini F, Tekalp AM, Moss AJ. A single-layer perceptron to discriminate non-sinus beats in ambulatory ECG recordings. In: *Proceedings of IEEE/EMBS Annual Conference, Paris*. New York: IEEE/EMBS, 1992: 521–2.
11. Badilini F, Moss AJ, Titelbaum EL. Cubic spline baseline estimation in ambulatory ECG recording. In: *Proceedings of IEEE/EMBS Annual Conference, Orlando*. New York: IEEE/EMBS, 1991: 584–5.
12. Pottala EW, Bailey JJ, Horton MR, *et al*. Suppression of baseline wander in the ECG using a bilinearly transformed null-phase filter. *J Electrocardiol* 1989; **22**(Suppl): 243–7.
13. Le HT, Van Arsdel WC, Makowski AM, *et al*. Automated analysis of rodent three-channel electrocardiograms and vectorcardiograms. *IEEE Trans Biomed Eng* 1985; **32**: 43–50.
14. Tayler DI, Vincent R. Artefactual ST segment abnormalities due to electrocardiograph design. *Br Heart J* 1985; **54**: 121–8.
15. Merri M, Moss AJ, Benhorin J, *et al*. Relation between ventricular repolarization duration and cardiac cycle length during 24-hour Holter recordings: findings in normals and patients with long QT syndrome. *Circulation* 1992; **85**: 1816–21.

20

Analysis of ST Segment Variability in Holter Recordings

Fabio Badilini, Wojciech Zareba, Edward L. Titlebaum and Arthur J. Moss

Introduction

The ST segment is the portion of the electrocardiogram that goes from the end of the QRS complex to the beginning of the T wave. This segment reflects the second phase of the transmembrane action potential (TAP) of ventricular myocardial cells. Phase 2, which is also called the 'plateau' phase, may last well over a hundred milliseconds and is characterized by a rather low membrane conductance to all ions. Since there is little change in TAP during this phase, the ST segment is usually isoelectric in normal subjects. Abnormalities of the ST segment are seen in several pathologic conditions, including myocardial ischemia,[1] hypertension[2] and pericarditis.[3] These abnormalities consist of displacements of the ST segment either above the isoelectric line (elevation) or below it (depression). During these situations the electrical equilibrium characteristic of the plateau phase is disturbed as ion currents are allowed to flow between the inside and outside of the cells.[4] Changes of the ST segment morphology can often be transient, as is the case with exercise-related myocardial ischemia. Consequently, the ambulatory recording is a useful tool for the monitoring and evaluation of transient episodes of pathological ST displacements.

Long-term ECG analysis of episodic ST segment displacement dates back to 1974.[5] The ambulatory approach deals with the monitoring of ST segment displacements during 24 hours.[6] Each value of deflection is generally obtained with averaging techniques; i.e. one measurement may be associated with many cardiac complexes. The trend of ST segment displacements is then compared with that of the heart rate to evaluate physiological correlations. The need for a more complete understanding of the cause and effect mechanisms that trigger transient ischemia and regulate its relationship with ST segment deflections is apparent. In this regard, a beat-to-beat approach is preferable since it allows direct evaluation of the dynamicity of the ST segment and of its direct relationship with other beat-to-beat series.

The advancements achieved in modern technology, and in particular the advent of high-sampling-rate digital recordings, have dramatically improved the quality of ST segment analysis. In particular, we can now apply a beat-to-beat approach to ST segment analysis. The ST segment can thus be treated as a discrete-time series as for the well-known time series of RR intervals. A classical approach for biological signals is the analysis of variability, either in the time domain (by means of standard deviation analysis), or in the frequency domain (study of signal variability at various frequencies). Analysis of variability of ST segment displacements has never been pursued before, the main reason being the difficulty of obtaining such signals in a reliable way.

This chapter describes a preliminary study that provided evidence for the presence of significant oscillatory components in the time series of beat-to-beat ST segment displacements. As with the time series of RR intervals, the autonomic nervous system plays a determinant role. The chapter is structured in three sections. The first section covers the crucial technical issues involved with the problem of the measurement of an appropriate ST level. These include the identification of reliable fiducial isoelectric points, the correction for baseline low-frequency drifts, and the selection of an opportune heart-rate adjusted ST segment. The second section deals with correction for the rotation-vector effect induced by respiratory activity. The ST segment displacement is a measurement strongly influenced by this phenomenon, and it needs to be removed. A model describing the behavior of the respiratory activity (based on amplitude modulation theory) is presented and a method for correcting it is shown. In the third section, the results of a dedicated experiment are reported, in particular the influence of vagal-tone on ST segment variability (STV). The importance of such findings in the general context of ambulatory recordings is discussed.

In this chapter, 'ECG amplitude-related measurements' will refer to all those variables derived from the amplitude of the ECG signal whose units are millivolts. The ST segment displacement is one of these, and this variable is extracted from the 'vertical domain' of the ECG. On the other hand, 'ECG time-related measurements' will refer to those variables derived from the time evolution of the ECG signal whose units are milliseconds. RR and QT belong to this 'horizontal domain' of the ECG.

Measuring a Reliable ST Segment Displacement Signal

Baseline estimation

Any ECG measurement involving amplitude relies on a clear definition of a zero voltage level, the so-called 'isoelectric line' (or baseline). This is the case for ST segment displacement, where the measurements are of amplitude shifts between the voltage levels of points in the ST segment and the physiologic zero of the ECG signal. The physiologic zero does not coincide with the electrical zero of the digitized ECG since the baseline may wander. In many studies found in the literature, the isoelectric level is estimated from the voltage level of a single point, the fiducial point, identified in the PR segment (the segment between the offset of the P wave and the onset of the subsequent QRS complex[7]). The rationale of this choice stems from the physiologic interpretation of the ECG, according to which the PR segment is thought to be the most reliable isoelectric reference of the electrocardiographic complex. The exact position of the fiducial point within the PR segment is generally found using minimization techniques. Any deviation measurement is then conventionally performed by taking the difference between the voltage level of the ECG signal in correspondence with the ST points of interest and the voltage level of the point selected in the PR interval.

One way to obtain better estimates of the baseline is to interpolate between consecutive fiducial points. Among the different types of interpolation, cubic spline (i.e. third-order polynomials fitted between consecutive fiducial points) seems to provide the best trade-off between accuracy and computation time. For short-time ECG recordings, as in an exercise test, a global baseline is generally estimated by interpolating all the available fiducial points. This approach becomes too computationally demanding for extended monitoring, and it would be impractical to identify a single baseline for an ambulatory recording. An elegant solution is to define a reference baseline specifically for each single

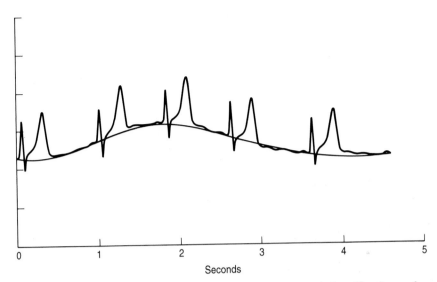

Figure 20.1 Example of baseline estimation with cubic-spline interpolation. The figure shows the baseline specifically estimated for the central beat. Six fiducial points are involved (three preceding and three following the ST segment considered).

ST segment. Low-frequency baseline wander usually lasts for a few seconds. Consequently, for a specific beat the baseline information can be gathered in the period immediately preceding and following the appropriate fiducial points. With this technique, the values of ST displacement of each beat are measured not with respect to the level of the preceding baseline (as is done in most commercially available Holter systems), but rather, with respect to an extrapolated baseline that is synchronous with each individual ST segment. Cubic-spline interpolation as a baseline estimator has been proposed in the past.[8,9]

The cubic spline, not being a filter, avoids the problem of phase distortion so critical in the analysis of ST segments.[10] Figure 20.1 shows an example of cubic-spline interpolation. Here, six fiducial points are considered, three preceding and three following the analyzed ST segment (the central one). The resulting interpolating splines are computed by matching first and second derivatives in the inner fiducial points. Since there are six fiducial points, a total of five splines (which means twenty parameters, each cubic spline being characterized by four parameters) are calculated. When the next ST segment is analyzed, one fiducial point (the last one backward in time) is discarded and the next one forward is introduced.

Mathematically, the beat-specific cubic-spline problem with N fiducial points requires the solution of an $N-2$ linear system.[11] This means that, for each beat, a linear system of order $N-2$ has to be solved. However, the characteristic matrix of the system is tridiagonal (i.e. it has elements only on the main, upper and lower diagonals) and the solution is generally fast to compute, since a tridiagonal matrix is easy to invert. By increasing the number of fiducial points, we could increase the amount of information used for a single baseline estimate; unfortunately this would also dramatically increase the computing time.

The reliability of the cubic-spline estimation of the ambulatory ECG baseline has been tested against the presence of white noise in the ECG and against variations in the segment length used to find the fiducial point.[12] This study suggested the use of a segment of about 900 ms prior the R wave peak. Moreover, evidence of the robustness of the method in the presence of noise was provided. The best value of N was six, as the accuracy of the estimate did not show significant improvements for larger values.

Beat-to-beat measurements

Ambulatory recording studies have not been consistent in defining the exact location on the ST segment to quantify the amount of deflection. Common practice is to use the end of the QRS complex as a reference point (the so-called J point), and to measure ST displacement at constant time intervals after the J point (typically 40, 60 and 80 ms). Mathematically, the J point is defined as the point following the QRS complex where *a sensitive decrease of ECG slope is observed.*[7] On high-frequency 12-lead ECGs, identification of the J point is a simple task, as the sensitive decrease in ECG slope can easily be identified visually. This is not true for most ambulatory ECGs. As a matter of fact, the J point is difficult to identify automatically (especially when working at low sampling rates) and, to the best of our knowledge, no algorithms have been proposed until now for automatic detection of the J point.

A better reference in ambulatory recordings may be found in the QRS peak (R wave peak). Indeed, various algorithms have been shown to detect this point accurately, among them parabolic interpolation and matched filtering. Choice of this point as opposed to the J point is further supported by the fact that the RJ interval is generally constant in subjects without particular conduction defects, the situation in which ST segment analysis is generally carried out. A second important factor usually not considered in conventional ST analysis is the effect of heart-rate dependency. The duration of the ST segment is not constant; rather, it is a function of the repolarization duration. It seems, then, reasonable 'to sample' ST displacements in points defined as a function of the heart rate. After a few attempts, we observed that a square-root dependence on the previous RR interval accurately achieves this task. In particular, an ST segment window could be defined as the time between two ECG points R–ST1 and R–ST2, expressed by the following empirical formulas:

$$R\text{–}ST1 = 40 + K1\sqrt{RR}$$
$$R\text{–}ST2 = 40 + K2\sqrt{RR}$$

$$(20.1)$$

where K1 and K2 are two constants to be determined *a priori* and R–ST1, R–ST2 and RR intervals are expressed in milliseconds. The constants K1 and K2 can be selected by forcing the intervals R–ST1 and R–ST2 for specific RR intervals. For instance, with a heart rate of 60 bpm (which corresponds to RR = 1000 ms), the intervals R–ST1 and R–ST2 could be set to 70 and 110 ms, respectively. These values set the constants K1 and K2 to 0.948 and 2.21 ms$^{\frac{1}{2}}$. Figure 20.2 shows the behavior of equations (20.1) for these values for K1 and K2. At a heart rate of 120 bpm (RR = 500 ms) the ST segment length is reduced to 28 ms, whereas at 40 bpm (RR = 1500 ms) the ST segment is enlarged to 49 ms.

Once a heart-rate-adjusted ST segment window has been defined, measurements of displacement can be taken in the two points ST1 and ST2 with respect to the previously estimated baseline. A global indicator of ST displacement could be identified in the average of all the possible displacements that can be measured within the ST window (including the two extremes). The number of measurable displacements depends on the sampling rate and on the window length that shortens at faster heart rates (as Figure 20.2 shows). We will refer to this average displacement (AVD) for the remainder of this chapter.

Other parameters that could be of clinical interest may be parameters relative to the ST slope and the area of the ST segment window below the baseline. An in-depth description of their calculation can be found in reference 13.

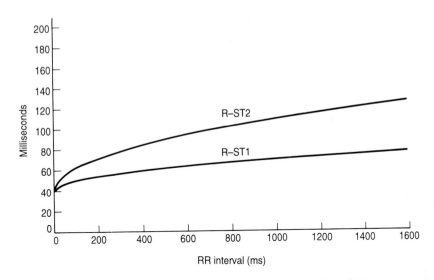

Figure 20.2 Curves describing the functions of equations (20.1).

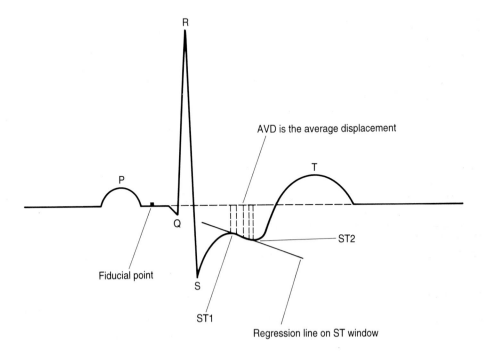

Figure 20.3 Measurements performed for each beat. ST segment window is defined by the heart-rate adjusted points ST1 and ST2. The value of AVD is the average of all the ST segment displacements that can be measured between the two points (inclusive). The number of available points depends on heart rate and sampling interval. A value of ST segment slope can also be calculated as the slope of the line fitted in the available samples.

Figure 20.3 shows a pictorial representation of the ST segment measurements of every beat. The correct unit for ST segment displacements is voltage (either millivolts or microvolts are appropriate). However, because of the way the deflections were initially measured on standard electrocardiographic paper, a more common unit is length, with 1 mm corresponding to 0.1 mV. As long as this voltage conversion is maintained, the unit of length can still be used.

Correction of Respiratory-Related Modulation

Introduction

Before performing an analysis of ST segment displacement variability, we must correct for motion-related respiratory modulation. To understand the rationale of this modulation, one can think of the ECG signal as the projection on an ideal line (the line connecting the surface leads) of a time-varying electrical vector. Indeed, as is well known in vectorcardiography, the electrical activity of the heart can be assessed in terms of an electrical dipole representing the vectorial summation of millions of micropotential differences associated with each single cardiac cell. The dynamic of this dipole reflects the time variations of the electrical status of the heart during the contraction phenomena. It is the different timing of depolarization and repolarization through different zones of the heart muscle that allows the inscription of the characteristic ECG waves.

In addition to these variations strictly related to the cellular activity of the heart, other noncardiac effects can cause the direction of the dipole to be shifted, thus influencing the projections on the exploring leads. The most typical undesired effect is caused by chest movements during inhalation and exhalation, which induce a relative motion between the surface leads and the heart.

In essence, the measured ECG can be characterized by modulations synchronous with the respiratory activity. This modulation causes 'shrinking and enlarging' phenomena; i.e. the amplitudes of the ECG characteristic waves are cyclically increased and decreased synchronously with the respiratory activity. Figure 20.4 depicts a portion of an ECG where this effect is evident. Variability of ST segment displacement time series is seriously influenced by this modulation, which may hide other physiological components.

The beat-to-beat time series of the RR intervals, or tachogram, is not affected by this modulation. The 'shrinking' and 'enlarging' phenomena are limited to the vertical (amplitude) domain, while the horizontal (time) domain is completely unaffected and no correction is necessary for time-related measurements. To give a better idea, the peak-to-peak changes of the R wave amplitude in precordial leads can vary as much as 0.5 mV (5 mm). In the ST segment the respiratory-induced amplitude shifts are smaller, but can still reach 0.2 mV (2 mm). The same is true for any other amplitude-derived time series.

Pulse amplitude modulation

The modulation evident in Figure 20.4 resembles a pulse train that has been amplitude-modulated by a lower-frequency carrier.[14] This is referred to as 'pulse amplitude modulation' (PAM). Let us denote the clean (unmodulated) ECG signal by $e(t)$ and the measured ECG by $y(t)$. The PAM model of the ECG can then be written as:

$$y(t) = e(t)[1 + \varepsilon r(t)] + b(t) \tag{20.2}$$

where $r(t)$ represents an electrical signal related to the respiratory activity and ε is the so-called modulating factor. This factor varies between zero (in which case no modulation is present and the measured ECG is corrupted only by the additive term $b(t)$) and

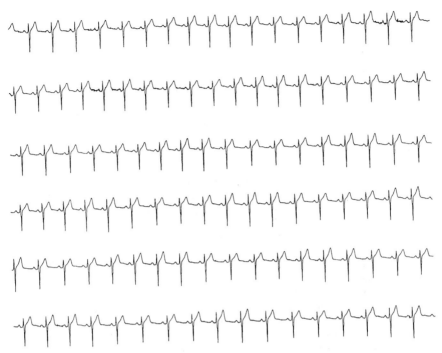

Figure 20.4 Example of 2 minutes of ECG (20 seconds per strip) with respiratory modulation evident. The shrinking and enlarging phenomena can be seen.

1 (in which case modulation is maximum). The additive term $b(t)$ is not part of the PAM model, but it has been introduced to account for the low-frequency components that are independent of the respiratory modulation present in ambulatory ECG. In the terminology of modulation theory, the ECG represents the pulse train (or carrier) and the respiratory signal represents the information signal. The pulse train (ECG) is not exactly periodic but has an intrinsic variability (the heart rate variability), and the information signal (respiration) resembles a sinusoid.

To verify the appropriateness of the PAM model, we can use the frequency domain. By taking the Fourier transform of equation (20.2) we obtain:

$$Y(\omega) = E(\omega) + \varepsilon E(\omega)*R(\omega) + B(\omega) \qquad (20.3)$$

where the symbol $*$ denotes convolution. According to equation (20.3), the spectrum of the modulated (measured) ECG, $Y(\omega)$, should be given by the spectrum of the original (unmodulated) ECG signal, $E(\omega)$, with two additional components overlapping.

The first such component is the convolution of the original spectrum with the spectrum of the respiratory signal scaled by the modulating factor ε. Since $R(\omega)$ is close to a sinusoid (whose spectrum is a plain impulse at the sinusoid frequency), this term should introduce sidebands around the peaks of $E(\omega)$ at distances equal to the respiratory frequency, the amplitude of these sidebands depending on the value of ε. In particular, sidebands around the DC component of the ECG component should be visible.

The second additional term, $B(\omega)$, represents low-frequency baseline wander and should simply contribute to power at the very low frequencies (even lower than the respiratory frequency).

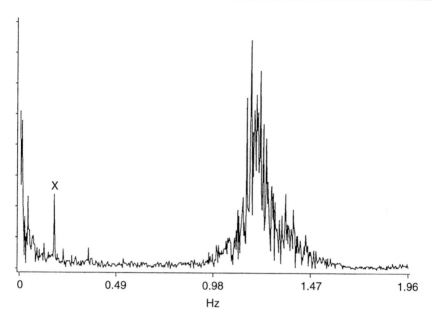

Figure 20.5 Spectrum of an ECG with respiratory modulation evident. The peak at 0.17 Hz (X) is the DC replica of the respiratory spectrum. The fundamental frequency of the heart rate is represented by the impulse shape centered at 1.22 Hz. Upper and lower sidebands produced by convolution of the fundamental component with the respiratory rate are visible at 1.04 Hz and 1.39 Hz. The power at very low frequencies (below 0.1 Hz) is produced by baseline wander.

Figure 20.5 shows the spectrum of 262 seconds of an ECG sampled at 1000 Hz with controlled breathing at 10 cycles per minute (0.17 Hz). Only frequencies up to 1.96 Hz are shown. The first peak, at exactly 0.17 Hz, represents the sideband caused by the convolution of the DC component of the ECG with the respiratory signal, which in this case is almost a perfect sinusoid. The large impulsive shape centered at 1.22 Hz is the first peak of the ECG spectrum (average rate of the period analyzed is 73 bpm). Sidebands 0.17 Hz from these peaks can be identified (the upper sideband is particularly clear). Similar sidebands can be seen in the higher harmonies of the ECG spectrum. The low-frequency component $B(\omega)$ is represented by the power very close to DC.

The demodulator

PAM demodulation (restoration of the *information signal*) is generally achieved by using lowpass filters with cutoff frequency between the frequency of the information signal and the frequency of the first harmonic of the train pulse. This is not appropriate in the hypothesized model, as the 'wanted' signal is not the information (respiratory) signal but rather the pulse train (the ECG). The clean ECG signal is recovered by solving equation (20.2) for $e(t)$:

$$e(t) = \frac{y(t) - b(t)}{1 + \varepsilon r(t)}. \tag{20.4}$$

To accomplish this, estimates of the respiratory signal $r(t)$, the modulating factor ε and of the additive component $b(t)$ must be determined.

The term $b(t)$ represents the baseline and, as described earlier, it can be estimated by means of the cubic-spline interpolation technique. Figure 20.6 shows the spectrum of the

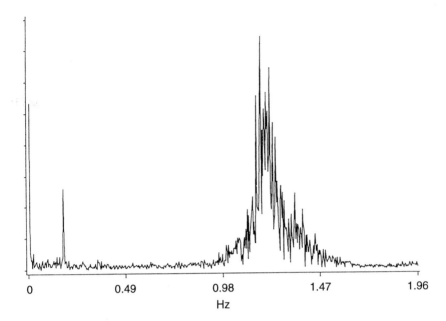

Figure 20.6   Spectrum of the ECG of Figure 20.5 after cubic-spline baseline removal. The VLF noise has disappeared.

ECG in Figure 20.5 after the removal of $b(t)$. It is clear that all the very-low-frequency noise has disappeared and everything else is practically the same.

After baseline removal, an estimate of the respiratory signal can be obtained by using an appropriate lowpass filter which must retain the DC replica of the respiratory spectrum while suppressing everything else (and in particular the first harmonic of the ECG spectrum). The recommendation is to apply a frequency-selective filter (e.g. a Butterworth filter[15]) with a cutoff frequency larger than the highest respiratory rate and lower than the minimum heart rate. For most cases (with the exclusion of hyperventilation and bradycardia) a cutoff of 0.4 Hz (which corresponds to 24 cycles per minute) should be appropriate. Details of a recursive and bidirectional Butterworth filter to accomplish this task are described in reference 13. In particular, the output of this filter is fully synchronized with the shrinking and enlarging phenomena, and highly correlated ($r = 0.99$) with an independently acquired respiratory signal. The capability of the lowpass filter to obtain a reliable estimate of the respiratory signal depends strictly on the prior baseline removal. If this is not done, low-frequency baseline wander can dramatically distort the respiration information embedded in the ECG signal.

An estimate of the modulating factor ε can be obtained quite easily by measuring the peak-to-peak variations of a generic point of the ECG. In particular, it can be shown that ε can be written as follows:

$$\varepsilon = V_{\text{pp}}/2x \tag{20.5}$$

where x is the average level of the selected point and V_{pp} is its peak-to-peak sweep value. In most of the cases we have analyzed the modulating factor was between 0.1 and 0.15, and was never more than 0.2 or less than 0.03. This reflects the fact that PAM-like modulation, even if weak, is consistently present. The modulating factor may also vary with time, as the conditions for the respiratory modulation may change (e.g. sitting versus standing). For this reason the modulation factor should be estimated continuously, for instance every 5 minutes.

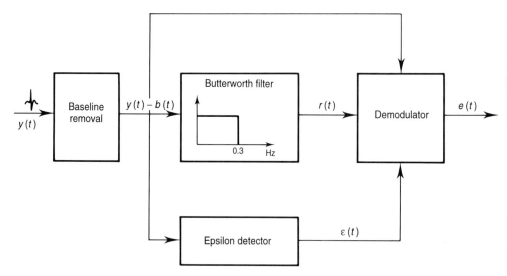

Figure 20.7 Schematic of the demodulator.

When all the above terms have been estimated, demodulation represented by equation (20.4) can be carried out. Figure 20.7 depicts the schematic of the global demodulator, and Figure 20.8 shows an example of one minute of measured ECG, the relative estimated respiratory waveform obtained by Butterworth lowpass filtering, and the demodulated ECG. The effect of demodulation is strongly evidenced in Figure 20.9. The sidebands at the respiratory frequency have totally disappeared.

To check for reliability, the demodulator was tested on simulated data.[13] The clean ECG was simulated with 100 replicas of a single beat extracted from a normal subject, and heart rate variability was introduced by varying the number of padding zeros between the replicas, in such a way that the series of RR intervals matched the one of another normal subject. PAM was applied with $r(t)$ approximated by a sinusoid at 0.17 Hz and the modulating factor fixed to 0.2. Baseline wander was finally added by means of two sinusoids at different frequencies and different amplitudes. The total root-mean-squared error between the original ECG and the one at the output of the demodulator was 6.27 μV which corresponds to a peak-signal-to-noise ratio of 180 (the peak of the simulated ECG was 1.12 mV).

ST Segment Displacement Variability

The autonomic nervous system (ANS) is known to influence the regulation of time series derived by the time evolution of the ECG signal, such as the heart rate and the repolarization duration variability signals.[16] For instance, heart rate variability is characterized by two spectral components, one in the band of respiration (which reflects the parasympathetic branch activity) and one at lower frequencies (thought to reflect aspects of sympathetic activity).[17] These ANS components are thought to act at the level of the myocellular channels, during phase 4 for heart rate and during phase 3 for repolarization. Evidence of ANS modulation of ion channel permeabilities during phase 2 has also been reported.[18] It is then reasonable to postulate that ANS-related oscillations may also affect the variability of ST segment displacement signals during phase 2 of the transmembrane action potential. Other types of modulation of the ST signal may be mechanically

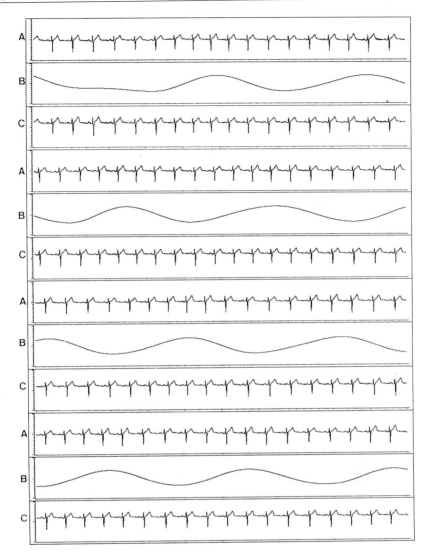

Figure 20.8 (a) One minute of ECG signal. (b) Lowpass filtered ECG. (c) Demodulated ECG. Each strip is 15 seconds long.

mediated by the respiratory activity as an indirect effect of the heart loading and unloading processes. Respiration may also influence the metabolic milieu of the myocardium with cyclic changes in oxygen and carbon dioxide that could produce cyclic changes in the ST segment.

Experiment protocol and data analysis

Nine normal volunteers (ages 22–35; 3 females) underwent the experimental procedure. The experiment was performed in the clinical Research Center of Strong Memorial Hospital, Rochester, NY. The test was divided into four periods, wherein the mechanical, metabolic and neurogenic parasympathetic factors were altered following a control

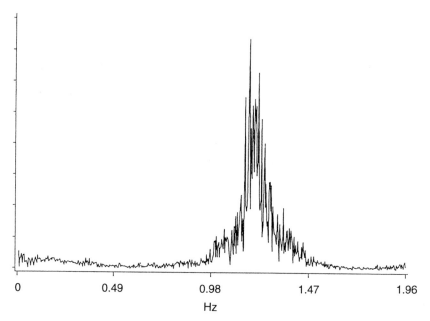

Figure 20.9 Spectrum of the ECG of Figure 20.5 after demodulation. The 0.17 Hz DC replica of the respiratory spectrum has been completely removed, as have the upper and lower sidebands around the ECG fundamental frequency.

period. The mechanical factor was altered by forcing the subject to breathe faster and with deeper intensity; the metabolic factor was altered by making the subject breath pure oxygen; and the neurogenic parasympathetic factor was altered with intravenous administration of atropine. During the test, the respiratory rate was controlled with the use of a metronome, and two channels of ECG (V2-like and V5-like) plus one channel of respiratory signal were simultaneously recorded with a dedicated recorder provided by DMI (Diagnostic Medical Instruments, Syracuse, NY) which utilized 1000 Hz sampling frequency. The recorder, which generally has three channels, was modified to receive into its third input a signal with the characteristics of the respiratory waveform. This was obtained by means of a nasal thermistor connected to a bridge circuit and fed to an operational amplifier. The four periods of the experiment can be summarized as follows:

1. *The control period*: The subject breathed room air (20% oxygen) at 10 cycles/min (0.17 Hz) for approximately 5 minutes.
2. *The fast respiration period*: The respiratory rate with room air was increased to 15 cycles/min (0.25 Hz) for another 5 minutes.
3. *The metabolic period*: The subject breathed 100% oxygen at the control rate of 10 cycles/min for about 8 minutes.
4. *The neurogenic period*: After 10 minutes of breathing pure air, atropine was administered intravenously, and the subject breathed room air at the control rate of 10 cycles/min for another 10 minutes.

The three channels of digitized data from the output of the DMI recorder were downloaded to a PC computer and transferred to a SUN SparcServer 4/470 for signal processing. The two ECG channels were first demodulated as described previously to correct for motion-induced variability. All the beat-to-beat time series, and in particular the time series of the RR intervals and time series of the AVD values, were extracted. In addition, a beat-to-beat respiratory time series was obtained by sampling the respiratory signal in correspondence with each detected QRS complex. The power spectral density (PSD) of the two series were calculated both with autoregressive modeling and fast Fourier transform (averaged periodogram) approaches. The cross-spectral densities and squared-coherence functions between the various time series were calculated using the fast Fourier transform method. For the autospectra, attention was focused on the values of total and relative power in the respiratory band (as determined by the spectrum of the measured respiratory signal). In the same way, the squared-coherence functions were evaluated in the respiratory band. As is generally done with beat-to-beat time series, the frequency units of cycles/beats were transformed into 'equivalent hertz' by dividing them by the average RR interval of the period being analyzed.[14] The adjective 'equivalent' highlighted the fact that the units obtained are not effective hertz but rather their estimate performed assuming constant heart rate.

All parameters described were compared between the four periods. The same was done for the squared-coherence function between the AVD and RR time series and between the AVD and the respiratory time series. Statistical comparison between the four periods was performed with a Wilcoxon signed-rank test.

Results of the experiment

Table 20.1 summarizes the results of the Wilcoxon rank-test applied to the relative change in the total variability of the power spectral density of the AVD. The relative change is calculated as the difference between the variability after the intervention and the variability during the control period P1, normalized with respect to the variability in P1. The relative decrease between periods P1 and P4 is statistically significant (estimated median decrease is 44%, $p = 0.014$). The change between P1 and P2 is also significant (estimated median change 14%, $p = 0.03$); the oxygenation period P3 is not associated with a significant change when compared with control.

Table 20.2 shows the results of the same test applied to the change in the relative (normalized) power of the respiratory component of the PSD of the AVD. The relative

Table 20.1 Results of Wilcoxon rank-test on relative changes of total variability in the AVD signal when comparing control versus atropine (P1/P4), control versus hyperventilation (P1/P2), and control versus breathing 100% oxygen (P1/P3). A positive value for mean and median indicates a decrease.

Comparison periods	Mean relative change	Wilcoxon test *p*-value	Estimated median change
P1/P2	0.16	0.03	0.144
P1/P3	−0.42	0.813	−0.118
P1/P4	0.43	0.014	0.445

Table 20.2 Results of Wilcoxon rank-test on relative changes of relative power in the respiratory band of the PSD of the AVD when comparing control versus atropine (P1/P4), control versus hyperventilation (P1/P2), and control versus breathing 100% oxygen (P1/P3). A positive value for mean and median indicates a decrease.

Comparison periods	Mean relative change	Wilcoxon test *p*-value	Estimated median change
P1/P2	0.05	0.142	0.050
P1/P3	0.05	1.000	0.020
P1/P4	0.26	0.035	0.282

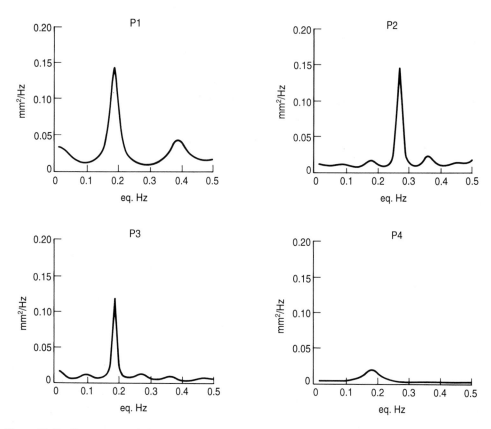

Figure 20.10 Power spectral densities of the AVD signal during the four periods of the experiment. The effect of atropine administration (P4) is evident.

power significantly decreases only with atropine intervention (estimated median change 28%, $p = 0.035$).

Figure 20.10 shows the PSD of the AVD time series during the four periods for one of the subjects; in this, the decrease of total variability after atropine is apparent, as is the change of relative power.

These results suggest that the parasympathetic nervous system plays a role in the regulation of ST segment variability, the mechanical respiratory activity plays a lesser but still significant role, and 100% oxygen inhalation does not influence AVD variability. Similar results were observed for heart rate variability, thus suggesting that the mechanisms influencing the evolution of these time series are similar. In particular, the median decrease of total HRV was 84% ($P = 0.014$), thus confirming the well-known strong effect of atropine on heart rate.[19]

Table 20.3 shows the results of the test on the changes relative to the squared-coherences. There are no significant changes for periods P2 and P3. During the first three periods, the mean squared-coherences at respiratory frequency were respectively 0.81, 0.83 and 0.83, showing a strong association between the peaks of the spectra. The strong significance in the relative decrease (median 20%, $p = 0.014$) of the squared-coherence between P1 and P4 suggests that the association between AVD and RR is significantly decreased. Actually, it may be said that the relationship had disappeared, as the mean coherence during P4 was reduced to 0.61 (high values of squared-coherence are required

Table 20.3 Results of Wilcoxon rank-test on relative changes of squared-coherence function evaluated at the respiratory frequency between AVD and RR variability signals (STV–HRV) and between AVD and respiration (STV–RES), when comparing control versus atropine (P1/P4), control versus hyperventilation (P1/P2), and control versus breathing 100% oxygen (P1/P3). A positive value for mean and median indicates a decrease.

Comparison periods	STV–HRV		STV–RES	
	Median	p	Median	p
P1/P2	0.01	1.00	−0.005	1.00
P1/P3	−0.015	0.86	−0.01	0.95
P1/P4	0.2	0.014	0.12	0.05

to state association between two signals). An interpretation of this result is that the common source that ties the respiratory peak in the PSD of the HRV and AVD time series is essentially related to vagal tone. Other residual mechanisms, such as mechanical influences, are probably unrelated to each other. A significant decrease in the squared-coherence between HRV and AVD signals provides proof that the variability of the ST displacement is not an artifactual consequence of the heart rate. If this were the case, there should be no decrease in the squared-coherence. On the contrary, we conclude that the coherence between the two signals is mostly due to vagal tone.

Quite interestingly (but with no surprise), the outcome of the experiment described depends strictly on the ECG signal being demodulated first. In other words, all the significant differences ceased to be so when the measured ECG was not demodulated. The logical explanation is that in this case the variability of the AVD signal was dominated by the motion-related phenomena (which was not modified by the administration of atropine) and that physiologic variability is at least an order of magnitude inferior. To give a more concrete figure, the AVD standard deviations before the demodulation ranged between 0.31 and 0.42 mm whereas after demodulation they were between 0.1 and 0.2 mm. The demodulator could be further improved, but the effect of its application is clear. In conclusion, the following can be stated:

1. The ANS has an important role in regulation of the AVD time series.
2. Mechanical hyperventilation is associated with a reduction of variability. However, this action is significantly milder than the one of atropine, and it is associated with no significant changes in the normalized power.
3. Inhalation of 100% oxygen does not have an effect on AVD variability.

Comments

The experiment described here is the first of its kind and further trials need to be performed to obtain a more complete assessment of the physiological variables that influence the dynamics of ST segment displacement. A specific limitation of the experiment was that the three interventions cannot be put on the same level in terms of intensity. In other words, the neurogenic environment was stressed much more than the metabolic and mechanical environments.

Nevertheless, the presence of a physiologic variability in the ST segment displacement signal is a new and important finding that strengthens the importance of the autonomic nervous system in regulation of the ventricles. Furthermore, the presence of physiologic variability should extend the domain of ST segment analysis from a simple detector of ischemia to that of an important component of the comprehensive cardiovascular equilibrium. The ability to remove the vector-rotation effect induced by the respiratory activity opens, by itself, new frontiers in the field of ambulatory ECG recordings. The demodulated ECG must be seen in a context wider than ST segment analysis, as it allows the development of other amplitude-derived beat-to-beat time series such as R wave amplitudes and T wave areas. As a secondary effect, the ability to obtain a reliable estimate of the respiratory waveform can further be used in those cases where breathing can play a determinant cardiovascular role (hyperventilation, sudden infant death).

In conclusion, analysis of the variability of ST segment displacement beat-to-beat time series is possible, but its accomplishment is still complex owing to the signal processing required to cleanse the measured ECG signal of motion-related modulations. Modern technology should permit the application of demodulators directly to digital recorders, and the analysis of any amplitude-related ECG variables should be feasible.

References

1. Armstrong WF, Morris SN. The ST segment during ambulatory electrocardiographic monitoring. *Ann Intern Med* 1983; **98**: 249–50.
2. Cosby RS, Herman LM. Sequential changes in the development of the electrocardiographic pattern of left ventricular hypertrophy in hypertensive heart disease. *Am Heart J* 1962; **63**: 180.
3. Hull E. The electrocardiogram in pericarditis. *Am J Cardiol* 1961; **7**: 21.
4. Nelson SD, Kou WH, Annesley T. Significance of ST segment depression during paroxysmal supraventricular tachycardia. *J Am Coll Cardiol* 1989; **13**: 804.
5. Stern S, Tzivoni D, Early detection of silent ischemic heart disease by 24-hour electrocardiographic monitoring of active subjects. *Br Heart J* 1974; **36**: 481–6.
6. Biagini A, Mazzei MZ, Carpeggiani C, *et al*. Vasospastic ischemic mechanism of frequent asymptomatic transient ST–T changes during continuous electrocardiographic monitoring in selected unstable patients. *Am Heart J* 1982; **103**: 4–12.
7. Akselrod S, Norymberg M, Peled I, *et al*. Computerized analysis of ST segment changes in ambulatory electrocardiograms. *Med Biol Eng Comput* 1987; **25**: 513–19.
8. Meyer CR, Kaiser HN. Electrocardiogram baseline noise estimation and removal using cubic splines and state–space computation techniques. *Comput Biomed Res* 1977; **10**: 459–70.
9. Pottala EW, Bailey JJ, Horton MR, Gradwohl JR. Suppression of baseline wander in the ECG using a bilinearly transformed, null-phase filter. *J Electrocardiol* 1989; **22**(Suppl): 243–7.
10. Tayler DI, Vincent R. Artefactual ST segment abnormalities due to electrocardiograph design. *Br Heart J* 1985; **54**: 11–28.
11. Badilini F. *Myocardial Ischemia in Ambulatory ECG Recordings*. Master thesis, College of Engineering and Applied Science, Rochester, NY, 1991.
12. Badilini F, Moss AJ, Titlebaum EL. Cubic spline baseline estimation in ambulatory ECG recordings. In: *Proceedings of the IEEE/EMBS Annual Conference*. New York: IEEE/EMBS, 1991: 584–5.
13. Badilini F. *Time and Frequency Analysis of ST Segment Displacement Signals in Ambulatory ECG Recordings*. Doctoral thesis, College of Engineering and Applied Science, Rochester, NY, 1994.
14. Oppenheim AV, AS Wilsky. *Signals and Systems*. Englewood Cliffs, NJ: Prentice-Hall, 1983.
15. Oppenheim AV, Shafer RW, *Discrete-Time Signal Processing*. Englewood Cliffs, NJ: Prentice-Hall, 1989.
16. De Boer RW, Karemaker JM, Strackee. Comparing spectra of a series of point events, particularly for heart rate variability data. *IEEE Trans Biomed Eng* 1984; **31**: 384–7.
17. Cerutti S, Alberti M, *et al*. Automatic assessment of the interaction between respiration and heart rate variability signal. *Med Prog Tech* 1988; **14**: 7–19.
18. Trautwein W, Osterriede W. Mechanisms of beta-adrenergic modulation and cholinergic control of Ca and K currents in the heart. In: Nathan RD (ed.), *Cardiac Muscle: the Regulation of Excitation and Contraction*. London: Academic Press, 1986: 87–128.
19. Alcalay M, Israeli S, Wallach RK, *et al*. Paradoxical pharmacodynamic effect of atropine on parasympathetic control: a study by spectral analysis of heart rate fluctuations. *Clin Pharm Ther* 1992; **52**: 518–527.

21

Clinical Utility of ST Segment Monitoring

Arthur J. Moss

Background

Clinical and laboratory observations suggest that asymptomatic ST segment depression on ambulatory Holter recordings may be an important indicator of silent myocardial ischemia reflecting advanced and potentially unstable coronary occlusive disease. These concerns are derived from the ST segment shifts that occur with acute coronary disease, with vasospastic coronary disease (Prinzmetal's variant angina), and with exercise testing. In 1969, Parker *et al.*[1] reported that anginal pain was a late event during pacing-induced ischemia in coronary patients with typical effort angina. ST depression accurately reflected the onset, presence, and disappearance of metabolically defined myocardial ischemia (lactate production). Clinical episodes of spontaneous myocardial ischemia reflect an imbalance of myocardial oxygen supply and demand. The overwhelming evidence indicates that the pathogenetic mechanism involved in spontaneous ischemia during daily life is similar to that responsible for exercise-induced ischemia; i.e. increased myocardial oxygen demand in the setting of restricted coronary flow.[2] Vasospastic reduction in myocardial oxygen supply is thought to play only a minor contributing role to myocardial ischemia in chronic coronary disease.

In 1974, Stern *et al.*[3] reported the detection of silent ischemic heart disease with 24-hour Holter monitoring during everyday activities in 80 patients with angina pectoris and normal resting 12-lead electrocardiograms. Holter monitoring was interpreted as positive for ischemia if transient ST depression or elevation of at least 1 mm and/or major T wave inversion were detected for several beats.[4] Ischemic ST–T changes were observed in 37 of the 80 patients during Holter monitoring. The authors concluded that '24-hour monitoring of the electrocardiogram under normal everyday activity is a reliable and convenient method for detecting ischemic changes at an early stage'. The era for Holter monitoring for the detection of silent myocardial ischemia was ushered in. During the course of the next 20 years many descriptive studies using the Holter technology for the detection of transient myocardial ischemia (ST segment shifts) were reported, with only a few prospective studies reporting on the prognostic significance of Holter-detected ST segment depression in stable coronary patients.

Technical Considerations

The criteria for defining an episode of transient myocardial ischemia on the Holter recording were derived from exercise-testing criteria and from clinical experience with the Holter technique. A conventional definition evolved, and most Holter investigators utilize the following criterion for 'ischemia': an episode of transient ST segment depression of ≥ 1 mm (0.1 mV) at 80 ms after the J point from the baseline ST segment position, lasting for ≥ 1 minute in consecutive beats. This conventional definition has never been validated as truly indicating myocardial ischemia.

At present, most Holter systems utilize 2-lead 24-hour ECG tape-recordings, although high-quality digital recordings are now becoming available. The techniques for quantitating ST depression involve technician-interactive high-speed (60–120 × real time) scan analysis and partial automatic processing according to certain prespecified parameters. Most systems also provide a complete record of every complex in compressed time and voltage scales. The resolution of these 'full disclosure' records is insufficient to accurately detect morphologic ST segment shifts. No technique provides perfect discrimination between physiologic signals and noise or artifact. Transient ST segment depressions are, for the most part, due to myocardial ischemia, but physiologic events other than ischemia may produce similar ST segment shifts (postural changes, tachycardia, hypertension, sympathetic activity, hyperventilation, left ventricular dimension and pressure changes, alterations in intraventricular conduction, and drug-level fluctuations).

The test–retest reliability of quantitating Holter-recorded ST segment shifts has not been adequately documented in the literature. The reliability or reproducibility of identifying ST segment depression episodes using standard prespecified criteria when the same tracing is reread has been reported in only one publication. Moss et al.,[8] in a multicenter myocardial ischemia study, evaluated the agreement between blinded duplicate analyses of Holter recordings by the *kappa statistic*. The kappa statistic evaluates the degree of agreement between rereads with adjustment for chance-expected agreement.[9] Kappa values range from +1 (perfect agreement) to −1 (perfect disagreement), with positive kappa values indicating agreement better than chance. For most purposes, values between +0.40 and +0.70 represent fair to good agreement beyond chance, and values greater than +0.70 represent excellent agreement beyond chance. In the multicenter myocardial ischemia study,[8] the kappa statistic for blinded reanalysis of 55 Holter recordings for ischemia by the same core laboratory was +0.51 (fair agreement).

New and improved approaches are needed to detect ischemic-type ST segment depression episodes reliably. Chapter 20 in this volume highlights a new direction, for it involves digital processing of Holter tapes, utilizes several statistical-based criteria for abnormal ST depression for each individual subject, incorporates automatic computerized beat-by-beat ST segment analyses resulting in a kappa retest statistic of +1.0 (perfect agreement), and validates the new ischemic-type ST abnormalities against conventional Holter analysis in a population with documented coronary disease and spontaneous ischemic episodes.

Risk Stratification in Coronary Disease

Acute coronary syndromes

In 1986, Gottlieb et al.[10] showed that silent ischemia on Holter recordings is associated with an unfavourable short-term (1-month) outcome in patients with unstable angina receiving intensive medical therapy in the coronary care unit. Similar findings were reported by Langer et al.[11] These articles were published before the routine use of intravenous heparin, early angiography, and aggressive revascularization procedures in this high-risk group. Clinically, physicians are not routinely using Holter recordings for risk assessment of patients with unstable angina during the early hyperacute phase of their illness. In similar manner, the time dependence for thrombolytic intervention in the early phase of acute myocardial infarction precludes the use of Holter monitoring for risk assessment in this patient group.

Subacute coronary syndromes

Holter monitoring before hospital discharge has been used to evaluate the likelihood of early (3–6 month) recurrent coronary events in patients convalescing from unstable angina and acute myocardial infarction. In most of the studies, frequent and/or prolonged durations of myocardial ischemia were associated with an increased probability of an adverse short-term outcome.[12,13] However, the limited sensitivity of Holter-detected ischemia for predicting future coronary events in convalescent postcoronary patients is such that this technique cannot be recommended as a routine screening procedure in this patient population.

Coronary angioplasty is being widely performed, and coronary restenosis with symptomatic angina occurs in 30–40% of the angioplasty population within 6 months of the initial procedure. Routine Holter monitoring at a month or so after the angioplasty has been recommended for detecting those at risk for restenosis. However, there have been no reported studies demonstrating the usefulness of Holter-detected silent ischemia for predicting who will and who will not develop restenosis.

Chronic coronary disease

Several Holter monitoring studies have been carried out to determine if the detection of silent ischemia in patients with stable chronic coronary disease (i.e. after full recovery from myocardial infarction or unstable angina) is a harbinger of future coronary events. Although there is some controversy in this area,[8,14–18] the accumulating data in properly conducted prospective studies indicate that Holter-detected silent ischemia is relatively frequent in these stable coronary patients and has little or no prognostic value. In the multicenter study of silent myocardial ischemia involving 936 patients, 2–6 months after recovery from myocardial infarction or unstable angina, Holter-detected ST segment depression, similar to other noninvasive tests employed including thallium stress testing, was not associated with a significant increase in subsequent coronary events (coronary death, nonfatal myocardial infarction, or unstable angina, whichever occurred first) during a 2-year follow-up.[8] It should be emphasized that this study utilized only naturally occurring endpoints and did not include physician-determined endpoints such as bypass surgery or angioplasty.

Time interval after an acute coronary event

It is clear that the prognostic value of Holter-recorded ST segment depression is related to the pretest risk exhibited by the patient (Bayes' theorem). In practical terms, this means that the prognostic significance of Holter-recorded ST segment depression is a function of when the Holter is obtained after the index coronary event. Figure 21.1 shows a schematic of the inverse relationship between the prognostic value of Holter-identified ischemia and the time interval after the event.

Coronary bypass surgery

Holter monitoring has been used to evaluate the prognostic significance of silent ischemia after coronary bypass surgery. The studies have yielded conflicting results,[19–21] and it is not clear that residual ischemia detected by Holter monitoring in this population has an adverse effect on prognosis, at least in the short term. In the Coronary Artery

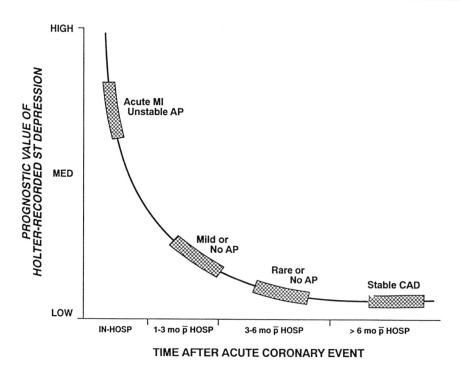

Figure 21.1   Schematic of the inverse relationship between the prognostic value of Holter-recorded ST segment depression and the pretest risk category of the patient in terms of the time interval after an acute coronary event. MI = myocardial infarction; AP = angina pectoris; CAD = coronary artery disease.

Surgery Study, 6-month postoperative exercise-induced ischemia was associated with reduced survival, but the effect was not evident until the tenth year of follow-up.[22]

It should be noted that, in patients with normal left ventricular function and one- or two-vessel coronary artery disease, severe exercise-induced ischemia (ST-segment depression at a low workload and decrease in ejection fraction) was not associated with reduced survival during 5-year follow-up.[23] It is unlikely that Holter monitoring would have provided different results in this carefully defined low-risk subgroup.

Screening patients for vascular surgery

Patients who undergo peripheral vascular surgery are difficult to assess preoperatively because of physical limitations, yet these patients are at increased risk for perioperative and postoperative cardiac arrests. Several studies have shown that Holter-detected preoperative ischemia is useful in predicting perioperative and postoperative cardiac events,[24–28] and Holter monitoring can be recommended for the assessment of risk in this group of patients.

Evaluating Efficacy of Antianginal Therapy

Since the Holter recording can detect episodes of asymptomatic ST depression (silent ischemia) in coronary patients, it has been hypothesized that the frequency and overall time duration of the ST depression episodes during 24-hour recordings reflect the 'myocardial ischemic burden'. Several studies have been and are being carried out to determine whether anti-ischemic therapy with nitrates, beta-blockers or calcium-channel blockers reduces Holter-detected ischemic episodes during daily life, and whether this reduction in silent ischemia is associated with a more favorable outcome. The recently published Asymptomatic Cardiac Ischemia Pilot (ACIP) study found that 40% of patients with angiographically documented coronary artery disease and asymptomatic ischemia were free of Holter-detected ischemia after 12 weeks of anti-ischemic therapy.[29] The ACIP study is the forerunner of a large, prospective anti-ischemia trial to determine whether treatment of silent ischemia is, in fact, beneficial. Until that study is completed, Holter monitoring cannot be recommended for evaluation of the efficacy of anti-ischemia therapy in patients with ischemic heart disease.

Diagnosis of Coronary Vasospasm

Prinzmetal's variant angina relates to the occurrence of classical angina pectoris, usually at rest or during inactivity, in association with transient ST segment elevation suggesting a hyperacute myocardial infarction. It is important to record an electrocardiogram during the episode of chest discomfort since exercise testing is frequently nondiagnostic. The variant anginal episodes are due to coronary vasospasm and may occur in patients with normal coronary arteries or in patients with partially obstructive coronary lesions. Holter monitoring is clearly indicated in such clinical cases when Prinzmetal's variant angina is suspected. Not infrequently, multiple 24-hour recordings are required in order to obtain an electrocardiographic tracing during a symptomatic episode.

Conclusions

Transient ST depression on the Holter recording is due, in part, to transient episodes of myocardial ischemia, but other physiologic events and artifact may produce similar ST segment shifts. The magnitude of the false-positive ST segment depression rate for myocardial ischemia is uncertain.

The criteria for an ischemic ST segment depression response during exercise-testing may not be fully transferable to Holter monitoring because the conditions affecting repolarization may be quite different in the two recording situations. New, improved, and validated criteria for Holter-detected ischemia are required.

The reproducibility (test–retest reliability) for identifying ST depression on a given Holter recording is currently only fair, at best. The impaired reproducibility severely reduces the diagnostic and prognostic power of this technique in clinical cardiology.

Holter technology for detecting ischemic-type ST segment shifts is being improved with the advent of digital real-time recorders and computer analysis. This new Holter technology should significantly enhance the clinical usefulness of this methodology for accurate detection of transient myocardial ischemia.

Existing knowledge indicates that transient ST segment depression on the Holter recording relates in part to the severity of the coronary disease, and the findings are analogous to the significance of ST segment changes with exercise-testing. Thus, Holter monitoring may be equivalent to a low-level exercise with low diagnostic sensitivity in low-risk patients. Only in high-risk coronary patients is the test likely to add diagnostic information. Screening of low-risk patients for silent ischemia is not recommented.

The prognostic significance of asymptomatic ST depression on Holter recordings relates, in part, to Bayes' theorem. The predictive accuracy of a positive test (ST depression) to identify patients at risk for having a subsequent cardiac event is strongly influenced by the prior probability of experiencing such events; i.e. the severity of the pre-existing coronary heart disease.

Transient ST segment depression on the Holter recording may reflect the extent and severity of obstructive coronary disease, but it surely does not provide information about the 'activity' of the coronary lesion or the propensity of the coronary lesion to subsequent thrombotic occlusion. Thus, even if ischemic ST segment depression episodes are detected, it is unlikely that the identification of such episodes will accurately predict cardiac death or nonfatal myocardial infarction during the subsequent few years in stable coronary patients.

References

1. Parker JO, Chiong MA, West RO, Case RB. Sequential alterations in myocardial lactate metabolism, ST segments, and left ventricular function during pacing induced angina. *J Am Coll Cardiol* 1983; **1**: 934–9.
2. Deedwania PC, Nelson JR. Pathophysiology of silent myocardial infarction during daily life: hemodynamic evaluation by simultaneous electrocardiographic and blood pressure monitoring. *Circulation* 1990; **82**: 1296–304.
3. Stern S, Tzivoni D. Early detection of silent ischaemic heart disease by 24-hour electrocardiographic monitoring of active subjects. *Br Heart J* 1974; **36**: 481–6.
4. Wolf E, Tzivoni D, Stern S. Comparison of exercise tests and 24-hour ambulatory electrocardiographic monitoring in detection of ST–T changes. *Br Heart J* 1974; **36**: 90–5.
5. Nademanee K. Intarachot V, Josephson MA, Rieders D, Mody FV, Singh BN. Prognostic significance of silent myocardial ischemia in patients with unstable angina. *J Am Coll Cardiol* 1987; **10**: 1–9.
6. Deedwania PC, Carbajal EV. Silent ischemia during daily life is an independent predictor of mortality in stable angina. *Circulation* 1990; **81**: 748–56.
7. Yeung AC, Barry J, Orav J, Bonassin E, Raby KE, Selwyn AP. Effects of asymptomatic ischemia on long-term prognosis in chronic stable coronary disease. *Circulation* 1991; **83**: 1598–604.
8. Moss AJ, Goldstein RE, Hall WJ, Bigger JT, Fleiss JL, Greenberg H, Bodenheimer M, Krone RJ, Marcus FI, Wackers FJT, Benhorin J, Brown MW, Case R, Coromilas J, Dwyer EM, Gillespie JA, Gregory JJ, Kleiger R, Lichstein E, Parker JO, Raubertas RF, Stern S. Tzivoni D, Van Voorhees L. Detection and significance of myocardial ischemia in stable patients after recovery from an acute coronary event. *JAMA* 1993; **269**: 2379–85.
9. Fleiss JL. *Statistical Methods for Rates and Proportions*, 2nd edn. New York: John Wiley, 1981: 217.
10. Gottlieb SO, Weisfeldt ML, Ouyang P, Mellits ED, Gerstenblith G. Silent ischemia as a marker for early unfavourable outcomes in patients with unstable angina. *New Eng J Med* 1986; **314**: 1214–19.
11. Langer A, Freeman MR, Armstrong PW. ST segment shift in unstable angina: pathophysiology and association with coronary anatomy and hospital outcome. *J Am Coll Cardiol* 1989; **13**: 1495–502.
12. Gottlieb SO, Gottlieb SH, Achuff SC, Baumgardner R, Mellits ED, Weisfeldt ML, Gerstenblith G. Silent ischemia on Holter monitoring predicts mortality in high-risk postinfarction patients. *JAMA* 1988; **259**: 1030–5.
13. Langer A, Minkowitz J, Dorian P, Casella L, Harris L, Morgan CD, Armstrong PW. Pathophysiology and prognostic significance of Holter-detected ST segment depression after myocardial infarction. *J Am Coll Cardiol* 1992; **20**: 1313–17.
14. Hands ME, Sia STB, Shook TL, Anderson K, Stone PH, Levy D, Castelli WP, Rutherford JD. Silent myocardial ischemia in asymptomatic survivors of unrecognized myocardial infarction and matched controls. *Am Heart J* 1988; **116**: 1488–92.
15. Tzivoni D, Gavish A, Zin D, Gottlieb S, Moriel M, Keren A, Banai S, Stern S. Prognostic significance of ischemic episodes in patients with previous myocardial infarction. *Am J Cardiol* 1988; **62**: 661–4.
16. Gandhi MM, Wood DA, Lampe FC. Characteristics and clinical significance of ambulatory myocardial ischemia in men and women in the general population presenting with angina pectoris. *J Am Coll Cardiol* 1994; **23**: 74–81.
17. Deedwania PC. Does myocardial ischemia portend poor prognosis? *J Am Coll Cardiol* 1994; **23**: 229–32.
18. Chang J, Atwood JE, Froelicher V. Prognostic impact of myocardial ischemia. *J Am Coll Cardiol* 1994; **23**: 225–8.
19. Crea F, Kaski JC, Fragasso G, *et al*. Usefulness of Holter monitoring to improve the sensitivity of exercise testing in determining the degree of myocardial revascularization after coronary artery bypass grafting for stable angina pectoris. *Am J Cardiol* 1987; **65**: 225–41.
20. Kennedy HL, Seiler SM, Sprague MK, *et al*. Relation of silent myocardial ischemia after coronary artery bypass grafting to angiographic completeness of revascularization and long-term prognosis. *Am J Cardiol* 1989; **65**: 14–22.
21. Egstrup K. Asymptomatic myocardial ischemia as a predictor of cardiac events after coronary artery bypass grafting for stable angina pectoris. *Am J Cardiol* 1988; **61**: 248–52.
22. Wiener DA, Ryan TJ, Parsons L, Fisher LD, Chaitman BR, Sheffield LT, Tristani FE. Prevalence and prognostic significance of silent and symptomatic ischemia after coronary bypass surgery: a report from the Coronary Artery Surgery Study (CASS) randomized population. *J Am Coll Cardiol* 1991; **18**: 343–8.
23. Miller TD, Christian TF, Taliercio CP, Zinsmeister AR, Gibbons RJ. Severe exercise-induced ischemia does not identify high-risk patients with normal left ventricular function and one- or two-vessel coronary artery disease. *J Am Coll Cardiol* 1994; **23**: 219–24.
24. Raby KE, Goldman L, Creager MA, Cook EF, Weisberg MC, Whittemore AD, Selwyn AP. Correlation between preoperative ischemia and major cardiac events after peripheral vascular surgery. *New Eng J Med* 1989; **321**: 1296–300.

25. Raby KE, Goldman L, Cook EF, Rumerman J, Barry J, Creager MA, Selwyn AP. Long-term prognosis of myocardial ischemia detected by Holter monitoring in peripheral vascular disease. *Am J Cardiol* 1990; **66**: 1309–13.
26. Fleisher LA, Rosenbaum SH, Nelson AH, Barash PG. The predictive value of preoperative silent ischemic cardiac events in vascular and nonvascular surgery patients. *Am Heart J* 1991; **122**: 980–6.
27. Pasternack PF, Grossi EA, Baumann FG, Riles TS, Lamparello PJ, Giangola G, Yu AY, Mintzer R, Imparato AM. Silent myocardial ischemia monitoring predicts late as well as perioperative cardiac events in patients undergoing vascular surgery. *J Vasc Surg* 1992; **16**: 171–9.
28. Raby KE, Barry J, Creager MA, Cook EF, Weisberg MC, Goldman L. Detection and significance of intraoperative and postoperative myocardial ischemia in peripheral vascular surgery. *JAMA* 1992; **268**: 252–3.
29. Knatterud GL, Bourassa MG, Pepine CJ, Geller NL, Sopko G, Chaitman BR, Pratt C, Stone PH, Davies RF, Rogers WJ, Deanfield JE, Goldberg AD, Ouyang P, Mueller H, Sharaf B, Day P, Selwyn AP, Conti CR. Effects of treatment strategies to suppress ischemia in patients with coronary artery disease: 12-week results of the Asymptomatic Cardiac Ischemia Plot (ACIP) study. *J Am Coll Cardiol* 1994; **24**: 11–20.

SECTION VI

The QT Interval

Introduction by Philippe Coumel

The ECG is the preferred tool of cardiologists after a century of use, and short- and long-term recordings of the ECG provide considerable information about the physiology both of the heart and of the autonomic nervous system (ANS). This information can be obtained if we do our analysis using appropriate algorithms. It is important to use various approaches jointly rather than studying them in isolation. For example, the temporal–spatial behavior of heart rate (HR) and ventricular repolarization (VR) should be analyzed together when using the ECG in the analysis of heart rhythm. Looking for relationships between the various electrophysiologic parameters is important when investigating the dynamics of the heart rhythm.

The Holter technique added a new dimension to electrocardiography. We realize now how important it is to monitor the dynamicity of the HR. The instantaneous HR value obtained from a few cardiac cycles of the routine surface ECG recording is a static parameter with only limited relevance when viewed alone. The short- and long-term modulations of HR were recognized as important parameters, to the point that the attention paid to heart rate variability (HRV) was at the expense of interest in HR itself. HRV and HR are intimately linked, and ignoring this relationship will compromise our ability to understand basic principles of cardiac electrophysiology.

Looking at the sinus rhythm, we are not exploring the heart itself, but rather the ANS activity through its effects on the sinoatrial node. Many aspects of the heart function are dependent on ANS modulation, and dysfunction of the cardiovascular system may provoke a reaction from the ANS which tends to re-establish homeostasis. We can consider the ANS behavior as a mirror which reflects an image of the heart, as the ANS sees it. The information conveyed by the ANS to the heart may be more reliable than information we obtain directly. For instance, measuring the left ventricular ejection fraction is a global and simplistic way to assess the complex mechanical functions of the heart. The simple index of HRV, the standard deviation of the RR intervals over 24 hours which evaluates the ANS influence on the heart, may be a more reliable prognostic index than the ejection fraction. It is important to keep these notions in mind when shifting from the sinoatrial node and HR modulation to VR and its dynamicity. The assessment of VR is technically more difficult, and the information obtained is more complex than that obtained from HR modulation. VR involves both the ANS and the ventricular myocardium where most of heart disease occurs. Discerning which information is relevant and which parameter is really important is the real challenge.

The knowledge and know-how of quantitative electrocardiology should be transferred into the domain of dynamic electrocardiology. Following dynamically the QRS–T morphology is not simple, and the first step is to discern which criteria of evaluation are pertinent. For example, in vectorcardiography, the spatial T wave loop is dispersed in 3-dimensional space. What appears at first glance to be a loss of information becomes, curiously, enhanced information relative to quantitative analysis of 3-dimensional QT dispersion.

QT dispersion and QT dynamicity are apparently quite different. QT dispersion is fundamentally static, although there might be some time-dependent changes in QT dispersion over 24 hours. The QT interval is dynamic and it certainly changes over time. It would be inadequate to limit the investigation of VR to the QT interval itself. Although the QT interval on the ECG reflects the action potential duration at the cellular level, in a strict sense the QT duration expresses the group of cells with the longest repolarization. This prolonged depolarization may be due to later activation, longer action potential duration, or special physiological/pathological behavior. The QT duration and QT dynamicity may represent an extreme situation since in both cases the duration and dynamicity characteristics may simply quantitate the last small group of cells to be repolarized.

It is not sufficient to limit investigations to simply the end of the T wave. The dynamicity of the interval from the Q to the apex of the T wave differs from that of the Q wave to the end of the T wave. This discrepancy varies with circadian influences and may also be different in patients with the long QT syndrome. QT dynamicity may have more importance than the QT interval itself. The T wave apex is the fiducial point of VR, and it does not represent the beginning or the end of the repolarization process in the ventricular myocardium. In other words, the time and space exploration of VR should encompass the entire repolarization process, from the first to the last cell.

An important aspect of repolarization is its rate dependency, but it is also influenced by the ANS. As VR obviously depends on HR, it is most important to differentiate as clearly as possible what is related to HR and what to ANS when analyzing VR. This problem and others involving the complex relationships between HR, sinus node function, VR and ANS are addressed in the chapters in this section.

22

QT Interval, Heart Rate and Ventricular Arrhythmias

Pierre Maison Blanche, Didier Catuli, Jocelyne Fayn and Philippe Coumel

Introduction

On the body-surface ECG, the QT interval corresponds to the time elapsed between depolarization of the first myocardial ventricular cell (beginning of the Q wave) and the end of repolarization of the last ventricular cell (end of the T wave). Often, it is referred to as the repolarization-duration interval. Assessment of the QT interval from ECG recordings is important because an abnormally prolonged QT interval has become an increasingly accepted marker of malignant ventricular arrhythmias, such as torsades de pointes. However, until now, no upper limit of acceptable QT prolongation has been identified. In certain situations, an increase in the ventricular action potential duration actually constitutes an antiarrhythmic mechanism, but the circumstances under which prolongation of ventricular repolarization is beneficial or dangerous are unknown.[1] QT interval prolongation alone is probably not the best quantitative ECG feature of ventricular repolarization.[2] Recently, it has been shown that QT interval dispersion measured on a 12-lead ECG (QTmax–QTmin) is a reliable predictor of life-threatening arrhythmias. T-wave alternans (beat-to-beat subtle changes of the surface ECG) is also associated with severe rhythm disorders in many clinical situations. These features are examined in detail in Chapters 23 and 25.

Failure of adaptation of the QT interval to changes in the heart rate may also be a more meaningful parameter than the QT prolongation itself. Numerous formulas for heart rate adjustment of QT, based on 12-lead resting ECG or on exercise-testing, have been proposed: their hallmark is that they correlate the QT interval duration to the immediately preceding RR interval alone. Unfortunately, these formulas do not provide a complete correction for all of the rate influences involved since there is evidence of a 'memory phenomenon'; i.e. there is a time delay between a change in heart rate and the subsequent change in QT interval.[3,4] One way to overcome this phenomenon is to use atrial pacing at a constant cycle length until QT has reached its steady state.[5] But pacing is an invasive procedure and therefore it cannot be tested in large populations. Provided that automatic identification of stable heart rate periods is feasible, an alternative approach is to use the spontaneous heart rate changes in 24-hour Holter ECG data. Another advantage of Holter recordings is that the modulating effects of the autonomic nervous system (ANS) on cycle length dependency of QT interval can also be evaluated without any drug administration by analyzing separately the diurnal and the nocturnal periods, which are characterized by different sympathovagal influences.

Rate Dependency of the QT Interval from Resting ECG and Exercise-Testing Recordings

Investigation of the rate dependency of ventricular repolarization is still a very active field, suggesting that no satisfactory or widely admitted alternative to Bazett's equation has yet been proposed. The relations between QT and RR intervals have been extensively explored either by resting 12-lead ECG or by exercise-testing.

Relationship Between QT and RR Intervals from a Resting ECG

A resting ECG is the most classic approach. In 1920, the data obtained from only 39 young normal men led to the well-known Bazett's formula: $QTc = QT/\sqrt{RR}$.[6] In the same year Fridericia proposed the cubic-root equation, based on measurements in 50 normal subjects. Strikingly, it has not been as popular as Bazett's correction formula. Actually, Bazett's square-root formula has been criticized for more than 30 years, even by investigators using the same static ECG approach. Puddu et al.[7] compared ten QT prediction equations in 881 middle-aged men (manual measurements in lead 2, range of RR intervals 420–1280 ms) and concluded that the cubic-root equation provided the best fit to the QT/RR relation. Multiparameter equations did not improve the fit. Puddu confirmed that Bazett's formula overcorrected the QT interval at high heart rates and undercorrected it at low heart rates.[7]

Sagie et al.[8] evaluated the heart rate dependency of the QT interval from ECG data of the Framingham Heart Study, which included 5018 subjects, 2239 men and 2779 women (manual measurements from the lead with the longest QT, range of RR intervals 500–1470 ms). These authors proposed a linear regression equation [$QTc = QT + 0.154(1-RR)$] which applied for both men and women, and which corrected QT more reliably than Bazett's formula.[8] Sagie et al. also tested the models used by Puddu and confirmed that the linear regression models (except Bazett's) were not inferior to the others.

As with exercise-testing, a resting ECG only takes into account the immediately preceding cycle length. Sagie et al. used stepwise regression to differentiate the influences on QT from the preceding RR interval, sex, and age. As a single variable, the RR interval explained only 42% of the QT variance. The sex variable explained 3.6% of the variance. These authors concluded that the QT interval is related not only to this preceding cycle length, but also to other factors such as the ANS.[8] They emphasized this limitation by constructing 95% confidence intervals for QT at different RR cycle lengths: it was clear that individual variability was large. Hence, extrapolating an adjustment formula obtained from the resting ECG to explore QT dynamicity in single individuals is highly debatable.

In addition, the range of heart rates spanned in the resting ECG approach is generally narrow. Karjalainen et al.[9] evaluated the relation between QT and RR intervals at extreme heart rates in the resting ECGs of 324 healthy young men (manual measurement from the lead with the longest QT, range of heart rate 39–120 bpm). They found that a single adjustment equation was inadequate at the lowest and the highest heart rates.[9] The QT/RR relation was determined by three linear regressions: the slope values were 0.116 for a heart rate less than 60 bpm, 0.156 from 60 to 100 bpm, and 0.384 for more than 100 bpm. Karjalainen et al. also suggested that their findings could be explained by the probable influences of other modulators of the QT duration.

More recently, by using a modified treadmill protocol that produces small workload increments, Lax et al.[10] also found that it was not valid to apply the same correction formula over a wide range of exercise heart rates.

An obvious drawback of all these QT correction formulas is that, following a sudden sustained modification of the RR cycle length, the changes in QT interval lag behind the heart rate changes.[3,4,11,12] By analyzing recordings of the monophasic action potential (MAP), Franz *et al.* showed that after a sudden increase of heart rate, rapid action potential duration (APD) changes were followed by a slower adaptation phase.[3,4] The mean time to reach steady state was about 3 minutes. These authors concluded that if heart rate was not constant for at least 3 minutes, any correction of QT interval might not be valid. Lau and Ward[11] confirmed these fast and slow adaptation phases of QT intervals, with 90% of QT changes achieved in approximately 2 minutes.

Relationship between QT and RR Intervals from an Exercise-Testing ECG

More recently, exercise-testing has been proposed to investigate the QT/RR relation over a wide range of RR intervals. With the conventional resting ECG, the QT/RR paired data are collected from a group of individuals, which means that each RR value corresponds to the spontaneous resting heart rate of one subject. With exercise-testing, many RR interval changes are collected for each individual. Thus, this approach may explore more accurately the dynamicity of ventricular repolarization. However, as already mentioned, this technique does not overcome the limitation of the use of a single RR interval value. Furthermore, it mixes the respective influences of heart rate changes and the increase of the autonomic drive during exercise, as pointed out by many authors.[13–17]

Rickards and Norman analyzed 9 patients in complete heart block with ventricular pacemakers set at 70 bpm. They found that, during an exercise test, the time interval between the stimulus and the end of the T wave decreased.[13] When the atrial rate reached 100 bpm, the decrease in QT interval was 95 ms. Milne *et al.* also demonstrated that, in 11 patients who were pacemaker-dependent, exercise shortened the paced QT interval from a mean of 433 ms to 399 ms.[14] Fananapazir *et al.* determined that the contribution of the heart rate changes to the QT interval shortening during exercise varied from 26% to 75%.[15] Coghlan *et al.* reported that, in response to exercise, the QT interval during fixed-rate ventricular pacing initially lengthened;[16] after the first minute, however, the typical QT linear response was evident. Oda also found this behavior in 3 out of 9 of his reported cases.[17] Some experiments demonstrated that a brief sympathetic nerve stimulation or a rapid injection of catecholamine resulted in transient QT prolongation, and not in QT shortening. To reduce QT interval duration, sympathetic nerve stimulation had to be prolonged.[18]

The lack of separation of heart rate and ANS influences may explain why the measures of repolarization duration with respect to cycle length do not show a linear behavior. Sarma and coworkers showed that an exponential model fitted the QT/RR relation during exercise.[19,20] They also found that this exponential formula did not fit the data of the recovery phase (hysteresis phenomenon). Lecocq *et al.*[21] later confirmed this monoexponential relation:

$$QT = A - B \exp(-k\text{RR}).$$

Despite the confusion of these two influences, significant clinical conclusions have been drawn from this noninvasive electrophysiologic approach. Funck-Brentano *et al.* studied the rate-dependent effects of sotalol during a maximal exercise test.[22] They showed that the rate dependence of this class III drug was the inverse of the rate dependence of sodium-channel blockade: QT prolongation with sotalol was more pronounced when the RR interval increased, but it was concealed during exercise-induced sinus tachycardia. Vincent *et al.* used treadmill exercise to enhance the cardiac sympathetic activity in both Romano–Ward patients and normal controls.[23] They showed that the QT interval in long QT syndrome shortened through the initial phase of exercise, but did not further shorten after a threshold of approximately 115 bpm. This failure of the QT interval to shorten normally might be a helpful diagnostic criterion to implement in a scoring approach. More recently, Gill *et al.* examined the shortening of ventricular repolarization during exercise in patients with idiopathic ventricular tachycardia and compared it with patients with ischemic heart disease.[24] In patients with a structural cardiac abnormality the slope of the QT/RR relation was lower than in patients with normal hearts.

Noninvasive Electrophysiology and the Rate Dependency of the QT Interval

The use of ambulatory 24-hour recordings as a tool to evaluate the dynamicity of ventricular repolarization provides an ideal environment for a dynamic analysis. Indeed, in recent years its application has increased although not as much as could be expected. One reason for this is most probably related to the technical difficulty in quantifying the QT interval duration on ambulatory ECG data. The number of cardiac complexes (around 100 000 beats for a 24-hour recording from an adult subject) is not compatible with a manual or even a semiautomatic method. Furthermore, the reduced number of leads, the data corruption by artefacts and the presence of noise do not allow implementation of conventional quantitative ECG algorithms.

Conventional Use of Ambulatory 24-Hour Recordings

Despite the relatively poor quality of the ECG in Holter recordings, many investigators considered that it was essential to obtain a large number of QT/RR paired data per subject to investigate the QT interval dynamicity. A fully computerized method to perform a beat-to-beat quantification of ventricular repolarization duration remains a very difficult technical endpoint.

To achieve this goal, Merri *et al.* used the RTm interval (the time interval between the peak of the R wave and the peak of the T wave) instead of the global QT interval, because exact determination of Q wave onset and T wave offset was difficult.[25] This group had shown previously that the rate dependency of ventricular repolarization was located mainly in its early phase.[26] They obtained in their study more than 90 000 cardiac beats per tape. But the noise level inherent in ambulatory data resulted in critical modifications of the QRST complexes and therefore in aberrant values after the quantification procedure. A further filtering of the RR and RTm time series was needed to eliminate the outlying values. This data filtering was based on setting upper and lower limits for RR, RTm and even slope values. On average, 74% of the RR/RTm pairs were accepted following this procedure.

Laguna *et al.* presented a challenging approach to defining automatically, on a beat-to-beat basis, the end of the T wave.[27] The algorithm calculated the first derivative of the ECG signal, and its comparison with a threshold value. This approach also required the removal of nonphysiological data. The procedure for doing so was rather complex. In a set of 5 beats, the highest and the lowest QT intervals were rejected, together with the values of more than 15% from a current average.

However, the ECG segments that are most likely to contain artefacts are precisely those corresponding to daily activities, and specifically to exercising. Thus, a possible consequence of using some rejecting procedures is to eliminate the data that are most interesting clinically.

Investigators have managed this difficulty most often by performing only an intermittent sampling of the 24-hour ECG recordings (i.e. a measurement every n minutes is taken). This sampling has generally been done in real time, at large intervals such as every 30 or even 60 minutes,[29,30] or more frequently every 5 minutes.[31] The RR and QT intervals were defined on paper ECG strips, obtained at various speeds, with the help of a digitized board which also stored the data in a computer. The criteria used for determination of the T wave offset were generally those of Lepeschin and Surawicz:[28] from the steepest point of the downslope of the T wave, a tangent is drawn and its crossing with the isoelectric line is considered as the end of the T wave.

Whatever the quantity of the paired QT/RR data obtained (from a few dozen up to a hundred thousand), QT intervals have been plotted against RR intervals and the equation which best described the relation has been calculated. It has been found to be linear[25] or monoexponential,[31] and normalization of the QT intervals by this equation has been compared with the results obtained from Bazett's formula (although it had never been recommended in this situation). Holter studies confirmed that the formula overestimated QT at short RR intervals, and underestimated it at long RR, because the normalized points did form a nonrandom pattern.[31] On the contrary, a random distribution around a horizontal line was interpreted as an accurate removal of the cycle-length dependence of the QT interval.

Nevertheless, despite some technical limitations of these studies, some interesting issues have been raised. First, the waking and the sleeping periods had to be considered separately[29,30] because the QT dynamicity does not behave similarly in the two periods. Second, direct comparison of QT intervals at identical heart rates was proposed to avoid the use of any correction formula.[29,30,32,33] Finally, the concept of selection of stable heart rate segments for QT analysis has been introduced,[32] even if these stable segments were identified by visual inspection of the RR tachograms. Observed heart rate values were also used to perform intermittent sampling of the Holter data.[32–35]

In conclusion, it is apparent that a noninvasive electrophysiologic investigation of QT dynamicity from Holter recordings should consider many factors. Above all, the observation period of the heart rate should include more than one RR interval, and the ANS influences should be separated from the rate effects. A reproducible computerized analysis of ventricular repolarization has still to be defined.

QT Interval, Heart Rate and the Autonomic Nervous System

The philosophy of our method is to go beyond the conventional beat-to-beat approach where each single RR/QT couple is considered regardless of any other cardiovascular variable. We assess the QT interval in a more complex environment that attempts to take into account the heart rate and the ANS influences. One of the mandatory tools to fulfilling these goals is selective beat-averaging. Two of the major advantages of this technique are the following:

1. By 'averaging', a higher signal-to-noise ratio (SNR), which is often necessary for an accurate quantitative analysis, can be obtained. In addition, the amount of digital data to be stored/transmitted can be substantially reduced.
2. By 'selecting', the environment can be controlled. This can be done by averaging only those beats meeting specific criteria regardless of their time occurrence during the recording.

Selective beat-averaging

In conventional Holter analysis, a long-term ECG is first recorded either with a cassette or with a digital recorder. In both cases, the analysis is subsequently carried out on a dedicated computer with appropriate software. The computer platform can vary from a single PC to a multiuser workstation. Generally, the users do not have direct access to the internal information (ECG data), but simply to the standard diagnostic tools. To obtain research-oriented applications, most of the Holter systems are moving towards a more flexible environment where internal data can be accessed easily. In particular, thanks to the availability of fully digitized Holter systems, most physicians have direct access to the raw-data ECG file (ECG data constitute a relatively large file depending upon the sampling rate, the number of leads and the coding procedure) and to the so-called annotation file. The latter file (whose size is generally less than 1 Mbyte) usually includes a time series of the RR intervals (time distance between consecutive QRS complexes) and the beat label associated with the next QRS complex (normal, ventricular, ...). An annotation file is extracted from the ECG data by detection and classification processes with a perfectly superposed time track. The annotation file is the tool to perform a selective averaging of the ECG data. For instance, depending on the occurrence of normal complexes in relation to ventricular beats (VBs), one can select two different types of beats: sinus beats preceding a VB, and sinus beats following a VB. Two low-noise templates can then be computed by averaging selectively each type of normal beat.[36]

By using the same tool, all normal complexes can be classified according to the preceding heart rate. Many parameters can characterize the preceding heart rhythm, but the most accurate is the RR interval, either considered individually or averaged. The length of the observation period may vary from only a few RR intervals up to 1 or 2 minutes, or more. The standard deviation of RR intervals over that period can also be calculated as well as other descriptive parameters. Low-noise templates can be obtained by averaging selectively normal beats fitting these parameters. In our laboratory, the RR interval variables during the observation periods were stratified into intervals of 25 ms in a stepwise fashion (for instance, a range of RR intervals between 700 and 1200 ms generated 20 templates). The effects of the ANS were evaluated by processing separately the diurnal and the nocturnal periods. To enhance the sympathovagal balance differences between the two periods, we defined the diurnal period as the eight active consecutive hours with the highest heart rate and the nocturnal period as the four sleeping consecutive hours with the lowest heart rate. Hence, a single selective averaging protocol led to approximately 40 templates (20 for each of the two circadian periods).

Quantification of ventricular repolarization in Holter recordings

As long as an averaging procedure is implemented, low-noise templates can be obtained even from ambulatory ECG data containing artefacts. In Figure 22.1(a), approximately 10 seconds of Holter ECG data are shown. The corrupting muscle noise level is relatively high, but the quality of the resulting averaged template (from 78 beats) shown in Figure 22.1(b) is quite good even in the Z lead. In our experience, as in other studies,[37] a lower limit of 50 accepted beats is generally acceptable.

As far as the T wave is concerned, a crude alignment of the beats on the QRS fiducial points obtained from the RR annotation files in digitized Holter systems can be performed. It is well known that in Holter ECG data this fiducial point is not very stable (at least ± 1 sample point, or ± 7.8 ms at 128 Hz sampling rate). A significant trigger jitter phenomenon is clear in Figure 22.2(b), where the sinus beats were aligned on this QRS onset sample. In Figure 22.2(a), alignment was improved by fitting a parabola through the samples of the peak of the R wave, and one can observe the differences between the QRS waveforms when the beats are aligned on the vertex of the parabola; however, the T waveforms look similar.

By reducing random noise and by increasing the SNR, signal-averaging makes the Holter data convenient to any quantitative ECG analysis. However, because the averaging procedure is selective, the number of templates generated from a 24-hour recording is

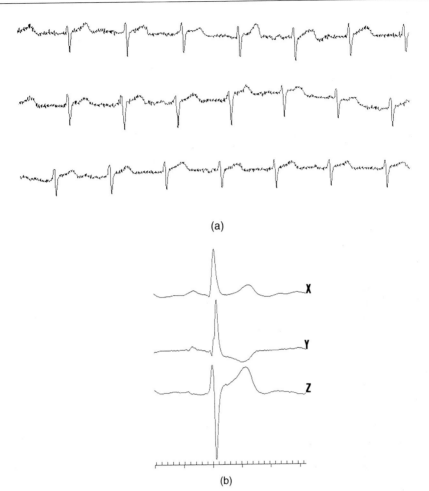

(a)

(b)

Figure 22.1 Noise reduction in Holter ECG data. (a) Ten seconds of daytime Holter ECG data (in the Z lead) corrupted by muscle noise. Digital ECG data are synchronized with the annotation file made up by beat labels and RR intervals. (b) A low-noise template obtained by averaging 78 sinus beats, including those in (a). Even in the Z lead, the signal-to-noise ratio is suitable for manual measurement or any quantitative analysis. The XYZ configuration allows the use of both scalar and spatial algorithms.

limited, and manual measurement remains feasible. Two-channel ambulatory ECG monitoring is the most commonly available system, but expanded devices that record three instead of two ECG leads are now commonly used. Consequently, patients can be hooked-up in the orthogonal bipolar XYZ-lead configuration.

The potential clinical applications of 3-lead systems are numerous, for three main reasons:

1. Three-dimensional quantitative ECG algorithms can be implemented in digitized Holter systems. This combination introduces the field of dynamic quantitative ECG analysis.
2. The vector magnitude of the orthogonal ECG data can be computed. Provided that the sampling rate and the amplitude resolution are sufficient (1000 Hz, $5\,\mu$V resolution even on short segments), high-resolution analysis can be performed.[38]

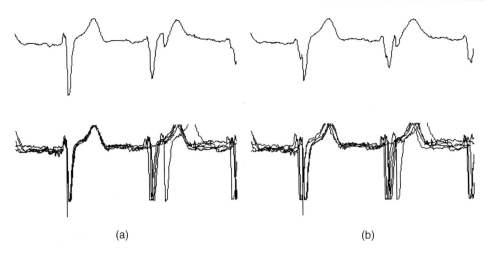

(a)   (b)

Figure 22.2   The importance of the alignment point. Five consecutive sinus beats have been averaged from a Holter recording. In (b), the alignment point is the QRS onset point provided by the annotation file: a major trigger jitter phenomenon is obvious (bottom traces). In (a), alignment has been made on a more stable point calculated by fitting a parabola through the samples of the peak of the QRS complex. Note that the averaged T waves (upper traces) have a similar pattern in both tracings.

3. The 3-lead dispersion can now be evaluated. If a good correlation with 12-lead data is confirmed, it will be possible to explore the rate-dependency of QT dispersion (see Chapter 23).

   Two different automatic quantification procedures can be used reliably. The first uses a conventional approach that determines only the apex of the T wave.[25] This scalar algorithm can be applied on single-, dual- or 3-channel ECG data. This parameter can also be computed on the vector magnitude of $\sqrt{(A^2+B^2)}$ or $\sqrt{(A^2+B^2+C^2)}$, in order to reduce the postural rotation of the heart. The peak amplitude of ECG samples in a time window following the previous QRS waveform is identified (Figure 22.3), and then a parabola is fitted through 10 samples centered in the maximum amplitude (at 200 Hz sampling frequency). The vertex of the parabola is used as the fiducial point for the apex of the T wave (QTa time interval). Many other quantitative variables of the repolarization could be computed.[26]

   However, scalar determination of the end of the T wave remains difficult even from low-noise templates. An alternative approach is to use a 3-D quantitative ECG analysis, which, by definition, can only process data originated from 3-lead recordings. A 3-D software named CAVIAR (Comparative Analysis of VCGs and their Interpretation with Auto-Reference to the patient) is preferred; it is a serial algorithm, dedicated to compare two spatial loops rather than to quantify a single complex (it can be applied to QRS or T loops but data only on the T loop will be presented). The implementation of CAVIAR has been described in detail elsewhere.[39] Briefly, the two loops to be compared are not projected in the conventional Frank XYZ system, but in a new orthogonal system UVW, related to a preferential space made up by the two maximum inertia axes of the loops. The aim of this procedure is to free the loops from extracardiac factors like thorax anatomy, respiratory phase, and heart position. The deviation between the loops (see Figure 22.4) is quantified by their mean quadratic deviation (MQD), which is the mean of the squared differences between homologous points on the two loops. The key feature of this program is the systematic assumption that there is no intrinsic change between the two loops superimposed in their preferential space. This statement results in an iterative procedure with the aim of minimizing the MQD. The program carries out geometric

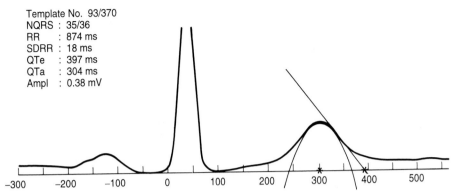

Figure 22.3 Determination of a T wave apex. The validated sinus complexes from 30 seconds of Holter ECG data have been averaged. This selective procedure, on a time basis only, leads to 2880 templates for a 24-hour recording. The peak of the T wave has been determined by fitting a parabola through the samples of a window following the QRS complex. The end of the T wave is calculated by the method described by Lepeschkin and Surawicz. The corresponding numerical data are shown in the left part of the figure. They include the number of sinus complexes within the template, the mean and the standard deviation of the RR intervals. Both annotation list and raw ECG data are used simultaneously to construct a 30-second template.

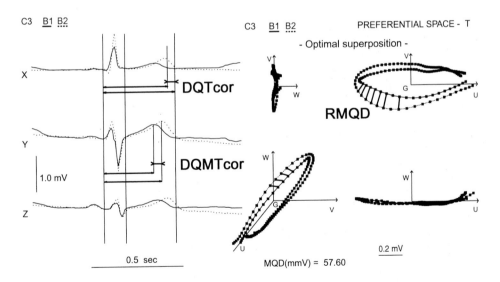

Figure 22.4 Quantitative comparison of two cardiac beats by the 3-D approach. The XYZ scalar representation of two beats B1 and B2 to be compared is shown in the left part of the figure. The two corresponding T loops are projected in their preferential space and the MQD between the two loops is calculated (right part). Then an iterative procedure tends to minimize the MQD by using time-resynchronization and geometric transformations. When the MQD is stabilized, the time-interval differences between B1 and B2 are calculated from the newly obtained fiducial points. MQD = mean quadratic deviation; RMQD = mean quadratic deviation of the repolarization loop; DQTcor = difference in QT corrected for resynchronization; DQMTcor = difference in Q to maximum (apex) of the T wave, corrected for resynchronization.

transformations, such as rotation and translation, as well as a time-related synchronization in order to correct the T wave delineation errors (Figure 22.4). The procedure reaches stability (i.e. MQD is stabilized) after approximately 15 iterations. Of note, the values of the MQD obtained from low-noise Holter-averaged templates are in the range 20–50 μV, which is equivalent to or even less than the values obtained from resting ECG.[40,41] Finally, the changes in both morphology and chronology between the two complexes can be quantified. In this chapter, only the differences in the time interval variables calculated by CAVIAR will be reported, excluding other morphologic indexes such as, for instance, the planarity of the loops. It is noteworthy that, either by means of the parabola method or by using a *serial* 3-D approach, the resolution of the QT quantification procedure is in the range of 1 millisecond, higher than the ECG sampling rate.

Since the implementation of this link between Holter data and a conventional quantitative analysis, significant improvements in signal processing have been achieved in our laboratory. At the very beginning, Holter analog data were sampled at 128 Hz; then the analog tapes could be digitized at 256 samples per second and the amplitude resolution reached 5 μV. More recently, fully digital recorders have been developed, with user-defined parameters.[42] At the time of writing, we can easily record six consecutive hours at 1000 Hz sampling rate with a 5 μV amplitude resolution, and it is clear now that the specifications of ambulatory recorders will match in the very near future those of diagnostic devices.

The main characteristic of a quantitative approach based on an averaging process is that beat-to-beat changes of ventricular repolarization and their relationship with RR variability are deliberately ignored. Actually, both the parabola method and the 3-D program can be applied on individual consecutive beats and on low-noise averaged templates.[39] However, from the experience of Merri and Laguna with such data,[25,27] it appears that the removal of aberrant data is a crucial issue. Moreover, most of the published works investigating this aspect of ventricular repolarization flexibility refer to short-duration ECG segments, and not to continuous 24-hour data.[34]

Heart Rate Dependency of the QT Interval

To follow different aspects of the rate dependency of the ventricular repolarization duration, three selective averaging protocols were designed. Our rationale was that a mean RR interval and other descriptors of the cardiac rhythm, calculated over 1 or 2 minutes or even longer, could be much more representative of the cycle length influences on QT interval duration than the value of the single preceding RR interval as in Bazett's formula. This is a simple way to track noninvasively the memory phenomenon of the T wave.

These protocols were carried out in 17 young male healthy subjects aged 20–25 years. All had a normal physical examination, and were free of any medication. They underwent a resting 12-lead ECG and 2-dimensional echocardiography to eliminate any cardiac abnormality. A 24-hour Holter recording was then performed by a 3-channel analog tape-recorder (Del Mar Avionics, model 459) with an XYZ pseudo-orthogonal electrode configuration. We studied the effects of the following selective averaging protocols:

1. The preceding sinus cycle (RR-1) before a target complex was fixed but the mean preceding RR interval was variable.
2. This preceding cardiac rhythm was programmed to be stable or unstable.
3. The mean preceding RR interval could be further filtered by its standard deviation.

Here we report the rate dependency of the QT apex interval duration, measured either by the 3-D program or by the scalar parabola approach. We deal later with the respective dynamic behavior of the global QT interval duration and of its early phase QTa.

The role of the mean preceding heart rate

The first selective averaging protocol was designed to study the respective influences of the immediately preceding RR-1 interval and of the mean value of the preceding RR intervals, calculated over 1 minute (RRMN-1). For each beat, labeled as normal in the annotation file, the software examined the value of the RR-1. If this single value was equal (± 15 ms) to the mean RR value of the corresponding circadian period (the mean diurnal and nocturnal RR cycle lengths varied from one subject to another), this beat was extracted from the ECG file. The RRMN-1 value was then used as a second criterion to classify in steps of 25 ms the selected normal beats in a template (Figure 22.5).

The rationale for this approach was that, if conventional correction formulas were accurate, the QTa interval duration should not vary significantly from one 25 ms class to

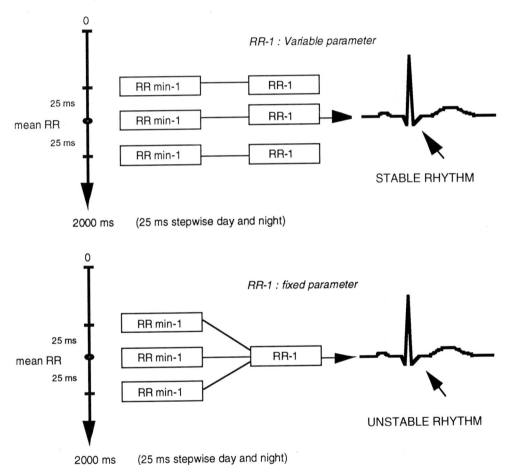

Figure 22.5 A rate-basis selective averaging protocol can be used to mimic a stable or an unstable heart rate environment before a target complex. *Lower panel*: First, the single RR-1 interval before the complex has to be identical (± 15 ms) to the mean RR of the explored circadian period. The mean RR value has been chosen to obtain a large number of beats. All beats obtained from the first filter are further classified according to the value of RRMN-1 (left vertical scale). Consequently, the cardiac rhythm must include a recent modification, either a decreasing or an increasing trend. *Upper panel*: The RR-1 and the RRMN-1 are always set at the same value and classified in 25 ms steps. The cardiac rhythm which precedes the target complex is relatively stable. QTa and global QT intervals will be plotted against RRMN-1.

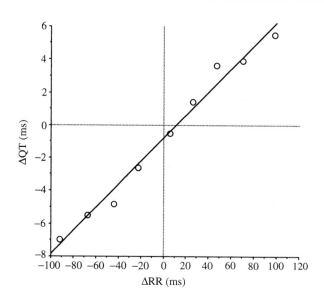

RR-1	RR min-1	ΔRR	ΔQT
670	578	-92	-7
669	602	-67	-5,5
668	624	-44	-4,8
669	647	-22	-2,6
672	678	6	-0,5
672	698	26	1,4
673	720	47	3,6
672	742	70	3,9
672	770	98	5,5

Figure 22.6 Respective influences of RR-1 and RRMN-1 intervals on QT dynamicity. The QT interval differences between templates (ΔQT) are plotted against the differences in milliseconds between RR-1 and RRMN-1 (see Figure 22.5, lower panel). Although RR-1 was very stable (668–673 ms), the QT differences were positively correlated ($r^2 = 0.98$) with the recent RR interval variations (ΔRR). In this subject, the range of ΔRR was −92 ms to +98 ms.

another, as long as the RR-1 interval was programmed to be stable. But if the memory phenomenon of the T wave does exist, then the QTa interval might vary according to another RR interval time-scale. Even when RR-1 was fixed, we found a significant linear relation between the QTa interval duration and the value of RRMN-1. The correlation coefficient was high in both circadian periods ($r = 0.86$ during the day and $r = 0.84$ at night). The slope of this relation was steeper during the diurnal period than during the nocturnal one (0.110 versus 0.094 respectively) but it did not reach statistical significance.

Figure 22.6 is a graphic representation of the results obtained from the diurnal data in one representative subject. The corresponding numerical values from this example are displayed in the lower part of the figure. It becomes obvious that the larger the variation between the two cycle-length variables RR-1 and RRMN-1, the larger the QT interval modification.

The role of the preceding heart rate stability

Since the influence of the mean RR value of the preceding minute seems of major importance, the effects of an unstable rhythm, including short-term changes of the RR cycle length, might be different from those of a stable rhythm with a more constant RR interval. To explore this rather unusual aspect of the rate dependency of the ventricular repolarization duration, the averaging protocol described above was modified. The RR-1 cycle length could be set either as a fixed parameter or as a variable one, always identical to the RRMN-1 value (Figure 22.5). In that case, both RR-1 and RRMN-1 were classified 25 ms stepwise.

According to this simple algorithm, when RR-1 was a fixed parameter differing from RRMN-1, the target normal beat was considered to be preceded by an unstable cardiac rhythm; on the other hand, when RR-1 and RRMN-1 were equal, the normal beat was considered to be preceded by a stable rhythm. These definitions of stability and instability remain to be improved on. When the preceding RR interval was considered as constant for 1 minute, the relation between QTa and RRMN-1 was linear ($r = 0.92$ during the day, $r = 0.86$ at night) and the value of the diurnal slope was higher than the nocturnal one (0.162 versus 0.120, $p = 0.02$). In 15 subjects, we could select normal beats preceded by a stable heart rate as defined previously for 2 and even for 3 minutes (only for the diurnal period). The slopes of the relation at 2 and 3 minutes were respectively 0.146 and 0.154, and they were not different from the QTa/RRMN-1 relation. Moreover, we compared the results obtained from the two models (stable and unstable rhythm simulation). In both cases, the mean values of the preceding RR intervals calculated over 1 minute (25 ms classified) were identical, but the regression lines were higher in a stable environment (0.160 versus 0.115 during the day, $p < 0.001$; and 0.126 versus 0.094 at night, $p < 0.01$).

The role of the standard deviation of RR intervals

The variance of beat-to-beat RR interval fluctuations is a time-domain parameter which describes the global variability of the signal. It is mathematically equivalent to the total power spectrum of the RR time-series. As a simple model of stability strikingly modified the QTa/RRMN-1 relation, a third selective averaging procedure was implemented, aimed at filtering the cardiac complexes by both the mean preceding RR interval and its standard deviation. However, for various technical reasons (mainly time consumption), we slightly modified our method.

After a careful validation of all morphologic classes, all sinus complexes were averaged on a 30-second time basis, excluding artifacts, supraventricular and ventricular beats, to obtain low-noise templates. The QT apex interval was determined automatically for each template by the scalar approach (parabola fitted through the peak of the T wave, see above). The resulting 2880 templates (for a complete 24-hour recording) were then classified according to their corresponding mean RR interval computed over 1, 2 or 3 minutes, separately for the two circadian periods (Figure 22.7). We used a cutoff value of 50 ms for the standard deviation (SD) of RR intervals within the corresponding period to filter the RR classes. The relation between the QTa interval duration of a 30-second template and the mean RR interval was calculated consecutively with and without the SD filtering criterion. This allowed us to differentiate the QTa/RR relation in a low heart-rate-variability environment.

Our results are shown in Table 22.1. The QTa/RR relation was linear ($r = 0.99$ during the day and $r = 0.94$ at night for a 1-minute observation period) and the regression line was higher again during the waking period (0.142 versus 0.093, $p < 0.01$). When the SD filtering criterion was applied, we did not observe any significant changes in the diurnal

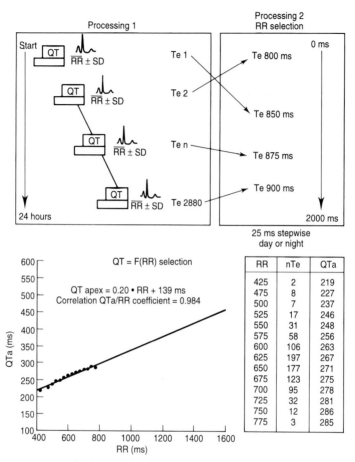

Figure 22.7 Calculation of the standard deviation of RR intervals. 2880 templates can be computed by means of a time-basis selective protocol (left part). Their mean RR interval is used to organize them into RR classes from 25 ms to 25 ms (middle part). The standard deviation is also calculated at this step. Note that the number of templates (nTe) within each RR class varies (right table). The equation is then computed from the 25 ms classification table. The standard deviation of RR intervals associated with each template can be used to select ECG data in a low-HRV environment.

relations. However, the nocturnal slope values were higher in a low-HRV environment. In this situation the circadian trend was no longer evident.

Figure 22.8 shows the effects of a filtering procedure of the templates by means of the SD value in one subject. Only the nocturnal slopes significantly changed, although the percentage of reduction of the number of templates was nearly identical for the two periods.

The role of long-term circadian modulation

Whatever the selective averaging protocol used, we consistently found that the QTa/RR relations were dependent on the circadian period (Table 22.2). All regression lines were lower during sleep. Browne *et al.* were the first to describe this circadian trend.[29] In their study, the values of the slopes were quite similar to those obtained from our different

Table 22.1 Role of the standard deviation of RR intervals on the QTa/RR regression lines. QT interval values have been plotted against the mean RR interval, calculated over 1, 2 and 3 minutes (left day and night columns). The QTa/RR relation is then computed only from minutes with a low HRV environment (right day and night columns).

Filter	Day QTa/RR slopes			Night QTa/RR slopes		
	$\overline{RR}$		$\overline{RR}$ SD < 50 ms	$\overline{RR}$		$\overline{RR}$ SD < 50 ms
1 min	0.142	NS	0.144	0.093*		0.129
2 min	0.144	NS	0.137	0.092*		0.131
3 min	0.139	NS	0.141	0.094**		0.129

*$p < 0.05$; **$p < 0.01$.

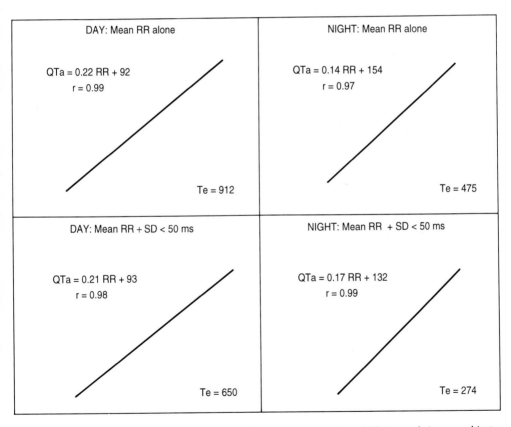

Figure 22.8 Effects of selective averaging using the standard deviation of RR intervals in one subject. First, the 2880 templates were classified (upper panel) according only to their mean RR intervals, separately for the two circadian periods. Then the SD is set at a 50 ms cutoff value and the templates fitting this criterion are selected (lower panel). During the day, the regression lines do not differ, but at night the QTa/RR relation is steeper in a low-HRV environment. The number of templates (*n*Te) obtained from each selective averaging protocol is indicated in the right bottom part of each plot. All the correlation coefficients are over 0.96.

Table 22.2 Circadian modulation of the QTa/RR relation. Whatever the averaging protocol used, the regression lines are lower during the nocturnal period.

Model	Day	Night
Unstable HR	0.11	0.094
Stable HR	0.162	0.120*
Mean RR	0.142	0.093**

*$p < 0.05$; **$p < 0.01$.

models (0.134 the diurnal and 0.113 the nocturnal). Furthermore, they emphasized that the regression lines for daytime and nighttime were significantly different from the global QT/RR relation calculated by merging the 24-hour data.

The group from Zipes' laboratory was also the first to show from Holter data that the ventricular repolarization duration was prolonged during the nocturnal period. To demonstrate this phenomenon, they proposed to make a direct comparison on QT intervals at similar RR interval levels between the two states, by means of the regression lines provided that there was a sufficient overlap of RR intervals. At an RR value of 1000 ms, Browne *et al.* reported a 19 ms QT prolongation during sleep.[29] Alexopoulos *et al.* applied the same approach in denervated transplanted human hearts and did not find any difference in the QT between awake and sleep states in transplant patients.[30]

Viitasalo and Karjalainen later improved this method by selecting spontaneous stable heart rates before calculating the nocturnal lengthening of QT intervals. They found, at a stable heart rate of 60 bpm that was common to the two states, an 18 ms QT prolongation at night.[32]

The long-term modulating influences of the circadian periods were demonstrated by Bexton *et al.*, who assessed the changes of the QT interval from Holter recordings in patients totally pacemaker-dependent, but with normally innervated hearts. QT intervals were longer during sleep than during waking hours (the pacemakers were programmed to a pacing rate of 70 bpm), and the largest changes occurred during morning hours.[43] In contrast, in diabetic patients with proven autonomic neuropathy, there was no diurnal variation of the QT intervals (the hourly variations in heart rate were almost absent in these patients).

Our data are in good accordance with these previous findings. For instance, in our study population the QTa duration increased by 19 ms at a common RR interval of 900 ms ($p < 0.01$). Furthermore, this result was obtained by a fully automatic procedure.

The Respective Dynamic Behavior of QTa and QT Interval Durations

To date, Holter studies dealing with the rate dependency of ventricular repolarization duration have considered either the QT apex interval alone[25] or (most often) the global QT interval.[27,29–35] Choice of the QTa interval as a surrogate of the global repolarization duration was based on the work of O'Donnell, Rubel and Merri.

O'Donnell *et al.* found that the terminal part of the repolarization decreased between rest and maximal exercise in normal men.[44] However, when measurements were made separately during two stages (at standing rest and maximal exercise, over a wide range of heart rates between individuals), the terminal phase of the QT interval was not rate-dependent.

Rubel *et al.* showed that the terminal segment of the ventricular repolarization measured by the CAVIAR program was very stable in a cohort of 242 healthy national

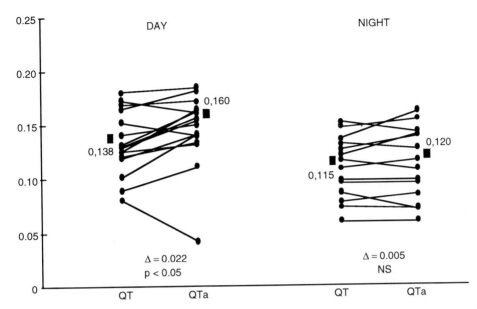

Figure 22.9 Respective dynamic behavior of QTa and QT intervals. The vertical axis corresponds to the slope values of the QTa/RR and QT/RR relations. Comparisons between the two repolarization variables have been made separately for day and night. The QTa/RR regression line is higher than the QT/RR one, but only during the day.

servicemen recorded twice with a 3-month delay.[40] Although this segment was the most stable ECG variable, only a weak correlation with the RR interval was found.

Merri *et al.* reported that, among seven repolarization variables excluding the total QT duration, only the SoTm interval duration (between the S wave offset and the peak of the T wave) was dependent on heart rate. The TmTo interval (between Tm and the T wave offset) notably was RR independent.[26] When compared, the linear regression lines between the QT and SoTm intervals were not found to be identical. In the total population, the slope (after logarithmic transformation of QT and RR values) was 0.40 for the QT interval and 0.46 for SoTm. This difference was even more pronounced according to gender: 0.40 versus 0.59 in women and 0.44 versus 0.53 in men.

In these three studies, each RR interval value was obtained from a single patient. This is slightly different from any usual Holter approach to the rate dependency of any ECG variable, where a wide range of RR values can be spontaneously observed in each recording. The use of a 3-D quantitative analysis (see above) allowed us to quantify separately the duration of the total QT interval and the duration of its different time components. The respective rate dependencies of the QTa and of the QT intervals in our patient population are presented in Figure 22.9. In a stable HR environment, the QTa/RR regression lines were higher than the QT/RR ones, but the difference reached statistical significance only during the day (0.160 versus 0.138, $p = 0.02$). Comparison of the slopes in an unstable environment did not evidence any variation between the dynamicity of QT and QTa intervals. Figure 22.10 shows the circadian QTa and QT dynamicities in a typical case.

Physiological and Pathophysiological Behavior of QT Dynamicity

Our data demonstrate clearly that the rate dependency of the QT interval cannot be described accurately by a single equation. We found strong linear correlations between

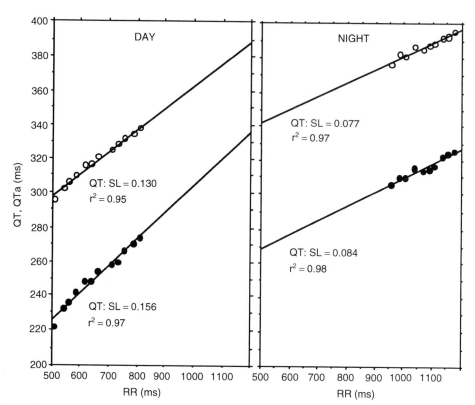

Figure 22.10 The respective behaviors of QTa and QT intervals in one representative subject. The diurnal and the nocturnal regression lines were obtained in a stable HR environment. The time intervals are plotted against RRMN-1 (and not RR-1). It is noteworthy that the slopes of the QTa/RR relations are steeper than the QT/RR ones. All the correlation coefficients are over 0.94.

the QT interval measurements and the mean RR interval calculated over 1 minute. No other mathematical approach improved the goodness of fit of the relation. However, the discussion about the respective drawbacks and advantages of some equations appears to be much less meaningful since we showed that multiple physiological factors may influence the QT/RR relation. No formula for rate correction of QT intervals can be applied equivalently during the day and at night. Within each circadian period, the choice of the cycle-length variable to describe the relationship between QT and heart rate is crucial. Our results indicate that a mean RR interval performs better than the usual single preceding RR interval. Nevertheless, an identical averaged RR value can be obtained from various cardiac rhythms. The presence of a decreasing or increasing trend in this rhythm will lead to a significantly different formula, when compared with a stable rhythm. Similarly, a mean RR interval will influence the QT interval according to its heart rate variability environment.

Another interesting finding in our study is that the implications drawn from the rate dependency of the early phase of ventricular repolarization (QTa interval) are not valid for the total duration of the repolarization, at least for the diurnal period. Consequently, one has to be cautious about the clinical significance of QT interval adaptation in response to changes in heart rate. A normal or abnormal dynamic behavior may be highly dependent on the choices of the rate and repolarization variables.

Physiological Behavior of QT Dynamicity

The long-term circadian modulation of QT interval duration has been related to both the increase of the parasympathetic activity and the decrease of the sympathetic tone occurring at night. Aging tends to decrease this circadian flexibility: a comparison of 11 young (31 ± 6 years) and 15 older (58 ± 10) normal subjects showed that the nocturnal lengthening was significantly greater in the young group (33 versus 19 ms).

The influence of the parasympathetic nervous system on the electrophysiologic properties of the ventricle has been assessed in many studies *in vitro* and *in vivo*. Litovsky and Antzelevitch have demonstrated that acetylcholine prolonged action potential duration (APD) in canine ventricular epicardium.[45] This direct effect was reversed with atropine. In humans, parasympathetic influence has often been studied by autonomic blockade with atropine. Prystowsky *et al.*[46] and Morady *et al.*[47] have shown that cholinergic blockade shortened ventricular refractoriness regardless of background sympathetic activity. Eckberg and coworkers explored the direct effects of enhanced vagal tone using neck suction or phenylephrine infusion; they found that vagal stimulation significantly prolonged ventricle refractoriness.[48]

In contrast, as previously said, a sympathetic stimulation has complex effects on the physiology of APD:[18] brief adrenergic stimulation increases the QT interval whereas prolonged stimulation shortens APD. Results of studies have suggested that chronic beta-blockade prolongs the QT interval in man but not acute administration.[46,47,49,50] Sarma *et al.* evaluated the effects of a single oral dose of propranolol (40 mg) on the QT/RR relation during exercise; propranolol exhibited a 'biphasic' effect on this relation, as it significantly prolonged the QT interval at long RR cycle lengths, and shortened it at shorter cycle lengths.[51]

The circadian modulation of QT dynamicity first evidenced by Browne *et al.*[29] and confirmed in our experiments has not been clearly explained. Cappato *et al.* found no significant differences between QT/RR slopes during basal state and after the administration of intravenous propranolol.[5] However, after autonomic blockade (propranolol plus atropine) the mean slope was significantly lower than in the basal state. These authors concluded that the rate-dependent changes in QT were influenced essentially by the vagal tone. In contrast, in patients with implanted pacemakers programmed in atrial synchronized mode, Fananapazir *et al.* showed that when the heart rate was increased at rest, the QT interval shortening was lower than during exercise.[15] Furthermore, the QT interval shortening was reduced by beta-adrenergic blockade with 100 mg atenolol given orally 1 hour before exercise tests. Opposite conclusions about the potential role of the sympathetic nervous system on the QT interval dynamicity could be drawn from these studies. This discrepancy could be explained on the basis of 'accentuated antagonism'. Both the hemodynamic and electrophysiologic effects of the parasympathetic nervous system have been found to be accentuated in the setting of a beta-adrenergic stimulation.[45,47]

Finally, the differences between the QTa and QT interval dynamicities might be related to the heterogeneity within the ventricular wall.[45,52] The rate dependence of APD is more pronounced in epicardium than in endocardium: at short cycle lengths, the epicardium APD is less prolonged than in endocardium, but it is more prolonged at long cycle lengths. Furthermore, a subpopulation of cells has been identified by Sicouri and Antzelevitch in the deep subepicardium, named 'M cells'.[52] Their rate dependence is even higher than that of epicardium and endocardium. The differences in the electrophysiologic characteristics of these tissue types might contribute to the electrocardiographic aspects of the T wave.

Pathophysiological Behavior of QT Dynamicity

Recent data have shown that the lack of circadian flexibility of the QT interval duration is a very sensitive index of the presence of underlying cardiac disease. Alexopoulos et al.[30] and Bexton et al.[43] had already demonstrated that in denervated hearts the QT interval was no longer prolonged during the nocturnal period. Murakawa et al.[33] later showed that the relative increase of the QT interval at night was larger in healthy subjects than in patients with coronary artery disease ($4.2 \pm 2.1\%$ versus $2.2 \pm 1.8\%$ at a heart rate of 60 bpm, $p < 0.01$). The same significant reduction of the circadian flexibility of the QTa interval was found in two groups of patients with left ventricular hypertrophy and with heart failure (7.4 ± 10.3 ms and 8.0 ± 10.5 ms, respectively, versus 19.9 ± 6.7 ms in an age-matched control group). Impairment of vagal activity, which is frequently associated with ischemic heart disease and heart failure, probably explains the loss of QT nocturnal lengthening in these settings.

The LQTS is characterized by exercise- or stress-induced ventricular arrhythmias, syncope and sudden death. However, it probably has an electrophysiologic substrate. Recent genetic studies have emphasized the limitations of a resting QTc cutoff value of 440 ms (in lead II) for the diagnosis of LQTS patients. In these patients, determination of the rate dependency of the QT interval may be helpful. Our preliminary results confirm the complexity of this approach. Indeed, we found the expected impairment of QT interval adaptation only during the diurnal period. But, to detect this diurnal impairment, it was mandatory to observe the QT variations following a recent modification in heart rate (unstable selective protocol), and furthermore to quantify separately the QTa and global QT durations. Indeed, when the cycle length was stable for 1 minute (stable selective protocol), the QTa and QT intervals in a group of 20 LQTS patients (with a mean age of 23 ± 15 years) behaved as in the age- and sex-matched controls. After a short-term change of the heart rate, the diurnal QTa/RR slope was lower than in controls (0.096 versus 0.128, $p < 0.01$), but the QT/RR slope was nearly identical in both groups (0.99 versus 0.104, NS). During the nocturnal period, our findings were the opposite: the regression lines between any ventricular repolarization parameters and heart rate were always higher in LQTS patients than in normal subjects. In other terms, the rate dependency of the QT interval in the long QT syndrome is a polymorphic phenomenon, necessitating a flexible tool to be handled accurately.

References

1. Singh BN. When is QT prolongation antiarrhythmic and when is it proarrhythmic? *Am J Cardiol* 1989; **63**: 867–9.
2. Franz MR. Time for yet another QT correction algorithm? Bazett and beyond. *J Am Coll Cardiol* 1994; **23**: 1554–6.
3. Franz MR, Swerdlow CD, Liem BL *et al*. Cycle-length dependence of human action potential duration *in vivo*: effects of single extrastimuli, sudden sustained rate acceleration and deceleration, and different steady-state frequencies. *J Clin Invest* 1988; **82**: 972–9.
4. Franz MR, Swerdlow CD, Liem BL *et al*. Cycle-length dependence of human ventricular action potential duration in the steady and non-steady state. In: Butrous GS, Schwartz PJ (eds), *Clinical Aspects of Ventricular Repolarization*. London: Farrand Press, 1989: 163.
5. Cappato R, Alboni P, Pedroni P *et al*. Sympathetic and vagal influences on rate-dependent changes of QT interval in healthy subjects. *Am J Cardiol* 1991; **68**: 1188–93.
6. Bazett HC. An analysis of the time relations of electrocardiograms. *Heart* 1920; **7**: 353–70.
7. Puddu PE, Jouve R, Mariotti S *et al*. Evaluation of ten QT prediction formulas in 881 middle-aged med from the seven countries study: emphasis on the cubic-root Fridericias' equation. *J Electrocardiol* 1988; **21**: 219–29.
8. Sagie A, Larson MG, Goldberg RJ *et al*. An improved method for adjusting the QT interval for heart rate (the Framingham Heart Study). *Am J Cardiol* 1992; **70**: 797–801.
9. Karjalainen J, Viitasalo M, Manttari M *et al*. Relations between QT intervals and heart rates from 40 to 120 beats/min in rest electrocardiograms of men and a simple method to adjust QT interval values. *J Am Coll Cardiol* 1994; **23**: 1547–53.
10. Lax KG, Okin PM, Kligfield P. Electrocardiographic repolarization measurements at rest and during exercise in normal subjects and in patients with coronary artery disease. *Am Heart J* 1994; **128**: 271–80.

11. Lau CP, Ward DE. QT hysteresis: the effects of an abrupt change in pacing rate. In: Butrous GS, Schwartz PJ (eds), *Clinical Aspects of Ventricular Repolarization*. London: Farrand Press, 1989: 175.

12. Arnold L, Page J, Attwell D et al. The dependence on heart rate of the human ventricular action potential duration. *Cardiovasc Res* 1982; **16**: 547–51.

13. Rickards AF, Norman J. Relation between QT interval and heart rate: new design of physiologically adaptive cardiac pacemakers. *Br Heart J* 1981; **45**: 56–61.

14. Milne JR, Ward DE, Spurrell RAJ et al. The ventricular paced QT interval: the effects of rate and exercise. *PACE* 1982; **5**: 352–8.

15. Fananapazir L, Bennett DH, Faragher EB. Contribution of heart rate to QT interval shortening during exercise. *Eur Heart J* 1983; **4**: 265–71.

16. Coghlan JG, Madden B, Norrell MN et al. Paradoxical early lengthening and subsequent linear shortening of the QT interval in response to exercise. *Eur Heart J* 1992; **13**: 1325–8.

17. Oda E. Changes in QT interval during exercise testing in patients with VVI pacemakers. *PACE* 1986; **9**: 36–41.

18. Abildskov JA. Adrenergic effects on the QT interval of the electrocardiogram. *Am Heart J* 1976; **92**: 210–16.

19. Sarma JSM, Sarma RJ, Bilitch M et al. An exponential formula for heart rate dependence of QT interval during exercise and cardiac pacing in humans: reevaluation of Bazett's formula. *Am J Cardiol* 1984; **54**: 103–8.

20. Sarma JSM, Venkataraman K, Samant DR et al. Hysteresis in the human RR–QT relationship during exercise and recovery. *PACE* 1987; **10**: 485–91.

21. Lecocq B, Lecocq V, Jaillon P. Physiologic relation between cardiac cycle and QT duration in healthy volunteers. *Am J Cardiol* 1989; **63**: 481–6.

22. Funck-Brentano C, Kibleur Y, Lecoz F et al. Rate dependence of sotalol-induced prolongation of ventricular repolarization during exercise in humans. *Circulation* 1991; **83**: 536–45.

23. Vincent GM, Jaiswal D, Timothy KW. Effects of exercise on heart rate, QT, QTc and QT/QS2 in the Romano–Ward inherited long QT syndrome. *Am J Cardiol* 1991; **68**: 498–503.

24. Gill JS, Baszko A, Xia R et al. Dynamics of the QT interval in patients with exercise-induced ventricular tachycardia in normal and abnormal hearts. *Am Heart J* 1993; **126**: 1357–63.

25. Merri M, Moss AJ, Benhorin J et al. Relation between ventricular repolarization duration and cardiac cycle length during 24-hour Holter recordings: findings in normal patients and patients with long QT syndrome. *Circulation* 1992; **85**: 1816–21.

26. Merri M, Benhorin J, Alberti M et al. Electrocardiographic quantitation of ventricular repolarization. *Circulation* 1989; **80**: 1301–8.

27. Laguna P, Thakor NV, Caminal P et al. New algorithm for QT interval analysis in 24-hour Holter ECG: performance and application. *Med Biol Eng Comput* 1990; **28**: 67–73.

28. Lepeschkin E, Surawicz B. The measurement of the QT interval of the electrocardiogram. *Circulation* 1952; **6**: 378–88.

29. Browne KF, Prystovsky E, Heger JJ et al. Prolongation of the QT interval in man during sleep. *Am J Cardiol* 1983; **52**: 55–9.

30. Alexopoulos D, Rynkiewicz A, Yusuf S et al. Diurnal variations of QT interval after cardiac transplantation. *Am J Cardiol* 1988; **61**: 482–5.

31. Sarma JSM, Venkataraman K, Nicod P et al. Circadian rhythmicity of rate-normalized QT interval in hypothyroidism and its significance for development of class III antiarrhythmic agents. *Am J Cardiol* 1990; **66**: 959–63.

32. Viitasao M, Karjalainen J. QT intervals at heart rates from 50 to 120 beats per minute during 24-hour electrocardiographic recordings in 100 healthy men: effects of atenolol. *Circulation* 1992; **86**: 1439–42.

33. Murakawa Y, Inoue H, Nozaki A et al. Role of sympathovagal interaction in diurnal variation of QT interval. *Am J Cardiol* 1992; **69**: 339–43.

34. Sarma JSM, Singh N, Schoenbaum MP et al. Circadian and power spectral changes of RR and QT intervals during treatment of patients with angina pectoris with nadolol providing evidence for differential autonomic modulation of heart rate and ventricular repolarization. *Am J Cardiol* 1994; **74**: 131–6.

35. Sadanaga T, Ogawa S, Okada Y et al. Clinical evaluation of the use-dependent QRS prolongation and the reverse use-dependent QT prolongation of class I and class III antiarrhythmic agents and their value in predicting efficacy. *Am Heart J* 1993; **126**: 114–21.

36. Narayanaswamy S, Berbari EJ, Lander P et al. Selective beat signal averaging and spectral analysis of beat intervals to determine the mechanisms of premature ventricular contractions. In: *Computers in Cardiology 1993*. Los Alamitos: IEEE Computer Society Press, 1993: 81–4.

37. Schmidt G, Barthel P, Kreuzberg H et al. Flecainide, mexiletine and propafenone: QRS width in Holter ECGs. *J Am Coll Cardiol* 1993; **21**: 171A.

38. Kelen G, Henkin R, Lannon M et al. Correlation between the signal-average electrocardiogram from Holter tapes and from real-time recordings. *Am J Cardiol* 1989; **63**: 1321–5.

39. Fayn J, Hamidi S, Maison-Blanche P et al. Quantitative assessment of changes in the repolarization phase in Holter recordings using CAVIAR. In: *Computers in Cardiology 1992*. Los Alamitos: IEEE Computer Society Press, 1992: 171–4.

40. Rubel P, Fayn J, Mohsen N et al. New methods of quantitative assessment of the extent and significance of serial ECG changes of the repolarization phase. *J Electrocardiol* 1988; **21**(Suppl): S177–81.

41. Fayn J, Rubel P, Mohsen N. An improved method for the precise measurement of serial ECG changes in QRS duration and QT interval: performance assessment on the CSE noise testing database and on a healthy 720-case-set population. *J Electrocardiol* 1992; **24**(Suppl): S123–7.

42. De Maso J, Myers S, Nels D *et al.* Ambulatory high-resolution ECG recorder using disk storage. *J Ambul Monit* 1992; **5**: 317–22.

43. Bexton RS, Vallin HO, Camm AJ. Diurnal variation of the QT interval: influence of the autonomic nervous system. *Br Heart J* 1986; **55**: 253–8.

44. O'Donnell J, Knoebel SB, Lovelace DE *et al.* Computer quantitation of QT and terminal T wave (aT–eT) intervals during exercise: methodology and results in normal men. *Am J Cardiol* 1981; **47**: 1168–72.

45. Litovsky SH, Antzelevitch C. Differences in the electrophysiological response of canine ventricular subendocardium and subepicardium to acetylcholine and isoproterenol: a direct effect of acetylcholine in ventricular myocardium. *Circ Res* 1990; **67**: 615–27.

46. Prystowsky EN, Jackmann WM, Rinkenberger RL *et al.* Effect of autonomic blockade on ventricular refractoriness and atrioventricular nodal conduction in humans: evidence supporting a direct cholinergic action on ventricular muscle refractoriness. *Circ Res* 1981; **49**: 511–18.

47. Morady F, Kou WH, Nelson SD *et al.* Accentuated antagonism between beta-adrenergic and vagal effects on ventricular refractoriness in humans. *Circulation* 1988; **77**: 289–97.

48. Ellenbogen KA, Smith ML, Eckberg DL. Increased vagal cardiac nerve traffic prolongs ventricular refractoriness in patients undergoing electrophysiology testing. *Am J Cardiol* 1990; **65**: 1345–50.

49. Edvardsson N, Olsson SB. Effects of acute and chronic beta-receptor blockade on ventricular repolarization in man. *Br Heart J* 1981; **45**: 628–36.

50. Browne KF, Zipes DP, Heger JJ *et al.* Influence of the autonomic nervous system on the QT interval in man. *Am J Cardiol* 1982; **50**: 1099–1103.

51. Sarma JSM, Venkataraman K, Samant DR *et al.* Effect of propranolol on the QT intervals of normal individuals during exercise: a new method for studying interventions. *Br Heart J* 1988; **60**: 434–9.

52. Antzelevitch C, Sicouri S, Litovsky SH *et al.* Heterogeneity within the ventricular wall: electrophysiology and pharmacology of epicardial, endocardial, and M cells. *Circ Res* 1991; **69**: 1427–49.

23

Dispersion of Repolarization: Noninvasive Marker of Nonuniform Recovery of Ventricular Excitability

Wojciech Zareba, Arthur J. Moss and Fabio Badilini

Measurement of the QT interval duration is routinely performed in clinical electrocardiology. Assessment of repolarization duration has gained particular clinical attention since the first cases of idiopathic long QT syndrome (Jervell–Lange–Nielsen and Romano–Ward syndromes) were reported. During the past three decades, several studies have demonstrated that QT interval duration is representative for an overall ventricular refractory time, and have also documented that prolongation of repolarization can be associated with an increased risk of ventricular arrhythmias.[1-4] The group at risk includes not only patients with the idiopathic long QT syndrome, but also those with secondary QT interval prolongation caused, for example, by myocardial infarction or ischemia, electrolyte or metabolic imbalance, or the action of various drugs.[1-3] Nevertheless, QT interval prolongation is not a unique factor contributing to arrhythmia triggering. Current theories of arrhythmogenesis emphasize that the heterogeneity of local recovery periods throughout the myocardium may be responsible for arrhythmia generation. This heterogeneity (or nonuniformity) of recovery periods may be evaluated noninvasively by measuring repolarization durations in several ECG leads; i.e. analyzing dispersion of repolarization.

The Electrophysiology of Dispersion of Repolarization

First observations that the pattern of repolarization may vary in relation to recorded ECG leads were made in the 1930s.[5] Later, in the 1950s, Lepeschkin and Surawicz, in their pioneer work on QT interval measurements, noted a 40 ms difference in the QT duration between just three (I, II and III) limb leads.[6] These preliminary observations and pioneer investigations on nonuniform recovery of excitability in the myocardium have opened an entire field of research on dispersion of repolarization that is now flourishing in electrocardiology.

Nonuniform recovery of excitability and ventricular arrhythmias

In the early 1960s, Han and Moe[7,8] demonstrated that a nonuniform (asynchronous) recovery of excitability in the myocardium is an important factor in the triggering of

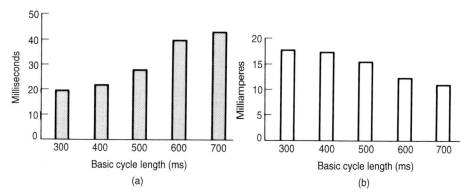

Figure 23.1   Dispersions of (a) ventricular refractory period and (b) ventricular fibrillation threshold, for various basic cycle lengths. (Reproduced with permission from reference 8)

ventricular arrhythmias. They found that even adjacent (atrial or ventricular) myocardial fibers may demonstrate a meaningful difference in refractory period durations. A maximal observed value of temporal dispersion for atrial refractory periods was 55 ms (at the cycle length of 600 ms) and for ventricular refractory periods was 43 ms (at a cycle length of 700 ms). This asynchrony of recovery of excitability was associated with an increased vulnerability to ventricular fibrillation. As shown in Figure 23.1, an increasing dispersion of ventricular refractory periods was associated with a lowered ventricular fibrillation threshold.

These early observations were further confirmed by experimental and clinical electrophysiologic studies[9–11] which supported the idea that nonuniform recovery of excitability plays an important role in arrhythmogenesis. However, nonuniform recovery of excitability should not be identified only with dispersion of refractoriness because both dispersion of local activation times and dispersion of local refractory periods augment the dispersion of total recovery times.[11] The relative contribution of these factors may depend on the underlying myocardial abnormality. Dispersion of recovery times creates suitable conditions for the mechanism of re-entry, which may be responsible for arrhythmia generation. A unidirectional block, required to promote a re-entry phenomenon, can be created by a prolongation of the local recovery time which restricts propagation of the electrical wavefront. A higher magnitude of dispersion of the adjacent recovery periods and a smaller area of this nonuniformity can facilitate induction of re-entry and further perpetuate a circus movement tachycardia.

The heterogeneity of action potentials

The concept of the crucial role of heterogeneous repolarization in generating arrhythmias also finds support in a number of investigations analyzing the morphology of myocardial action potentials.[9,12,13] Kuo *et al.*[9] demonstrated that dispersion of monophasic action potentials throughout the myocardium creates suitable conditions for ventricular arrhythmia to be induced. However, an increased magnitude of dispersion was not sufficient to induce ventricular tachycardia. In addition, stimulation at the site of short (not long) monophasic action potentials was also necessary. This observation suggests that even a marked dispersion of repolarization may not be associated with arrhythmias unless premature beats originating from the region of shorter repolarization begins a circus movement tachycardia.

Different distribution and activity of cellular ionic currents between adjacent areas is a potential reason for changes in action potential morphology which may create dispersion

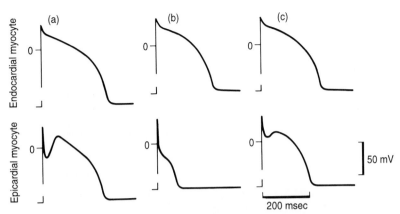

Figure 23.2 Endocardial and epicardial action potential morphology in (a) control conditions, (b) during ischemia, and (c) during ischemia with 4-aminopyridine (4-AP) administered. (Reproduced with permission from reference 12: © American Heart Association)

of repolarization.[12–14] Even in a normal myocardium, the morphology of the endocardial action potential differs from a pattern of epicardial action potential[12] (Figure 23.2(a)).

Different activity of potassium outward and calcium inward currents could be a reason for action potential changes. For example, a large and active transient outward current (I_{to}) has been found in the epicardium, but in the endocardium its activity is very weak. These differences can be further exacerbated by ischemia (Figure 23.2(b)). Under ischemic conditions, the action potential of epicardial cells demonstrates more intensive changes than the action potential of endocardial cells. An ischemia-related increase of outward repolarizing currents, especially transient outward current, leads to major changes of epicardial action potentials. The use of 4-aminopyridine, a transient outward current blocker, reverses ischemia-induced depression of epicardial action potential (Figure 23.3(c)), further confirming an important role of I_{to} in ischemia-related changes of the action potential pattern.

The transient outward current is not the only current involved in the process of action potential changes. The role of other currents, like ATP-regulated potassium or calcium currents, is under further investigation. As suggested recently by Antzelevich's group,[13] M cells may have an additional contribution to repolarization heterogeneity. The M cells, considered to be abundant in the mid-myocardium, were found to have an excessive prolongation of action potential duration in comparison with endocardial and epicardial cells. They hypothesize that M-cell activity may be responsible for the manifestation of late deflections (notches) of T wave and for the origin of U waves in a surface ECG. These cellular electrophysiology findings have major clinical significance, not only because they improve our understanding of the cellular background of arrhythmias, but also because they open new directions for pharmacological antiarrhythmic interventions.

Dispersion of Repolarization in Clinical Studies

A significant relationship between nonuniform recovery of excitability and lowered ventricular fibrillation threshold guided the directions of further clinical application of the dispersion of repolarization, which can be noninvasively evaluated on a standard surface ECG. First of all, dispersion of repolarization may be used as a tool in the stratification of risk for malignant ventricular arrhythmias or cardiac death. Also, analysis of dispersion may be a practical method of evaluating safety and efficacy of treatment.

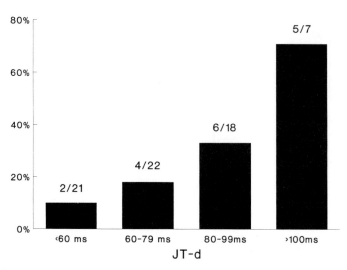

Figure 23.3   Cardiac death rates in relation to the magnitude of dispersion (JT-d). Fractions above bars represent the number of arrhythmic cardiac deaths per number of patients for each JT-d category. (Reproduced with permission from reference 15)

Dispersion of repolarization as risk factor for cardiac death

A relationship between heterogeneity of recovery times and increased vulnerability for ventricular tachycardia or ventricular fibrillation has been shown in experimental studies and also during some clinical studies with ventricular tachycardia induction protocol.[7–11] However, there are few data on the relationship between the dispersion of repolarization and cardiac death naturally occurring during a follow-up.

Recently, we studied the prognostic significance of dispersion of repolarization in a group of 68 ischemic patients after an acute coronary event (myocardial infarction or episode of unstable angina).[15] The magnitude of dispersion of repolarization, evaluated in 12 standard ECG leads, was compared between the 17 patients who died from arrhythmic cardiac death during a mean 2-year follow-up and the 51 matched survivors. We found that an increased dispersion of repolarization made an independent and significant contribution to the risk of arrhythmic cardiac death in patients with ischemic heart disease. A gradually increased dispersion of repolarization was associated with a stepwise increase in a cardiac death risk (Figure 23.3).

This clinical observation further supports previous experimental findings on the potential arrhythmogenic role of an increased dispersion of repolarization. In trying to establish a practically useful cutoff, we found that JT interval dispersion of at least 80 ms effectively identifies patients at increased risk of arrhythmic cardiac death (Figure 23.4).

The long-term prognostic value of dispersion of repolarization was also recently reported by Barr et al.[16] in 44 patients with chronic heart failure secondary to ischemic heart disease. During a mean 3-year follow-up, 12 patients died due to progression of heart failure and in 7 the mechanism was sudden cardiac death. The QTc dispersion was significantly higher in sudden cardiac death patients than in patients who died from progressive heart failure and in survivors (mean $98.6 \pm 19.4\,\mathrm{ms}^{1/2}$ versus $66.7 \pm 14.9\,\mathrm{ms}^{1/2}$ and $53.1 \pm 11.2\,\mathrm{ms}^{1/2}$, respectively; $p < 0.05$).

There are no published data on the long-term prognostic value of dispersion parameters in patients with nonischemic, dilated or hypertrophic, cardiomyopathy. Nevertheless, patients with these cardiomyopathies who experienced episodes of ventricular tachycardia or ventricular fibrillation have been shown to exhibit a higher dispersion

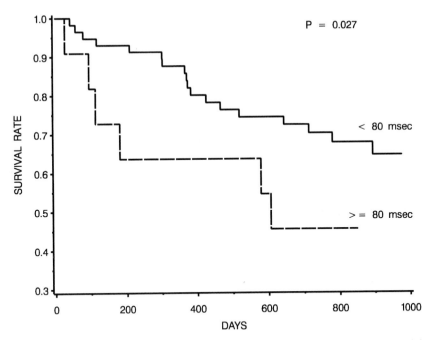

Figure 23.4 Cumulative survival rate in coronary artery disease patients with the JT interval dispersion <80 ms and ≥80 ms (*p* value calculated with a log-rank test).

than those without these arrhythmias.[17,18] In patients with hypertrophic cardiomyopathy, Buja *et al.*[17] found that QT dispersion was 115 ± 2 ms in 13 patients with documented ventricular tachycardia or fibrillation, and 43 ± 9 ms in 13 without history of arrhythmias ($p < 0.001$). A similar observation was recently made by Pye *et al.*[18] in patients with dilated cardiomyopathy. Nine patients with sustained ventricular tachycardia had QT dispersion of 76 ± 18 ms versus 40 ± 11 ms in 10 patients without sustained ventricular tachycardia ($p < 0.01$). In the same study, a group of eight patients with otherwise normal hearts but with sustained ventricular tachycardia also exhibited an increased QT dispersion in comparison with controls (65 ± 7 ms versus 32 ± 8 ms, respectively; $p < 0.05$). Patients with the idiopathic long QT syndrome are particularly prone to exhibit an increased dispersion of repolarization[19-22] which also may be considered as a marker of arrhythmic risk in these patients. However, an analysis of larger patient populations during a long-term follow-up is needed to evaluate the prognostic significance of dispersion in these patients.

The preliminary data presented above indicate that dispersion of repolarization evaluated on a standard 12-lead ECG may be a useful and easily accessible parameter to estimate the risk of cardiac death and life-threatening ventricular arrhythmias in various patient populations. However, further large studies, particularly with an automatic (observer-independent) analysis of dispersion, are needed to verify the real clinical usefulness of this parameter.

Analysis of dispersion for therapy monitoring

Usefulness of the assessment of dispersion of repolarization should not be limited only to its prognostic value in patients at risk of cardiac death. The other potential clinical applications of dispersion analysis may include the monitoring of treatment that is particularly pertinent to antiarrhythmia drugs. Since nonuniform recovery of excitability is thought to play a major role in arrhythmogenesis, the action of various drugs (especially those likely to affect the homogeneity of recovery periods) may influence the magnitude of dispersion of repolarization. Hii et al.[23] demonstrated that patients who experienced torsade de pointes during therapy with class Ia antiarrhythmia drugs (quinidine, procainamide, disopyramide) had a significantly higher precordial QT interval dispersion than those without this drug-induced arrhythmia. These findings suggest that a careful monitoring of the magnitude of dispersion during the first days of antiarrhythmia therapy may identify patients with a potential proarrhythmic effect from the drug. However, of note is that a baseline QT dispersion, evaluated in an ECG recorded before the beginning of treatment, was not useful in predicting a drug-related increase of dispersion. In the same study, chronic amiodarone therapy (implemented after class Ia antiarrhythmia drugs were withdrawn) did not increase the magnitude of dispersion when compared with the baseline values. Another class III drug, sotalol, has been shown to reduce the magnitude of dispersion in postinfarction patients during long-term therapy.[24] Recently, beat-blockers were also shown to reduce the magnitude of dispersion in patients with long QT syndrome.[22] These preliminary observations suggest that modification of dispersion by antiarrhythmia drugs could be used to evaluate the safety and efficacy of antiarrhythmic therapy. Nevertheless, further studies in larger patient populations are required to substantiate this captivating concept.

Another possible application of dispersion analysis was recently reported by Moreno et al.[25] who demonstrated that successful thrombolytic therapy can reduce the magnitude of dispersion of repolarization. In that study, 244 patients after acute myocardial infarction (recruited from the second trial of Thrombolysis with Eminase in Acute Myocardial Infarction; TEAM-2) were treated with streptokinase or antistreplase and had angiographic evaluation of the TIMI perfusion grade of the infarct-related coronary artery. Dispersion of repolarization was evaluated from a 12-lead ECG at hospital discharge.

As shown in Figure 23.5, the mean magnitude of dispersion was higher in patients with TIMI grade 0 and 1 (occluded infarct-related artery), than in those with TIMI grade 2–3 (reperfused infarct-related artery); the QTc dispersion was 104 ± 35 ms versus 61 ± 24 ms, respectively ($p < 0.0001$), and JTc dispersion was 108 ± 36 ms versus 69 ± 25 ms, respectively ($p < 0.0001$). These observations indicate that in patients with acute myocardial infarction treated with thrombolysis, the assessment of QT or JT dispersion could be used to predict patency of the infarct-related artery.

Dispersion of repolarization: its relationship to heart rate and repolarization duration

Repolarization duration is highly dependent on heart rate. Thus, when evaluating dispersion, a major concern involves the possible influence of heart rate on the magnitude of dispersion. Experimental studies showed that dispersion of repolarization can be increased at lower and decreased at higher heart rates.[7–9] However, this phenomenon is not consistently observed in clinical studies, which usually describe physiological, spontaneous or exercise-induced, changes in heart rate.[15,19,20,26] Merri et al.,[26] studying 423 normal subjects, did not find a significant correlation between RR interval and the magnitude of dispersion. In our previously mentioned 68 ischemic patients,[15] we did not find an association between the magnitude of dispersion and heart rate which ranged in these patients between 44 and 100 bpm (Figure 23.6).

Recently, we investigated the influence of incremental atrial pacing on the magnitude of dispersion in two LQTS patients with implanted atrial (AAI) pacemakers. In both individuals, the magnitude of dispersion decreased gradually but only at heart rates above 90–100 bpm. These observations suggest that the magnitude of dispersion of

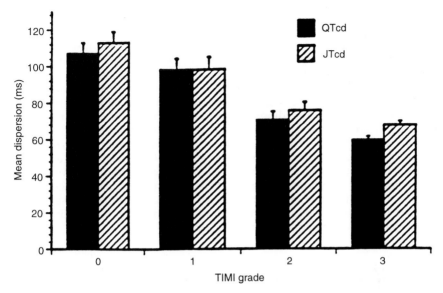

Figure 23.5 Dispersion of repolarization (QTcd and JTcd) in relation to the TIMI perfusion grade of the infarct-related artery in acute myocardial infarction patients treated with thrombolysis. (Reproduced from reference 25 with permission: © American Heart Association)

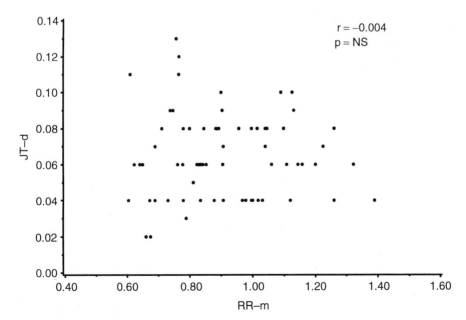

Figure 23.6 Dispersion of repolarization (JT-d) in relation to the mean RR interval in 68 patients with recent coronary events.

repolarization does not change significantly at normal heart rates usually observed in clinical practice.

Another consideration relates to a potential relationship between the overall duration of repolarization and the magnitude of dispersion. Do patients with longer durations present with increased or decreased dispersion of repolarization? In our ischemic patients with QTc values ranging from 0.34 to 0.48 s, there was no association between the overall QTc duration and the magnitude of dispersion ($r = 0.09$; NS). Another pattern may be expected in patients with idiopathic long QT syndrome since they are particularly likely to exhibit an increased magnitude of dispersion. However, in our recently reported[27] small group of LQTS patients who had QTc values ranging from 0.45 to 0.70 s, we did not observe a significant association between QTc length and automatically computed dispersion of repolarization ($r = 0.13$; NS). Earlier studies did not find this association either.[20,21] Although LQTS patients frequently have an increased magnitude of dispersion, there is not enough proof to state that a magnitude of dispersion is directly related to the magnitude of repolarization duration. Some other factors like autonomic nervous system imbalance may affect this relationship.

Methodology for Evaluation of Dispersion of Repolarization

Since dispersion of repolarization was found to be a clinically and prognostically useful tool in electrocardiology, a number of methodological approaches have been described. Various ECG measures of repolarization duration and different statistical approaches can be applied to evaluate the magnitude of dispersion in chosen numbers and configurations of electrocardiographic leads.

ECG parameters to describe dispersion of repolarization

The duration of repolarization can be measured in the ECG as an absolute value of the QT or JT interval and is usually corrected for heart rate with the Bazett formula (QTc or JTc). The same variables, expressed in absolute or heart-rate corrected values, are also measured to evaluate dispersion of repolarization; i.e. the difference in duration of repolarization between multiple ECG leads.[15–18,21–24] When analyzing dispersion of repolarization, the use of heart-rate corrected values instead of absolute values provides similar results but does not have a particular advantage. First, since the durations of repolarization are usually evaluated in simultaneously recorded leads, at the same or similar heart rate, a correction for heart rate would not be expected to improve analysis. Second, the weak correlation between the magnitude of dispersion and heart rate (in normally observed heart rate ranges; see Figure 23.6), does not support the use of heart-rate corrected measures of dispersion.

The question may be raised whether the QT or JT interval should be used for evaluation of repolarization duration and dispersion. Current studies demonstrate that evaluation of either of these parameters appears to reliably represent dispersion of repolarization.[15,23,25] Nevertheless, in some clinical circumstances (i.e. in patients with a prolongation of QRS duration) JT interval better describes repolarization duration.[28] This seems to be also relevant for postinfarction patients, since QT interval encompasses the duration of ventricular depolarization and repolarization together and the QRS duration can contribute to the risk of cardiac death independently of repolarization abnormalities.[15] The analysis of dispersion parameters in our ischemic patients[15] revealed that JT dispersion and a mean QRS duration were independent and significant predictors of subsequent arrhythmic cardiac death, whereas the QT dispersion was a less effective predictor of subsequent cardiac death (Figure 23.7).

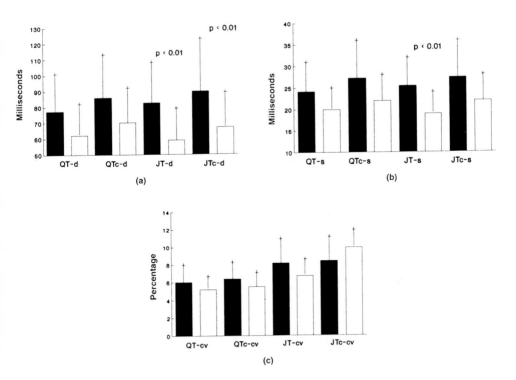

Figure 23.7 Parameters of dispersion of repolarization in patients who subsequently died of arrhythmic cardiac death (black bars) and in survivors (open bars). (a) Maximal dispersion between 12 ECG leads (QT-d, QTc-d, JT-d, JTc-d). (b) Standard deviation of the mean from 12 ECG leads (QT-s, QTc-s, JT-s, JTc-s). (c) Coefficient of variation of the mean for 12 ECG leads (QT-cv, QTc-cv, JT-cv, JTc-cv). (Reproduced with permission from reference 15)

Statistical measures of dispersion

Various statistical measures of the spread (or dispersion) can be applied to analyze repolarization dispersion in electrocardiology. A maximal dispersion (i.e. a maximal difference between duration of repolarization interval in evaluated leads) is the most commonly used parameter, representing the widest spectrum of repolarization heterogeneity in a studied ECG. A standard deviation or coefficient of variation (standard deviation/mean × 100%) of repolarization duration calculated in a number of evaluated leads are also in use.[29] These parameters are less useful for a manual evaluation of dispersion, but they may be applied for a computerized analysis. Although standard deviation and coefficient of variation are less sensitive to erroneous measurements of a single QT or JT interval, they may not represent wide ranges of repolarization durations, especially if a smaller number of leads are evaluated.

Predictive effectiveness of the three parameters (maximal dispersion, standard deviation, and coefficient of variation) may be different, as shown in Figure 23.7, for dispersion of QT, QTc, JT, and JTc in the study referred to above.[15] The maximal dispersion of JT or JTc and standard deviation of JT intervals provided the best and the most significant separation between cardiac death patients and survivors. The maximal dispersion and standard deviation of QT or QTc interval were less predictive, whereas coefficient of variation was not a useful predictor in this study.

Choice of ECG leads to assess dispersion

Evaluation of repolarization dispersion involves the analysis of various numbers and configurations of recorded ECG leads, from multilead body-surface mapping[30–33] through a standard 12-lead ECG[15–18,21–25,34] to a 3-channel Holter recording.[27,35] A proper evaluation of repolarization duration does not require a multilead analysis, as evidenced by Sylven et al.[30] who showed that the average QT duration computed from orthogonal Frank's leads correlates highly ($r = 0.885$; $p < 0.001$) with the average QT duration assessed from 120-lead body surface mapping. Dispersion of repolarization is usually evaluated in a standard ECG from either all 12 or 6 precordial leads.[15–18,21–25,34] The magnitude of dispersion represented by these configurations may differ, but they represent a similar pattern of observed dispersion. Some authors[16,21] have also used measures of dispersion with additional adjustment for the number of leads evaluated (QTc dispersion square-root of number of leads). However, this adjustment does not have a rationale in the electrophysiologic basis of dispersion. Attention has to be paid to the choice of assessed leads rather than their total number. Our recent observations (see below) suggest that even three orthogonal-type leads (I, aVF, V2) are sufficient to substantiate 12- or 6-lead configurations in order to identify patients with an increased dispersion of repolarization. This observation is particularly relevant for potential applications for recording dispersion of repolarization in a 3-channel Holter or exercise ECG testing.

Automatic Detection of Dispersion of Repolarization

A visual (manual) evaluation of repolarization duration from a standard paper copy of a 12-lead ECG (the most widely used approach) is a time-consuming process and has some limitations. The degree of precision may be influenced by paper speed, signal amplification, and by distortions caused by enlargements (if used). Additional inaccuracies may come from reader bias, further contributing to a decreased reproducibility of the measurements.[36] A digital processing of ECG signal and computerized analysis of QT interval measurements may overcome these difficulties.[19,26,31,37]

Body-surface mapping

During the past decade, multilead body-surface mapping (Table 23.1) has been demonstrated as a successful method of evaluating the interlead variation of repolarization duration in experimental animal studies and in various patient populations.[30–33]

These studies showed that dispersion of repolarization can be measured reliably from the body surface and they further confirmed an association between increased dispersion of repolarization and lowered ventricular fibrillation threshold. However, body-surface mapping is not a clinically useful method to evaluate larger groups of patients. Thus, a standard 12-lead ECG recording has to be considered a more practical approach for evaluating automatically dispersion of repolarization in clinical settings.

Table 23.1 Dispersion of repolarization in clinical studies with body-surface mapping

Authors	Body-surface ECG mapping	Patient population and number of patients
Sylven et al.[30]	120 leads	Prolonged QT (14 pts)
Mirvis[31]	150 leads	Acute myocardial infarction (30 pts)
DeAmbroggi et al.[32]	117 leads	Long QT syndrome (40 pts)

Standard 12-lead ECG

In 1988–89, Merri, Alberti and coworkers[19,26] developed a computerized algorithm to evaluate automatically the pattern of the repolarization segment and to determine heterogeneity of repolarization from a digital 12-lead ECG (Marquette ECG format; 256 samples per second per channel). Among several repolarization variables, early (SoTm = interval between S offset and T wave maximum) and late (TmTo = interval from the peak to the offset of the T wave) components of repolarization were computed automatically and compared between precordial leads to measure the magnitude of repolarization heterogeneity. Computerized measures of heterogeneity included standard deviations of early and late components and standard deviation of the time interval to accumulate 50% of the total absolute repolarization area (that includes the area from the S wave offset to the T wave or U wave offset). This approach, tested in 423 normals and further validated in 37 patients with LQTS,[19,20,26] showed that automatically computed measures of repolarization were highly correlated with the manual assessment of repolarization made in the same ECG leads. An additional, meaningful observation by these authors was that dispersion of repolarization is mainly due to a heterogeneity of the early component of repolarization (SoTm), whereas the late part (TmTo) contributes less to repolarization heterogeneity. This study demonstrated that a standard digital ECG recording can be used to evaluate automatically dispersion of repolarization.

If there is no access to digital ECG recordings and an analysis of paper (hard) copy ECGs is needed, a computerized method to automatically detect dispersion of repolarization from a hard-copy ECG can be an alternative approach, despite some limitations.[29] Nevertheless, since the majority of currently produced electrocardiographs facilitate recording and storing ECG signals in a digital form, an automatic analysis of dispersion from a digital 12-lead ECG appears to be the method of choice in routine clinical practice.

Holter-Recorded Dispersion of Repolarization

Numerous patients who undergo ambulatory ECG Holter recordings may also have dispersion of repolarization evaluated automatically. Current Holter technology with precise digital ECG recordings may provide a useful approach to determining dispersion of repolarization not only in static conditions (the 12-lead ECG) but also in dynamic conditions. This novel application of digital Holter technology was the subject of our recent investigation.[27,35]

Are three ECG leads sufficient to evaluate dispersion of repolarization?

Earlier studies reported 6- or 12-lead standard ECG configurations to evaluate a magnitude of dispersion. Since Holter technology supports 3-lead configurations, questions may be raised about whether three leads are sufficient to demonstrate reliably the pattern of repolarization heterogeneity. Studying this, in the 68 ischemic heart disease patients, we evaluated the predictive value of dispersion parameters calculated from three, orthogonal-like ECG leads (I, aVF, V2) in comparison with measures computed from six or twelve ECG leads.

As shown in Figure 23.8, the analysis of dispersion in just three orthogonal-type ECG leads was an effective way of identifying patients who had arrhythmic cardiac death during follow-up. This observation indicated that the X, Y and Z orthogonal leads may be considered as a potential approach for Holter recording of dispersion of repolarization. Therefore, we developed an algorithm to compute dispersion of repolarization automatically from a 3-channel Holter recording.

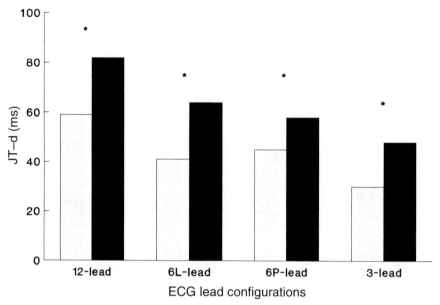

Figure 23.8   Dispersion of repolarization (JT-d) evaluated in four ECG lead configurations in 68 ischemic heart disease patients. Black bars show cardiac death patients, open bars show survivors. The 12-lead, 6-precordial (6P), 6-limb (6L) and 3-lead (orthogonal-type; i.e. I, avF, V2) ECG lead configurations were used. * $p < 0.05$ when comparing cardiac death patients and survivors.

Computer algorithm for analysis of dispersion in Holter recordings

Standard Holter recordings are usually made with a 128 Hz sampling frequency per channel. This translates to an analysis of consecutive samples approximately every 8 ms, which may affect the results of computed dispersion of repolarization. To increase precision, we chose to acquire the ECG signal using a digital recorder (DMI AltairDisc Holter; Diagnostic Medical Instruments Inc., Syracuse, NY) set at a sampling frequency of 1000 Hz per channel which permits analysis of the ECG signal every 1 ms.[38] The X, Y and Z bipolar, orthogonal ECG leads which can demonstrate 3-dimensional changes in repolarization pattern were chosen for Holter recordings. After ECG acquisition, the digital data was transferred to a SUN WorkStation 4/470 for further analyses. Four-minute time series of acquired ECG signals were analyzed to evaluate the duration and configuration of repolarization in X, Y and Z leads. After QRS detection, a beat-specific baseline was estimated for low-frequency drift adjustment, and the repolarization segment (1-second window after the peak of the R wave) was smoothed with a moving-average filter (main-lobe cutoff 20 Hz). Thereafter, first and second derivatives of the filtered signals within the repolarization segment were computed to define the peak, the beginning and the end of the T wave. The duration of repolarization was computed in each lead from the peak of the R wave to the end of the T wave (RT). The heart-rate adjusted (with preceding RR interval) RTc was also calculated for each beat. A U wave, when apparent, was not included in the measured duration of repolarization. Dispersion of repolarization was computed as a maximal difference in repolarization durations between simultaneously recorded X, Y and Z leads for each recorded beat. The median values of maximal RT differences (RTd) were used as measures of the dispersion magnitude.

Table 23.2 Duration and dispersion of repolarization measured automatically in 10 long QT syndrome patients compared with 10 normal subjects

Automatic ECG variables		Controls	LQTS
RR interval (ms)		925 ± 114	1019 ± 192
Duration of repolarization	RTc (ms)	328 ± 13	450 ±43*
	RTmc (ms)	257 ± 8	364 ± 35*
Dispersion of repolarization	RT-d (ms)	13 ± 6	44 ± 11*
	RTm-d (ms)	15 ± 11	60 ± 23*

RTc = interval between the peak of the R wave and the end of the T wave, corrected for heart rate; RTmc = interval between the peak of the R wave and the maximum of the T wave, corrected for heart rate; RT-d = dispersion of RT intervals; RTm-d = dispersion of RTm intervals; *significantly higher than in controls ($p < 0.01$).

Clinical application of Holter analysis of dispersion

The approach described above was tested in 10 patients with long QT syndrome, with Bazett's heart-rate corrected QTc of 520 ± 78 ms, and in 10 control subjects with normal QTc values (QTc of 372 ± 14 ms). Patients with long QT syndrome were chosen because they are extremely likely to exhibit an increased magnitude of dispersion. Table 23.2 summarizes the data on Holter-recorded duration and dispersion of repolarization in long QT syndrome patients and controls.

Heart rate was similar in both groups (mean RR interval 1019 ± 192 and 925 ± 114 ms, respectively), and RTc value was significantly higher in LQTS patients than in controls. Holter-derived RTc values were highly correlated with QTc values calculated from the standard 12-lead ECG which was recorded immediately before Holter recording ($r = 0.89; p < 0.001$). Dispersion of repolarization (RTd), computed in three Holter-recorded leads, ranged in controls from 7 to 22 ms (average 13 ± 6 ms), whereas in LQTS patients RTd values were on average three times higher (44 ± 11 ms). In one LQTS patient (with QTc = 494 ms$^{1/2}$) the magnitude of dispersion (RTd = 23 ms) approached values observed in controls, whereas in the other 9 patients RTd values varied between 35 and 56 ms. Dispersion evaluated in 3-lead Holter recording showed a high correlation with measures of dispersion derived from 12 leads of a standard ECG ($r = 0.82; p < 0.001$).

Figure 23.9 shows the relationship between dispersion parameters computed from 3-

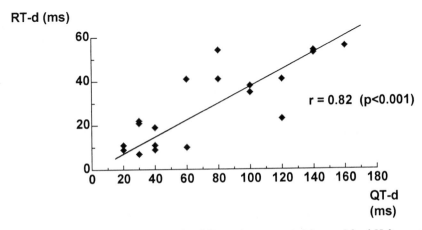

Figure 23.9 Relationship between magnitude of dispersion computed from a 3-lead Holter recording (RT-d) and calculated in a 12-lead standard ECG (QT-d).

channel Holter recording and those from a standard 12-lead ECG for a pooled data of LQTS patients and controls. Evaluation of this association in each studied group separately further proves our previous observations that dispersion evaluated from 3-lead Holter recordings may be used to assess reliably the magnitude of dispersion in a studied patient. The clinical usefulness of Holter-recorded dispersion of repolarization requires further studies in various patient populations. Nevertheless, it appears that the current development of digital Holter technology creates an opportunity to retrieve information on dispersion of repolarization automatically from ambulatory ECG recordings, enhancing diagnostic capabilities of this common noninvasive technique.

Dispersion of repolarization provides information only on a spatial (recorded during the same heart beat) heterogeneity of repolarization. However, ventricular recovery of excitability may also exhitit dynamic (beat-to-beat) changes expressed in an ECG as T-wave alterans (see Chapter 25). We recently demonstrated[27] that digital Holter ECG recording enables automatic detection of both spatial and dynamic aspects of heterogenous repolarization by simultaneous evaluation of dispersion of repolarization and T-wave alterans. This comprehensive approach further improves diagnostic potentials of modern Holter technology.

Summary

Dispersion of repolarization, a measure of interlead variation in repolarization duration, is a noninvasive approach to evaluate nonuniform recovery of ventricular excitability which may contribute to an increased risk of ventricular arrhythmias. Recent clinical studies indicate that this simple method, which consists of measuring and comparing QT or JT interval durations in several recorded leads, may be useful in identifying patients at risk for life-threatening ventricular arrhythmias or cardiac death. Besides that, assessment of dispersion of repolarization may be considered a promising method to evaluate efficacy and safety of therapy, particularly with antiarrhythmia drugs.

Nevertheless, a manual evaluation of dispersion in several leads is impractical, time-consuming, and sometimes may be inaccurate. Therefore, novel computerized approaches are being developed to provide automatic analysis of dispersion from a digital 12-lead ECG and from a digital 3-lead Holter monitoring. The latter approach provides an opportunity to monitor dynamic changes in repolarization dispersion (heterogeneity) over a longer period of time, which further increases potential diagnostic possibilities of ECG Holter monitoring in everyday clinical practice.

References

1. Moss AJ, Schwartz PJ. Delayed repolarization (QT and Q-U prolongation) and malignant ventricular arrhythmias. *Mod Concepts Cardiovasc Dis* 1982; **51**: 85–90.
2. Schwartz PJ, Wolf S. QT interval prolongation as predictor of sudden death in patients with myocardial infarction. *Circulation* 1978; **57**: 1074–7.
3. Surawicz B, Knoebel SB. Long QT: good, bad or indifferent? *J Am Coll Cardiol* 1984; **4**: 398–413.
4. Moss AJ, Schwartz PJ, Crampton RS *et al.* The long QT syndrome: prospective longitudinal study of 328 families. *Circulation* 1991; **84**: 1136–44.
5. Wilson FN, Macleod AG, Barker PS, Johnston FD. Determination of the significance of the areas of the ventricular deflections of the electrocardiogram. *Am Heart J* 1934; **10**: 46–61.
6. Lepeschkin E, Surawicz B. Measurement of the QT interval of the electrocardiogram. *Circulation* 1952; **6**: 378–88.
7. Han J, Moe GK. Nonuniform recovery of excitability in ventricular muscle. *Circ Res* 1964; **14**: 44–60.
8. Han J, Millet D, Chizzonitti B, Moe GK. Temporal dispersion of recovery of excitability in atrium and ventricle as a function of heart rate. *Am Heart J* 1966; **71**: 481–7.
9. Kuo CS, Munakata K, Reddy CP, Surawicz B. Characteristics and possible mechanism of ventricular arrhythmia dependent on the dispersion of action potential durations. *Circulation* 1983; **67**: 1356–67.
10. Gaugh WB, Mehra R, Restivo M, Zeller RH, El-Sherif N. Reentrant ventricular arrhythmias in the late myocardial infarction period of the dog. 13: Correlation of activation and refractory maps. *Circ Res* 1985; **57**: 432–42.

11. Vassalo JA, Cassidy DM, Kindwall KE, Marchlinski FE, Josephson ME. Nonuniform recovery of excitability in the left ventricle. *Circulation* 1988; **78**: 1365–72.
12. Lukas A, Antzelevich C. Differences in the electrophysiological response of canine ventricular epicardium and endocardium to ischemia: role of the transient outward current. *Circulation* 1993; **88**: 2903–15.
13. Antzelevich C, Sicouri S. Clinical relevance of cardiac arrhythmias generated by afterdepolarization. Role of M cells in the generation of U waves, triggered activity and torsade de pointes. *J Am Coll Cardiol* 1994; **23**: 259–77.
14. Noble D. Ionic mechanisms determining the timing of ventricular repolarization: significance for cardiac arrhythmias. *Ann NY Acad Sci* 1992; **644**: 1–22.
15. Zareba W, Moss AJ, leCessie S. Dispersion of ventricular repolarization and arrhythmic cardiac death in coronary artery disease. *Am J Cardiol* 1994; **74**: 550–3.
16. Barr CS, Naas A, Freeman M, Lang CC, Struthers AD. QT dispersion and sudden unexpected death in chronic heart failure. *Lancet* 1994; **343**: 327–9.
17. Buja G, Miorelli M, Turrini P, Melacini P, Nava A. Comparison of QT dispersion in hypertrophic cardiomyopathy between patients with and without ventricular arrhythmias and sudden death. *Am J Cardiol* 1993; **72**: 973–6.
18. Pye M, Quinn AC, Cobbe SM. QT interval dispersion: a noninvasive marker of susceptibility to arrhythmia in patients with sustained ventricular arrhythmias? *Br Heart J* 1994; **71**: 511–14.
19. Alberti M, Merri M, Benhorin J, Locati E, Moss AJ. Electrocardiographic precordial interlead variability in normal individuals and patients with long QT syndrome. In: Murray A, Ripley KL (eds), *Computers in Cardiology*. Los Alamitos, CA: IEEE Computer Society, 1990: 475–8.
20. Benhorin J, Merri M, Alberti M, Locati E, Moss AJ, Hall WJ, Cui L. Long QT syndrome: new electrocardiographic characteristics. *Circulation* 1990; **82**: 521–7.
21. Day CP, McComb JM, Campbell RWF. QT dispersion: an indication of arrhythmic risk in patients with long QT intervals. *Br Heart J* 1990; **63**: 342–4.
22. Priori SG, Napolitano C, Diehl L, Schwartz PJ. Dispersion of the QT interval: a marker of therapeutic efficacy in the idiopathic long QT syndrome. *Circulation* 1994; **89**: 1681–9.
23. Hii JTY, Wyse DG, Gillis AM, Duff HJ, Solylo MA, Mitchell LB. Precordial QT interval dispersion as a marker of torsade de pointes: disparate effects of class Ia antiarrhythmic drugs and amiodarone. *Circulation* 1992; **86**: 1376–82.
24. Day CP, McComb JM, Matthews JJ, Campbell RWF. Reduction in QT dispersion by sotalol following myocardial infarction. *Eur Heart J* 1991; **12**: 423–7.
25. Moreno FL, Villanueva T, Karagounis LA, Anderson J. Reduction in QT interval dispersion by successful thrombolytic therapy in acute myocardial infarction. *Circulation* 1994; **90**: 94–100.
26. Merri M, Benhorin J, Alberti M, Locati E, Moss AJ. Electrocardiographic quantitation of ventricular repolarization. *Circulation* 1989; **80**: 1301–8.
27. Zareba W, Badilini F, Moss AJ. Automatic detection of heterogenous repolarization. *J Electrocardiol* 1994; **27**: 65–71.
28. Zareba W, Moss AJ, and the LQTS Study Group. Criteria for delayed repolarization in patients with wide QRS complex. *J Am Coll Cardiol* 1994; **23**: 37A.
29. Bhullar HK, Fothergill JC, Goddard WP, deBono DP. Automated measurement of QT interval dispersion from hardcopy ECGs. *J Electrocardiol* 1993; **26**: 321.
30. Sylven JC, Horacek BM, Spencer CA, Klassen GA, Montague TJ. QT interval variability on the body surface. *J Electrocardiol* 1984; **17**: 179–88.
31. Mirvis DM. Spatial variation of QT intervals in normal persons and patients with acute myocardial infarction. *J Am Coll Cardiol* 1985; **5**: 625–31.
32. DeAmbroggi L, Negroni MS, Monza E, Bertoni T, Schwartz PJ. Dispersion of ventricular repolarization in the long QT syndrome. *Am J Cardiol* 1991; **68**: 614–20.
33. Abildskov JA, Lux RL. Distribution of QRST deflection areas in relation to repolarization and arrhythmias. *J Electrocardiol* 1991; **24**: 197–203.
34. Cowan JC, Yusoff K, Moore M, Amos PA, Gold AE, Bourke JP, Transuphaswadikul S, Campbell RWF. Importance of lead selection in QT interval measurement. *Am J Cardiol* 1988; **61**: 83–7.
35. Zareba W, Badilini F, Moss AJ. Dispersion of repolarization: automatic detection from three-channel Holter recorded ECG. *J Amb Monitoring* 1994; **7**: 98.
36. Murray A, McLaughlin NB, Bourke JP, Doig JC, Furniss SS, Campbell RWF. Errors in manual measurement of QT intervals. *Br Heart J* 1994; **71**: 386–90.
37. Puddu PE, Bernard PM, Chaiyman BR, Bourassa MG. QT interval measurement by a computer assisted program: a potentially useful clinical parameter. *J Electrocardiol* 1982; **15**: 15–22.
38. De Maso J, Myers S, Nels D, Sellers C. Ambulatory high-resolution ECG recorder using disk storage. *J Ambul Monit* 1992; **5**: 317.

24

QT Variability

Mario Merri

The QT interval is an electrocardiographic parameter that quantifies the duration of ventricular repolarization. This chapter presents two techniques that provide insight into the mechanisms and the malfunctioning of the neurological and/or electrical functions of the heart. These two techniques are complementary and both consider as initial input the ventricular repolarization duration (RD) as measured from the surface electrocardiogram (ECG). The first technique analyzes its space (interlead) variability, the second one addresses its time and frequency variability.

The space variability represents the variability of RD when measured from several electrocardiographic signals simultaneously acquired on the same individual from different leads. The time and frequency variability is the variability of RD when measured from a single electrocardiographic signal acquired from a single lead over a period of time of at least a few minutes.

Despite these differences, some of the basic ECG preprocessing steps needed before studying the RD are similar and constitute the starting point of our data analysis.

Quantitation of Repolarization Duration

Ventricular repolarization is a complex electrical phenomenon that has been studied theoretically and experimentally. The TU wave complex on the ECG is the integrated signal of this repolarization process, and it has several distinct morphological features.[1] Conventionally, RD is quantified by measuring the QT interval or the heart-rate corrected form (QTc),[2] both of which are used clinically to assess the propensity to ventricular arrhythmias in certain subsets of patients.[3,4]

The results published in references 1 and 4 on quantitation of repolarization in normal individuals and in long QT syndrome (LQTS) patients have shown that the cardiac cycle-length dependency of RD is concentrated mainly in the first portion of the QT interval (ending at the peak of the T wave), and that the static relationship of repolarization duration to cardiac cycle length is best fitted linearly.

This conclusion brought us to move away from the classical QT interval towards other electrocardiographic measurements that could be at the same time highly representative of RD and more practical from a data processing point of view.

New Repolarization Duration Variables

As noted, most of the heart-rate dependent information in the RD is contained in early repolarization. Early RD can be quantified on the ECG by the interval SoTm; that is, the

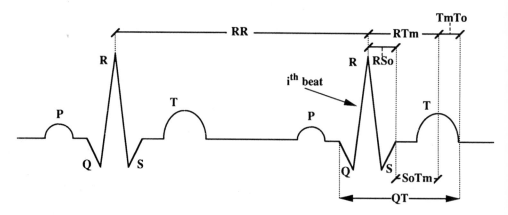

Figure 24.1 Schematic ECG with variables of interest. The QT interval is also indicated for comparison purposes.

interval between the offset of the S wave (So) and the peak of the T wave (Tm).[1,4] SoTm removes many of the problems associated with the automatic identification of both Q wave onset and T wave offset that are intrinsic in the measurement of the traditional QT interval.

On the other hand, the interval TmTo – that is, the interval between Tm and the offset of the T wave – is representative of late repolarization. Figure 24.1 defines these intervals graphically for the *i*th heart beat and describes the conventions that were used during analysis of the data.

In later work,[5] quantitation of early RD was further improved by introducing the interval RTm; that is, the time between the R wave peak and Tm. In fact, as opposed to SoTm, RTm does not require identification of the fiducial point So that is usually very difficult to locate automatically. Besides, the interval RSo does not contain relevant information as it is basically invariant to changes in the heart rate.

In addition to the fact that they are more easily measured automatically, SoTm and RTm present other advantages. Franz *et al.* have demonstrated that they represent a less diluted measurement of ventricular repolarization duration (Figure 24.2), as opposed to

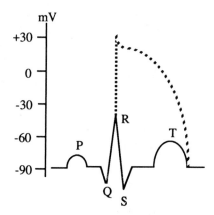

Figure 24.2 Simultaneous recordings of surface ECG (bold line) and ventricular cell monophasic action potential (dotted line). The close relation between action potential duration and the RTm interval is evident.

Table 24.1 Correlation coefficients of repolarization duration measurements (from lead V5) in 376 normal individuals

	QT	SoTm	RTm
SoTm	0.70		
RTm	0.79	0.94	
RSo	0.12	−0.34	−0.01

Reproduced from reference 7.

the QT interval which measures both depolarization and repolarization. In particular, they may be given a more precise physiological meaning as the duration of the average action potential of the ventricular cell.

For historical reasons, the sections below provide results in terms of SoTm and TmTo for the space variability, and in terms of RTm for the time and frequency variability. This should not confuse the reader as SoTm and RTm provide a virtually identical quantitation of RD. This is demonstrated by Table 24.1.

ECG Preprocessing

A procedure, implemented in a validated software package, was developed to preprocess the ECG and to measure the variables of interest. Note that the heart rate, quantified by the classical RR interval (that is the interval between two successive R wave peaks), was also measured. The software performs the following steps:

1. Access to the digitized ECG.
2. Measurement of electrocardiographic variables.
3. Removal of nonphysiological data.

Access to the digitized ECG

Data acquisition and digitization were carried out using a commercial electrocardiographic device. In order to gain external access to the digitized ECG, it was necessary to establish the appropriate hardware and software interfaces between the commercial device and the computer on which the preprocessing software was to run.

The ECGs that were to be used to study space variability were recorded and digitized using a MAC12 system digital electrocardiographer (250 Hz ECG sampling frequency), which provided lead-specific median beats over the 10-second acquisition period. A single beat for each lead was obtained by first synchronizing the R waves detected in the 10-second acquisition period in that lead, and then applying a median filter to obtain the median beat.[8]

The ECGs that were to be used to study time and frequency variability were obtained using an analog cassette recorder Series 8500 and digitized with the Laser Holter system (128 Hz ECG sampling frequency). All the equipment mentioned above was manufactured by Marquette Electronics Inc.

Measurement of electrocardiographic variables

With reference to Figure 24.1, measurement of the RR interval was carried out by looking for the R wave using an adaptive threshold on the amplitude of the first derivative of the electrocardiogram. Once the threshold was reached, the time of occurrence of the maximum of the R wave was identified.

Since the accuracy of the time measurements on the ECG was limited by the sampling rate of the commercial system,[9] a parabola was fitted through the R wave maximum value itself and the previous and the successive samples. The parabola vertices were then used as fiducial points to identify the peaks of two consecutive R waves. The RR interval was computed as the difference between the occurrences of two consecutive parabolic vertices.

After detection of the second R wave, the algorithm analyzed the portion following the R wave, looking for the maximum of the T wave. One second (or whatever was available) of ECG following the peak of the R wave was passed through a digital lowpass filter (FIR filter, 15 Hz cutoff), and the maximum value of the signal was searched within a time window starting from the previous R wave to 15% and 75% of the running RR interval mean (in the case of space variability, the mean RR was provided by the MAC12). A parabola was then fitted through seven samples centered about the maximum, and the abscissa of its vertex was taken as the fiducial point for the occurrence of the maximum amplitude of the T wave (Tm). Finally, To was defined as the location after Tm where a specific combination of signal, its derivative and its integral values was satisfied. RTm was measured as the difference between two consecutive fiducial points for R and Tm. SoTm and TmTo were calculated as the difference between the fiducial points of Tm and those of So and To, respectively. Note that So was provided by the MAC12. Full details of the measurement algorithm can be found in references 7 and 8.

Removal of nonphysiological data

For the time and frequency variability analysis, the values of RTm and RR were obtained from every heart beat in a Holter ECG. Exclusion of any one of these values resulted in the exclusion of the entire beat. In particular, if $350 < RR < 1500$ ms and $200 < RTm < 600$ ms, then the beat was considered physiologic and the variables accepted for further analysis. Otherwise it was labeled as 'nonphysiologic' and the variables discarded. Note that this criterion, although crude, was able to detect and eliminate several signal distortions including noise in the ECG and some kinds of arrhythmias.

Also for the space variability analysis, outlying values of SoTm and TmTo were identified via predefined lower and upper thresholds. In addition, a baseline shift larger than 15 μV was considered as a criterion for beat exclusion.

Space Variability of Repolarization Duration

The condition and functioning status of an individual's heart are often deduced by a cardiologist on the basis of ECG waveforms. It is therefore important to establish how electrocardiographic morphological features appear different when measured from a different location on the body surface; or, in other words, from a different lead.

Here we shall concentrate on the ECG morphological feature that defines the duration of the ventricular repolarization process; in particular, the variability of RD when measured on the same heart beat but from different precordial leads. Figure 24.3 gives the approximate positions of the precordial leads on the horizontal plane of the human chest. Other morphological characteristics of the ECG ventricular repolarization and their variability are discussed elsewhere.[1,4]

Figure 24.4 shows an example of the computer-processed ECGs of a normal individual (upper panel) and an LQTS patient (lower panel), in which five superimposed precordial leads (V2–V6) are aligned by the peaks of the R waves. In addition to prolongation of the repolarization signal, the electrocardiogram of the LQTS patient exhibits random wave shapes and a more pronounced malalignment of the five precordial T waves.

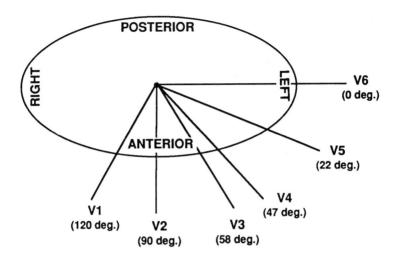

Figure 24.3 Distribution on the human chest of the six precordial leads (V1–V6). The figure represents schematically the transversal section of the chest. The angles, in degrees, of V1–V5 are also provided with respect to V6.

Method

The study population

The population for this phase of the work consisted of 229 normal individuals and 25 LQTS patients, aged 17–60 years, who had 12-lead ECG recordings digitized on a MAC12 recorder. The normal individuals were asymptomatic, with no cardiovascular medical history, with normal physical examination, and normal 12-lead ECG. The LQTS patients were all participants in the International Long QT Syndrome Registry.[10] All these patients belonged to well-defined LQTS-affected families and had a QTc > 0.44 s.

Data processing

For each individual, normal or patient, and for each of the five precordial leads that were considered (V2–V6), SoTm and TmTo were measured. Both variables were expressed in milliseconds. The precordial lead V1 was excluded because it usually presents a downward biphasic T wave owing to its location on the body surface, as opposed to the monophasic upward T wave that characterizes all other precordial leads.

To quantify the malalignment of the five precordial T waves, a new parameter was introduced: the *precordial sequence index* (PSI). The PSI was computed for both variables, SoTm and TmTo, to quantify the disorder in the repolarization sequence with respect to a predefined, variable-specific, template sequence. A template sequence was defined in the population of 229 normal individuals as the sequence that the mean values of the variable in question assumed across the precordial leads after the mean values were arrayed in increasing order of magnitude. As an example, if the mean value of SoTm monotonically increases from V2 to V6, then the V2–V6 template sequence for SoTm is 1,2,3,4,5.

Disorder was defined as follows. For $i = 2, \ldots, 6$, let M_i be the values of a given variable in the ith precordial lead of a given individual, and X_i the corresponding sequence number. In practice, X_i corresponds to the position of M_i after sorting M_i in increasing

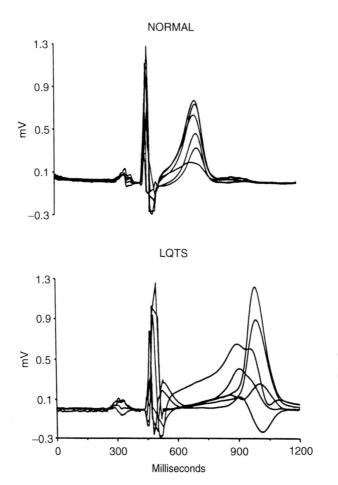

Figure 24.4 An example of computer-processed ECGs of a normal individual (upper panel) and an LQTS patient (lower panel). The five precordial leads are superimposed and aligned by the peaks of the R waves.

order. As an example, assume that SoTm of an individual is measured with the following results in milliseconds: V2, $M_2 = 180$; V3, $M_3 = 184$; V4, $M_4 = 170$; V5, $M_5 = 175$; V6, $M_6 = 190$. From this it follows that $X_2 = 3$, $X_3 = 4$, $X_4 = 1$, $X_5 = 2$ and $X_6 = 5$.

Finally, assume that $\underline{X}_i$, $i = 2,...,6$, is the template sequence relative to that ECG variable; that is, the order the variable under consideration should follow in a normal situation. Note that both X_i and $\underline{X}_i$ could only assume values from 1 to 5. For a given individual, the PSI is defined as:

$$PSI = \sum_{i=2}^{6} (X_i - \underline{X}_i)^2.$$

A value of PSI equal to zero indicates that the repolarization sequence is identical to the template sequence, while a value of PSI different from zero identifies interlead disorder with respect to the template sequence. The bigger the PSI, the bigger the disorder.

Statistical analysis

The statistical analysis was organized in two steps: (1) evaluation of the presence of significant differences among the mean values of each variable from lead to lead within the same population; and (2) where significant differences were found, construction of a mathematical model to describe the interlead changes.

Analysis within the study populations. The first step was organized as a two-way mixed analysis of variance (ANOVA) model, the two factors being the leads (fixed effect) and the subjects (random effect).[11] The presence of patterns in the variables' mean values was assessed qualitatively from scatter diagrams and quantitatively from regression models. The scatter diagrams gave a visual indication of the type of the regression model that would be most appropriate, and the direction of the relationship.

Analysis between the study populations. Student's *t*-test was applied to both variables to identify significant differences between the study populations as follows: (1) on the lead-specific mean values; and (2) on the PSI. The tests were done on the transformed row data, in order to correct for skewness in the distributions. In particular, SoTm and the PSI were square-root transformed while TmTo was log-transformed.

Results

Analysis within the study populations. For the two populations, Table 24.2 shows lead-specific means and standard errors of SoTm and TmTo.

The ANOVA applied to these data showed that, for the normal population, there was a relationship between the ECG variables and the locations of precordial electrodes on the body surface. For both variables, the effects due to the leads on the variability of the transformed variable were significant ($p < 0.0001$) and, consequently, the existence of a pattern was assessed. In particular, moving from V2 to V6, the mean values of SoTm monotonically increased, while the mean values of TmTo monotonically decreased. In both cases, the patterns were statistically significant. Both patterns were modeled using a linear regression model as shown in Figures 24.5 and 24.6, which gave $r^2 = 0.955$ for SoTm and $r^2 = 0.97$ for TmTo.

Table 24.2 Lead-specific descriptive statistics of SoTm and TmTo (milliseconds) in the normal and LQTS populations

	Precordial lead Mean (SE)				
	V2	V3	V4	V5	V6
Normal (n=229)					
SoTm	191.6	199.3	207.4	211.7	214.2
	(1.78)	(1.82)	(1.87)	(1.80)	(1.77)
TmTo	123.8	121.3	115.9	111.3	106.1
	(1.89)	(0.99)	(1.03)	(1.16)	(1.21)
LQTS (n=25)					
SoTm	266.9	279.4	305.0	312.0	312.3
	(16.0)	(17.5)	(16.4)	(15.4)	(14.7)
TmTo	153.1	167.2	152.8	134.4	129.8
	(14.5)	(14.1)	(10.3)	(7.3)	(7.4)

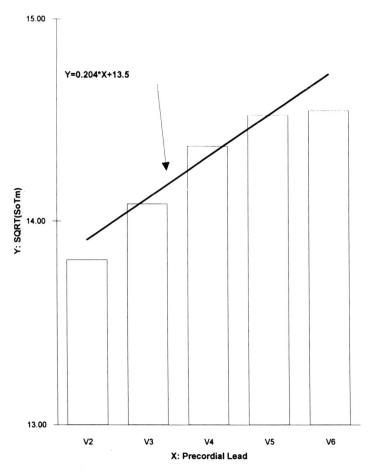

Figure 24.5 Mean values of the square-root-transformed SoTm versus precordial leads for the normal population ($n = 229$). The regression line is also shown and its equation given (V2: $X = 2$; V3: $X = 3$; ...).

Table 24.3 Comparison between the precordial sequence indexes of SoTm and TmTo with respect to their template sequence, for normal individuals and LQTS patients

Precordial sequence index	Normals ($n=229$)		LQTS ($n = 25$)		
	Mean	SE	Mean	SE	p-value
PSI_{SoTm}	2.01	0.35	0.51	0.086	0.0003
PSI_{TmTo}	3.82	0.37	2.27	0.12	0.0007

P-values refer to the square-root-transformed PSI data and were calculated via the t-test. The V2–V6 template sequences were '1,2,3,4,5' and '5,4,3,2,1' for SoTm and TmTo, respectively.

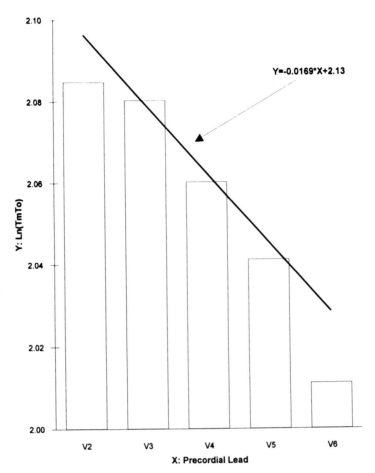

Figure 24.6 Mean values of the log-transformed TmTo versus precordial leads for the normal population (*n* = 229). The regression line is also shown and its equation given (V2: *X* = 2; V3: *X* = 3; . . .).

On the other hand, for the LQTS population, the results of the ANOVA test on both variables showed that the effect of the leads was not significant and, consequently, no pattern could be identified.

Analysis between the study populations. Lead-by-lead comparisons between the variables' mean values in the two populations revealed significant differences for all the leads ($p < 0.005$) except for TmTo in lead V2. As shown in Table 24.3, Student's *t*-test was used to compare the precordial sequence indexes between normal individuals and LQTS patients.

Time and Frequency Variability of Repolarization Duration

Study of the time variability of some cardiovascular parameters (typically the heart rate) has traditionally been used as a diagnostic tool in cardiology. In most cases, these parameters have been evaluated over a very short time (a few seconds). Recent advances in technology, above all in ECG recording capabilities and in the ability to process large amounts of data (e.g. the 24-hour Holter), have opened new frontiers for longer-term analysis of these parameters.

On the other hand, analysis of the frequency variability of cardiovascular parameters is a relatively new and promising technique that has been used to quantify the sympatho-vagal balance at the sinus node. This analysis has been developed mostly for the heart rate variability (HRV) signal. It has been shown that, in normal individuals, the power spectral density (PSD) of the HRV presents a well-defined pattern with low-frequency (0.02–0.15 Hz) and high-frequency (0.15–0.40 Hz) components.[12]

Experiments with pharmacologic blockade, surgical denervation, and mechanical stimulation have demonstrated the predominant role of the parasympathetic nervous system in the HF component (respiratory sinus arrhythmia) and the concomitant actions of both sympathetic and parasympathetic activities in the LF component.[13,14] It has also been shown that a convenient parameter to quantify the sympathovagal balance at the sinus node is the ratio between the powers of the LF and HF components of the PSD of the HRV. In fact, this ratio changes in a consistent manner with selective stimulation of parasympathetic and sympathetic limbs of the autonomic nervous system (ANS).

In contrast to the large number of studies assessing the mechanisms that control sinus node activity, only a few studies have evaluated the influence of the ANS on ventricular repolarization duration. The present work was designed to test the hypothesis that, in normal individuals, both RD and cardiac cycle length (CL, the reciprocal of the heart rate) are controlled by the ANS in a tonic and parallel manner.

It is well known that an abnormal RD may be associated with an increased propensity for fatal arrhythmias.[3] In this context, the ability of the control mechanisms to alter the duration of cardiac repolarization in response to changes in the heart rate is an essential component of the cardiovascular control. Increases in heart rate that are not accompanied by an appropriate decrease in the RD may lead to conduction disturbances that may predispose to ventricular re-entry and fibrillation.

In this perspective, the beat-to-beat study of synchronous series of RD and CL intervals could provide insight into the long-term (24 hours) and the short-term (3–4 minutes) regulation of these intervals. Long-term monitoring (over 24 hours) of the short-term RD variability under different physiologic conditions could reveal the role of tonic autonomic influences on ventricular RD.

Method

Study population and experimental protocol

The population consisted of 10 young healthy individuals (ages 23–31 years; 2 females) who volunteered to participate in the study. All were asymptomatic, medication-free and with no cardiovascular history suggestive of any organic heart disease. All underwent a baseline 24-hour Holter recording in which they were asked to act normally but to avoid maneuvers that could compromise the quality of the recording (e.g. heavy sport activity). They were instructed to keep a diary of their activities and to observe a period of passive standing for about 10 minutes immediately after waking up in the morning.

Six male subjects volunteered also for the second part of the experiment, which required treatment with beta-adrenergic blocking (BB) medication. The protocol was approved by the Committee on Investigations Involving Human Subjects of the University of Rochester and included, after cardiologic examination, oral treatment with the long-acting beta-blocker, nadolol (80 mg/day), for three consecutive days, and recording of the second Holter ECG on the third day. There were at least 22 days between the first and the second recordings, and the recording under treatment was always taken after the baseline one.

Data processing

Regression estimation. For all the subjects, the linear regresion equation RTm = a*RR + b, and the power regression equation RTm = a*RR^b, were estimated from all physiological RR–RTm pairs found in the entire 24-hour period.

Spectral estimation. Here, the time series involving consecutive values of RR and RTm intervals are referred to as HRV and repolarization duration variability (RDV) signals, respectively.

As shown in Figure 24.7, a data segment was defined as a sequence of 256 consecutive and synchronous couples of physiological RR and RTm intervals (approximately 3.5 minutes of ECG) that did not contain outliers according to prespecified subject-dependent thresholds. These thresholds were determined after visual inspection of the 24-hour RR and RTm histograms. A software program was developed to extract as many data segments as possible from the 24-hour Holter recordings of each individual.

Each data segment was tested for the presence of outliers, and abnormal values were replaced by linear splines with the values in the boundary regions. This correction technique permits a reliable estimate of power in the low- and high-frequency bands of the HRV signal power spectral density.[15] The linear trend was also calculated for each data segment and removed from the data segment itself.

Short-term (i.e. data segment) stationarity was assumed for both HRV and RDV signals. Each data segment was divided into seven subsegments of 64 values each that overlapped on each other for 50% of their lengths (32 values). For each subsegment, the data were weighted with a Hanning window, and the periodogram was estimated via the fast Fourier transform algorithm.[16,17] Finally, the data segment PSD was obtained by averaging the seven subsegment periodograms rescaled to take into account the power loss due to windowing. This technique provides statistically significant spectral estimates by limiting the leakage problem introduced by the implicit windowing of the data, and by giving stability to the estimate secondary to the reduction of the variability due to the tapering.

The cross-spectrum between HRV and RDV signals was quantified via the 'squared coherence spectrum' (SCS) and the 'phase spectrum' (PS) from the previously defined

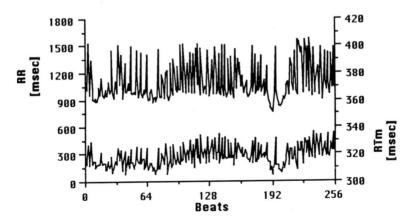

Figure 24.7 A data segment of 256 consecutive and synchronous values of RR and RTm intervals. The scales of the vertical axes are in milliseconds. The horizontal axis is in beat number. The left vertical scale refers to the HRV signal (top trace), while the right vertical scale refers to the RDV signal (low trace). (Reproduced with permission from reference 5: © IEEE)

overlapping subsegments. Considering a given data segment, and letting $X_i(f)$ and $Y_i(f)$, $|f| < 0.5$, be the periodograms of the HRV and the RDV signals, respectively, from the ith subsegment, we have:

$$S_x(f) = c \sum_{i=1}^{7} |X_i(f)|^2$$

$$S_y(f) = c \sum_{i=1}^{7} |Y_i(f)|^2$$

$$S_{xy}(f) = c \sum_{i=1}^{7} X_i^*(f)Y_i(f) \exp[-j2\pi(i-1)(P'/P)]$$

where $S_x(f)$ and $S_y(f)$ are the PSD of the HRV and RDV signals, respectively, and $S_{xy}(f)$ is the cross-spectrum. The frequency, f, originally expressed in cycles/beat, was success-fully converted to hertz.[13] The symbol * indicates a complex conjugate, the constant c is equal to $1/(7f_sP)$, where f_s is the time series' sampling frequency (1 in our case); P is the number of data points in each subsegment (64 in our case); and P' is the number of data points that are overlapped (32 in our case).

The PS is given by the phase of $S_{xy}(f)$, while the SCS is obtained as:

$$K_{xy}(f) = \frac{|S_{xy}(f)|^2}{S_x(f)S_y(f)}.$$

The SCS always ranges between 0 and 1, zero indicating no correlation between the signals $x(n)$ and $y(n)$. For a linear system, the SCS can be interpreted as the fractional portion of the mean-square value at the output $y(n)$ that is contributed by the input $x(n)$ at frequency f, or vice versa.

Statistical analysis

Two experiments were designed to investigate the effect of the autonomic nervous system on the RDV. The first, which we called 'night versus morning', was a mechanical maneuver; the second, called 'control versus beta-blocker', was a pharmacological stimulation.

In the *time-domain analysis*, classical statistical descriptors (mean, standard deviation) were used for RR and RTm. Furthermore, the 24-hour regression equations were also estimated for the available population and their coefficients were statistically compared using the ANOVA.

In the *frequency-domain analysis*, for all spectral and cross-spectral measurements, two main frequency bands were considered as specified earlier. The ratio, LH$_{RR}$, between the powers in LF and HF of the HRV power spectrum was used to estimate the instantaneous autonomic activity on the sinus node as suggested in reference 13.

The cross-spectrum between HRV and RDV was studied via the 'average maximum squared coherence' (AMSC) and the 'average phase delay' (APD) in the LF and HF bands. For each individual and for each of the two frequency bands, the AMSC was obtained by averaging, for all data segments under consideration, the maximum values of the SCS in that frequency band. Analogously, the APD was calculated by averaging the phase delays measured corresponding to the frequencies where the AMSCs were calculated. According to our conventions of Figure 24.1, a negative value of the phase delay indicated that HRV led RDV.

As for the HRV, the spectral distribution of the RDV was investigated via the parameter LH_{RTm}; that is, the ratio between the powers in LF and HF in the RDV power spectrum.

Night versus morning. For each individual, this experiment aimed at comparing the auto- (RDV) and cross- (HRV versus RDV) spectra between two data segments, one taken during the night and the other during the morning.

To avoid bias in data segment selection, the following criteria were established. The night segment was defined as the data segment with the smallest value of the LH_{RR} ratio between 3am and 5am, provided that the subject was sleeping as documented in her/his diary. If the subject was not sleeping, or if there were technical problems that prevented any reliable utilization of the data in that time period, the first 2 hours in which the subject was asleep were considered and the data segment with the smallest LH_{RR} ratio was chosen. REM sleep may have occurred during the selected nocturnal segment, and if so, it might compromise the steady state to some degree.

The morning segment was taken during the passive standing period defined as the interval between the first and the second tags electronically marked on the Holter tape via the event-button available on the Marquette Holter recorder.

Significant differences between night and morning in basic HRV and RDV parameters and in the previously described cross-spectral characteristics were calculated via a paired t-test. A p-value larger than 0.05 was considered not significant. Variances and LH ratios were log-transformed to make the respective distributions normal.

Control versus beta-blocker. For each of the six subjects who underwent treatment with a beta-blocker, this experiment aimed at comparing the following points before and after pharmacologic treatment: (1) the 24-hour RTm–RR regression equation coefficients over the entire 24-hour period; (2) the auto- (RDV) and cross- (HRV versus RDV) spectra with the modality explained below.

In order to account for the natural circadian variability of the ANS drive, the LH_{RR} ratio was computed in the 24-hour period for all the available data segments. The first (Q1) and the third (Q3) quartiles of the LH_{RR} ratio distribution were calculated. Each data segment was then classified into one of three possible 'autonomic activity classes' (AACs) according to the following criterion:

- autonomic activity class 1 (AA1), when $LH_{RR} > Q3$;
- autonomic activity class 2 (AA2), when $Q1 < LH_{RR} < Q3$;
- autonomic activity class 3 (AA3), when $LH_{RR} < Q1$.

As a result, each data segment was assigned a label indicating a particular spectral activity level: AA1 indicated prevalence of LF activity in the HRV power spectral density, AA2 a balanced situation, and AA3 prevalence of HF activity. Note that this labeling procedure was purposely subject-dependent to reduce the effect of the subject-to-subject variability.

For each individual participating in the experiment, 30 data segments in each of the three AACs were randomly selected from both the control and the BB-treated recordings (hence 90 (control) + 90 (BB) = 180 data segments in total per subject). Significant differences between controls and those treated with BB in basic HRV and RDV parameters and in the previously described cross-spectral characteristics were calculated via a paired t-test. A p-value larger than 0.05 was considered not significant. Variances and LH ratios were log-transformed to make the respective distributions normal.

The effect of a beta-blocker on the parameter LH_{RTm} was also investigated via a mixed three-way ANOVA model that was fitted through the log-transformed LH_{RTm} ratio. Main effects were the drug (fixed effect), the AAC (random effect), and the subject (random effect). This was done to isolate the variation in LH_{RTm} due to the beta-blocker from those due to the subject-to-subject variability and to natural circadian variation in the ANS drive. Both first- and second-order interactions were also considered in the model.

Results

24-hour analysis

Time-domain analysis. For each individual in the study population, an average of 93 044 cardiac beats were detected, 68 201 RR and RTm measurements (74% of the total number) were accepted for further analysis, 266.4 data segments were obtained, and 0.8 and 2.4 spline corrections per data segment in the HRV and RDV signals were performed, respectively.

The 24-hour mean linear regression equation was estimated for the entire population ($n = 10$) by averaging slopes and intercepts weighted by the inverse of the respective estimated variances. The equation found was:

$$RTm = 0.138 * RR + 0.154$$

where both RTm and RR are expressed in seconds. The mean correlation coefficient was 0.83 (ranging from 0.69 to 0.89) and all slopes were significantly different from zero ($p < 0.001$). Figure 24.8 shows the 24-hour regression line fitted through the data of subject 6.

A similar good fit was found when the regression line was estimated from the log-transformed data (power equation). All slopes were significantly different from zero ($p < 0.001$), and the mean correlation coefficient was again 0.83 (minimum 0.69, maximum 0.89). The mean regression line, expressed in terms of a power equation, was:

$$RTm = 0.291 * RR^{0.423}$$

where both RTm and RR are expressed in seconds. It is interesting to note that the exponent of this second equation is reasonably close to the value 0.5 used in Bazett's formula.[2] The reason why an equally good fit was obtained from both linear and power functions is that the range of variation of the independent variable (RR interval) between 500 and 1300 ms was far from zero; that is, from the region in which the power curve shows most of its nonlinearity.

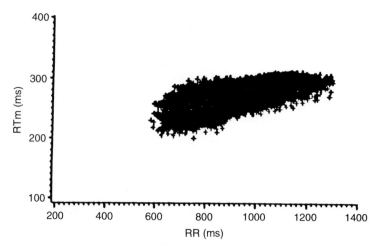

Figure 24.8 Scattergram between RTm and RR intervals in the 24-hour period for subject 6. The plot is obtained from 59 392 certified beats. The vertical and horizontal axes represent RTm and RR intervals, respectively and are expressed in milliseconds.

Frequency-domain analysis. Graphical representation of the 24-hour HRV and RDV power spectra was attained via three-dimensional clockplots as shown for subject 3 in Figures 24.9(a) and (b). Visual comparison alone suggests the qualitative identification of common spectral contributions.

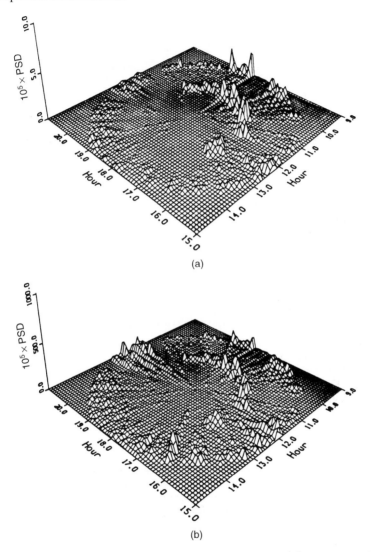

(a)

(b)

Figure 24.9 Three-dimensional clockplot as 24-hour representation of the power spectral density of (a) the HRV and (b) the RDV signals for subject 3. The clockpot is a diagram that is plotted in a 'mixed' coordinate system: the two independent variables, the time of the day and the frequency, are transformed in polar coordinates, while the dependent variable, the power spectral density, is left untouched. The base of the diagram, the polar part, can be considered as the face of a clock with 24 hours instead of the regular 12. As for a conventional clock, the time is a function of the angle with respect to a fixed radius and increases clockwise. As an example, the lower corner of the diagram represents hour 15:00, or 3pm. The frequency axis coincides with the radius: a frequency of 0 Hz corresponds to the largest radius attainable in the diagram, while a frequency of 0.5 Hz corresponds to radius zero, that is the center of the diagram. The vertical axis represents the power spectral density and is expressed in ms²/Hz. (Reproduced with permission from reference 5: © IEEE)

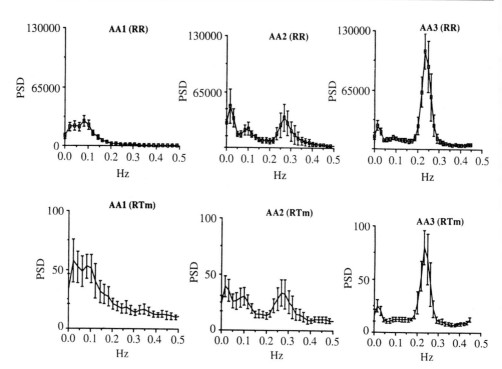

Figure 24.10   Averaged power spectral densities of HRV and RDV in different autonomic activity classes for subject 3. The vertical axes represent PSD and are expressed in ms²/Hz; the horizontal axes represent frequency and are expressed in Hz. The vertical bars indicate 95% confidence intervals.

Quantitative analysis showed that the mean AMSC for the entire untreated population (10 individuals, 90 data segments per individual: $n=900$) was 0.67 in LF and 0.61 in HF. Figure 24.10 shows for subject 3 the average PSDs of HRV and RDV in the three AACs. Here too, common spectral contributions are evident.

Night versus morning

Time-domain analysis. Table 24.4 presents the results of the 'night versus morning' experiment for the entire population (10 individuals, 1 data segment per individual and per experimental condition: $n=10$). The differences between night and morning were highly significant ($p < 0.005$) for all the HRV and RDV parameters considered.

Frequence-domain analysis. Figure 24.11 shows results from the night and morning experiment for subject 3. In particular, the HRV and RDV power spectra are given together with their SCS and PS. Differences are evident between the night and the morning segments. In particular, HF components dominated during the night, LF periodicities in the morning.

As quantitatively shown in Table 24.4, the LH_{RTm} ratio measured in the night was significantly smaller than the one in the morning. The AMSC calculated in the LF differed significantly between night and morning, while the AMSC calculated in the HF as well as the APD for both LF and HF did not. The average frequencies where AMSC and APD were measured were 0.09 Hz and 0.3 Hz and did not significantly change between night and morning.

Table 24.4 Comparison between night and morning for time-domain and frequency-domain variables

	Night (n=10)		Morning (n=10)		
	Mean	SE	Mean	SE	p-value
Time-domain analysis					
RR(ms)	1052	27.86	725	26.32	<0.0001
σ^2_{RR} (ln(ms^2))	7.69	0.33	8.84	0.22	<0.005
RTm (ms)	310	6	257	5.6	<0.0001
σ^2_{RTm} (ln(ms^2))	2.156	0.18	4.10	0.15	<0.0001
Frequency-domain analysis					
LH$_{RR}$(ln(.))	−0.77	0.25	2.50	0.17	<0.0001
LH$_{RTm}$(ln(.))	−0.884	0.12	0.63	0.18	<0.0001
AMSC LF	0.48	0.041	0.71	0.061	<0.006
AMSC HF	0.58	0.065	0.48	0.048	N S
APD LF (beats)	−0.8	0.67	0.6	1.7	N S
APD HF (beats)	0.6	0.14	−0.08	0.3	N S

The natural-logarithm transformation was used to normalize some of the distributions, and p-values were calculated via the paired *t*-test. As only one segment per individual and per experimental condition was used, the AMSC and APD figures were averaged only among subjects.
AMSC = average maximum squared coherence (dimensionless); APD = average phase delay; HF = high-frequency band; LF = low-frequency band; LH.. = LF/HF power spectral ratio (dimensionless); NS = not significant (p-value > 0.05); σ^2 = variance.

Control versus beta-blocker

Time-domain analysis. Table 24.5 provides basic time-domain measurements. The mean regression equations for the beta-blocked situation were:

$$RTm = 0.095 \text{ RR} * 0.189$$
$$RTm = 0.284 * RR^{0.342}$$

where both RR and RTm intervals are expressed in seconds.

It is interesting to note that, for the available population, Bazett's formula was no longer the best approximation, as found before in the untreated cases. In particular, Bazett's formula would have underestimated the repolarization duration for short RR intervals (RR < 800 ms) and overestimated it for long RR intervals (RR > 1200 ms). Table 24.6 shows the effect of the beta-blocker on the linear regression equation parameters.

A two-way mixed ANOVA model with no replications was fitted through the slopes of the regression lines (linear function) obtained before and during treatment with the beta-blocker. The two main factors were drug (fixed effect factor), and subject (random effect factor). Because of the absence of replications, the sum of squares of the error included also the possible interaction effects between drug and subject. Table 24.7 shows the results of the ANOVA.

The effect of the drug on the regression line slope was significant considering both the linear (p = 0.001) and the power (p = 0.005) regressions. Furthermore, for the linear function, the intercepts and the Fisher's z-transformed correlation coefficients were also significantly different (p < 0.01) before and during treatment with beta-blocker. Conversely, for the power function, only the slope (the exponent) and the correlation coefficient were significantly different (p < 0.01) before and during treatment with beta-blocker, while the intercept (the multiplicative factor) was not. In particular, slopes and

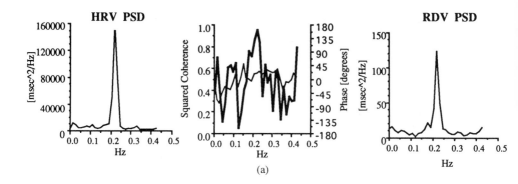

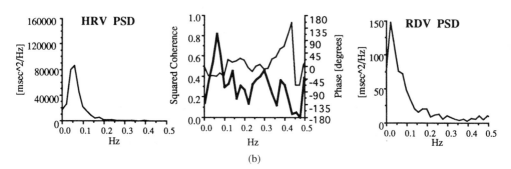

Figure 24.11 (a) Night segment and (b) morning segment. The left and the right charts represent the power spectra of the HRV and RDV, respectively. The y-axes are in ms^2/Hz, the x-axes are in HZ. The central chart represents the squared coherence spectrum (bold line) and the phase spectrum (light line) superimposed. The SCS is dimensionless (y-axis scale on the left) while for the PS the y-axes are in degrees (y-axis scale on the right). The x-axes are in HZ. The data are from subject 3. (Reproduced with permission from reference 5: © IEEE)

correlation coefficients for both functions decreased with treatment with beta-blocker, while the intercept of the linear function was increased by beta-blocker.

Frequency-domain analysis. Table 24.5 presents the results of the 'control versus beta-blocker' experiment for the available population (6 individuals, 90 data segments per individual and per experimental condition: $n = 540$). Also for this experiment the differences between control and treatment with BB were highly significant ($p < 0.0001$) for all the HRV and RDV parameters considered. The AMSC calculated in both LF and HF were significantly different between control and treatment with BB, while the APD for both LF and HF were not. The average frequencies where AMSC and APD were measured were 0.1 Hz and 0.3 Hz and did not significantly change between control and treatment with BB.

The ANOVA model shown in Table 24.8 confirmed that BB significantly reduces the LH$_{RTm}$ ratio. (The different levels of significance can be explained by the fact that, because of the nature of the model, no exact F-test could be calculated for the effect of the drug.) Furthermore, the ANOVA details the complexity of the relationships among the three main effects (Drug, AAC, and Subject), which was highlighted by the significance of all the interaction factors.

Table 24.5 Effect of beta-adrenergic blockade on time-domain and frequency-domain variables

	Control $(n=540)$		Beta-blocker $(n=540)$		
	Mean	SE	Mean	SE	p-value
Time-domain analysis					
RR (ms)	894	6.3	1087	6.6	<0.0001
σ^2_{RR} (ln(ms^2))	8.74	0.038	9.26	0.041	<0.0001
RTm (ms)	271	1.4	294	1.4	<0.0001
σ^2_{RTm} (ln(ms^2))	3.31	0.037	3.54	0.028	<0.0001
Frequency-domain analysis					
LH$_{RR}$ (ln(.))	1.01	0.043	0.52	0.045	<0.0001
LH$_{RTm}$ (ln(.))	−0.141	0.027	−0.490	0.019	<0.0001
AMSC LF	0.66	0.008	0.56	0.007	<0.0001
AMSC HF	0.58	0.008	0.54	0.007	<0.0001
APD LF (beats)	−1.3	0.13	−1.4	0.10	N S
APD HF (beats)	0.36	0.03	0.30	0.03	N S

The natural logarithm transformation was used to normalize some of the distributions, and p-values were calculated via the paired t-test. See also notes to Table 24.4.

Table 24.6 Slopes and correlation coefficients of the regression lines (linear equation), estimated for six normal males during control and beta-adrenergic blockade (the total number of heart beats that were used to estimate the regression equations is also given)

Subject	Control			Beta-blocker		
	Slope	r	Beats	Slope	r	Beats
1	0.09	0.69	90 802	0.08	0.69	85 248
2	0.11	0.79	94 109	0.07	0.63	75 349
3	0.13	0.86	102 166	0.09	0.81	91 877
4	0.13	0.84	77 173	0.10	0.78	75 907
5	0.14	0.84	90 939	0.11	0.72	76 847
6	0.16	0.89	75 122	0.12	0.81	78 102

Slope and r are dimensionless.

Conclusions

Preprocessing of the ECG

In this work, data acquisition and digitization were carried out using commercial electrocardiographic devices. In cardiologic research this approach has several potential advantages over *ad hoc* acquisition equipment. In fact, it provides a standard data acquisition procedure that allows scientists to concentrate on the data processing phase. As a consequence, it also contributes to the reproducibility of the results.

The use of new ECG variables, SoTm and RTm, as alternatives to the conventional QT interval, has proved to be feasible and has many advantages. RTm appears to be the most reliable RD measurement. In fact, RTm is a well-defined measurement in the majority of cases because it is limited by two sharp edges in the ECG (the R and T waves).

Table 24.7 Effect of beta-adrenergic blockade on the slope of the regression line (linear equation): two-way mixed ANOVA model with no replications (drug fixed effect factor, subject random effect factor). The population was six normal males each having two Holter ECGs (control and treatment with BB)

Source	DF	SS	MS	F	p-value
Drug	1	0.0042	0.0042	41.75	0.001
Subject	5	0.0041	0.0008	8.05	0.019
Error	5	0.0005	0.0001		
Total	11	0.0088	0.0008		

DF = degrees of freedom; F = F-statistic; MS = mean squares; SS = sum of squares.
Reproduced from reference 7.

Table 24.8 Effect of beta-adrenergic blockade on the LH_{RTm} ratio: three-way mixed ANOVA model with $n = 30$ replications per treatment (drug fixed effect factor, autonomic activity class and subject random effect factors)

Source	DF	SS	MS	F	p-value
Drug	1	32.863	32.863	8.69*	0.032
AAC	2	80.385	40.193	20.71	<0.001
Subject	5	40.322	8.064	4.16	0.026
Drug × AAC	2	3.680	1.840	4.08	0.051
Drug × subject	5	11.961	2.392	5.31	0.012
AAC × subject	10	19.405	1.940	12.27	<0.001
Drug × AAC × subject	10	4.508	0.451	2.85	0.002
Error	1044	165.045	0.158		
Total	1079	358.169	0.332		

AAC = autonomic activity class; DF = degrees of freedom; F = F-statistic; MS = mean squares; SS = sum of squares; × = interaction; * = approximate F-statistic.

Space variability

This work has described the precordial interlead variability of RD in normal individuals and LQTS patients. It implicitly assumed that minor errors in the placement of the electrodes were purely random and their effect on mean values cancels out.

A pattern dependent on lead location was identified in normal individuals for both SoTm and TmTo. The precordial sequence index, based on lead-location-dependent patterns, was introduced to represent the degree of disorder in the repolarization sequence of the variables with respect to a predefined template sequence.

Comparison between patterns obtained for the same variable in normal individuals and LQTS patients showed that the normal individuals had interlead changes that followed an identifiable pattern, while the LQTS patients did not show this pattern. The absence of this lead-location-dependent pattern in the LQTS population may be attributed to a disorder in the sequence of the underlying ventricular repolarization process that might be quantified by the precordial sequence index. The ability of this index to separate the two populations was shown for both variables.

The pattern of these two ECG variables, SoTm and TmTo, across the precordial leads in combination with the corresponding precordial sequence index might be clinically useful to identify patients with repolarization disorders.

Time and frequency variability

In the past two decades, many authors have studied the control of ventricular RD. The general conclusion has been that both CL and autonomic activity affect the RD, but it was not clear whether they act in parallel or whether the CL is the major determinant.[18,19] It is also known that sympathetic and parasympathetic innervations affect the ventricular myocardium as well as the sinus node.

A point common to most earlier studies has been that the measurements of both RD and CL were averaged over several beats. Hence, it was possible to refer to that technique as a 'static' approach. Conversely, with the hypothesis of a tonic autonomic influence on RD, our interest focused on the beat-to-beat variations of RD. According to this hypothesis, if the autonomic nervous system controls RD in a tonic manner, then this should produce periodicities in the RDV with periods reflecting the time responses of the neural systems involved in the control process.[7]

Time-domain analysis. This work has presented a computerized method to analyze automatically the 24-hour relationship between RD and CL. In particular, the increased accuracy in the RD measurement that follows from the RTm definition allows the use of noninteractive software to analyze 24-hour Holter recordings. As a consequence, for each individual, quantitation of the CL dependency of RD can be obtained on a large number of heart beats and, taking advantage of the physiological variations during the 24-hour period, over a wide range for both CL and RD.

A linear equation describes the relationship between RD and CL. An increase in regression equation complexity by log-transforming the data does not improve the goodness of the fit.

It was shown that treatment with a beta-blocker produces a significant reduction in the slope of the regression line in normal individuals. In other work,[20] it was demonstrated that patients with long QT syndrome have significantly increased RTm/RR slope when compared with normal individuals, indicating an exaggerated delay in repolarization following prolonged CLs. These pieces of evidence seem to indicate the appropriateness of a BB-based therapy for LQTS patients.

These findings provide additional insight into pause-dependent mechanisms of arrhythmic vulnerability of patients with delayed repolarization. It is hoped that this approach to the quantitative analysis of ventricular repolarization might improve the identification of patients at risk for malignant ventricular arrhythmias.

Frequency-domain analysis. SCS was used to assess common variations in the RDV and HRV signals on a frequency basis, and it may be interpreted as the squared correlation coefficient used in regression analysis. AMSCs of 0.67 and 0.61 were found in the LF and HF bands, respectively, for the entire untreated population. This means that more than half of the variability in one signal can be explained by the other. Note that this result alone does not imply causality between the two signals. Further, it was shown that the phase delay between RDV and HRV signals was small for LF and nearly zero for HF. These results suggest that there are tonic oscillations in RDV that are synchronously or nearly synchronously related to those in HRV.

The 'night versus morning' experiment provided two very different and meaningful patterns. In the spectra of both HRV and RDV, the predominant vagal influence of the night was well defined by a sharp peak in the HF band. In the morning, during passive standing, the spectra were dominated by the LF band. The pattern was consistent in all

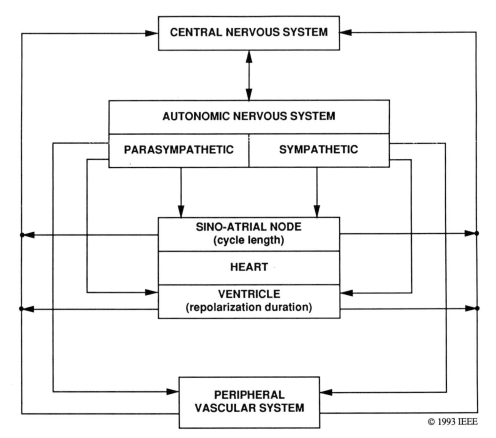

Figure 24.12   Schematic of the control of the autonomic nervous system on the heart. (Reproduced with permission from reference 5: © IEEE)

subjects. The beta-blocker, besides significantly lengthening the RTm and the RR intervals, had a marked effect on both RDV and HRV. In fact, the BB significantly increased their variances and shifted their power spectral densities towards the HF band.

These results suggest that the RDV has an autonomic origin and that both limbs of the ANS are involved on a beat-to-beat basis in RD control. More specifically, it is possible to assess the existence of a relationship between the power in the LF band and the sympathetic control of RD, and between the power in the HF band and the parasympathetic control of RD.

In normal individuals, the frequency contents of the RDV and HRV are qualitatively very similar, both having power contributions around 0.1 and 0.3 Hz. Attwell *et al.*[19] have shown a long-term response of the RD (similar to the response of a lowpass filter with cutoff frequency of about 0.007 Hz) to abrupt changes in the HR in an isolated portion of human ventricle devoid of neural input. If shorter-term periodicities in the HRV (e.g. 0.1 and 0.3 Hz) were transmitted to the RDV through this mechanism, they would be filtered out because they are at frequencies largely above the system cutoff frequency. This finding argues against a direct influence of HRV on RDV.

Figure 24.12 presents the basic conclusions of this study. In fact, at least for the short-term variability, for the range of normal variability in the HR (emergency situations such as sudden reduction of the HR have not been considered in this study), and for a population of normal individuals, our results suggest that both neural limbs of the ANS act in parallel and in similar ways to control the HR and the RD. In particular, the ANS controls HR by acting on the sinoatrial node and controls RD by acting directly on the ventricle. It is reasonable to speculate that some pathological conditions might uncouple the normal autonomic balance acting on the sinoatrial node (HR) and on the ventricle (RD), with resultant ventricular arrhythmias.

The possibility of having a quantitative measure of the autonomic factors affecting the sinus node and the ventricle could contribute to a better understanding of the autonomic influences involved in ventricular arrhythmias.

Finally, since LQTS is known to be a hereditary disease, the possibility of identifying more precisely affected individuals by RDV could be important in gene linkage studies.

Acknowledgement

The author would like to thank Michela Alberti, MS, for the material provided on the space variability of ventricular repolarization duration. This work was performed while the author was with the Department of Electrical Engineering, University of Rochester, New York.

References

1. Merri M, Benhorin J, Alberti M, Locati E, Moss AJ. Electrocardiographic quantitation of ventricular repolarization. *Circulation* 1989; **80**: 1301–8.
2. Bazett HC. An analysis of the time-relations of electrocardiograms. *Heart* 1920; **7**: 353–69.
3. Moss AJ, Schwartz PJ. Delayed repolarization (QT or QTU prolongation) and malignant ventricular arrhythmias. *Mod Conc Cardiovasc Dis* 1982; **51**: 85–90.
4. Benhorin J, Merri M, Alberti M, Locati E, Hall WJ, Moss AJ. The long QT syndrome: new electrocardiographic characteristics. *Circulation* 1990; **82**: 521–7.
5. Merri M, Alberti M, Moss AJ. Dynamic analysis of ventricular repolarization duration from 24-hour Holter recordings. *IEEE Trans Biomed Eng* 1993; **40**: 1219–25.
6. Franz MR, Bargheer K, Rafflenbeul W, Haverich A, Lichtlen PR. Monophasic action potential mapping in human subject with normal electrocardiogram: direct evidence for the genesis of the T wave. *Circulation* 1987; **75**: 379–86.
7. Merri M. *Static and Dynamic Analyses of Ventricular Repolarization Duration*. PhD thesis, University of Rochester, NY, 1989.
8. Alberti-Merri M. *Electrocardiographic Precordial Interlead Variability in Normal Individuals and Patients with Long QT Syndrome*. MS thesis, University of Rochester, NY, 1989.
9. Merri M, Farden DG, Mottley JG, Titlebaum EL. Sampling frequency of the electrocardiogram for spectral analysis of the heart rate variability. *IEEE Trans Biomed Eng* 1990; **37**: 99–106.
10. Moss AJ, Schwartz PJ, Crampton RR, Locati E, Carleen E. The long QT syndrome: a prospective international study. *Circulation* 1985; **71**: 17.
11. Neter J, Wasseman W, Kutner MH *Applied Linear Statistical Models*. Homewood, IL: R.D. Irwin Inc., 1985.
12. Baselli G, Cerutti S, Civardi S, Lombard F, Malliani A, Merri M, Pagani M, Rizzo G. Heart rate variability signal processing: a quantitative approach as aid to diagnosis in cardiovascular pathologies. *Int J Biomed Comp* 1987; **20**: 51–70.
13. Pagani M, Lombardi F, Guzzetti S, Rimoldi O, Furlan R, Pizzinelli P, Sandrone G, Malfatto G, Dell'Orto S, Piccaluga E, Turiel M, Baselli G, Cerutti S, Malliani A. Power spectral analysis of heart rate and arterial pressure variabilities as a marker of sympatho-vagal interaction in man and conscious dog. *Circ Res* 1989; **59**: 178–93.
14. Cerutti S, Alberti M, Baselli G, Rimoldi O, Malliani A, Merri M, Pagani M. Automatic assessment of the interaction between respiration and heart rate variability signal. *Med Prog Techn* 1988; **14**: 7–19.
15. Albrecht P, Cohen RJ. Estimation of heart rate power spectrum bands from real-world data: dealing with ectopic beats and noisy data. In: *Computers in Cardiology*. Bethesda, MA: IEEE Computer Society, 1988.
16. Oppenheim AV, Schafer RW. *Digital Signal Processing*. Englewood Cliffs, NJ: Prentice-Hall, 1975.
17. Bendat JS, Piersol AG. *Random Data: Analysis and Measurement Procedures*. New York: John Wiley, 1986.
18. Ahnve S, Vallin H. Influence of heart rate and inhibition of autonomic tone on the QT interval. *Circulation* 1983; **65**: 435–9.
19. Attwell D, Lee JA. A cellular basis for the primary long QT syndromes. *Lancet* 1988; 1136–1139.
20. Merri M, Moss AJ, Benhorin J, Locati E, Alberti M, Badilini F. Relation between ventricular repolarization duration and cardiac cycle length during 24-hour Holder recordings: findings in normal patients and patients with long QT syndrome. *Circulation* 1992; **85**: 1816–21.

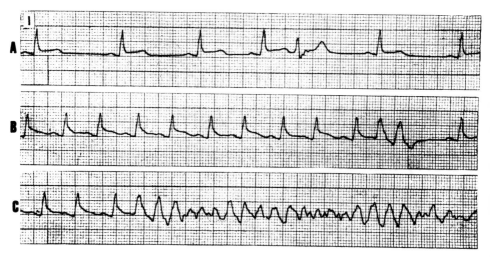

Figure 25.1 Tracing of a patient with acute myocardial ischemia in the early phase of anterior myocardial infarction shows a significant degree of alternans in lead I associated with ventricular premature beats. Following administration of atropine (0.6 mg IV), there was a significant increase in alternans level which culminated in ventricular fibrillation. We would anticipate, based on our canine studies of myocardial ischemia and our angioplasty studies, that the magnitude of alternans in the precordial leads overlying the ischemic zone would have been more marked than in the lead-I ECG depicted in the tracing. The top tracing shows sinus bradycardia (rate 55 bpm) with ventricular ectopics. The middle is a record 2 minutes after atropine administration, showing sinus tachycardia (rate 110/min) with consecutive ventricular ectopics. The bottom is a record 3 minutes after atropine, showing development of ventricular fibrillation. (Reproduced with permission from reference 31)

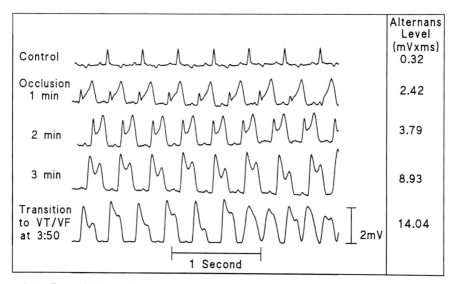

Figure 25.2 Precordial V5 ECG recorded during control and left anterior descending coronary artery occlusion in a representative canine experiment which culminated in ventricular fibrillation (VF). A progressive increase in the alternans level reached a maximum value just prior to onset of ventricular tachycardia (VT) which subsequently degenerated into ventricular fibrillation. (Reproduced with permission from reference 7)

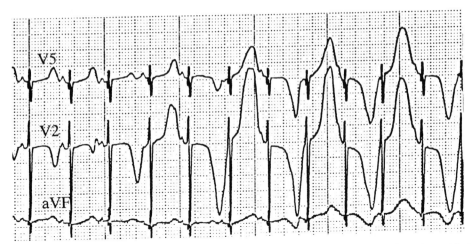

Figure 25.3   T-wave alternans recorded in a 3-channel ambulatory Holter recording of a patient with the long QT syndrome. Note beat-to-beat changes in shape, amplitude and phase of the T wave. (Reproduced with permission from reference 23)

2. What are the relative advantages of the current techniques for alternans analysis, namely fast Fourier transformation and complex demodulation?
3. In which pathologic conditions is alternans predictive of ventricular tachyarrhythmias and arrhythmic death?
4. What have been the technical and conceptual limitations to clinical use of alternans as a measure of vulnerability?
5. In which respects is electrocardiographic ambulatory recording uniquely suited to exploiting the prognostic potential of T-wave alternans, and how is digital technology superior to conventional AM recording?
5. What are the main hurdles in the application of ambulatory monitoring of T-wave alternans to assess risk for ventricular tachycardia and fibrillation?

T-Wave Alternans as a Marker of Vulnerability to Spontaneous Ventricular Arrhythmias

Reports by several investigators of a strong association between the occurrence of visible T-wave alternans and susceptibility to spontaneous ventricular tachycardia and fibrillation in experimental animals have been recently reviewed.[1] Russell and coworkers found in a canine study of 20 LAD occlusions which resulted in ventricular fibrillation that T-wave alternans was evident in 19 (95%). Dilly and Lab found in 7 intact porcine hearts which succumbed to fibrillation that in 5 (71%), alternans heralded the arrhythmias. In the acutely ischemic porcine heart, Downar and associates observed alternation to precede spontaneous ventricular fibrillation in 17 of 25 (68%) cases. These significant associations were observed without the benefit of quantification of alternans magnitude. T-wave alternans was simply approached by visual inspection of the electrocardiogram and treated as a qualitative parameter deemed to be 'present' or 'not present'.

Quantitative tracking of T-wave alternans during myocardial ischemia and reperfusion

Adam *et al.*[3] and Smith *et al.*[4] were the first investigators to show a close correlation between the magnitude of alternans and changes in fibrillation threshold produced by myocardial ischemia and rapid atrial pacing. This evidence that alternans, at least in the setting of myocardial ischemia, is a continuous function spawned a number of studies in which computerized methods were employed to evaluate alternans magnitude numerically and provided the opportunity to delineate its predictive potential.

Two general analytical techniques have been applied. The first involves fast Fourier transformation, which treats the alternans signal as a sine wave of constant magnitude and phase. This technique yields an average measure of T-wave alternans over as few as 128 beats.[3,4,6] In the more recent studies, a matrix method, which averages Fourier transforms obtained from 100 points across the ST segment and T wave, was used.[4,6] This type of signal-averaging generally reduces random noise in the power spectral estimate as a result of cancellation. Both methods carry the general intrinsic disadvantage of requiring a high degree of data stationarity and no changes in alternation pattern (i.e. ABAB to BABA), as may occur during abrupt cycle-length changes and arrhythmias. Unless adapted, these methods are not suited to tracking rapid changes in cardiac electrical stability such as those which occur during post-ischemia reperfusion and surges in autonomic activity.

The second category of techniques comprises dynamic methods, which are well-suited for analyzing ambulatory recordings of the transitory arrhythmogenic stimuli of daily life. The techniques include complex demodulation, estimation by subtraction, least-squares estimation, autoregressive (AR) estimation, and autoregressive moving-average (ARMA) estimation. The dynamic method which has been most extensively employed is complex demodulation.[5,7,11] This spectral analytical technique estimates the alternans signal as a sine wave whose amplitude and phase may vary with time and thus provides a continuous measure of T-wave alternans on a beat-by-beat basis. This technique has been described in detail.[11] The mathematical transformations essentially provide a measure of the changing area under successive T waves. The technique is relatively tolerant of nonstationary data, independent of phase-shift perturbations, and requires less than 30 seconds of data. These performance characteristics make it suitable for quantifying the effects of transient events, such as abrupt release-reperfusion and surges in autonomic nervous system activity, which may occur reflexly or in response to behavioral stress, and which exert a profound influence on cardiac vulnerability but may last less than a minute.

In a recent study, Nearing, Oesterle and Verrier[7] applied complex demodulation to analyze over 150 000 beats on a beat-to-beat basis. This database was obtained from 61 chloralose-anesthetized dogs during 122 ten-minute LAD coronary occlusions followed by abrupt reperfusion. A close temporal relationship between the spontaneous occurrence of ventricular tachycardia and fibrillation and the magnitude of T-wave alternans was demonstrated (Figure 25.4). A close linear relationship was discovered between the magnitude of T-wave alternans ($r^2 = 0.98$; $p < 0.06$) and the incidence of ventricular fibrillation and tachycardia. By contrast, there was no evident relationship between the incidence of these arrhythmias and the degree of ST segment depression in the left ventricular ECG ($r^2 = 0.26$; NS) or the prevalence of ventricular premature beats ($r^2 = 0.24$; NS). ST segment depression declined during the reperfusion-induced surge in vulnerability. The capacity of T-wave alternans to track vulnerability to arrhythmias during both coronary artery occlusion and reperfusion is particularly significant because it is well-established that differing mechanisms are responsible for vulnerability during these two events, and any suitable method for predicting susceptibility to fibrillation must be sensitive to both events.

Optimum lead system for detecting T-wave alternans

Ischemia-induced alternans. Recent evidence suggests that the precordial leads are well-suited to detect ischemia-induced T-wave alternans. Nearing, Oesterle and Verrier

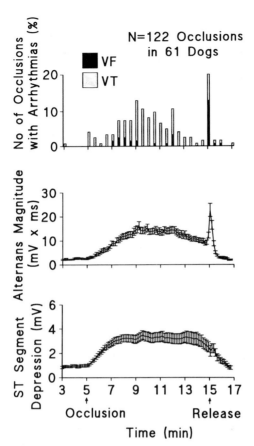

Figure 25.4 Simultaneous time course of spontaneous ventricular fibrillation (VF) and tachycardia (VT), T-wave alternans, and ST segment depression during 10 minutes of left anterior descending coronary artery occlusion and reperfusion in 61 chloralose anesthetized dogs monitored with a left ventricular (LV) ECG catheter. Two occlusion/release sequences were performed in each dog. Incidence of spontaneous VT and VF was summed for each 30 s period. T-wave alternans and ST segment changes were summed for each 10 ms interval. The waxing and waning of T-wave alternans magnitude closely parallels the spontaneous occurrence of malignant ventricular arrhythmias during both occlusion and reperfusion. By contrast, the ST segment changes were dissociated from arrhythmogenesis during the initial and latter minutes of the occlusion and upon reperfusion. The alternans and ST segment values are means, error bars = SEM. VT was defined as four or more successive ventricular ectopic beats. (Reproduced with permission from reference 7)

demonstrated in the 61 experimental animals described above that alternans is regionally specific and is linearly projected to the precordium.[7] The precordial lead system provides the maximum proximity of the recording electrode to the cardiac signal source, namely, the ischemic zone, which is the site of alternans generation.[1] T-wave alternans measured from the precordial ECG overlying the ischemic zone exhibited a statistically significant linear relationship to the left ventricular ECG ($r^2 = 0.86$; $p < 0.01$), detected the waxing and waning of T-wave alternans during occlusion and reperfusion, and correctly reproduced the period of maximum alternans during the vulnerable phase of the cardiac cycle.

The precordial leads were also found to detect the greatest magnitude of T-wave

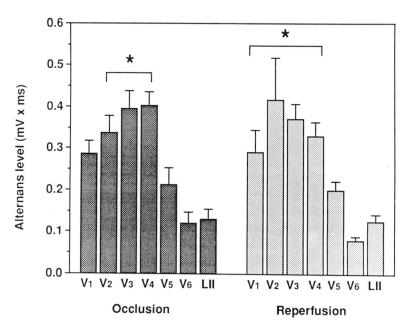

Figure 25.5 Magnitude of T-wave alternans as a function of recording site in seven patients at 3 minutes of angioplasty-induced occlusion and upon balloon deflation. Alternans detected during occlusion in leads V2–V4, the sites overlying the ischemic zone, was significantly greater ($p < 0.05$) than in leads II, V1, V5 and V6. During reperfusion, alternans levels in leads V1–V4 were significantly greater than in leads II, V5 and V6 ($p < 0.05$). Values are means, error bars = SEM. (Reproduced with permission from reference 7)

alternans in patients during angioplasty-induced ischemia of the LAD region. In seven patients it was found that leads V2 to V4, which overlie the ischemic zone, are superior to the other precordial leads and to the limb leads in detecting the extent of alternans (Figure 25.5). Precordial alternans was concentrated during the first half of the T wave, coinciding with the vulnerable period of the cardiac cycle. Alternans was not present in the Frank leads. These findings are congruent with clinical reports indicating that exercise stress testing,[1] attacks of Prinzmetal's angina,[9] and angina due to total LAD coronary occlusion[12] can provoke alternans in the precordial leads. In the latter case, T-wave alternans was most prominent in leads V2 to V5 during the first 3 minutes of the anginal attack (Figure 25.6).

Studies in experimental animals utilizing multiple epicardial electrograms during coronary occlusion[1,7] and human monophasic action potential recordings during coronary bypass graft occlusion[1] indicate that T-wave alternans is largely restricted to the ischemic region. These studies suggest that T-wave alternans will be most prominent in the ECG leads which have the ischemic injury within the field of view, namely V5–V6 for lateral ischemia, aVF for inferior, and V7–V9 for posterior ischemia.

Alternans during nonischemic states. The most appropriate leads for detecting alternans under nonischemic conditions remain to be determined. It has been demonstrated in the long QT syndrome that large-magnitude T-wave alternans can be detected using

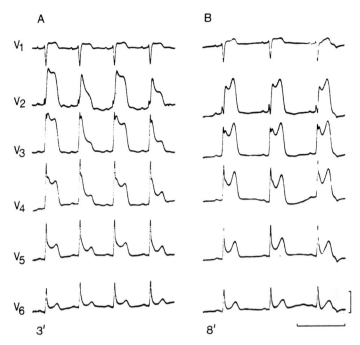

Figure 25.6 The left tracings show alternation in precordial leads V2–V5, 3 minutes after onset of chest pain due to complete left anterior descending coronary occlusion. In the right tracings, recorded 8 minutes after beginning of pain, alternation has disappeared, coinciding with lessening of ischemia and abatement of pain. (Reproduced with permission from reference 12)

various lead configurations, including the precordial, limb, and X,Y,Z orthogonal-type bipolar lead systems. This may be a consequence of complex sympathetic innervation and variations in regional sensitivity of the myocardium to catecholamines. In the population referred for electrophysiologic studies, the myocardial substrate may be highly varied and complex. Rosenbaum *et al.*[6] found in a mixed group of 83 patients with and without organic heart disease, at rest and in the absence of acute myocardial ischemia, that the Frank lead system was capable of disclosing microvolt levels of T-wave alternans.

The autonomic nervous system and T-wave alternans

Because autonomic influences play an important role in the genesis of ventricular tachyarrhythmias during ischemia and reperfusion, it was essential to demonstrate that T-wave alternans is capable of detecting the influence of both divisions of the autonomic nervous system. Stellectomy, which reduces sympathetic innervation, significantly diminished alternans during LAD coronary artery occlusion but enhanced its magnitude during reperfusion.[5] This observation concurs with the finding that sympathetic influences play a key role during ischemia, whereas washout products of cellular ischemia are largely responsible for susceptibility to fibrillation during reperfusion. The augmentation in vulnerability during reperfusion is probably due to the fact that stellectomy reduces coronary tone, thereby augmenting the reactive hyperemic response to release-reperfusion. This in turn leads to greater liberation of ischemic constituents, which enhances alternans.

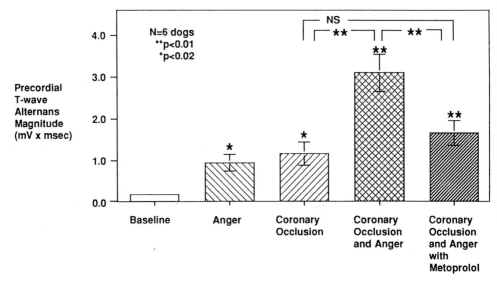

Figure 25.7 Effects of inducing aggressive arousal in canines on T-wave alternans before and during a 3-minute period of LAD coronary artery occlusion.[14] The behavioural paradigm consisted of a confrontation over access to food. The precordial V5 ECG demonstrates that, even in the absence of coronary occlusion, aggressive arousal elicits a significant degree of T-wave alternans (0.92 ± 0.2 mV ms, as quantified by complex demodulation). When aggressive arousal was superimposed on coronary occlusion, the alternans magnitude was nearly twice that observed with occlusion alone. The stress-related effects were significantly lessened by intravenous administration of metoprolol (1.5 mg/kg). The results were obtained during spontaneous rhythm. (Reproduced with permission from reference 14)

Stellate ganglion stimulation elicited a moderate increase in T-wave alternans prior to occlusion and a major enhancement throughout the 10-minute period of acute ischemia.[5] This finding is consistent with the existing literature on spontaneous ventricular fibrillation and on vulnerable period threshold testing. Simultaneous assessment by complex demodulation of heart rate variability and T-wave alternans demonstrates that the maximum level of T-wave alternans during occlusion coincides temporally with the maximum increase in reflex sympathetic activity.[13]

Particularly important in the context of assessment of the arrhythmogenic influences of daily life activities is the recent demonstration that T-wave alternans magnitude is sensitive to the effects of behavioural stress.[14] Using the precordial V5 ECG and a standardized paradigm in canines of aggressive arousal involving confrontation over access to food, it was found that stress elicited a significant enhancement in T-wave alternans prior to occlusion and increased by twofold the level of alternation elicited by a 3-minute period of occlusion alone. The stress-induced changes were significantly blunted by intravenous administration of metoprolol (1.5 mg/kg), further implicating a primary role of beta$_1$-adrenergic receptors in sympathetically induced vulnerability and T-wave alternans (Figure 25.7).

The mechanisms whereby enhanced sympathetic activity increases T-wave alternans and cardiac vulnerability in the normal and ischemic heart are complex as they result from both indirect and direct influences. Among the major indirect effects are an increase in heart rate which compromises diastolic coronary perfusion time, changes in coronary vasomotor tone, impairment of oxygen supply–demand ratio due to increased metabolic activity, and alterations in preload and afterload. The direct effects on cardiac electrophysiologic function include derangements in impulse formation, conduction, or both. The precise ionic bases for catecholamine-induced T-wave alternans remain to be elucidated.

Table 25.1 Ability of T-wave alternans to predict antifibrillatory efficacy of agents in current clinical use

Metoprolol reduces alternans induced by anger superimposed on myocardial ischemia[14]

Muscarinic blockade with glycopyrrolate enhances alternans associated with anger and myocardial ischemia (unpublished observations)

Nitroglycerin with blood pressure control prevents alternans during ischemia and reperfusion[15]

Calcium-channel blockade with diltiazem, verapamil or LU-49938 protects against ischemia- and reperfusion-induced alternans[1,9,32]

Nifedipine not effective in suppressing alternans or arrhythmias[22]

Vagus nerve stimulation is also capable of modulating the magnitude of T-wave alternans during acute coronary artery occlusion.[15] This is consistent with the finding that vagus nerve excitation is antifibrillatory during acute myocardial ischemia.[1] However, parasympathetic stimulation did not reduce reperfusion-induced alternans or fibrillation when heart rate was kept constant. The likely basis for these differing effects of vagal activity on alternans during occlusion and reperfusion is that the antifibrillatory influence of this pathway is dependent on accentuated antagonism of adrenergic activity during ischemia but not during release-reperfusion.

Other physiologic interventions which have been tested include rapid atrial pacing and hypothermia, and the results obtained with respect to T-wave alternans are concordant with the influence of these interventions on vulnerability to ventricular fibrillation.[3]

Pharmacologic interventions

There have been a limited number of studies of the effects of pharmacologic agents on T-wave alternans. The available data suggest that those drugs which suppress alternans appear to be antifibrillatory during both coronary artery occlusion and reperfusion. These results are summarized in Table 25.1. Whereas the findings are encouraging in indicating that alternans may be a useful guide for antifibrillatory therapy, considerable work remains to be performed.

Electrophysiologic Mechanisms Underlying T-Wave Alternans as an Index of Vulnerability

This issue has been addressed in detail in recent review articles,[1,2] and so the essential considerations will be summarized in this chapter.

Dispersion of repolarization

The bulk of the evidence indicates that regional disturbances in repolarization rather than in activation sequence are the basis for the link between ischemia-induced T-wave alternans and cardiac vulnerability. This concept is supported by studies utilizing diverse methodologic approaches ranging from intracellular recordings in isolated ischemic tissue to intracellular and extracellular recordings in intact preparations both with and without isopotential maps. Using monophasic action potential recordings, Kurz and coworkers demonstrated that both the amplitude and duration of action potentials alternate within the region of ischemia and exhibit regional heterogeneity. Smith and

Cohen have provided evidence using finite-element analysis that dispersed subpopulations of cells could give rise to macroscopic electrical alternans by creating transitory barriers to conduction leading to wavefront fractionation and re-entry.

Konta and coworkers employed epicardial mapping of electrograms to study the pattern of regional ST-segment alternans during LAD coronary artery occlusion in canines. They found that the amplitude of ST-segment alternans, measured as the difference in ST segment elevation in two consecutive electrograms, was significantly greater in dogs which fibrillated than in those which did not. The alternans was restricted to the ischemic and border zones and did not appear in normal tissue. No relationship was found between the area and magnitude of ST segment elevation and the occurrence of ventricular fibrillation. It was concluded that increased magnitude of ST-alternans during acute ischemia provides a measure of risk for ventricular fibrillation because alternans is an indicator of temporal and spatial unevenness of ventricular repolarization, properties which have been integrally linked to ventricular vulnerability.

Disturbances in recovery of excitability have also been implicated as a potential basis for the link between T-wave alternans and vulnerability to ventricular fibrillation. The main mechanisms appear to be post-repolarization refractoriness leading to unidirectional block and re-entry and the occurrence of ventricular tachycardia. Others have suggested a role of triggered activity in the form of early afterdepolarizations as a basis for T-wave alternans.[16]

Ionic basis for ischemia- and reperfusion-induced T-wave alternans

There is growing evidence that alterations in transmembrane or intracellular calcium movement play a major but not exclusive role in the genesis of T-wave alternans during acute myocardial ischemia. This is based on investigations involving calcium channel blockers, including verapamil and diltiazem, which suppress T-wave alternans and prevent ventricular fibrillation during myocardial ischemia and reperfusion. In patients with Prinzmetal's variant angina, Salerno *et al.*[9] found that pretreatment with diltiazem was capable of abolishing both T-wave alternans and ventricular arrhythmias precipitated by the ischemic attacks. Whereas these drugs do alter myocardial perfusion as well as cardiac electrical properties, based on TQ segment data, it appears that the capability to suppress T-wave alternans is independent of the influence of the drug on the extent of the ischemic insult. Utilizing the fluorescent calcium indicator Indo 1, Lee and colleagues demonstrated that alternans in the ischemic area is associated with spatial heterogeneity of calcium transients. Moreover, ryanodine, a drug which blocks calcium release from the sarcoplasmic reticulum, can suppress ischemia-induced alternans and the accompanying transients in calcium ion flux. The precise mechanisms whereby ionized calcium induces alternans, the specific intracellular compartments involved, and the role of sodium–calcium exchange require further exploration.

It is also important to consider the role of potassium in ischemia-induced T-wave alternans, because extracellular accumulation of this ion is thought to be responsible for post-repolarization refractoriness and is likely to contribute to the well-established depression of electrical restitution of action potential duration. Recently, Lucas and Antzelevitch[17] observed that the transient outward current is prominent mainly in epicardial but not endocardial tissue, a divergence which may contribute to differences in action potential morphology. During ischemia they found electrical alternans of epicardial action potential with a 2:1 or 3:1 pattern (Figure 25.8). This observation further emphasizes that a relationship between ionic channel kinetics, which can be determined by density or number of channels and by the time needed for channel opening, and the RR interval can be responsible for the observed pattern of T-wave alternans. In a pilot study, it has been shown that glibenclamide, which blocks the ATP-sensitive potassium

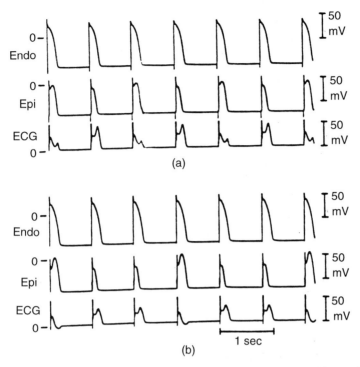

Figure 25.8 Typical patterns of electrical alternans obtained during simulated ischemia. In each panel, the upper and middle traces are microelectrode recordings from the endocardium (Endo) and epicardium (Epi), respectively, and the lower trace is the simulated ECG obtained by differential recording of the endocardial and epicardial voltages. (a) A 2:1 pattern of alternans obtained at a basic cycle length (BCL) of 800 ms. The action potentials in epicardium show an alternating sequence of long and short durations caused by the alternate presence and absence of the dome. Action potential duration is relatively constant in endocardium, so that the changes in the T wave are due entirely to the changes occurring in the epicardium. (b) A 3:1 pattern of alternans obtained during ischemia in a different set of epicardial and endocardial preparations at a basic cycle length of 800 ms. In this example, an action potential with a dome in epicardium is followed by two action potentials where the dome is suppressed. Changes in both the amplitude and polarity of the T wave were obtained in the ECG under these conditions. Action potential duration remained constant in endocardium during the period over which the record was taken. (Reproduced with permission from reference 17)

channel, prevents reperfusion-induced as well as ischemia-induced shortening of action potential and re-entrant arrhythmias.

Pathologic Conditions in which Alternans is Predictive of Arrhythmic Death

T-wave alternans has been observed under diverse clinical conditions,[16] including pericardial tamponade,[1] acute ischemia and infarction,[1,7,12] Prinzmetal's angina,[9,10,18,19] and the long QT syndrome.[20-22] It is essential to recognize that the electrophysiologic basis for alternans may differ depending on the specific disease state, and consequently may or may not indicate vulnerability to malignant ventricular arrhythmias. For example, during pericardial tamponade, the mechano-electrical interaction due to the swinging motion of the heart appears to be the primary cause of alternans[16] and is not associated with heterogeneity of repolarization or vulnerability to ventricular fibrillation. Thus, in this pathophysiologic context, alternans does not reflect heightened risk for arrhythmic death. By comparison, during acute myocardial ischemia, extensive experimental evidence reviewed above indicates that the magnitude of alternans does estimate the likelihood of impending fibrillation because it is a measure of nonuniformity of repolarization. The clinical relevance of this concept is supported by several studies which point to a link between alternans and the appearance of malignant arrhythmias in patients with ischemic heart disease, with Prinzmetal's angina, or with QT prolongation.

Myocardial ischemia and T-wave alternans in humans

Repolarization alternans has been observed under conditions conducive to myocardial ischemia,[1,12] including Prinzmetal's angina,[9,10,18,19] angioplasty,[1,7,23] bypass graft occlusion,[1] myocardial infarction,[1] and the post-exercise period.[1]

T-wave alternans and ischemia-induced arrhythmogenesis in Prinzmetal's angina

There have been numerous reports of the occurrence of visible T-wave alternans during attacks of variant angina. A reasonable possibility is that the occurrence of alternans in this condition is not a peculiarity of the syndrome but is rather a direct consequence of ischemia-induced conduction delay and heterogeneity of repolarization. In several large group studies of variant angina, Kleinfeld and Rozanski,[18,19] Salerno *et al*,[9] and Turitto and El-Sherif,[10] found a statistically significant association between the occurrence of visible T-wave alternans and ventricular arrhythmias during ischemic attacks. Both Salerno and colleagues and Turitto and El-Sherif based their analyses on ambulatory monitoring records, demonstrating the feasibility of this approach. However, in none of the studies was the degree of alternans quantified.

In Salerno's investigation involving 86 patients, visible alternans was observed in the ambulatory monitor record in 16 (35%) of 46 patients with Prinzmetal's variant angina who exhibited ventricular arrhythmias during ischemia, whereas the phenomenon was never observed in the remaining 40, who were arrhythmia-free during their ischemic attacks. It is noteworthy that in two recordings of ischemia in a single patient, one with and one without arrhythmia, the episode leading to arrhythmia exhibited a considerably greater magnitude of alternans (Figure 25.9). Based on data obtained from iso-area measurements of chest electrodes, Salerno and colleagues concluded that the induction of T-wave alternans in arrhythmogenesis was probably due to impaired conduction and heterogeneity of repolarization.

Turitto and El-Sherif[10] found in 65 patients that the incidence of arrhythmias in the ambulatory record was significantly higher in patients with visible ST-segment alternans (78%) than those (32%) without ST-alternans ($p < 0.05$). The statistical correlation between alternans and arrhythmogenesis pertained only to the occlusion and not the reperfusion phases. The frequency of ischemic attacks accompanied by angina, the magnitude of ST segment elevation at the peak of the ischemic attack, and the duration of the attack were all significantly greater in patients with visible T-wave alternans. They concluded that alternans of the ST segment represents an index of the severity of ischemia and is a precursor of ventricular arrhythmias.

In studies of Prinzmetal's angina patients in the hospital setting, Kleinfeld and Rozanski[18,19] noted that visible T-wave alternans was a concomitant of significant arrhythmias including ventricular fibrillation and tachycardia. In a study of 93 patients, 28 (30%) showed visible T-wave alternans during their ischemic attacks and these

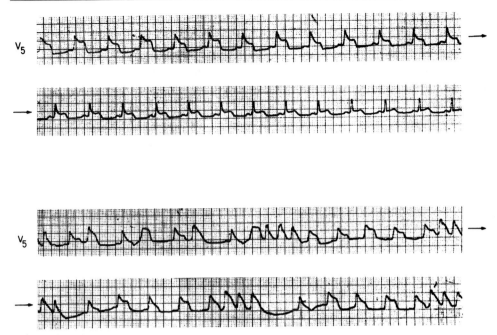

Figure 25.9 In the upper tracings, the resolution of an ischemic episode of Prinzmetal's angina with ST segment elevation of 5-minute duration is shown; no arrhythmias appear despite the presence of an evident ST-segment alternans. In the lower tracings, the electrocardiogram of the same case during another ischemic episode of 8-minute duration is reported; ST-segment alternans is associated with malignant ventricular arrhythmias. (Reproduced with permission from reference 9)

patients also experienced a greater frequency of arrhythmias during the attacks (95% versus 41% in patients without alternans), especially ventricular tachycardia and fibrillation (36% versus 4% in patients without alternans), along with more severe ischemia (5 mm versus 3 mm maximum elevation).[19]

T-wave alternans and idiopathic long QT syndrome

T-wave alternans has long been recognized as an integral component of the idiopathic long QT syndrome, in which it reflects heightened electrical instability[16,20,21] (Figure 25.3). Schwartz and colleagues have reproduced T-wave alternans in the cat by stimulating either the left stellate ganglion alone or both stellate ganglia with a greater intensity applied to the left.[20] They have also suggested that this phenomenon may be precipitated clinically by imbalances between right- and left-sided sympathetic nervous system activity which impinge on the myocardium hypersensitized by catecholamines, especially in response to physical and emotional stresses. Schwartz, Moss and colleagues[20] have established that pharmacologic or surgical blockade of the sympathetic nervous system has been effective in protecting patients against life-threatening arrhythmia, primarily in the form of torsades de pointes. An important precipitant of alternation and arrhythmias in the long QT syndrome is abrupt changes in cycle length.[16,20,21] Rosenbaum has proposed that the rate-dependency of T-wave alternans in patients with the long QT syndrome is due to disparities in action potential duration in response to rate of stimulation and in electrical restitution characteristics in subendocardial versus subepicardial fibers.[21] His hypothesis is that these regional differences in electrophysiologic

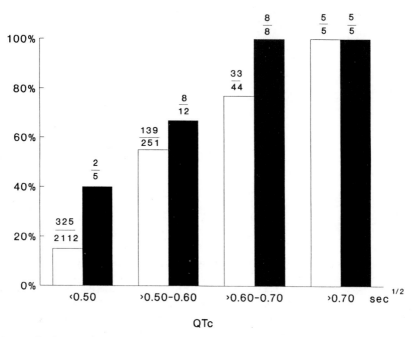

Figure 25.10   Cardiac event rates in patients with long QT syndrome with (solid bars) and without (open bars) T-wave alternans in relation to the repolarization delay (QTc interval length). Fractions above bars represent the number of patients with cardiac events in relation to the total number of subjects in each QTc category. (Reproduced with permission from reference 23)

properties account for the crossover in action potential durations on a beat-to-beat basis and this, in turn, is responsible for the dramatic reversion in polarity of the T wave which is often observed in the syndrome.

Zareba and colleagues observed a strong association between QTc prolongation and T-wave alternans among 1171 affected patients and the 1271 unaffected family members enrolled in the International Long QT Syndrome Registry.[23] They compared the events in the group of 30 patients who had visible T-wave alternans (2.6%) in a standard 12-lead ECG tracing to events in 583 patients whose ECG tracing showed no evidence of T-wave alternans. The incidence of cardiac events was significantly higher in members with (77%) than in those without (21%) visible T-wave alternans (Figure 25.10). In patients with QTc $\geq 0.60\,\text{s}^{1/2}$, visible alternans was also identified with increased cardiac vulnerability as seen in a greater number of episodes of torsades de pointes or ventricular fibrillation and runs of syncope. Because alternans magnitude was not assessed, its independent predictive value in this syndrome was not defined.

A critical issue is that gross T-wave alternans in the long QT syndrome is a highly transient and episodic phenomenon[20] which is unlikely to be recorded by chance in a routine 12-lead ECG generally taken over a 30-second period. There is a considerable risk that this snapshot approach will lead to a sizeable percentage of false negatives and inadequately represent the prevalence of the phenomenon. Ambulatory monitoring in these patients over a 24-hour period would provide a more adequate measure of the frequency of the phenomenon and the extent to which vulnerability may be precipitated by sympathetic activity such as occurs during behavioral arousal, phasic rapid eye movement sleep and exercise. Thus, the predictive value of alternans might have been augmented if the degree of T-wave alternans had been quantified, if continuous

Table 25.2 Limitations of standard clinical approaches for T-wave alternans analysis

Technical limitations
Low sensitivity and inadequate amplification of surface lead signals
Limited number of complexes recorded on standard 12-lead ECG
Poor fidelity and frequency response characteristics of certain AM ambulatory recordings

Conceptual limitations
Phenomenon viewed as 'present' or 'not present' rather than as a continuum requiring quantitative analysis
Inadequate recognition of the regional specificity of T-wave alternans, whose detection is optimized in the leads overlying the ischemic zone
Lack of use of provocative testing to expose latent cardiac electrical instability and T-wave alternans

Reprinted with permission from reference 2.

precordial rather than 12-lead electrocardiograms had been used (see Table 25.2), and if the patients had been recorded at or following periods of exertion or behavioral stress, which, as discussed above, are known to provoke alternans and cardiac vulnerability.

Zareba and coworkers have reported preliminary results of T-wave alternans recorded in long QT syndrome patients.[24,25] ECGs were acquired using a digital, 3-channel DMI AltairDisc Holter recorder (Diagnostic Medical Instruments Inc., Syracuse, NY), set at a sampling frequency of 1000 Hz per channel.[26] The magnitude of T-wave alternans was computed in each lead to obtain a specifically derived T-wave alternans index.[24] The maximum of median T-wave alternans index values in any of three leads was used to measure the extent of T-wave alternans in certain time series. They applied both autocorrelation and fast Fourier transform methods and found, in two-thirds of long QT syndrome patients studied, that T-wave alternans magnitude exceeded maximum values of age-matched controls[25] (Figure 25.11).

T-wave alternans and inducibility of ventricular tachycardia

In patients experiencing acute myocardial ischemia and those with the long QT syndrome, T-wave alternans may be sizeable on the surface ECG, occurring in the millivolt range and thus clearly visible. Recently, Rosenbaum *et al.*[6] found that nonvisible alternans in the microvolt range during atrial pacing at 100 bpm was a significant and independent predictor of inducible arrhythmias in 83 patients referred for electrophysiologic testing. They also observed in 66 of these patients that the presence of alternans and arrhythmia inducibility were significant and essentially equivalent predictors of arrhythmia-free survival ($p < 0.001$) (Figure 25.12). The patient population was diverse, including individuals with coronary artery disease, dilated cardiomyopathy, mitral valve prolapse and those without organic disease. It is likely that there are differing electrophysiologic bases for alternans under these varying conditions. Nevertheless, it is reasonable to infer that a common element underlies the ability of T-wave alternans to assess risk for arrhythmias under varying clinical conditions. This may be that alternans reflects nonuniform recovery of excitability, a prevalent and fundamental factor which predisposes to re-entrant tachyarrhythmias.

Technical and Conceptual Limitations

Decisive proof that T-wave alternans may be an index of cardiac vulnerability to fibrillation in humans has been elusive. This probably is attributable to several technical and conceptual limitations which have possibly underrepresented the occurrence and

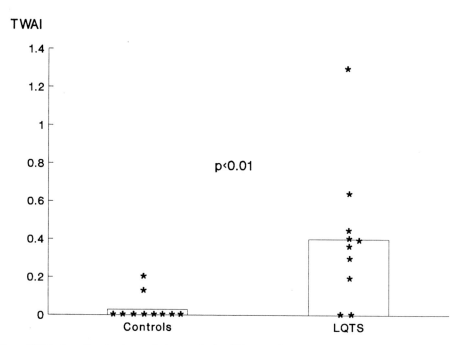

Figure 25.11   Results of autocorrelation analysis of T-wave alternans in digital Holter recordings of 10
· long QT syndrome patients and 10 age-matched controls. T-wave alternans index expresses the
magnitude of T-wave alternans. TWAI = T-wave alternans index. (Adapted with permission from
reference 24)

clinical significance of the phenomenon (Table 25.2). At least three important technical
limitations inherent in standard electrographic analysis contribute to the underestimation of T-wave alternans:

1. Surface leads have low sensitivity and are subject to cancellation of up to 90% of the
   electrocardiographic signal from the heart. In canines there is a 6- to 8-fold attenuation
   of the magnitude of T-wave alternans during occlusion in the surface leads overlying
   the ischemic zone, when compared with the simultaneous intracavitary ECG (Nearing and Verrier, unpublished observations).
2. Only a limited number of complexes are displayed in the standard 12-lead ECG,
   making visual detection of an alternation pattern virtually impossible.
3. Ambulatory monitors, a major potential resource for documenting alternans, exhibit
   limited fidelity and frequency response characteristics. The poor performance of
   certain AM recording units in accurately reproducing the content of the ECG in the
   low-frequency range is especially significant as this can critically distort recordings of
   ST segments or T waves and thus prevent accurate detection of alternans. Recent
   studies by Nearing and Verrier involving experimental animals, human subjects
   undergoing angioplasty, and computer simulations confirm this supposition and
   indicate furthermore that the distortion of T-wave alternans exhibits a rate-
   dependency (Figure 25.13). The distortion is most significant with heart rates in the
   range 60–120 bpm because of head resonance interference with low-frequency ECG
   components between 0.05 and 2.0 Hz. This observation carries important implications
   as it suggests that archival data of T-wave alternans from ambulatory monitors must
   be interpreted with caution.[33]

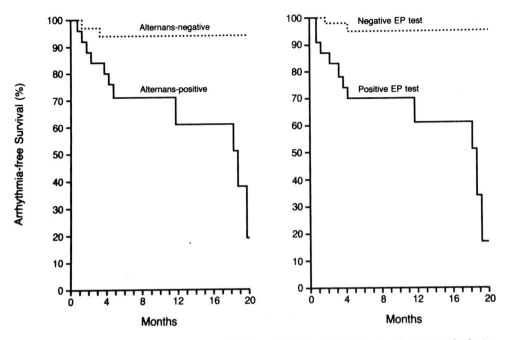

Figure 25.12 T-wave alternans and results of electrophysiologic (EP) testing in relation to arrhythmia-free survival among 66 patients. On the left, arrhythmia-free survival according to Kaplan–Meier life-table analysis is compared in patients with microvolt T-wave alternans (alternans ratio >3.0) and without it (ratio ≤3.0). Note that the presence of T-wave alternans is a strong predictor of reduced arrhythmia-free survival. On the right, arrhythmia-free survival among patients with positive EP tests is compared with that among patients in whom ventricular arrhythmias were not induced on EP testing (negative EP test). The predictive value of EP testing and T-wave alternans is essentially the same in this group of patients. (Reproduced with permission from reference 6)

The major conceptual limitations to the development of T-wave alternans as a marker of vulnerability to ventricular tachycardia and fibrillation relate to the need for improved quantitative methods for alternans detection, the regional specificity of the phenomenon, and the requirement of provocative testing to disclose latent cardiac electrical instability.

Except in a few recent studies, T-wave alternans has been regarded as being 'present' or 'not present' rather than as the continuous function indicated by the experimental studies. Power spectral analysis has revealed a quantifiable level of alternans in tracings in which it was not detectable by visual inspection.[6] The superiority of precordial electrodes for monitoring ischemia-induced alternans has only recently been demonstrated,[7] although diverse experimental and clinical studies have underscored the regional nature of the phenomenon.[1] To date, T-wave alternans has not been studied systematically in conjunction with provocative testing by exercise or behavioral stress. This shortcoming is especially significant since induction of major arrhythmia often requires not only the presence of a vulnerable myocardial substrate but also a physiologic precipitant.

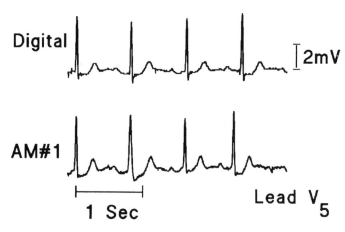

Figure 25.13 Representative tracing demonstrating overestimation of T-wave alternans magnitude by AM ambulatory monitor in an angioplasty patient in spontaneous rhythm. The probable basis for the electronic distortion is resonance of the signal with the recorder. (Reproduced with permission from reference 33)

Digital Monitoring and the Prognostic Potential of T-Wave Alternans

Technically, digital monitoring avoids electronic distortion associated with AM recorders and provides a ready interface with personal computers for signal enhancement, noise reduction, and quantification of T-wave alternans using a variety of spectral analytical methods in the time and frequency domains.

As a source of insights into pathophysiologic mechanisms of natural stressors, ambulatory monitoring of T-wave alternans permits detailed study of the interaction between potential arrhythmogenic triggers and the vulnerable cardiac substrate. Many of the daily life events which have been investigated with respect to silent myocardial ischemia are probably germane because of the close link between ischemia and the occurrence of T-wave alternans. Particularly relevant potential triggers are physical exertion and mental stress, which enhance sympathetic activity while reducing vagal tone. Several reports have documented the occurrence of T-wave alternans in patients with coronary artery disease during and after an exercise stress test,[1] but there have been no systematic studies of this relationship. The advent of standardized behavioral stress testing in humans represents a significant opportunity to determine whether behavioral interventions could be utilized in humans to uncover latent cardiac electrical instability as measured by T-wave alternans analysis. In experimental animals, it has been shown that induction of an anger-like state is capable of producing a high degree of alternans in the normal heart, an effect which is markedly enhanced when anger is superimposed on acute myocardial ischemia[14] (Figure 25.7).

Certain sleep states have been implicated in the genesis of myocardial ischemia and arrhythmic death. There is evidence linking rapid eye movement (REM) sleep to the exacerbation of nocturnal ischemia, and it has been suggested that this state may play a role in arrhythmic death in patients with severe congestive heart failure.[27] Finally, ambulatory monitoring of T-wave alternans may provide important insights into the mechanisms which account for the circadian pattern of sudden cardiac death in patients with ischemic heart disease and severe heart failure.[27,28] This issue is particularly germane in light of the recent evidence of circadian patterns in the discharge frequency of implantable cardioverter/defibrillators[29] and in the occurrence of ventricular tachycardia.[30]

Conclusions

T-wave alternans analysis is a promising method for assessing risk for ventricular tachycardia and fibrillation under diverse pathologic conditions. In the most extensively studied conditions, namely acute myocardial ischemia, Prinzmetal's angina, and the long QT syndrome, there is substantial evidence indicating that the predictive power is based on heterogeneity of repolarization, a central factor in re-entrant tachyarrhythmias. Several analytical techniques, including fast Fourier transform analysis, autocorrelation, and complex demodulation permit automated assessment of T-wave alternans magnitude. Digital recorders are highly preferable because they avoid electronic distortion of T-wave morphology associated with AM recorders. Thus, digital ambulatory ECG monitoring of T-wave alternans magnitude provides an attractive method for automated assessment of risk for ventricular tachyarrhythmia for use in routine clinical practice. This approach may also help to guide therapy, as there is encouraging evidence that T-wave alternans also predicts antifibrillatory efficacy of drugs and is able to disclose propensity to proarrhythmic responses.

Acknowledgement

The authors thank Sandra S. Verrier for her editorial contributions. The work was supported by grants HL33567, HL50078 and HL33843 from the National Heart, Lung and Blood Institute of the National Institutes of Health, Bethesda, Maryland, USA.

References

1. Verrier RL, Nearing BD. Electrophysiologic basis for T-wave alternans as an index of vulnerability to ventricular fibrillation. *J Cardiovasc Electrophysiol* 1994; **5**: 445–61.
2. Verrier RL, Nearing BD. T-wave alternans as a harbinger of ischemia-induced sudden cardiac death. In: Zipes DP, Jalife J (eds), *Cardiac Electrophysiology: From Cell to Bedside*, 2nd edn. Philadelphia: W.B. Saunders, 1995: 467.
3. Adam DR, Smith JM, Akselrod S, *et al*. Fluctuations in T-wave morphology and susceptibility to ventricular fibrillation. *J Electrocardiol* 1984; **17**: 209–18.
4. Smith JM, Clancy EA, Valeri CR, *et al*. Electrical alternans and cardiac electrical instability. *Circulation* 1988; **77**: 110–21.
5. Nearing BD, Huang AH, Verrier RL. Dynamic tracking of cardiac vulnerability by complex demodulation of the T-wave. *Science* 1991; **252**: 437–40.
6. Rosenbaum DS, Jackson LE, Smith JM, *et al*. Electrical alternans and vulnerability to ventricular arrhythmia. *New Engl J Med* 1994; **330**: 235–41.
7. Nearing BD, Oesterle SN, Verrier RL. Quantification of ischaemia-induced vulnerability by precordial T-wave alternans analysis in dog and human. *Cardiovasc Res* 1994; **28**: 1440–49.
8. Deedwania P, Carbajal E. Silent ischemia during daily life is an independent predictor of mortality in stable angina. *Circulation* 1990; **81**: 748–56.
9. Salerno JA, Previtali M, Panciroli C, *et al*. Ventricular arrhythmias during acute myocardial ischaemia in man: the role and significance of R–ST–T alternans and the prevention of ischaemic sudden death by medical treatment. *Eur Heart J* 1986; **7**: 63–75.
10. Turitto G, El-Sherif N. Alternans of the ST segment in variant angina: incidence, time course and relation to ventricular arrhythmias during ambulatory electrocardiographic recording. *Chest* 1988; **93**: 587–91.
11. Nearing BD, Verrier RL. Personal computer system for tracking cardiac vulnerability by complex demodulation of the T wave. *J Appl Physiol* 1993; **74**: 2606–12.
12. Cinca J, Janse MJ, Morena H *et al*. Mechanisms and time course of the early electrical changes during acute coronary artery occlusion: an attempt to correlate the early ECG changes in man to cellular electrophysiology in the pig. *Chest* 1980; **77**: 499–505.

13. Nearing BD, Verrier RL. Simultaneous assessment of autonomic regulation and cardiac vulnerability during coronary occlusion and reperfusion by complex demodulation of heart rate variability and T-wave alternans (abstract). *Circulation* 1992; **86**[Suppl I]: 639.

14. Kovach JA, Nearing BD, Verrier RL. Effect of aggressive arousal on precordial T-wave alternans magnitude in the normal and ischemic canine heart with and without beta$_1$-adrenergic blockade with metoprolol (abstract). *J Am Coll Cardiol* 1994; **23**: 329A.

15. Nearing BD, Verrier RL. Evaluation of antifibrillatory interventions by complex demodulation of the T-wave (abstract). *Circulation* 1991; **84**: II-499.

16. Surawicz B, Fisch C. Cardiac alternans: diverse mechanisms and clinical manifestations. *J Am Coll Cardiol* 1992; **20**: 483–99.

17. Lukas A, Antzelevitch C. Differences in the electrophysiologic response of canine ventricular epicardium and endocardium to ischemia: role of the transient outward current. *Circulation* 1993; **88**: 2903–15.

18. Kleinfeld MJ, Rozanski JJ. Alternans of the ST segment in Prinzmetal's angina. *Circulation* 1977; **55**: 574–7.

19. Rozanski JJ, Kleinfeld M. Alternans of the ST segment and T wave: a sign of electrical instability in Prinzmetal's angina. *PACE* 1982; **5**: 359–65.

20. Schwartz PJ, Zaza A, Locati E, *et al*. Stress and sudden death: the case of the long QT syndrome. *Circulation* 1991; **83**(Suppl 4): II-71–90.

21. Rosenbaum MB, Acunzo RS. Pseudo 2:1 atrioventricular block and T wave alternans in the long QT syndromes. *J Am Coll Cardiol* 1991; **18**: 1363–6.

22. Zareba W, Moss AJ, le Cessie S, *et al*. T wave alternans in idiopathic long QT syndrome. *J Am Coll Cardiol* 1994; **23**: 1541–6.

23. Sochanski M, Feldman T, Chua KG, *et al*. ST segment alternans during coronary angioplasty. *Cathet Cardiovasc Diag* 1992; **27**: 45–8.

24. Zareba W, Badilini F, Moss AJ. Automatic detection of spatial and dynamic heterogeneity of repolarization. *J Electrocardiol* 1994; **27**: 65–71.

25. Zareba W, Badilini F, Moss AJ. Holter identification of non-visible T-wave alternans in the long QT syndrome (abstract). *J Ambul Monit* 1994; **7**: 97.

26. DeMaso J, Myers S, Nels D, Sellers C. Ambulatory high-resolution ECG recorder using disk storage. *J Ambul Monit* 1992; **5**: 317–22.

27. Moser DK, Stevenson WG, Woo MA, *et al*. Timing of sudden death in patients with heart failure. *J Am Coll Cardiol* 1994; **24**: 963–7.

28. Muller JE, Ludmer PL, Willich SN, *et al*. Circadian variation in the frequency of sudden cardiac death. *Circulation* 1987; **75**: 131–8.

29. Tofler GH, Gebara OCE, Mittleman MA, *et al*. Morning peak in ventricular tachyarrhythmias detected by time of implantable cardioverter/defibrillator therapy. *Circulation* 1995 (in press).

30. Lampert R, Rosenfeld L, Batsford W, *et al*. Circadian variation of sustained ventricular tachycardia in patients with coronary artery disease and implantable cardioverter–defibrillators. *Circulation* 1994; **90**: 241–7.

31. Pantridge JF. Autonomic disturbance at the onset of acute myocardial infarction. In: Schwartz PJ, Brown AM, Malliani A, Zanchetti A (eds), *Neural Mechanisms in Cardiac Arrhythmias*. New York: Raven Press, 1978: 7.

32. Nearing BD, Hutter JJ, Verrier RL. Potent antifibrillatory effect of combined blockade of calcium channels and serotonin 5-HT$_2$ receptors with LU-49938 during myocardial ischemia and reperfusion in canines (abstract). *J Am Coll Cardiol* 1994; **23**: 42A.

33. Nearing BD, Barbey JT, Verrier RL, Potential limitations of AM Holter monitoring for tracking cardiac electrical instability by T-wave alternans magnitude (abstract). *PACE* 1995; **18**: 891.

26

Clinical Utility of QT Interval Monitoring

Peter J. Schwartz and Silvia G. Priori

Introduction

How impressive has been the change in the level of clinical interest for ventricular repolarization is best exemplified by the sentence 'The measurement of the QT interval has little usefulness', found in a respected textbook of electrocardiography published in 1957.[1] The clinical evidence accumulated primarily in the 1970s has largely convinced cardiologists that abnormal prolongation of the QT interval on the surface ECG is associated with an increased risk of arrhythmic death under a variety of conditions.[2–6] It is thus not surprising that there is now growing interest in the possibility that dynamic recording of the QT interval by Holter monitoring may also provide information of clinical relevance. However, in contrast to the mass of data based on surface ECGs, clinical data on the QT interval based on Holter recordings are scanty and several different methodologies are being evaluated, as is evident from earlier chapters.

In this chapter we discuss briefly some of the main methodological issues involved in the analysis of the QT interval based on ambulatory monitoring and what might be the clinical relevance today of the studies that focus on ventricular repolarization, thus including the QT interval and the morphology of the T wave.

Methodological Problems

The greatest weakness in all studies of the QT interval has been the subjective nature of its measurement, and specifically identification of the point considered to be the end of the T wave. This may not be a problem in most normal individuals because the return of the T wave towards the baseline is quite abrupt; nor in patients with marked pro-longation of repolarization because, despite the potential error, the measurement will show an abnormal value. However, there is a major problem in all borderline cases and in those with a definite but modest prolongation of the QT interval.

Most automated programs used to determine the end of the T wave involve either drawing a tangent to the steepest portion of the descending limb of the T wave, or the use of the peak of the T wave.

To draw such a tangent, the method proposed by Browne *et al.*[7] is acceptable when there is a uniform return to baseline. However, when the descending limb of the T wave has two components, the first quite rapid and the second slower, use of the tangent method leads to an underestimation of the length of the QT interval. It is important to remember that, particularly with neurally mediated alterations of ventricular repolariz-ation, it is indeed the last part of the T wave that is affected. Furthermore, the effect of the most important repolarizing current, the delayed rectifier I_k, becomes maximal towards the end of repolarization; it follows that abnormalities, secondary either to a disease or to a drug with potassium-channel blocking activity, will predominantly if not exclusively affect the last portion of the T wave. Use of the tangent method may portray as normal or mildly abnormal a repolarization that is actually grossly abnormal.

Use of the peak of the T wave results, of course, in an exaggeration of the consequences of drawing a tangent, because the entire final part of the T wave is left out. This may be acceptable when dealing with individuals with normal repolarization, but it presents a major problem when dealing with patients with abnormal repolarization. Even though the cycle-length dependency of repolarization is concentrated primarily in the first part of the QT interval ending at the peak of the T wave,[8] the arrhythmogenic substrate inherent in prolonged repolarization is largely confined to the second part of the T wave corresponding to phase 3 of action potential repolarization, the phase with the highest probability of early after-depolarizations.

Computerized analysis requires points to be mathematically defined, but caution is necessary when this may be at the expense of biologically relevant information. The temptation to adapt an analysis to the parameters most easily identifiable should not overrule the necessity to resist 'the tyranny of the great simplifiers', a message given long time ago by the Swiss philosopher Burkhardt. The crucial point here is that the last part of repolarization contains biologically important information that should not be neglected by any analysis. These considerations imply that some of the methods in current use may generate rapidly a large mass of data, but with a degree of oversimplification that, particularly when dealing with individuals with an abnormal repolarization, might lead to incorrect conclusions.

Current Approaches and Clinical Utility

The availability of 24-hour Holter monitoring has allowed the introduction of dynamic analysis in the evaluation of ECG recordings. Whereas the dynamicity of the RR interval has been widely explored in both the time and frequency domains, the concept of dynamic evaluation of the QT interval is relatively new.

Most current methods of analysis of ventricular repolarization from Holter recordings can be considered to belong to one of two groups. The first group deals largely with the analysis of the QT–RR relationship, with its own subdivisions. The second group deals primarily with beat-to-beat T wave fluctuations. As the field is rapidly evolving and several new techniques are already looming, it is likely that a critical reappraisal of this entire issue will soon become necessary.

Even though there have been few publications on QT dynamicity, several techniques have been proposed. Here, we will review the most promising approaches to the study of repolarization using Holter recording.

Analysis of the QT/RR Interval Relation

The vexed question of which formula best reflects the adaptation of the QT interval to heart rate has not yet produced a method that can be considered satisfactory under most conditions. As a consequence, it is unlikely that a simple adjustment equation could correctly reflect the QR/RR relationship. To avoid limitations inherent in the use of a 'correction' formula, the relationship between QT and RR intervals over a large range of rates is usually studied by identifying the regression line that best fits the distribution of

QT and RR intervals. However, this approach has the inherent limitation of assuming that a linear relationship exists between heart rate and QT, a concept which has been challenged[9,10] and which is probably true only within a limited range of frequencies.

Holter-recorded ECGs may provide access to a relatively large range of cycle lengths occurring spontaneously over the 24 hours and may permit investigation of the QT/RR relationship in individual subjects and its expression as the slope of the best-fitting line. Alterations in this QT/RR relationship have been shown to exist in clinical conditions associated with ventricular arrhythmias, and some examples are cited below.

Viñolas *et al.*[11] reported that post-MI patients with life-threatening arrhythmias have an altered QT/RR interval relationship. The slope of the best-fit linear regression equation between QT and RR in the control group of healthy individuals ($n = 10$) was 0.4, while in the post-MI patients with life-threatening arrhythmias it was 0.8. Fei *et al.*[12,13] found an altered slope of the linear regression line in patients with idiopathic ventricular tachycardia (0.24 versus 0.27 in control subjects) and in survivors of cardiac arrest (0.19 versus 0.12 observed in control subjects). Merri *et al.*[8] showed that the relationship between duration of ventricular repolarization and cycle length is altered in patients affected by the long QT syndrome. In the control group ($n = 11$) the slope was 0.14, while in LQTS patients ($n = 16$) it was 0.21.

Although the authors of all these studies conclude that under pathologic conditions there is an abnormal QT/RR relationship, large discrepancies exist even on the value that the QT/RR should have in control subjects (Table 26.1). These discrepancies may be due to the small sample size of the populations under study or to methodological differences in the measurement of the QT interval.

Merri *et al.*[8] measured the adaptation of ventricular repolarization to cycle-length changes not by measuring the QT interval, but using the RTm interval which extends from the peak of the R wave to the apex of the T wave. It is true that RTm can be more easily identified by an automatic computerized system than can the QT interval; however, as discussed earlier, this method neglects the final component of the T wave which is often the site of electrophysiologic abnormalities, particularly in patients affected by the long QT syndrome.[14,15]

In the two papers by Fei *et al.*,[12,13] the slope of the QT/RR regression line presents larger variations between the two control groups (0.12 versus 0.27) than between each control group and its respective patients group (0.12 versus 0.19 and 0.27 versus 0.24). Furthermore, whereas patients resuscitated from sudden cardiac death had a steeper slope than controls, patients with ventricular tachycardia had a flatter slope than controls. These conflicting results should call for extreme caution before drawing strong conclusions with this method.

Rasmussen *et al.*[16] studied 60 normal individuals in what is probably the largest study so far. The average value of the slope of the QT/RR regression line was 0.14, which is close to the normality values reported by Merri *et al.*[8] and by one of the two studies by Fei *et al.*[13] However, these values are remarkably different from those found by Viñolas *et al.*[11]

The lack of consistency between the results published on the cycle-length dependency of ventricular repolarization requires an explanation. Besides the very limited number of

Table 26.1 Slope of the best-fit linear regression equation between QT and RR intervals

Author	Controls	Patients	
Merri *et al.*[8]	0.14	0.21	(long QT syndrome)
Viñolas *et al.*[11]	0.40	0.80	(ventricular tachycardia)
Fei *et al.*[12]	0.12	0.19	(survivors of ventricular fibrillation)
Fei *et al.*[13]	0.27	0.24	(ventricular tachycardia)
Rasmussen *et al.*[16]	0.14	—	

individuals involved in each study, there are also oversimplifications in the data collection that may have contributed to the overall result.

Elharrar and Surawicz, in an *in vitro* study,[17] developed a quantitative method for the analysis of steady-state and kinetic properties of the rate-dependency of repolarization (restitution curves). When Franz et al.[18] and Zaza et al.[19] applied these methods *in vivo*, they confirmed the existence of a slow adaptation process of ventricular repolarization to changes in cycle length. These findings call for caution in interpreting data on the QT/RR relationship when they are not obtained in steady-state conditions (at least 3 minutes of constant heart rate). It follows that when data from Holter recordings are used, care should be taken to use only steady-state conditions for the evaluation of the QT/RR relationship. None of the studies discussed above has specified if these conditions were indeed met. When non-steady-state values are considered, or when averaging of consecutive beats is used, as happens with several examples of commercially available software, it is not surprising that large variability is observed. This may help to explain the inconsistencies currently present in the literature.

Despite the limitations listed above, the concept that an abnormal adaptation of the QT interval to RR changes may constitute an arrhythmogenic substrate has sound foundations. However, its clinical use for diagnostic or prognostic evaluations will have to wait until controlled studies are performed, first in a large cohort of normal individuals and then in well-defined patient populations.

Time-Domain and Frequency-Domain Assessment of Autonomic Modulation of the QT Interval

The autonomic nervous system plays an important role in the modulation of ventricular repolarization, not only by affecting heart rate but also through a direct action on the duration of the action potential.[20,21] Indeed, the QT interval may be shortened by atropine and by autonomic blockade in steady-state conditions.[7] Browne et al.[22] have shown that during sleep the QT interval is prolonged independently of heart rate changes, probably as a consequence of vagal stimulation.

Holter monitoring is already used to quantify the sympathetic and parasympathetic influences on heart rate and it may become a very suitable technique to study autonomic influences also on repolarization.

With the goal of discriminating the sympathetic and vagal effects on repolarization, several investigators are studying circadian variations of the QT interval. The underlying idea is that QT dynamics during the day may be an index of predominant sympathetic activity, while at night they may reflect a predominant vagal activity. Here there is a degree of oversimplification because sleep is not a homogeneous state, and it is well established that REM sleep is accompanied by bursts of sympathetic activity.

Benjoy et al.[23] recently showed the presence of a circadian variation in QT interval duration among normal individuals by comparing the QT interval at similar rates during the day and at night. The QT interval, measured at the apex of the T wave, was significantly longer during the night than during the day at all cycle lengths explored. By contrast, among patients affected by the long QT syndrome (LQTS), the diurnal variation observed in normal subjects was absent. An abnormal response to autonomic modulation among LQTS patients has been proposed to explain what was interpreted to be an impairment in the circadian variation of repolarization.

The slopes of the QT/RR regression line during the day and at night have been used to measure the autonomic modulation of repolarization. Tavernier et al.[24] reported that the slope is steepest during morning hours. Similar results were obtained using both the QT apex and the QT end. The authors concluded that autonomic modulation is responsible for the circadian variation of the QT/RR relationship.

Sarma *et al.*[25] used power spectral analysis of the QT interval to investigate the autonomic influences on repolarization. The QT interval variability in the frequency domain was smaller than the RR variability, it was highest at very low frequencies (0.05 Hz), and it decreased at higher frequencies. No day–night changes were observed in the QT variability, and this finding was interpreted as a demonstration of insensitivity of repolarization to vagal modulation. This interpretation is clearly in contrast with published data[7,22] obtained with other techniques, that suggest the presence of a parasympathetic modulation of the QT interval.

Lombardi *et al.*[26] also performed an analysis of RT spectral components in normal individuals and in patients with a previous myocardial infarction. The spectral profile of RT was characterized in both groups by a predominant high-frequency and a smaller low-frequency component. These findings are at variance with the data from Sarma *et al.*[25]

Caution is necessary when data on the frequency components of ventricular repolarization are interpreted as representing the counterpart of the activation of one limb of the autonomic nervous system. The correspondence between high frequencies and vagal activation and low frequency and sympathetic activation has proponents[27] and opponents,[28] even when dealing with the frequency components of RR variability. Whether the same will hold true for the spectral components of repolarization remains to be demonstrated.

Modulation of ventricular repolarization by the sympathetic nervous system may significantly modify the electrical stability of the heart. The availability of a technique that might help define the role and effect of the sympathetic and of the vagal components on ventricular repolarization would be very valuable. At the present time, however, too many unsettled aspects suggest that the clinical utility of Holter recording in this specific area still requires additional methodological progress before it could really be used to understand the autonomic modulation of the recovery of excitability.

Variability of QT Interval Dispersion

Dispersion of the QT interval (see Chapter 24) is an index of electrical instability that reflects dispersion of ventricular repolarization. QT dispersion is usually assessed as the difference between the longest and the shortest QT interval measured on the 12-lead ECG.

This index, originally proposed by Day *et al.*,[29] is abnormally increased in several conditions characterized by increased risk for arrhythmic death, such as the long QT syndrome,[29,30] myocardial infarction[31] and cardiac hypertrophy.[32] So far, QT dispersion has been assessed under static conditions; however, it would be very important to evaluate how QT dispersion is modified during daily activity under different conditions. A dynamic assessment of QT dispersion has been difficult to obtain given the limited number of leads used by traditional Holter recording systems. Recently, new solid-state cassette recorders have become available that can record from 12 leads, and these new systems will be ideal for the study of the dynamicity of QT dispersion.

The Electrophysiologic Effect of Antiarrhythmia Drugs

The electrophysiologic effect of antiarrhythmia drugs is affected by different heart rates and can be modulated by the autonomic nervous system. We recently reported that the electrophysiologic effect of potassium-channel blocking agents (i.e. the prolongation of action potential duration) is largely lost in the presence of beta-adrenergic activation.[33]

This finding, probably due to activation of the I_{ks} current which is not blocked by most of the available K^+-channel blockers, may account for the failure of some of these drugs to prevent lethal arrhythmias during acute myocardial ischemia associated with sympathetic hyperactivity.[34]

It is of obvious clinical relevance to evaluate the extent to which changes in autonomic output and in heart rate may modulate the electrophysiologic properties of antiarrhythmia drugs. Holter recording is the most suitable technique to assess dynamicity of drug effects and some studies have already been published. Sadanaga *et al.*[35] used it to demonstrate the presence of reverse-use dependency in the prolongation of QT induced by diisopyramide and by the potassium-channel blocker E4031. Laude *et al.*[36] reported a similar study in which the reverse-use dependency of dofetilide, another potassium-channel blocking agent, was demonstrated by Holter recording.

The quantification of the potential excessive prolongation of repolarization induced by drugs at slow heart rates may represent critical information in the assessment of the risk of proarrhythmic events during drug therapy, with special reference to the onset of torsades de pointes,[37] and should become a routine assessment of drug activity. This is an area where clinical utility of Holter analysis of ventricular repolarization can indeed be expected.

Beat-to-Beat Morphological Changes of the T Wave

Holter recordings offer, of course, ample opportunity to examine, and to quantify whenever appropriate, the morphology of the T wave and the duration of the QT interval in the periods immediately preceding the onset of important arrhythmic events. There are several examples of the immediate clinical utility of this relatively simple and unsophisticated analysis. We will present one in some detail because it exemplifies well the clinical potential of this approach.

Malfatto *et al.*[15] examined multiple recordings of a patient affected by the long QT syndrome who had a worsening of arrhythmias while on therapy with beta-blockers and who responded with long-term success to left cardiac sympathetic denervation. The initial recordings showed that this patient had long sinus pauses which were followed by the appearance of notches on the T wave, and that it was from these notches that premature ventricular beats, either isolated or repetitive, were taking off (Figure 26.1). The possibility that these notches, typical of LQTS,[38] are the electrocardiographic equivalent of early after-depolarizations is logical and attractive, albeit unproven. Analysis of the ratio between the amplitude of the T wave following sinus pauses and its amplitude in the beats preceding the pause (Figure 26.2) allowed the demonstration that beta-adrenergic blockade accentuated this phenomenon which was completely reversed by left cardiac sympathetic denervation (Figures 26.2 and 26.3). The striking concordance between post-pause changes in repolarization and therapeutic failure and success is a pointer to the validity and clinical utility of this type of analysis.

Another example is represented by current and still unpublished work by several groups to track the changes in the duration of the QT interval in the beats preceding the onset of torsades de pointes.

Verrier, Nearing and Huang[39,40] have demonstrated that it is now feasible to quantify the phenomenon of T-wave alternans in the microvolt range using Holter recordings (see Chapter 25). The relationship between T-wave alternans as a marker of prefibrillatory state, the autonomic nervous system, and the long QT syndrome had already been documented by our work in 1975.[41] The recent technical progress offers the chance of unmasking even T-wave alternans of small magnitude, and thus invisible to the naked eye, using Holter recordings. When adequate data have been published linking the presence of T-wave alternans to the subsequent occurrence of life-threatening

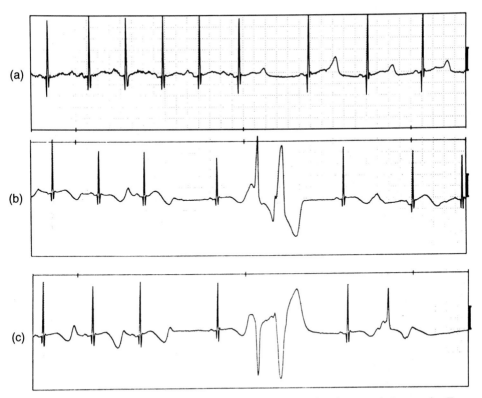

Figure 26.1 Strips taken from a Holter recording obtained in the absence of therapy for T-wave alternans. (a) shows a striking change in the T wave morphology induced by sinus pauses. (b) and (c) show the presence of ventricular arrhythmias in temporal relationship with the end of the T wave. (Reproduced with permission from reference 15)

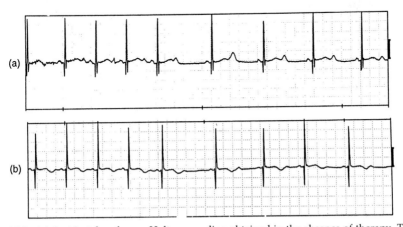

Figure 26.2 (a) A strip taken from a Holter recording obtained in the absence of therapy. The marked increase in the notch on the T wave after a sinus pause is clearly visible. (b) A strip recorded at follow-up after LCSD and during verapamil administration (2.5 mg/kg); sinus pauses persist. However, T morphology is changed, with a clear attenuation of the T notch (giving a flatter appearance to the T wave). Moreover, a pause of the same duration as the one in (a) is no longer followed by modifications of the T wave. (Reproduced with permission from reference 15)

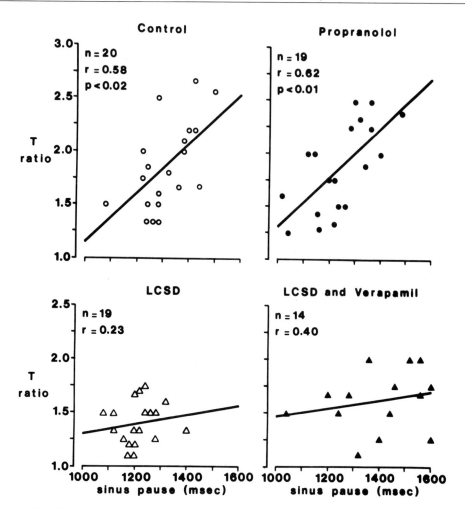

Figure 26.3 Relationship of the T ratio to the duration of the preceding sinus pause in the four clinical settings examined. In control (no therapy, $y = -1.17 + 0.0023x$) and during beta-blockade ($y = -1.13 + 0.0024x$), the magnitude of changes in the T notch after a pause (expressed as the T ratio) increased significantly with increases in the preceding RR interval (upper panels). In contrast (lower panels), after left cardiac sympathetic denervation (LCSD, $y = 0.28 + 0.0009x$) and after the administration of verapamil 2.5 mg/kg ($y = 0.529 + 0.0007x$), the T ratio was no longer related to the length of the preceding pause. (Reproduced with permission from reference 15)

arrhythmias in large populations, it will become possible to establish the clinical utility of this new approach that is now made possible by ambulatory monitoring.

Conclusions

Unlike the analysis of changes in the RR interval and in the ST segment, analysis of changes in ventricular repolarization during ambulatory monitoring has begun to receive considerable attention only during the last few years. The consequence is a considerable mismatch between the relatively large number of different techniques developed in the research laboratories and the very small number of published studies involving adequate patient populations.

The field is one of potentially great clinical value, but most of the data available so far are still of limited utility for a variety of reasons discussed in detail above. Automated programs currently available simplify analysis at the expense of important biologic information. Future technology, when it is able to combine rapid analysis with preservation of essential electrophysiologic information contained in the terminal portion of the T wave, will provide the cardiologist with measurements of considerable clinical utility.

References

1. Grant RP. *Clinical Electrocardiography*. New York: McGraw-Hill, 1957: 63.
2. Schwartz PJ, Wolf S. QT interval prolongation as predictor of sudden death in patients with myocardial infarction. *Circulation* 1978; **57**: 1074–7.
3. Schwartz PJ. Clinical significance of QT prolongation: a personal view. In: Butrous GS, Schwartz PJ (eds), *Clinical Aspects of Ventricular Repolarization*. London: Farrand Press, 1989: 343–56.
4. Moss AJ, Schwartz PJ, Crampton RS, Tzivoni D, Locati EH, MacCluer J, Hall WJ, Weitkamp L, Vincent GM, Garson A, Robinson JL, Benhorin J, Choi S. The long QT syndrome: prospective longitudinal study of 328 families. *Circulation* 1991; **84**: 1136–44.
5. Schouten EG, Dekker JM, Meppelink P, Kok FJ, Vandenbroucke JP, Pool J. QT interval prolongation predicts cardiovascular mortality in an apparently healthy population. *Circulation* 1991; **84**: 1516–23.
6. Algra A, Tijssen JGP, Roelandt JRTC, Pool J, Lubsen J. QTc prolongation measured by standard 12-lead electrocardiography is an independent risk factor for sudden death due to cardiac arrest. *Circulation* 1991; **83**: 1888–94.
7. Browne KF, Zipes DP, Heger JJ, Prystowsky EN. Influence of the autonomic nervous system on the QT interval in man. *Am J Cardiol* 1982; **50**: 1099–103.
8. Merri M, Moss AJ, Benhorin J, Locati EH, Alberti M, Badilini F. Relation between ventricular repolarization duration and cardiac cycle length during 24-hour Holter recordings. *Circulation* 1992; **85**: 1816–21.
9. Seed WA, Noble MIM, Oldershaw P, Wanless RB, Drake-Holland AJ, Redwood D, Pugh S, Mills C. Relation of human cardiac action potential duration to the interval between beats: implications for the validity of rate corrected QT interval (QTc). *Br Heart J* 1987; **57**: 32–7.
10. Karjalainen J, Viitasalo M, Mänttäri M, Manninen V. Relation between QT intervals and heart rates from 40 to 120 beats/min in rest electrocardiograms of men and a simple method to adjust QT interval values. *J Am Coll Cardiol* 1994; **23**: 1547–53.
11. Viñolas X, Homs E, Marti V, Guindo J, Bayés de Luna A. QT/RR relationship in postmyocardial infarction patients with and without life-threatening ventricular arrhythmias. *J Am Coll Cardiol* 1993; **21**: 94A.
12. Fei L, Statters DJ, Gill JS, Katritsis D, Camm AJ. Alteration of the QT/RR relationship in patients with idiopathic ventricular tachycardia. *PACE* 1994; **17**: 199–206.
13. Fei L, Statters DJ, Anderson MH, Katritsis D, Camm AJ. Is there an abnormal QT interval in sudden cardiac death survivors with a 'normal' QTc? *Am Heart J* 1994; **128**: 73–6.
14. Jackman WM, Friday KJ, Anderson JL, Aliot EM, Clark M, Lazzara R. The long QT syndromes: a critical review, new clinical observations and an unifying hypothesis. *Prog Cardiovasc Dis* 1988; **2**: 115–72.
15. Malfatto G, Rosen MR, Foresti A, Schwartz PJ. Idiopathic long QT syndrome exacerbated by beta-adrenergic blockade and responsive to left cardiac sympathetic denervation: implications regarding electrophysiologic substrate and adrenergic modulation. *J Cardiovasc Electrophysiol* 1992; **3**: 295–305.
16. Rasmussen V, Jensen G, Hansen JF. QT interval in 24-hour ambulatory ECG recordings from 60 healthy adult subjects. *J Electrocardiol* 1991; **24**: 91–5.
17. Elharrar V, Surawicz B. Cycle length effect on restitution of action potential duration in dog cardiac fibers. *Am J Physiol* 1983; **224**: H782–92.
18. Franz MR, Swerdlow CD, Liem LB, Schaefer J. Cycle length dependence of human action potential duration in vivo: effect of single extrastimuli, sudden sustained rate acceleration and deceleration and different steady state frequencies. *J Clin Invest* 1988; **82**: 972–9.
19. Zaza A, Malfatto G, Schwartz PJ. Sympathetic modulation of the relation between ventricular repolarization and cycle length. *Circ Res* 1991; **68**: 1191–203.
20. Kuo CS, Surawicz B. Ventricular monophasic action potential changes associated with neurogenic T wave abnormalities and isoproterenol administration in dogs. *Am J Cardiol* 1976; **38**: 170–7.
21. Priori SG, Corr PB. Mechanisms underlying early and delayed afterdepolarization induced by catecholamines in isolated adult ventricular myocytes. *Am J Physiol* 1990; **258**: H1796–805.
22. Browne KF, Prystowsky E, Heger JJ, Chilson DA, Zipes DP. Prolongation of the QT interval in man during sleep. *Am J Cardiol* 1983; **52**: 55–9.
23. Benjoy I, Maisonblanche P, Thomas O, Menabhi M, Malek S, Lucet Z, Coumel P. Circadian variation of ventricular repolarization in the congenital long QT syndrome (abstract). *Eur Heart J* 1994; **15**(Suppl): 158.

24. Tavernier R, DeBacker G, Jordaens L. Dynamic QT analysis in the 24-hour electrocardiogram in normal individuals (abstract). *Eur Heart J* 1994; **15**(Suppl): 160.

25. Sarma JSM, Singh N, Schoenbaum MP, Venkataraman, Singh BN. Circadian and power spectral changes of RR and QT intervals during treatment of patients with angina pectoris with nadolol providing evidence for differential autonomic modulation of heart rate and ventricular repolarization. *Am J Cardiol* 1994; **74**: 131–6.

26. Lombardi F, Sandrone G, Venturati M, Torzillo D, Porta A, Malliani A. Analysis of RR and RT variabilities after myocardial infarction (abstract). *Eur Heart J* 1993; **14**(Suppl): 255.

27. Pagani M, Lombardi F, Malliani A. Heart rate variability: disagreement on the markers of sympathetic and parasympathetic activities (letter). *J Am Coll Cardiol* 1993; **22**: 951–2.

28. Goldsmith RL, Bloomfield D, Rottman J, Bigger JT. Heart rate variability: disagreement on the markers of sympathetic and parasympathetic activities: reply (letter). *J Am Coll Cardiol* 1993; **22**: 952–3.

29. Day CP, McComb JM, Campbell RWF. QT dispersion: an indication of arrhythmia risk in patients with long QT intervals. *Br Heart J* 1990; **63**: 342–4.

30. Priori SG, Napolitano C, Diehl L, Schwartz PJ. Dispersion of the QT interval: a marker of therapeutic efficacy in the idiopathic long QT syndrome. *Circulation* 1994; **89**: 1681–9.

31. Moreno FL, Villanueva MT, Karagounis LA, Anderson JL, for the TEAM-2 Study Investigator. Reduction in QT interval dispersion by successful thrombolytic therapy in acute myocardial infarction. *Circulation* 1994; **90**: 94–100.

32. Miorelli M, Buja GF, Turrini P, Melacini P, Azzolini R, Nava A. Correlation between QT dispersion and signal-averaging electrocardiograms in hypertrophic cardiomyopathy patients with and without complex ventricular arrhythmias and sudden death. *New Trend Arrh* 1993; **9**: 121–4.

33. Napolitano C, Diehl L, Schwartz PJ, Priori SG. Modulation of the electrophysiologic effects of ambasilide induced by beta-adrenergic stimulation in isolated ventricular myocytes (abstract). *J Am Coll Cardiol* 1994; **23**: 444A.

34. Vanoli E, Priori SG, Nakagawa H, Hirao K, Napolitano C, Diehl L, Lazzara R, Schwartz PJ. Sympathetic activation, ventricular repolarization and I_{Kr} blockade: implications for the antifibrillatory efficacy of K^+ channel blockers. *J Am Coll Cardiol* 1995; **25**: 1609–14.

35. Sadanaga T, Ogawa S, Okata Y, Tsutsumi N, Iwanaga S, Yoshikawa T, Akaishi M, Handa S. Clinical evaluation of the use-dependent QRS prolongation and the reverse use-dependent QT prolongation of class I and class III antiarrhythmic agents and their value in predicting efficacy. *Am Heart J* 1993; **126**: 114–21.

36. Laude G, Maisonblanche P, Fuick Brentano C, Sayn J, Roubel P, Ghandafar N, Coumel P. Type III drug-induced reverse use dependence can be assessed from QT duration in Holter recordings (abstract). *Eur Heart J* 1994; **15**(Suppl): 191.

37. Napolitano C, Priori SG, Schwartz PJ. Torsade de pointes: mechanisms and management. *Drugs* 1994; **47**: 51–65.

38. Schwartz PJ, Locati EH, Napolitano C, Priori SG. The long QT syndrome. In: Zipes DP, Jalife J (eds), *Cardiac Electrophysiology: From Cell to Bedside*, 2nd edn. Philadelphia: W.B. Saunders, 1995: 788–811.

39. Nearing BD, Huang AH, Verrier RL. Dynamic tracking of cardiac vulnerability by complex demodulation of the T wave. *Science* 1991; **252**: 437–40.

40. Verrier RL, Nearing BD. Electrophysiologic basis for T wave alternans as an index of vulnerability to ventricular fibrillation. *J Cardiovasc Electrophysiol* 1994; **5**: 445–61.

41. Schwartz PJ and Malliani A. Electrical alternation of the T wave: clinical and experimental evidence of its relationship with the sympathetic nervous system and with the long QT syndrome. *Am Heart J* 1975; **89**: 45–50.

SECTION VII

Circadian Rhythms

Introduction by James Muller and Geoffrey Tofler

The advances in the field of noninvasive electrocardiography described in earlier sections have occurred in parallel with studies documenting a circadian variation in occurrence of sudden cardiac death. This fortuitus combination of progress in two fields creates new opportunities for research into the pathyphysiologic basis of lethal cardiac arrhythmias.[1]

The method of the new approach is to measure an electrocardiographic variable (QTc interval and ST segment depression are the two considered in the following chapters) and determine if the temporal characteristics of the variable match the daily pattern of occurrence of sudden cardiac death. If a variable peaks at the same time of day as sudden cardiac death, an association has been demonstrated that may, in some cases, be causal. In such cases, an intervention that decreased the electrocardiologic process might provide a new means to prevent sudden cardiac death. Our understanding of the mechanism of sudden cardiac death has also been advanced by studies demonstrating the role of thrombosis leading to sudden cardiac death, with or without a preceding myocardial infarction. Davies and Thomas,[2] Falk, and others building on the pioneering studies of Constantinides,[3] identified the pathoanatomic role of plaque disruption and thrombosis in sudden death, unstable angina, and myocardial infarction.

While a morning increase in cardiovascular risk has been postulated for many decades, the clear documentation of circadian rhythms of disease onset required a combination of improved epidemiologic methods and new technology. The use in 1985 of creatine kinase measures to objectively time the onset of myocardial infarction in the MILIS study identified 9–10 am as the peak period of disease onset. The availability and refinement of 24-hour ambulatory electrocardiographic monitoring, as described by Mulcahy and Quyyumi in this section, has permitted accurate and complete recording of ischemic activity.

Ambulatory monitoring has also facilitated accurate recording of arrhythmias and the exploration of mechanisms of arrhythmogenesis. Viñolas and colleagues use the presence of a morning peak of sudden cardiac death, as established by epidemiologic methods, as a springboard to investigate the role of autonomic imbalance as a triggering factor. Whereas alterations in sympathovagal balance have been primarily studied using measures of heart rate variability, Viñolas and colleagues focus on changes in the QT interval. The QT interval, which reflects changes in repolarization, is influenced by a number of factors, many of which are dependent on the autonomic nervous system.

Comparison of circadian patterns in various subgroups of patients can also suggest differences in pathophysiology of onset. Patients with prior beta-adrenergic blockade do not have the increase in infarction or sudden death in the hours after awakening observed in those not receiving such therapy, indicating the importance of sympathetic activation.

Adjustment for time of awakening and onset of activity has indicated that the morning peaks of transient ischemia, nonfatal myocardial infarction, and sudden cardiac death all occur after awakening and initiation of the activities of the day. This observation emphasizes the role of the activity/rest cycle rather than merely time of day, as playing a key role in the triggering of disease onset. Thus, the events can be said to follow an exogenous, as opposed to endogenous, circadian rhythm.

Many of the pathophysiologic changes that occur in the morning also occur following potential triggers such as heavy physical activity and mental stress. This leads to the concept that activities may trigger disease onset at any time of day – a more important idea than that of circadian variation.

It has now become possible to determine the relative risk of a stressful activity triggering a cardiac event. A new technique termed 'case-crossover analysis' has been developed.[4] This utilizes each patient as his or her own control for the expected frequency of the potential triggering activity in a defined hazard period consisting of the hours immediately prior to disease onset. Relative risk is determined by comparing the observed to expected frequencies in the hazard period. The method greatly decreases confounding encountered in traditional case–control studies.

In the Myocardial Infarction Onset Study, an interview study conducted in over 1500 patients with myocardial infarction, it was found that 4.4% of patients reported heavy physical exertion within one hour prior to the onset of infarction. With the use of the case-crossover method, it was possible to calculate that the relative risk of infarction in the hour after heavy physical exertion was 5.9. Mulcahy and Quyyumi indicate in their chapter that a direct cause/effect relationship between ischemia and onset of acute myocardial infarction and sudden death has not been proven. However, the common circadian pattern present for transient ischemia, on the one hand, and acute myocardial infarction and sudden cardiac death, on the other, strongly demonstrate an association. In a parallel manner, Viñolas and colleagues point out that clusters of prolongation of the QT interval may be merely a marker for increased risk of malignant ventricular arrhythmia and not a component of the causal pathway.

As in any new field, there are many unanswered questions. What proportion of the circadian rhythm of disease onset is due to activity/rest cycle versus endogenous circadian variation? What are the triggers of onset and how do they operate? What are the acute risk factors produced by the trigger? Is it possible to sever the link between a potential trigger and its pathophysiologic consequence? Can we prospectively identify and then treat plaques vulnerable to disruption, or myocardium vulnerable to induction of a lethal arrhythmia?

Progress in scientific methods on the epidemiologic, clinical, and basic science levels provides the opportunity to address these questions. On the epidemiologic level, the new devices and analytic techniques to study circadian rhythms and the case-crossover methodology to study triggers are available for population study. In the catheterization laboratory, intracoronary ultrasound may have the potential to detect lipid-rich plaques within the arterial wall that are vulnerable to disruption.[5] Intracoronary angioscopy may complement this information by identifying surface characteristics of the vulnerable plaque, such as yellow color.[6]

Thus, a broad new area of potential research is apparent, and the tools with which to address its major questions are available. Improved insight into the ECG changes that occur at various times of the day, and are produced by triggering activities, would offer a new approach to prevention. Disease could be prevented by finding measures to sever the linkage between a potential trigger, such as an activity producing ST segment depression or QTc prolongation, and its catastrophic consequences.

References

1. Muller JE, Abela GS, Nesto RW, Tofler GH. Triggers, acute risk factors and vulnerable plaques: the lexicon of a new frontier. *J Am Coll Cardiol* 1994; **23**: 809–13.
2. Davies MJ, Thomas AC. Thrombosis and acute coronary artery lesions in sudden cardiac ischemic death. *New Engl J Med* 1984; **310**: 1137–40.
3. Constantinides P, Chakravarti RN. Rabbit arterial thrombosis production by systemic procedures. *Arch Path* 1961; **72**: 197–208.
4. Mittleman MA, Maclure M, Tofler GH, Sherwood JB, Goldberg RJ, Muller JE, for the Determinants of Myocardial Infarction Onset Study Investigators. Triggering of acute myocardial infarction by heavy physical exertion: protection against triggering by regular exertion. *New Engl J Med* 1993; **329**: 1677–83.
5. Nissen SE, Gurley JC, Booth DC, De Maria AN. Intravascular ultrasound of the coronary arteries: current applications and future directions. *Am J Cardiol* 1992; **69**: 18H–29H.
6. Nesto RW, Sassower MA, Manzo KS, *et al*. Angioscopic differentiation of culprit lesions in unstable versus stable coronary artery disease (abstract). *J Am Coll Cardiol* 1993; **21**(Suppl): 195A.

27

Circadian Repolarization Patterns and Ventricular Arrhythmias

Xavier Viñolas, Antoni Bayés Genís, Josep Guindo,
Eduard Homs, Vicenç Martí, Lucia Dumaresq
and Antonio Bayés de Luna

Introduction

More than 80% of patients who suffer from ventricular arrhythmias, especially malignant ventricular arrhythmias (sustained ventricular tachycardia, ventricular fibrillation/flutter and torsades de pointes) have an underlying ischemic heart disease; many of them are after a myocardial infarction. In patients with other types of heart diseases (dilated cardiomyopathy, hypertrophic cardiomyopathy, right ventricular dysplasia etc.), this percentage is much smaller. Very few patients without an underlying organic cardiac disease have malignant ventricular arrhythmias.[1] Some but not all patients in the latter group suffer from a congenital long QT syndrome.

It is evident that the problem of malignant ventricular arrhythmias in most cases is closely linked to old ischemic heart disease, specially an old myocardial infarction. Malignant ventricular arrhythmia may occur in conjunction with acute ischemia as well, especially if this is transmural and prolonged, as it is in patients with acute myocardial infarction. In these patients, the malignant ventricular arrhythmia is generally ventricular fibrillation unheralded by ventricular tachycardia.

Malignant ventricular arrhythmias have a high risk of relapse (40% in 1 year if untreated) and subsequent risk of sudden death. In a study by Bayés de Luna *et al.*[2] of Holter tapes recorded in patients who died while wearing a Holter recorder, it was found that 80% of the deaths were caused by malignant ventricular arrhythmias, and it was a bradyarrhythmia in only 20% of the patients. The same study demonstrated that very few patients had a new ischemic crisis suggested by ST changes in Holter recordings before the episode of malignant ventricular arrhythmia. Several other studies have shown that fewer than 30% of patients resuscitated from sudden death present thrombotic occlusion of a coronary artery[3–5] which could have produced acute myocardial infarction and secondary ventricular fibrillation.

Circadian Rhythm in Malignant Ventricular Arrhythmias and Cardiac Sudden Death

It has long been known that the occurrence of sudden death and acute myocardial infarction shows a circadian rhythm, being higher between 6am and noon than at other times of the day,[6,7] but the rate of occurrence according to the days of the week and the month of the year appears to have a random distribution. It is interesting to note that the higher morning rate of occurrence is absent in patients who have taken beta-blockers before the episode and also during the weekend, suggesting that a factor independent of the time of day is also involved; for example, the time of awakening, initiation of physical activity. The onset of physical activity modifies many physiologic parameters, such as circulating catecholamine levels, sympathetic-parasympathetic tone, etc., that could be responsible for the higher incidence of infarction at certain times of the day. Other studies[8,9] have also demonstrated circadian rhythm in cardiac sudden death (in most cases due to malignant ventricular arrhythmia). The circadian curve of the rate of occurrence of cardiac sudden death is similar to that of infarction (Figure 27.1), the peak rate appearing between 7am and 11am. Therefore, circadian rhythm is also observed in cases in which sudden death does not involve an acute ischemic episode. This has been confirmed by analyzing the time of day at which a shock was delivered in patients who had an implanted automatic cardioverter–defibrillator, which can now record the severe ventricular tachycardia that induces the shock. When the ventricular arrhythmia is not linked to an acute ischemic episode, a trigger factor (disturbance of the sympathovagal balance, increased number of ventricular premature beats, depression of left ventricular function, etc.) acts upon a vulnerable myocardium (frequently a postinfarction scar) and produces a malignant ventricular arrhythmia. Nevertheless, a vulnerable myocardium

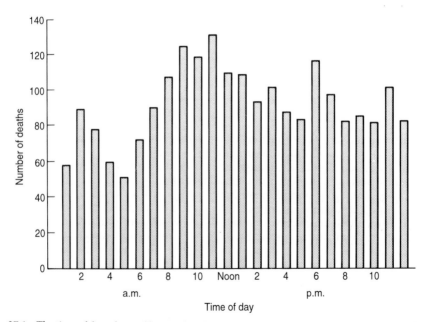

Figure 27.1 The time of day of out-of-hospital sudden cardiac death (<1 hour from onset of symptoms to death) for 2203 individuals dying in Massachussets in 1983. A statistically significant (*p* < 0.001) circadian rhythm is present with a peak between 7am and 11am, and a secondary peak between 5pm and 6pm. (Reproduced with permission from reference 8: © American Heart Association)

Table 27.1 Parameters and techniques used to stratify risk in postmyocardial infarction patients (see Figure 27.2)

	Parameters	Techniques
Electrical instability	Ventricular arrhythmias	Holter

	Autonomic nervous system
	  Heart rate variability
	  QT interval
		Holter

	Anatomic substrate	Late potentials (conventional or Holter techniques)
Ischemia	Coronary flow	Exercise testing Holter Imaging techniques
	Coronary stenosis	Coronariography MNR
	Prethrombolitic state	Blood test
Left ventricular dysfunction	Diastolic function	Echo–Doppler
	Systolic function	Echocardiography and isotopic techniques
	State of RAA axis	Blood test

may exist for days, months or even years with no complications. The occurrence of arrhythmia at a certain time during the follow-up depends on the appearance of a specific trigger or on the interaction of various trigger factors.

Study of the circadian rhythm of these triggers in relation to the circadian rhythm of malignant ventricular arrhythmias may provide very useful pathophysiological information.

Circadian variations in pathophysiologic processes related with malignant ventricular arrhythmias and sudden death

There is evidence of circadian rhythm in different pathophysiologic processes involved in the genesis of acute myocardial infarction. In the morning, increased platelet aggregability, decreased fibrinolytic activity, increased coronary tone, and increased blood pressure and dP/dT have been observed,[10–12] and these processes may favor the occurrence of coronary thrombosis and subsequent myocardial infarction, which can sometimes produce malignant ventricular arrhythmias. In other cases, malignant ventricular arrhythmia occurs without previous acute ischemic disturbance. The patients' prognosis depends on three main factors: ischemia, electrical instability, and left ventricular dysfunction; these factors interact, and disturbance or modification of any one of them leads to a change in the other two.

There are several parameters for evaluating the electrical instability of the heart, as ventricular late potentials, RR variability, programmed electrical stimulation, ECG disturbances, arrhythmias on Holter recordings, disturbances in the repolarization parameters, etc. Of these (Table 27.1), we will limit ourselves to evaluating the circadian behavior of repolarization parameters, particularly the behavior of the QT interval, an area of great recent interest.

QT Interval and Malignant Ventricular Arrhythmias

The relationship between the duration of the QT interval and presence of malignant ventricular arrhythmias is well known, and its maximum expression is the presence of the congenital long QT syndrome. In some cases, these patients have episodes of 'torsades de pointes' type ventricular tachycardia, which can lead to sudden death.

Interest in the QT interval also derives from observations that excessive prolongation of the QT interval with group I antiarrhythmic drugs is associated in some cases with proarrhythmia. But on the other hand, prolongation of the QT interval by amiodarone, within limits that have not yet been well established, is considered a good parameter of the drug's effectiveness.

The QT interval on the surface electrocardiogram is a simple measurement of an extremely complex process that is influenced by many factors: presence or absence of underlying organic heart disease, the autonomic nervous system, circulating catecholamines, electrolytes, drugs (cardiac and noncardiac), and others. Moreover, the QT interval varies with heart rate, being shorter in shorter cycles; this is an effect that is usually corrected by the Bazett formula,[13] which nevertheless somewhat distorts the results, especially at the upper and lower ranges of heart rate. It should be mentioned that isoproterenol infusion shortens the QT interval even at the same heart rate. Likewise, in patients with VVI pacemakers with a fixed heart rate, the QT interval becomes shorter with exercise. This indicates that the QT interval is influenced by a number of factors, many of them dependent on the autonomic nervous system – a subject discussed in Chapter 24.

QT variations in healthy persons

The QT interval reflects the duration of depolarization and repolarization. As repolarization is much more prolonged and variations in depolarization (except for the appearance of bundle branch block) are less variable, changes in the QT interval essentially reflect changes in repolarization. The QT interval becomes shorter as the cardiac cycle becomes shorter. Correction of the QT interval using Bazett's formula is known to be inexact and there are other correction formulas,[14] the most exact apparently being the normograms (based on analysis of the QT/RR ratio in each group) that show with how many milliseconds the QT should be corrected for each heart rate.[15] Bazett's correction for heart rate is still an important tool that allows changes in the QT interval to be evaluated with some, but not total, independence of changes in heart rate.

We studied the behavior of the QTc interval on the Holter tapes of 10 healthy people and compared these with those of postinfarction patients, with and without malignant ventricular arrhythmia. We used first a manual and thereafter an automatic measurement. The QTc interval was more prolonged between 11pm and 11am than during the other 12 hours of the day (Figure 27.2). The mean QT interval was shorter in the healthy subjects than in the postinfarction patients who had malignant ventricular arrhythmia, but similar to that of post infarction patients without malignant ventricular arrhythmia (Table 27.2). Ninety percent of the healthy subjects had QT intervals over 440 ms at some time of the day, but as none of the tapes analyzed showed peak QTc intervals in excess of 500 ms this value should be considered as the cutoff point for normality (Table 27.3).

Vervaet *et al.*[16] studied variations in the QT interval on the surface ECGs of 84 healthy subjects and also found a daily rhythm. They analyzed only ECGs recorded at different times of the day between 8am and 4pm. Although this restricts the possibility of studying circadian behavior, variations in the QT interval were found and the minimum QTc was between 10am and 12am.

Murakawa *et al.*[17] analyzed QTc interval values in different population groups (healthy subjects, postmyocardial infarction patients, and diabetic neuropathy patients). They manually analyzed sets of six QT intervals every 10 minutes throughout the day and night. Abrupt, transitory changes in the QT interval (QT peaks) may pass undetected with this method, in contrast with automatic analysis, but a sufficient number of QT intervals was studied to permit the circadian rhythm of the QT interval to be evaluated.

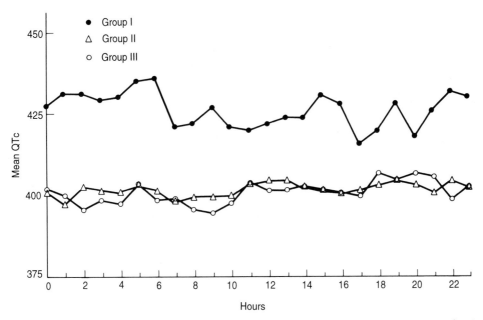

Figure 27.2 Mean hourly QTc in different groups of patients. Group I correspond to postinfarction patients with ventricular arrhythmias during follow-up. Group II correspond to postinfaction patients without ventricular arrhythmias during follow-up. Group III correspond to normal subjects. Circadian variations of QTc are similar in normal subjects and postinfarction patients without ventricular arrhythmias. Mean hourly QTc is longer during the day in postinfarction patients with malignant ventricular arrhythmias, specially during the night.

Table 27.2 Automatic QTc analaysis in the three groups studied

	Group I (n = 14)	Group II (n = 28)	Group II (n = 10)	p-value I vs II	p-value I vs III
Total of beats automatically analyzed	682 960	1 276 498	563 910	—	—
Global QTc (ms)	425 ± 15	408 ± 19	402 ± 20	<0.005	<0.001
Total number of peaks of QTc > 500 ms	11 114 (1.62%)	823 (0.06%)	0 (0%)	<0.005	<0.005
Patients with peaks of QTc >500 ms	7 (50%)	2 (7%)	None	<0.005	<0.03
Patients with clusters of peaks of QTc >500 ms	4 (28%)	None	None	<0.02	<0.02

Group I: Postmyocardial infarction patients who presented a secondary life-threatening arrhythmia; *Group II:* postmyocardial infarction patients who did not present life-threatening arrhythmias; *Group III:* healthy subjects.

Table 27.3 Healthy subjects (n = 10) with peaks of QTc lengthening measured automatically in Holter recordings according to a determined cutoff of QTc value

Peaks of QTc interval (ms)	Number
>440	9 (90%)
>460	4 (40%)
>480	3 (30%)
>500	0 (0%)

Instead of using the Bazett correction formula, the Murokawa study analyzed the regression of QT/RR using three different formulas. In the group of 23 healthy subjects, the nocturnal QTc interval was found to be longer than the diurnal QTc interval (38 ± 22 ms versus 400 ± 20 ms). This prolongation of the QT interval during the night coincided with periods of greater bradycardia; that is, with longer RR intervals. There was less variation and variability in the QTc intervals of patients with ischemic heart disease and of patients with diabetes mellitus.

Rasmusen et al.[18] analyzed variations in the QT interval in relation to time of day in 60 healthy subjects. They found that the QTc interval, corrected for heart rate using the Bazett formula or a regression equation, was longer in the measurements made between 2am and 6am. Correlations were found with heart rate, naturally, and with the time of day at which the ECG was recorded.

In patients with diabetic neuropathy, Ong et al.[19] studied the circadian variations in QT interval, QTc, and heart rate and compared these to healthy subjects. In the 13 healthy subjects they observed the longest QT interval between midnight and 6am, a period during which heart rate also was lower, suggesting vagal predominance during this period. A decreased RR variability, a higher heart rate, and a shorter QTc interval were seen in patients with diabetic neuropathy, suggesting disturbances in vegetative tone, in the form of increased sympathetic tone (or decreased vagal tone), which could trigger electrical instability and provoke malignant ventricular arrhythmias.

The effect of hypothyroidism on circadian variations in QT before and after tiroxine treatment was studied by Sarma et al.[20] QTc was prolonged in patients with hypothyroidism and remained so even at 8–12 weeks after normalization of biochemical indexes.

Merri et al.[21] analyzed Holter tapes of 10 healthy subjects using their own algorithm in order to try to identify variations of repolarization duration and cycle length and any correlation between the two phenomena. They used the frequency analysis of HRV, analyzing the low-frequency/high-frequency ratio as an index of sympathovagal balance. The repolarization duration was measured between the peak of the R wave and the peak of the T wave. Like other investigators, they also found that both cycle length and repolarization duration are longer during the night. All previous investigations had concluded that both the cycle length and the autonomic nervous system affected the repolarization duration, but it was not clear if they acted in parallel or whether the cycle length was a more major determinant of the repolarization duration. A main finding of this research is the similar frequency found both in HRV and repolarization variability. In the spectra of both HRV and repolarization duration variability (RDV), the predominant vagal effect during the night was reflected by an increase in the high-frequency band, while in the morning the spectrum was dominated by the low-frequency band. As the authors stated, the results suggest that repolarization duration variability has an autonomic origin and that both neural limbs of the autonomic nervous system are involved in the beat-to-beat repolarization duration control.

It seems now to be evident that there is circadian variation in the QTc interval of healthy subjects, although these changes are usually linked to changes in heart rate, with longer QT and QTc intervals occurring during periods of bradycardia. These variations are present regardless of the formula used to correct the QT interval, indicating that these changes are to some degree independent of heart rate. Circadian variations in the repolarization parameters are therefore a physiological phenomenon. The better understanding of the alterations in the circadian variations in patients who die suddenly will certainly provide information about possible triggers of sudden cardiac death. The study of circadian variations in the QT regulating factors using noninvasive methods (e.g. evaluation of changes in RR variability that reflect sympathovagal status) could clarify some of these mechanisms.

QT variations in postinfarction patients with and without malignant ventricular arrhythmias

In recent years, interest in the relationship between QT interval and postinfarction cardiac sudden death has grown. Various studies[22–29] have analyzed the relationship between the QT interval and the presence of malignant ventricular arrhythmias, all using surface ECGs. Some studies have shown that transient QT prolongation through the day could be more important than a single determination of its value at a given moment.

To determine if this hypothesis is correct, first we analyzed the value of QT variations in the Holter tapes of postinfarction patients with and without malignant ventricular arrhythmias. A manual measurement was made[30] of the QT intervals on the Holter tape and an algorithm was developed for automatic measurement of the QT interval. Manual measurement of the QTc intervals was done by selecting several beats per hour. These measurements did not provide information on the subtle and transitory changes in the QT/QTc interval.

We studied two groups of postinfarction patients. Group I consisted of 14 consecutive postinfarction patients with ventricular tachycardia (8 patients) or after an aborted sudden death episode (6 patients). Arrhythmia secondary to an acute ischemic episode was excluded in all patients. In 7 patients, ventricular arrhythmias occurred between the subacute phase and the second month of postinfarction, and in the rest of the patients it occurred after 2 months. Group II included 28 postinfarction patients 'matched' by clinical data, ejection fraction, and infarction site, and who did not have malignant ventricular arrhythmias during follow-up. There were no significant differences in the clinical characteristics of the two groups of patients (Table 27.4). Holter recordings were made routinely in all patients as a control before hospital release after myocardial infarction or as a routine 'screening' method during follow-up. At most, the Holter recording preceded the arrhythmic episode by one year. A 3-channel Holter recorder was used in all cases. The QT interval was analyzed on the channel that had the best signal-to-noise ratio.

We found no differences in mean QTc value between postinfarction patients with and without malignant ventricular arrhythmias. However, patients with malignant ventricular arrhythmias during the follow-up had QTc peaks >500 ms more frequently than patients without arrhythmic complications during the follow-up.

Table 27.4 Clinical characteristics of postmyocardial infarction patients with and without life-threatening arrhythmias

	Group I ($n = 14$)	Group II ($n = 28$)	p-value
Sex (M/F)	12/2	25/3	NS
Age (years)	59±13	57±10	NS
Anterior MI	9 (64%)	16 (57%)	NS
LV ejection fraction (%)	40±6	44±8	NS
LV ejection fraction <40%	6 (42%)	13 (46%)	NS
Angina	3 (21%)	7 (25%)	NS
Diabetes mellitus	3 (21%)	8 (28%)	NS
Hypertension	8 (57%)	15 (53%)	NS

Group I: Postmyocardial infarction patients with secondary life-threatening arrhythmia; *Group II:* postmyocardial infarction patients without life-threatening arrhythmias. MI = myocardial infarction; NS = not significant.

Automatic measurement of the QT interval

The mathematical algorithm for automatic measurement of the QT interval has been described in detail elsewhere.[28] To limit errors due to the presence of excessive noise, premature beats, or other abnormalities, a selection was made: QT intervals were grouped and the beats with the largest and smallest QT values were discarded. RR beats differing by more than 15% from the previous measurement were also discarded. The QT interval was later corrected using Bazett's formula. The data of the different QTc intervals were stored in digital form and represented as a trend that allowed exact assessment of the behavior of the QTc interval throughout the day in a practical form. In all, each point on the graph of the trend did not represent an isolated value of a QT interval but the mean of the QT intervals measured for 6 seconds.

The next step was to validate the algorithm. This was done by comparing the results obtained from manual measurements by two cardiologists on recordings printed at 25 mm/s with the results obtained by automatic analysis[32] (Table 27.5).

An analysis was made of 650 beats on 18 different tapes. The mean error between the manual and automatic measurements was 2.4 ± 17 ms and 2 ± 14 ms and the difference between the manual measurements by the two experts was 1.9 ± 10 ms. Therefore, the differences between automatic and manual measurements were similar to those of manual measurements by two experts. This validated the use of this method for analysis of larger population groups and, above all, the analysis of all QT values, which cannot be done manually. Automatic measurement seems to be the only valid means of evaluating transitory changes in the value of QT intervals, and thus analyzing 'peaks' of QT.

We analyzed mean QTc value, peaks of QTc (QTc values above a certain value), and clusters (groups of peak QT values lasting more than 1 minute). The mean QTc interval was longer in patients with malignant ventricular arrhythmias than in patients without these arrhythmias: 425 ± 20 ms versus 405 ± 17 ms (Table 27.2).

The behavior of the QT interval in relation to time of day is shown in Figure 27.2. This confirms the tendency towards longer QTc values from 11pm to 11am than from 11am to 11pm (430 ± 18 ms versus 425 ± 19 ms). These differences were not statistically significant, perhaps because of the small sample size, but they suggested a trend and concurred with findings in healthy subjects.

QT peaks. QT peaks were analyzed for different cutoff points: >440, >460, >480, and >500 ms. Statistically significant differences were found only when the group of patients with QT interval values above 500 ms were analyzed (Table 27.6). Fifty percent of the postinfarction patients who had malignant ventricular arrhythmias had QT values over 500 ms, compared with only 7% (2 of 28) of those who did not have malignant ventricular arrhythmias. None of the healthy subjects analyzed had peak QTc over 500 ms. When we examined the presence of clusters, we found that none of the postinfarction patients without malignant ventricular arrhythmias had clusters, but 28% of the postinfarction patients with malignant ventricular arrhythmias did (Table 27.2). When the number of beats with QTc >500 ms was analyzed, postinfarction patients with malignant ventricular arrhythmias had long QTc in 1.62% of beats compared with only 0.06% of beats in such patients without malignant ventricular arrhythmia. Figure 27.3 shows a graphic representation of postinfarction patients who had peak QTc >500 ms. It is important to note that these peaks sometimes occurred in groups and did not correspond to artifacts of automatic analysis.

As for the hourly distribution of QTc peaks, the number of QTc peaks per hour in postinfarction patients with malignant ventricular arrhythmias was 463 ± 315 (Table 27.7). The trend in QTc intervals is shown on a graph (Figure 27.3).

Circadian rhythm of peaks. QTc peaks over 500 ms exhibited circadian rhythm. The percentage of QT peaks per hour was higher between 11pm and 11am than during the

Table 27.5 Validation results with two manual measurements and between observers on 18 Holter tapes

Tape	n	Automatic − expert₁				Automatic − expert₂				expert₁ − expert₂	
		d^*	d	SD^*	SD	d^*	d	SD^*	SD	d^*	SD^*
1	34	4.3	2.4	33.9	16.9	7.0	−0.8	36.0	12.6	3.6	12.6
2	42	3.5	3.0	15.1	12.0	1.7	−0.1	11.5	9.8	−0.3	14.7
3	26	−5.9	−8.5	21.0	19.5	−7.7	−7.4	18.8	20.9	2.7	18.5
4	19	−2.3	−2.8	7.7	7.3	−7.2	−7.5	7.3	8.1	4.7	6.8
5	38	4.5	3.2	10.3	8.6	4.5	3.2	10.3	8.6	1.9	10.2
6	49	−21.0	−20.0	10.4	9.0	−22	−21.0	14.4	15.4	0.0	10.7
7	39	−7.2	−10.0	20.4	15.0	−26	−28.0	23.7	17.4	19.2	14.4
8	41	1.0	2.4	13.1	13.3	−1.1	−1.2	14.6	14.5	2.1	14.1
9	29	16.5	16.8	18.7	19.3	16.7	16.5	16.9	17.7	−1.0	5.5
10	39	−8.8	−8.5	13.1	12.4	−7.1	−7.3	14.1	14.9	−1.3	7.6
11	42	9.5	9.1	14.0	11.6	6.8	6.3	11.0	7.5	2.6	7.9
12	45	−17.0	−16.0	16.7	14.6	−18	−15.0	19.1	16.9	0.9	8.4
13	36	8.8	9.4	17.8	15.2	9.4	11.4	19.0	17.5	−0.6	5.7
14	34	−7.7	10.9	17.0	14.8	12.3	14.6	17.7	15.7	−4.4	7.3
15	37	8.2	5.1	44.7	22.1	6.1	5.8	39.8	21.9	2.2	15.4
16	35	11.7	11.7	16.0	16.0	9.7	8.5	12.5	11.5	1.7	12.8
17	40	19.6	17.9	13.2	12.9	21.9	21.6	12.3	11.9	−0.2	6.5
18	35	9.5	9.3	15.9	17.5	9.9	8.4	14.8	16.7	−0.3	5.0
Mean	37	2.4	2.0	17.7	14.3	0.9	0.4	17.4	14.4	1.9	10.2

n is the number of beats measured on each tape; d^* is the mean difference between automatic and manual QT interval measurements; SD^* is the standard deviation; d and SD are values after rejection of maximum and minimum QT values in each five-beat set; Units for d, SD, d^* and SD^* are milliseconds.

Table 27.6 Patients with peaks of QTc lengthening measured automatically in Holter recordings according to a determined cutoff of QTc value

Peaks of QTc interval (ms)	Group I (n = 14)	Group II (n = 28)	p-value
>440	14 (100%)	20 (71%)	NS
>460	10 (71%)	14 (50%)	NS
>480	7 (50%)	8 (28%)	NS
>500	7 (50%)	2 (7%)	<0.005

Group I: Postmyocardial infarction patients who presented a secondary life-threatening arrhythmia: *Group II:* postmyocardial infarction patients who did not present life-threatening arrhythmias.

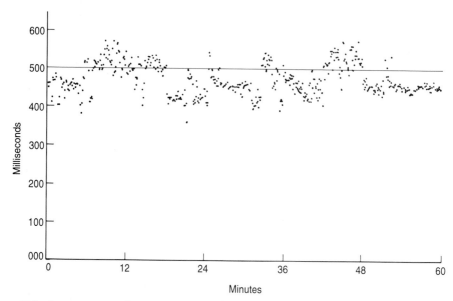

Figure 27.3 Representation of one hour of the trend of the QTc interval in a postinfarction patient with a ventricular tachycardia. Note the presence of peaks of QTc > 500 ms. There are peaks of QTc greater than 500 ms and also grouped peaks (clusters) at minutes 10 and 48.

Table 27.7 Circadian rhythm of the peaks and clusters of QTc lengthening over 500 ms in postmyocardial infarction patients with malignant ventricular arrhythmias (Group I)

	24-hours of Holter	11am–11pm	11pm–11am	p-value
Number of peaks of QTc > 500 ms, per hour	463 ± 315	336 ± 176	590 ± 375	<0.05
Percentage of peaks of QTc > 500 ms, per hour	4.17 ± 2.83	3.02 ± 1.58	5.31 ± 3.37	<0.05
Number of grouped peaks (clusters) with QTc lengthening > 500 ms, per hour	1.29 ± 1.17	0.84 ± 0.83	1.75 ± 1.48	NS
Mean duration (minutes) of the grouped peaks	7.41 ± 8.31	2.85 ± 1.95	10.60 ± 9.64	<0.04

Results represent mean ± SD taken from hourly Holter monitoring within the period of time indicated. The p-values relate to the differences between time comprised from 11am to 11pm versus from 11pm to 11am.

rest of the 24 hours. These findings coincide with hourly mean QTc values, which were longer during the same hours of the day. The QTc clusters also had circadian behavior, with a higher incidence between 11pm and 11am. If we analyze the total duration of QTc clusters, the duration was also longer during this period. The mean duration of clusters was 1.60 ± 9 minutes from 11pm to 11am and was 2.85 ± 1.95 from 11am to 11pm (Table 27.6). However, these data do not indicate whether the QT interval is a trigger factor of malignant ventricular arrhythmias or only an accompanying event.

The behavior of the QT and QTc intervals varied throughout the day in postinfarction patients with malignant ventricular arrhythmias: there was a longer mean QTc/hour, higher number of QTc values >500 ms in absolute terms and as a percentage of beats, and more frequent and prolonged QTc clusters in the period between 11pm and 11am.

Algra *et al.*[33] recently published a study in which QTc interval was analyzed automatically on Holter tapes. In this study, prolongation of the QTc interval to more than 440 ms doubled the patient's risk of sudden death. Moreover, the presence of a short QTc interval (<400 ms) was also predictive of arrhythmic complications during follow-up. However, this study is not entirely comparable to ours because only 50% of their very heterogeneous group of patients were postinfarction and many of them were taking drugs which may modify the QT interval.

As we mentioned at the beginning of the chapter, the rate of occurrence of sudden death and malignant ventricular arrhythmias is greater between 6am and noon. Although this may suggest a link between the two factors, it does not demonstrate a causal relation. Prolongation of the QT interval may be merely a marker of malignant ventricular arrhythmias, and not a trigger. Although some isolated cases have been reported we have been unable to confirm that a sudden prolongation of QTc is the triggering mechanism of sudden death. It may be only a manifestation of an underlying mechanism.

As noted, QT interval is influenced by sympathetic/parasympathetic tone. The QT and the RR interval also varies with sympathetic or parasympathetic stimulation. Variations in the QT interval may coincide with disturbances in the autonomic nervous system that may trigger malignant ventricular arrhythmias.

Conclusions

Both malignant ventricular arrhythmias and sudden cardiac death exhibit a circadian rhythm. Most of the presently known possible 'trigger' factors also show circadian patterns. In recent years a lot of attention has been focused on the important role of the autonomic nervous system as a trigger mechanism of malignant arrhythmias. Although we have not reviewed all the repolarization parameters of the sympathetic-parasympathetic balance, some of them, such as HRV, also show this circadian rhythm. QT and QTc intervals are other important parameters for autonomic nervous system analysis, although they can be also influenced by other factors (such as circulating catecholamines and drugs).

We have reviewed the circadian rhythm of QT interval in normal subjects. In postinfarction patients without malignant ventricular arrhythmias during follow-up, this circadian pattern remains but sudden prolongation of QTc values ('peaks') appears, usually grouped in a cluster form. The circadian rhythm of these peaks is quite similar to the circadian pattern of sudden death, although this is not a demonstration nor evidence that QTc prolongation is the triggering factor of sudden death. This QTc prolongation may merely be the evident manifestation of an underlying process, such as a sudden imbalance of the autonomic nervous system.

Many mechanisms, triggers and modulators are still unknown, and why an arrhythmia develops at a certain moment remains a mystery. Many questions are yet to be answered: Does the circadian pattern of these parameters have any clinical relevance? Is it only an external manifestation of an underlying mechanism or is it the real trigger? Is the loss of the circadian pattern a bad prognostic factor in postinfarction patients?

Without any doubt, technological improvements in Holter equipment in the future, with the possibility of studying not only circadian variations of HRV but also other repolarization parameters such as QT interval, T-wave alternans,[34] etc., and their modifications before an arrhythmic episode (using Holter recordings or AICD devices), will further our knowledge of the mechanisms leading to malignant ventricular arrhythmias.

References

1. Wellens HJJ. Pathophysiology of ventricular tachycardia in man. *Arch Int Med* 1975; **135**: 475.
2. Bayés de Luna A, Coumel P, Leclercq JF. Ambulatory sudden death: mechanisms of production of fatal arrhythmia on the basis of data from 157 cases. *Am Heart J* 1989; **117**: 151–9.
3. Baum RS, Alvarez H, Cobb LA. Survival after resuscitation from out-hospital ventricular fibrillation. *Circulation* 1974; **50**: 1231.
4. Schaffer WA, Cobb LA. Recurrent ventricular fibrillation and modes of death in survivors of out-of-hospital ventricular fibrillation. *New Eng J Med* 1975; **293**: 259.
5. Liberthson RR, Nagel EL, Hirschman JC, Blackbourne BD, Davis JH. Pathophysiologic observations in prehospital ventricular fibrillation and sudden cardiac death. *Circulation* 1974; **49**: 790.
6. Muller JE, Stone PH, Turi ZG, and the MILIS Study Group. Circadian variation in the frequency of onset of acute myocardial infarction. *New Engl J Med* 1985; **313**: 1315.
7. Roberts R, Croft C, Gold HK, *et al*. Effects of propranolol on myocardial infarct size in a randomized, blinded, multicenter trial. *New Engl J Med* 1984; **311**: 218.
8. Muller JE, Ludmer PL, Willich SN *et al*. Circadian variation in the frequency of sudden cardiac death. *Circulation* 1987: **75**: 131.
9. Willich SN, Levy D, Rocco MB, *et al*. Circadian variation in the incidence of sudden cardiac death in the Framingham Heart Study Population Study. *Am J Cardiol* 1987; **60**: 801–6.
10. Huber K, Resch I, Rose D, *et al*. Circadian variation of plasminogen activator inhibitor (PAI) and the incidence of severe ischemic attacks in patients with coronary artery disease. *Thromb Hemos* 1987; **58**: 66.
11. Tofler GH, Brezinski DA, Schafer AI, *et al*. Concurrent morning increase in platelet aggregability and the risk of myocardial infarction and sudden cardiac death. *New Engl J Med* 1987; **316**: 1514.
12. Millard-Craig MW, Bishop CN, Raftery EB. Circadian variation of blood pressure. *Lancet* 1978, **1**: 795.
13. Bazett HC. An analysis of the time-relation of the electrocardiogram. *Heart* 1920; **7**: 353–70.
14. Puddu PE, Jouve R, Mariotti S, *et al*. Evaluation of 10 QT prediction formula in 881 middle-aged men from seven country studies: emphasis on the cubic root Fridericia's equation. *J Electrocardiol* 1988; **21**: 219–29.
15. Karjalainen J, Viitasalo M, Mänttäri M, Manninen V. Relation between QT intervals and heart rates from 40 to 120 beats/min in rest electrocardiograms of men and a simple method to adjust QT interval values. *J Am Coll Cardiol* 1994; **23**: 1547–53.
16. Vervaet P, Amery W. Reproducibility of QTc measurements in healthy volunteers. *Acta Cardiol* 1993; **48**: 555–64.
17. Murakawa Y, Inoue H, Nozaki A, Sugimoto T. Role of sympathovagal interaction in diurnal variation of QT interval. *Am J Cardiol* 1992; **69**: 339–43.
18. Rasmusen V, Jensen G, Hansen JF. QT interval in 24-hour ambulatory ECG recordings from 60 healthy adult subjects. *J Electrocardiol* 1991; **24**: 91–5.
19. Ong J, Sarma J, Venkataraman K, Levin S, Singh B. Circadian rhythmicity of heart rate and QTc interval in diabetic autonomic neuropathy: implications for the mechanisms of sudden death. *Am Heart J* 1993; **125**: 744–52.
20. Sarma J, Venkataraman K, Nicod P, *et al*. Circadian rhythmicity of rate-normalized QT interval in hypothroidism and its significance for development of class III antiarrhythmic agents. *Am J Cardiol* 1990; **66**: 959–63.
21. Merri M, Alberti M, Moss A, Dynamic analysis of ventricular repolarization from 24-hour Holter recordings. *IEEE Trans Biomed Eng* 1993; **40**: 1219–25.
22. Schwartz PJ, Wolf S. QT interval prolongation as predictor of sudden death in patients with myocardial infarction. *Circulation* 1978; **57**: 1074–7.
23. Haynes RE, Hallstrom AP, Cobb LA. Repolarisation abnormalities in survivors of out-of-hospital ventricular fibrillation. *Circulation* 1978; **57**: 654–8.
24. Anhve S, Gilpin E, Madsen EB, Froelicher V, Henning H, Ross J. Prognostic importance of QTc interval at discharge after acute myocardial infarction: a multicenter study of 865 patients. *Am Heart J* 1984; **108**: 395–400.
25. Algra A, Tijsen JGP, Roeland J, Pool J, Lubsen J. QTc prolongation measured by standard 12-lead electrocardiography is an independent risk factor for sudden death due to cardiac arrest. *Circulation* 1991; **83**: 1888–94.
26. Moller M. QT interval in relation to ventricular arrhythmias and sudden cardiac death in post-myocardial infarction patients. *Acta Med Scand* 1981; **220**: 73–7.

27. Wheelam K, Mukharji J, Rude RE. Sudden death and its relation to QT prolongation after acute myocardial infarction: 2-year follow-up. *Am J Cardiol* 1986; **57**: 745–50.

28. Boudoulas H, Sohn YH, O'Neill WM, Brown R, Weissler AM. The QT<QS2 syndrome: a new mortality indicator in coronary artery disease. *Am J Cardiol* 1982; **50**: 1229–35.

29. Pohjola-Sintonen S, Siltanen P, Haapakosi J. The QTc interval on the discharge electrocardiogram for predicting survival after acute myocardial infarction. *Am J Cardiol* 1986; **57**: 1066–8.

30. Martí V, Guindo J, Homs E, Viñolas X, Bayés de Luna A. Peaks of QTc lengthening in Holter recordings as a marker of life-threatening arrhythmias in postmyocardial infarction patients. *Am Heart J* 1992; **124**: 234–5.

31. Homs E, Viñolas X, Guindo J, Martí V, Bayés de Luna A. Automatic QTc measurement in postmyocardial infarction patients with and without malignant ventricular arrhythmias (abstract), *JACC* 1993.

32. Laguna P, Thakor NV, Caminal P, Jané R, Bayés de Luna A, Marti V, Guindo J. New algorithm for QT interval analysis in 24-hour Holter ECG: performance and applications. *Med Biol Eng Comput* 1990; **28**: 67–73.

33. Algra A, Tijssen JGP, Roetlandt JRTC, Pool J, Lubsen J. QT interval variables from 24-hour electrocardiography and the two-year risk of sudden death. *Br Heart J* 1993; **70**: 43–8.

34. Rosembaum BS, Jackson L, Smith JM, *et al*. Electrical alternans and vulnerability to ventricular arrhythmias. *New Engl J Med* 1994; **330**: 235–41.

28

Clinical Implications of Circadian Rhythms Detected by Ambulatory Monitoring Techniques

David Mulcahy and Arshed A. Quyyumi

Introduction

Ambulatory monitoring has now been an investigative clinical and research device for over 30 years, during which time significant technical refinements have been made, followed closely by increasing practical applications. The original ambulatory monitoring devices were designed primarily for the recording of cardiac rhythm and the detection of arrhythmias. The discovery in the early 1970s that transient alterations in the ST segment could be detected during ambulatory monitoring in patients with coronary disease led to a major expansion in ambulatory monitoring hardware and software in order to accurately detect ST segment changes, thus allowing the investigation of ischemic activity during daily life. A particular stimulus to the development of ambulatory ST segment monitoring devices was the fact that most episodes of transient ST segment change, reflecting ischemia, occurred in the absence of symptoms, thus raising the possibility that detection of predominantly silent ischemia during daily life might allow for early treatment of patients at risk of a future adverse outcome. In the 1980s, devices were designed which accurately recorded systolic and diastolic blood pressure in the ambulatory setting, and recently the nuclear VEST has provided assessment of the left ventricular ejection fraction during daily activities, although to date this remains primarily of research interest.

Thus, using ambulatory monitoring, we now have the ability to accurately record heart rate, blood pressure, and both ischemic and arrhythmic activity outside the hospital environment. Because available equipment can record for at least a 24-hour period, it has been possible to investigate the circadian variation of all these parameters. In this chapter, we focus on discussion of the circadian variation in myocardial ischemia, correlate the findings with the known circadian variations in onset of acute myocardial infarction, ventricular arrhythmia, and sudden cardiac death, and discuss the clinical implications of circadian variations in cardiovascular physiological and pathophysiological parameters as detected using monitoring techniques during normal daily activities.

Circadian Variation in Ischemic Activity

Ambulatory ST segment monitoring in patients with stable coronary artery disease has confirmed that 30–50% have transient ischemic episodes during their daily lives, and approximately 70–90% of such episodes are unrecognized or 'silent'. Many studies have confirmed the ischemic nature of these transient ST segment alterations. Assessment of the timing of ischemic episodes using 24-hour ambulatory ST segment monitoring has shown that there is a distinct circadian variation in ischemic activity, with a surge in the morning waking hours that reaches a plateau at approximately 1pm, a possible secondary evening peak, a gradual decline in late evening, and a trough at night [1] (Figure 28.1).

Various factors may contribute to this circadian variation in ischemic activity in the presence of significant coronary stenoses. Myocardial ischemia results, to a greater or lesser extent, from increases in myocardial oxygen demand and reductions in myocardial oxygen supply. The factors which we must consider are those likely to alter the supply/demand ratio in an unfavorable way in the presence of coronary stenoses, and whether such factors themselves have identifiable circadian rhythms.

Heart rate and blood pressure, the two most measurable parameters of myocardial oxygen demand, both surge in the morning waking hours, thus resulting in a significant morning increase in myocardial oxygen requirement. Both have a circadian variation very similar to that of myocardial ischemia.[2] Mirroring these changes is a surge in plasma catecholamines in the morning waking hours[3] (Figure 28.2). This results in increased myocardial contractility primarily as a consequence of increased circulating epinephrine, and an increase in coronary and peripheral vascular resistance due to an increase in the alpha vasoconstrictor effects of norepinephrine. Plasma renin and cortisol, both of which peak in activity in the morning hours,[4,5] may further contribute to this phenomenon

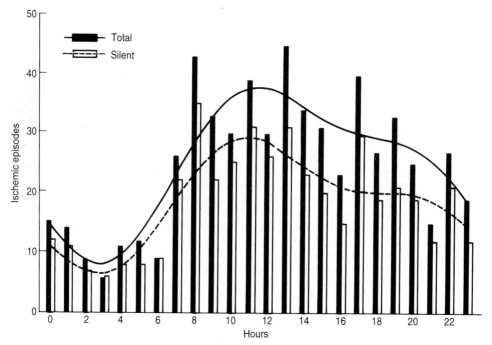

Figure 28.1 Circadian variation of total and silent ischemic episodes in 150 patients with coronary artery disease off therapy. (Reproduced with permission from reference 1)

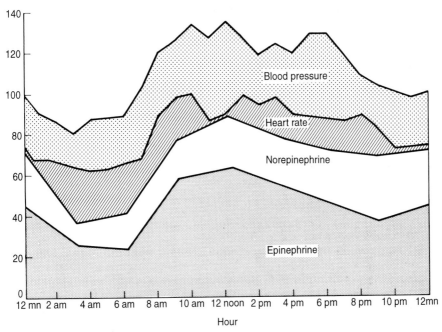

Figure 28.2   Circadian variation of heart rate, blood pressure, plasma epinephrine and plasma norepinephrine. Plasma norepinephrine levels have been reduced by 3.5 times for uniformity of scaling. (Heart rate and blood pressure data adapted with permission from reference 2; plasma catecholamine levels adapted with permission from reference 3)

either directly by vasoconstrictor effects (renin),[4] or directly, by their synergistic effects on the action of catecholamines (cortisol).[5] Coronary blood flow is lower in the morning hours compared with the afternoon period under resting conditions in dogs.[6] This increased coronary vasoconstriction in the morning hours has also been confirmed in humans: patients with coronary disease have been shown to have a reduced ischemic threshold on exercise-testing in the morning compared with the afternoon.[7] The combined results of all these changes are a reduction in myocardial oxygen supply due to coronary vasoconstriction and an increase in myocardial oxygen demand secondary to increase in heart rate, blood pressure, contractility and afterload. In addition, the surge in plasma catecholamines in the morning waking hours, by lowering the arrhythmia threshold, may contribute to ventricular arrhythmias that have been demonstrated to occur more frequently in the morning waking hours than at other times of the day.[8]

Platelet aggregability is highest in the morning waking hours, and appears to be triggered by assuming the upright posture.[9] This may potentially result in partial and transient obstruction to coronary blood flow at the sites of coronary stenoses either due to formation of microthrombi or from vasoconstriction resulting from release of vasoconstrictor substances from aggregating platelets. Furthermore, there is a distinct circadian variation in the fibrinolytic state, with a trough in the early morning hours, resulting from reduced activity of tPa (tissues plasminogen activator) and increased activity of PAI (plasminogen activator inhibitor).[10] It is likely, however, that these changes are more relevant to onset of acute thrombotic coronary syndromes than to transient ischemic activity during daily activities.

Pathophysiology of Transient Ischemic Episodes

The clinical significance and therapeutic implications of finding a distinct circadian variation in ischemic activity will depend to a large extent on the relation between ischemic activity and the endpoints of coronary disease, and on what the likely underlying mechanisms of ischemia are. Various researchers have noted the discrepancy between the heart rates at the onset of transient ischemic episodes during daily life and the heart rate at the onset of ischemia during formal exercise testing. [11,12] The finding that the heart rate at onset of ischemia during ambulatory monitoring was lower than that during exercise-testing prompted the suggestion that transient ischemia resulted predominantly from alterations in coronary vasomotor tone. Many studies have, however, confirmed that transient ischemia occurs almost exclusively in patients with a positive exercise test for ischemia, [13,14] and that the majority of ischemic episodes during daily activities are preceded by an increase in heart rate. [15–19] Panza *et al.*, in a study of exercise-testing using two different protocols, and ambulatory ST segment monitoring, reported that the heart rate at onset of ischemia during ambulatory monitoring was similar to that during formal exercise when using a gentle exercise protocol (NIH combined protocol) whereas it was lower than heart rate at onset of ischemia using the more aggressive Bruce protocol. [15] Deedwania and Nelson, in a study incorporating ambulatory ST segment and blood pressure monitoring in patients with coronary disease, have reported that the majority of transient ischemic episodes are preceded by significant increases in heart rate and systolic blood pressure. [16] They concluded that increases in myocardial oxygen demand played a significant role in the genesis of (silent) myocardial ischemia. McLenechan *et al.* have shown that, while there may be no significant increase in heart rate in the minute prior to onset of many ischemic episodes during daily life, important increases in heart rate occurred 5–30 minutes prior to most ischemic episodes. [17] Andrews *et al.* performed ambulatory ST segment monitoring on 50 patients with coronary disease who were treated with propranolol, diltiazem, nifedipine or placebo in randomized, double-blind crossover trial, and assessed mean minute heart rate activity. [18] They noted that 81% of all recorded ischemic episodes were preceded by an increase in heart rate of more than 5 bpm.

Thus, although underlying pathophysiological mechanisms of ischemia are likely to be complex and multifactorial, heart rate increases appear to play a pivotal role in the genesis of ischemic episodes in chronic stable angina.

The complexities involved in the genesis of ischemic episodes are, however, well reflected by the fact that the heart rate increases do not simply increase myocardial oxygen demand in patients with coronary artery disease. While coronary flow will increase in response to an increase in heart rate in those with normal coronary anatomy, paradoxical constriction can occur in those with significant coronary disease. [20] Many physiological stimuli which cause vasodilatation in normal coronary arteries have been shown to cause vasoconstriction in the presence of coronary artery disease; [21,22] these paradoxical responses result from endothelial dysfunction, due to partial or complete denudation at the sites of coronary stenoses.

Circadian variation in ischemic threshold

Ambulatory ST segment monitoring has allowed us not only to assess ischemic activity during daily life, but also to assess variations in pathophysiological mechanisms. In addition to establishing that there is a distinct circadian variation in ischemic activity, and that the majority of ischemic episodes are preceded by increases in heart rate, it has also been reported that there is a circadian variation in ischemic threshold during daily life.

Quyyumi *et al.*, using sequential exercise-testing throughout the day, have shown that ischemia occurs at lower levels of myocardial oxygen demand in the early morning and at night when compared with midday and 5pm, suggesting that coronary vascular resistance is higher in the morning and at night.[7] They also demonstrated, using forearm plethysmography, that peripheral vascular resistance was also increased at times when the ischemic threshold was reduced (Figure 28.3), indicating that the apparent increase in vascular resistance in the morning hours is a generalized phenomenon involving the coronary and peripheral vasculature.

Benhorin *et al.* performed serial ambulatory ST segment monitoring in 23 patients off all antianginal medications.[23] They noted that, in addition to a peak ischemic activity in the morning waking hours, there was also a distinct circadian variation in ischemic threshold (measured as heart rate at onset of ischemia), which was significantly less during the night hours (lowest between 1am and 3am and highest between 10am and 1pm) compared with the daytime (Figure 28.4). They suggested that the low ischemic threshold at night may indicate that the mechanism of ischemia during these hours is

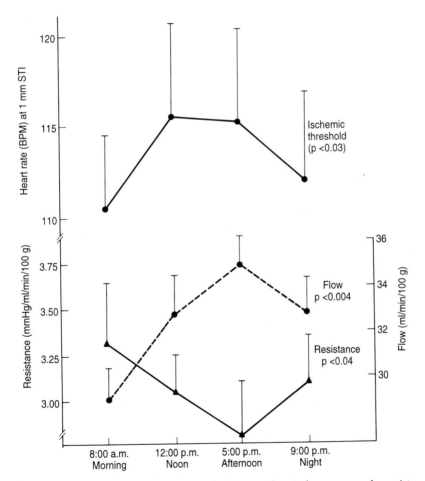

Figure 28.3 Circadian variation in ischemic threshold, postischemic forearm vascular resistance, and blood flow in patients with stable coronary artery disease. Ischemic threshold is lower in the morning waking hours and at night compared with during the day, and corresponds with higher forearm vascular resistance in the early morning and at night. (Reproduced with permission from reference 7: © American Heart Association)

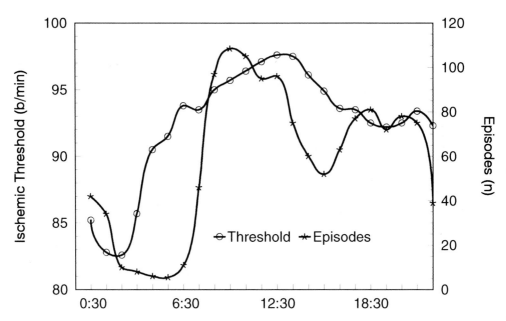

Figure 28.4 Diurnal distribution of ischemic episodes and threshold of ischemia (heart rate at onset of 1 mm ST segment depression) in 41 patients who had 1371 ischemic episodes on ambulatory ST segment monitoring. (Reproduced with permission from reference 23: © American Heart Association)

reduced coronary flow due to increased coronary tone. The increased frequency of ischemia during the day when the ischemic threshold was high pointed towards increases in the determinants of myocardial oxygen demand as being the predominant precipitating mechanism in most ischemic episodes.

It is, however, quite possible that there are similar increases in heart rate prior to ischemia at night; but in the presence of a lower resting heart rate and an increased basal coronary tone at this time, the ischemic threshold will be reached at a relatively lower overall heart rate.

Circadian variation of ischemic activity in variant angina

In 1959, Prinzmetal *et al.* described a variant form of angina from that described by Heberden, with pain occurring at rest or during times of the day or night that are not associated with effort. They noted that during an attack the ST segments are often transiently and markedly elevated, and that attacks almost invariably resolve spontaneously, or with nitrates. They also noted the tendency for such attacks to occur early in the morning, and observed that underlying coronary disease involving the artery subtending the ischemic area was invariably present. The authors clearly characterized what is now loosely referred to as coronary spasm, a condition reflecting an extreme degree of alteration in coronary vasomotor tone, usually at the sites of coronary lesions.

Continuous ambulatory ST segment monitoring has been particularly helpful in characterizing ischemic activity in such patients. Waters and his colleagues,[24] in a study of patients with classic variant angina, showed that spontaneous ischemic episodes (often asymptomatic) occurred significantly more often in the early morning hours (4–8am), and furthermore that ischemic episodes were more readily induced (by ergonovine) in the early morning (4am) compared with the afternoon (4pm). Araki *et al.*,[25] documented 364 episodes of ST segment elevation during 52 days of monitoring in 26 patients with variant angina, and reported that 72% of all episode occurred between midnight and 9am, with only a few episodes occurring between 10am and 6pm. Nademanee *et al.*,[26] in a study of both stable angina and variant angina patients, showed that, while the majority of ischemic episodes (predominantly ST segment depression) in patients with stable angina occurred during the daytime 'activity' hours, the majority of ischemic episodes in those with variant angina (predominantly ST segment elevation) occurred during the nocturnal hours (Figure 28.5). Furthermore, while there was a relation between peak frequency of ischemic episodes and maximal increases in heart rate in those with chronic stable angina, there was no correlation between heart rate changes and transient ischemic episodes in those with variant angina, suggesting spontaneous decreases in coronary blood flow as the primary underlying mechanism of ischemia in variant angina.

These reports confirm that, even at the sites of significant coronary stenoses, it is possible to at least partially alter luminal diameter in response to various dilator and constrictor stimuli. Brown has reported that the majority of coronary stenoses have an arc of normal arterial wall capable of such responses.[27] Ischemic episodes in variant angina result from transient coronary arterial occlusion due to extreme alterations in coronary vasomotor tone at the sites of such stenoses. The fact that this is more likely to occur at night and in the early morning hours supports the concept that there is an increased basal coronary tone at this time, resulting in a reduced ischemic threshold in those with 'stable angina' and frank occlusive ischemic episodes, representing the extreme of vasoconstrictor responses, in those with variant angina. These ambulatory monitoring findings, in addition to clarifying underlying pathophysiological mechanisms and the circadian variation in such mechanisms, have proven particularly useful in guiding therapy in the patient with variant angina.

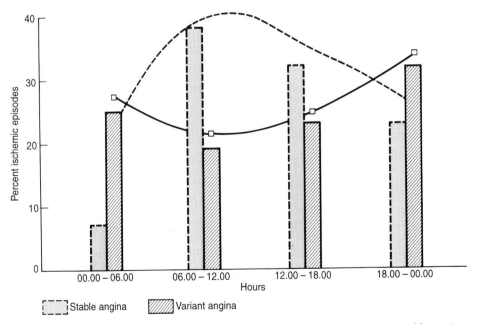

Figure 28.5 Circadian variation of ischemic episodes in patients with chronic stable angina and Prinzmetal's angina. There is a distinct circadian variation in transient ischemia in the setting of stable angina, with a peak in the morning waking hours and a trough at night. In Prinzmetal's angina, ischemic episodes are more likely to occur at night. (Adapted with permission from reference 26)

Relation of circadian variation in ischemic activity to time of waking

With the use of angina diaries during monitoring periods, and event buttons on the ambulatory ST segment monitoring devices, it has been possible to investigate, in detail, the relation between the morning peak in ischemic activity and specific time of awakening and commencing activities. This has confirmed that the morning surge in ischemic activity is particularly related to time of awakening and commencing activities, rather than more loosely, the morning waking hours. Rocco *et al.* demonstrated a distinct circadian variation in ischemic activity with a peak between 6am and noon.[28] When relating the occurrence of ischemic episodes specifically to time of awakening, however, they showed that the peak in ischemic activity occurred in the first 2 hours after waking and commencing activities (Figure 28.6). A recent study by Parker *et al.* has shown that, if patients with coronary artery disease rise and commence activities at 8am, the witnessed surge in heart rate and ischemic activity occurs at this time, whereas if the same patients arise and commence activities at 12 noon, the surge in both heart rate and ischemic activity is delayed until the later time[29] (Figure 28.7). The implication of these findings is that the 'circadian variation' in at least some physiological responses, and in ischemic activity, are not intrinsic circadian rhythms, but are primarily activity-related. However, it is clear that the period of rising and commencing activities, whenever that time happens to be, is associated with a series of physiological responses that can act adversely, either alone or more likely in combination, in the patient with coronary disease.

In addition, various studies using ambulatory monitoring have demonstrated that alterations in daily activity cycles can significantly alter the circadian variation in physiologic parameters which, in the setting of coronary stenoses, could precipitate ischemia. A study of continuous ambulatory heart rate and blood pressure monitoring in

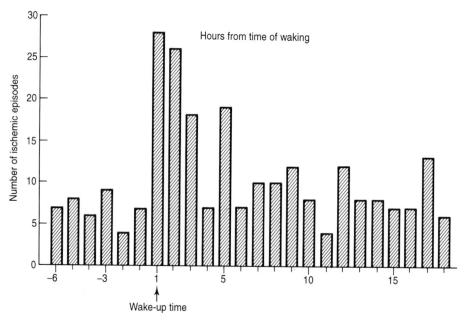

Figure 28.6 Circadian variation of transient ischemic episodes in patients with stable angina when corrected for time of awakening. (Adapted with permission from reference 28: © American Heart Association)

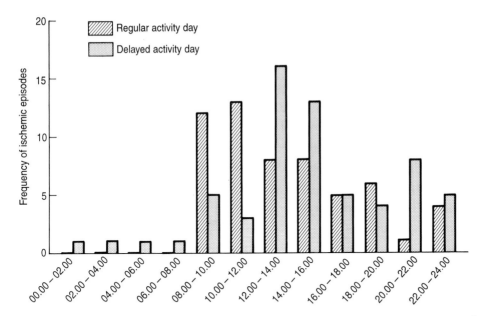

Figure 28.7 Frequency of episodes of ambulatory ischemia during placebo therapy on two activity days in patients with stable coronary artery disease. On the regular activity day, physical activities began at 8am; on the delayed activity day, they began at 12 noon. (Adapted with permission from reference 29: © American Heart Association)

normal subjects who include a siesta during their early afternoon activities has shown that the surge in myocardial oxygen demand following such a siesta is similar to that encountered on waking and commencing activities in the morning.[30] Subjects who rise in the morning but also perform their major body of work in the evening have their primary peak in heart rate activity in the evening rather than in the morning.[31] It is likely, therefore, that patients with coronary artery disease would show similar alterations in ischemic activity and indeed in timing of onset of acute cardiac events, under similar circumstances.

Circadian variation in ventricular arrhythmias

Using ambulatory monitoring, it has been possible to assess ventricular arrhythmic activity in detail in patients with coronary artery disease; to investigate the relation of such activity to both heart rate and ischemic change (as represented by ST segment alterations); and to investigate any underlying circadian periodicity in ventricular arrhythmic activity.

Raeder et al.,[32] in a study of patients with life-threatening ventricular arrhythmias who were refractory to medical therapy, performed periods of ambulatory monitoring off therapy, and demonstrated a distinct circadian variation in ventricular ectopic activity, with a peak between 10am and 12 noon, and a trough at 5am. They confirmed that the distribution of mean heart rate throughout the day followed a similar pattern. Lucente et al.,[33] in a study of ambulatory monitoring following acute myocardial infarction, confirmed that ventricular tachycardia in the stable phase following such an event also had a distinct circadian variation, with a primary peak in the late morning hours. Twidale et al.[34] investigated the circadian distribution of symptomatic ventricular arrhythmia from

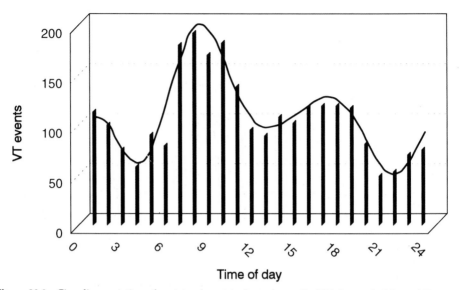

Figure 28.8 Circadian variation of sustained ventricular tachycardia (VT) for pooled data of 32 patients with coronary artery disease who have an AICD *in situ*. The bar graph shows time of day of occurrence of all VT events with superimposed fourth-order harmonic regression curve. (Reproduced with permission from reference 8: © American Heart Association)

the questioning of patients with documented ventricular arrhythmias during electro-physiological study, and their relatives. Syncope, presyncope, or palpitation was considered to reflect such an episode. They reported that the occurrence of VT centered around 9am.

In an attempt to assess the circadian variation of sustained ventricular arrhythmias (indirect representation of failed sudden death), Lampert *et al.* recently investigated 32 patients with documented coronary artery disease who had required prior insertion of an implantable cardioverter–defibrillator (Ventak PRX) device for sustained ventricular tachycardia.[8] These patients were followed longitudinally for up to 29 months (mean follow-up 14 months), and all had at least one episode of ventricular tachycardia terminated by their device. Among the 2558 episodes of ventricular tachycardia recorded by the device logs over the follow-up period, and requiring either ICD pacing or electrical discharge, VT occurrence peaked between 6am and 12 noon (Figure 28.8). In addition, 38% of all episodes recorded in patients with frequent episodes of ventricular tachycardia occurred within this time span. They showed that both high- and low-frequency subgroups showed significant aggregation of VT episodes in the morning time period, suggesting that the findings pertain to the population as a whole. D'avila *et al.* have reported that there is a similar morning peak in frequency of ventricular fibrillation or very rapid VT requiring termination by an ICD.[35]

An increasingly large body of evidence attests to the increased propensity to ventricular arrhythmias in the morning waking hours.

Clinical Implications of Circadian Variation in Myocardial Ischemia

The clinical implications of the morning increase in myocardial ischemia are both *prognostic and therapeutic*. The first issue concerns whether such ischemic activity,

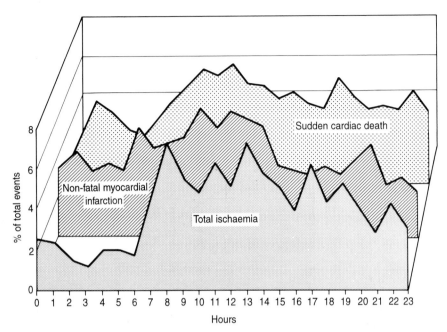

Figure 28.9 Circadian variation in transient myocardial ischemia, nonfatal myocardial infarction, and sudden cardiac death. (Reproduced with permission from reference 1)

particularly in the morning waking hours, leads to precipitation of acute coronary events. While relatively little direct evidence is available to support the belief that these ischemic episodes lead directly to onset of acute myocardial infarction or sudden cardiac death, study of the circadian variation of these cardiovascular endpoints has been carried out.

In 1985, Muller *et al.* reported, in an analysis of the MILIS study, that there was a circadian variation in onset of acute myocardial infarction, with a peak in the morning waking hours, and a trough at night.[36] Prospective studies have subsequently confirmed this finding.[37] In addition, it has been confirmed that there is a similar circadian variation in sudden cardiac death.[38] Available data therefore confirm that transient myocardial ischemia, onset of acute myocardial infarction and sudden cardiac death have very similar circadian variations (Figure 28.9) which, without necessarily implying a direct cause and effect relationship, strongly suggests a common association or 'trigger'.

It must also be considered that the witnessed surge in blood pressure, and the trough in fibrinolytic activity in the morning waking hours, might be causally related to the increased incidence in onset of acute myocardial infarction or sudden cardiac death, due to plaque rupture and thrombotic occlusion, and independent of its propensity to provoke ischemia. Likewise, it is possible that the increase in ventricular arrhythmic activity, and sudden cardiac death in the morning waking hours, may be at least partly explained by the increased propensity to ischemia at this time, although direct reduction in the arrhythmia threshold from the peak in catecholamine release in the morning may also be implicated. Overall it has not been established to date whether transient ischemia in stable coronary syndromes is a marker of coronary disease, or leads directly to the endpoints of such disease. Undoubtedly the relation between physiological responses, ischemia, infarction, arrhythmia and cardiac death is complex (Figure 28.10).

The therapeutic implications of finding a distinct circadian variation in myocardial ischemia are clearly reliant on the assumption that reduction or eradication of ischemia will improve the patient's outlook. To date this has not been shown to be the case. While

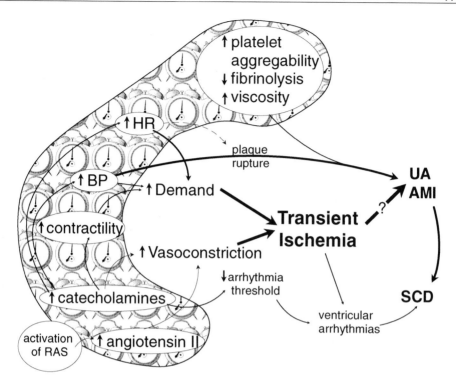

Figure 28.10 Possible inter–relationships between physiological processes occurring particularly in the morning waking hours and cardiovascular events in those with coronary atherosclerosis.

it might seem reasonable to assume that attempting to reduce or eradicate the total ischemic burden will be of benefit, this assumption must be balanced against the side-effects of aggressive pharmacological management.

Up until recent years, the majority of available anti-ischemic agents were short-acting, requiring administration 3–4 times a day. When patients awoke in the morning and commenced activities, the effects of the previous nighttime administration of antianginal agent would have worn off. The patient was potentially unprotected from the ischemia/angina viewpoint at the time of peak ischemic activity – the period soon after waking and commencing activities. The study of circadian rhythms has reflected the potential importance of long-acting anti-ischemic agents; ones that are still effective 'the morning after the night before'. Furthermore, ambulatory monitoring has shown that alterations in environmental stresses and activity patterns lead to significant alterations in physiological (and pathophysiological) responses, emphasizing the importance of '24-hour protection'. The explosion of new long-acting antianginal agents in recent years has clearly been driven partly by these concepts. Most available antianginal agents are effective in reducing ischemic activity during daily life,[39] and, perhaps particularly, those agents that exert at least some chronotropic control.[1,40,41] Long-acting nitrates present a unique difficulty in prescribing when considering the circadian variation in ischemic activity. Tolerance or 'an attenuated response' appears to develop in some patients when these agents are prescribed on a 24-hour basis.[42] It has been suggested that a nitrate-free interval at night, when ischemic activity is known to be very low, would overcome this problem. However, a nitrate-free interval at night means that when these agents are used as monotherapy, the patient will wake up and commence activity without any anti-ischemic protection until the morning dose is administered and absorbed. In view of this, many physicians will use nitrates in combination with another long-acting agent such as a beta-blocker, which does not suffer from such a problem. It has been suggested that, particularly for those who suffer morning waking angina, a short-acting nitrate preparation could be taken prophylactically prior to commencing activities, thus offering added protection at the recognized time of the surge in ischemic activity[43] (short-acting nitrates remain extremely effective even in that percentage of patients who develop an attenuated response to long-acting medications).

The study of circadian variation in ischemic activity has been particularly useful when planning therapy for the patient with variant angina. If these patients are taking medium-length acting calcium-channel blocking agents or nitrates, known to be very effective in preventing or reducing ischemic activity in variant angina, they should be encouraged to be compliant particularly with their nocturnal dosage, in view of the fact that the peak in ischemic activity is known to occur in the early morning. This is again of importance when considering a 'nitrate-free interval', as this interval should certainly not be at night in the patient with variant angina. A concomitant calcium-channel blocking agent should ideally be used. Again the potential attractions of a long-acting calcium-channel blocking agent are evident in such patients. Because of the potential for unopposed alpha vasoconstriction, beta-blockers have been avoided by many in treating variant angina.[44]

The clinical implications of the study of circadian variations in ventricular arrhythmic activity are similar to those for myocardial ischemia. As ventricular arrhythmias, both unsustained and sustained, are more likely to occur in the morning waking hours, also the time of increased incidence in sudden cardiac death, treatment should be designed to offer optimal protection at this time. Antiarrhythmic agents with a short half-life may not offer adequate protection at the time of waking and commencing activities in the morning. Long-acting antiarrhythmic agents which also combat the surge in sympathetic triggered activity in the morning waking hours may prove particularly useful in this regard, and indeed beta-blocking agents are effective in modifying both sympathetic activity and ventricular arrhythmic activity, and in significantly reducing the incidence of sudden cardiac death, at least in subsets of coronary patients.

The Use of Antianginal Agents

Heart rate, blood pressure, and catecholamine release peak in the morning waking hours, resulting in increased demands on the myocardium at a recognized time of decreased myocardial oxygen supply. The use of beta-blocking agents will modify these physiological responses, thus reducing the requirement of the myocardium for oxygen, and also reducing shear stresses, which may at least partly be responsible for plaque rupture and the increased frequency in onset of acute myocardial infarction in the morning hours. Beta-blockers have been shown to blunt the morning peak in myocardial ischemia,[1] onset of acute myocardial infarction [36,37] and sudden cardiac death;[45] whether this will translate into an overall reduction in such events, however, has yet to be clearly established.

The findings of the BHAT study indicate that beta-blockers reduce the incidence of sudden cardiac death following acute myocardial infarction,[45] suggesting that such agents may act in a beneficial way by increasing arrhythmia threshold. Calcium antagonists will oppose the increased peripheral vascular and coronary vascular resistance reported in the morning, in addition to exerting some control on the chronotropic response witnessed at this time (non-dihydropyridine agents). Their afterload-reducing effects will also modify the surge in systolic pressure in the morning waking hours, again helping to modify shear stresses, and rate of change in such stresses, which could potentially be associated with destabilization of atheromatous plaques. These agents, with their marked coronary vasodilator effects, are also particularly useful in managing the extreme alterations in coronary vasomotor tone known to occur in patients with variant angina, and, with nitrates, remain the treatment of choice in this condition.

Short-acting nitrate preparations remain excellent therapy for acute anginal attacks, in both its 'stable' and 'variant' forms. They are also excellent anti-ischemic agents, and their prophylactic use during expected periods of identifiable stress or exertion is becoming an increasingly popular therapeutic approach. They act rapidly as coronary vasodilators, and reduce venous return by venodilatation, reducing left ventricular end-diastolic volume and cardiac work. This effect is augmented by some reduction in afterload due to their arteriolar vasodilatory effects, reducing systolic pressure and shear stresses.

Conclusions

When addressing the issue of treatment of both transient ischemia and ventricular arrhythmic activity in patients with 'stable' coronary artery disease, we must urgently attempt to establish that treatment will indeed improve outcome. Until then we must intelligently prescribe, remembering that the morning waking hours are a time of particular threat, where the normal witnessed physiological responses can act adversely in the patient with coronary artery disease. Ambulatory monitoring has taught us a considerable amount about not only the pattern of normal physiological responses throughout the day, about patterns of ischemic and arrhythmia activity and their relationship to underlying pathophysiological mechanisms at play, but also about the detailed relationship between the sleep–wake period and the various 'circadian variations' which we witness when studying cardiovascular physiology or pathophysiology.

Should it be established that detection and treatment of transient myocardial ischemia during daily life results in an improved prognosis for the patient with coronary artery disease, or that modification in the circadian variation of myocardial ischemia, heart rate, blood pressure, or arrhythmic activity, particularly in the morning waking hours, is associated with a reduction in onset of acute cardiac events, ambulatory monitoring will become a mainstay in the investigative and therapeutic armamentarium of the cardiologist. Assessment of the effects of therapeutic interventions particularly on the morning peak in heart rate, blood pressure, ischemic and arrhythmic activity might prove useful in evaluating efficacy and further unravelling the mechanisms which trigger acute cardiac events.

References

1. Mulcahy D, Keegan J, Cunningham D, *et al*. Circadian variation of total ischaemic burden and its alteration with antianginal agents. *Lancet* 1988; **ii**: 755–9.
2. Millar–Craig MW, Bishop CN, Raftery EB. Circadian variation of blood pressure. *Lancet* 1978; **i**: 795–7.
3. Tofler GH, Brezinski DA, Schafer A, *et al*. Concurrent morning increase in platelet aggregability and the risk of myocardial infarction and sudden cardiac death. *New Eng J Med* 1987; **316**: 1514–18.
4. Gordon RD, Wolfe LK, Island DP, Liddle GW. A diurnal rhythm in plasma renin activity in man. *J Clin Invest* 1966; **45**: 1587–92.
5. Weitzman ED, Fukushima D, Nogeire C, Roffwarg H, Gallagher TF, Hellman L. Twenty–four hour pattern of the episodic secretion of cortisol in normal subjects. *J Clin Endocrinol Metab* 1971; **33**: 14–22.
6. Fugita M, Franklin D. Diurnal changes in coronary blood flow in conscious dogs. *Circulation* 1987; **76**: 488–91.
7. Quyyumi AA, Panza JA, Diodati JG, Lakatos E, Epstein SE. Circadian variation in ischemic threshold: a mechanism underlying the circadian variation in ischemic events. *Circulation* 1992; **86**: 22–8.
8. Lampert R, Rosenfeld L, Batsford W, Lee F, McPherson C. Circadian variation of sustained ventricular tachycardia in patients with coronary artery disease and implantable cardioverter–defibrillators. *Circulation* 1994; **90**: 241–7.

9. Brezinski DA, Tofler GH, Muller JE, *et al*. Morning increase in platelet aggregability: association with assumption of the upright posture. *Circulation* 1988; **78**: 35–40.

10. Andreotti F, Davies GJ, Hackett DR, *et al*. Major circadian variations in fibrinolytic factors and possible relevance to time of onset of myocardial infarction, sudden cardiac death, and stroke. *Am J Cardiol* 1988; **62**: 635–7.

11. Deanfield JE, Selwyn AP, Chierchia S, *et al*. Myocardial ischemia during daily life in patients with stable angina: its relation to symptoms and heart rate changes. *Lancet* 1983; **i**: 753–8.

12. Cohn PF, Lawson WE. Characteristics of silent myocardial ischemia during out–of–hospital activities in asymptomatic angiographically documented coronary artery disease. *Am J Cardiol* 1987; **59**: 746–9.

13. Mulcahy D, Keegan J, Sparrow J, Park A, Wright C, Fox KM. Ischemia in the ambulatory setting – the total ischemic burden: relation to exercise testing and investigative and therapeutic implications. *J Am Coll Cardiol* 1989; **14**: 1166–72.

14. Quyyumi AA, Mockus L, Wright C, Fox KM. Morphology of ambulatory ST segment changes in patients with varying severity of coronary artery disease: investigation of the frequency of nocturnal ischemia and coronary spasm. *Br Heart J* 1985; **53**: 186–93.

15. Panza JA, Quadri AA, Diodati JG, Callahan TS, Epstein SE. Prediction of the frequency and duration of ambulatory myocardial ischemia in patients with stable coronary artery disease by determination of the ischemic threshold from exercise testing: importance of the exercise protocol. *J Am Coll Cardiol* 1991; **17**: 657–63.

16. Deedwania PC, Nelson JR. Pathophysiology of silent myocardial ischemia during daily life: hemodynamic evaluation by simultaneous electrocardiographic and blood pressure monitoring. *Circulation* 1990; **82**: 1296–304.

17. McLenachan JM, Weidinger FF, Barry J, *et al*. Relations between heart rate, ischemia, and drug therapy during daily life in patients with coronary artery disease. *Circulation* 1991; **83**: 1263–70.

18. Andrews TC, Fenton T, Toyosaki N, *et al*. Subsets of ambulatory myocardial ischemia based on heart rate activity: circadian distribution and response to anti–ischemic medications. *Circulation* 1993; **88**: 92–100.

19. Panza JA, Diodati JG, Callahan TS, Epstein SE, Quyyumi AA. Role of increases in heart rate in determining the occurrence and frequency of myocardial ischemia during daily life in patients with stable coronary artery disease. *J Am Coll Cardiol* 1992; **20**: 1092–8.

20. Nabel EG, Selwyn AP, Ganz P. Paradoxical narrowing of atherosclerotic coronary arteries induced by increases in heart rate. *Circulation* 1990; **81**: 850–59.

21. Nabel EG, Ganz P, Gordon JB, Alexander RW, Selwyn AP. Dilation of normal and constriction of atherosclerotic coronary arteries caused by the cold pressor test. *Circulation* 1988; **77**: 43–52.

22. Gordon JB, Ganz P, Nabel EG, *et al*. Atherosclerosis influences the vasomotor response of epicardial coronary arteries to exercise. *J Clin Invest* 1989; **83**: 1946–52.

23. Benhorin J, Banai S, Moriel M, *et al*. Circadian variations in ischemic threshold and their relation to the occurrence of ischemic episodes. *Circulation* 1993; **87**: 808–14.

24. Waters DD, Miller DD, Bouchard A, Bosch X, Theroux P. Circadian variation in variant angina. *Am J Cardiol* 1984; **54**: 61–4.

25. Araki H, Koiwaya Y, Nakagaki O, Nakamura M. Diurnal distribution of ST–segment elevation and related arrhythmias in patients with variant angina: a study by ambulatory ECG monitoring. *Circulation* 1983; **67**: 995–1000.

26. Nademanee K, Intarachot V, Josephson MA, Singh BH. Circadian variation in occurrence of transient overt and silent myocardial ischemia in chronic stable angina and comparison with Prinzmetal angina in men. *Am J Cardiol* 1987; **60**: 494–8.

27. Brown BG, Bolsen EL, Dodge HT. Dynamic mechanisms in human coronary stenosis. *Circulation* 1984; **70**: 917–22.

28. Rocco MB, Barry J, Campbell S, *et al*. Circadian variation of transient myocardial ischemia in patients with coronary artery disease. *Circulation* 1987; **75**: 395–400.

29. Parker JD, Testa MA, Jimenez AH, *et al*. Morning increase in ambulatory ischemia in patients with stable coronary artery disease: importance of physical activity and increased cardiac demand. *Circulation* 1994; **89**: 604–14.

30. Mulcahy D, Wright C, Sparrow J, *et al*. Heart rate and blood pressure consequences of an afternoon SIESTA (Snooze-Induced Excitation of Sympathetic Triggered Activity). *Am J Cardiol* 1993; **71**: 611–13.

31. Mulcahy D, Keegan J, Fingret A, *et al*. Circadian variation of heart rate is affected by environment: a study of continuous electrocardiographic monitoring in members of a symphony orchestra. *Br Heart J* 1991; **64**: 388–92.

32. Raeder EA, Hohnloser SH, Graboys TB, Podrid PJ, Lampert S, Lown B. Spontaneous variability and circadian distribution of ectopic activity in patients with malignant ventricular arrhythmia. *J Am Coll Cardiol* 1988; **12**: 656–61.

33. Lucente M, Rebuzzi AG, Lanza GA, *et al*. Circadian variation of ventricular tachycardia in acute myocardial infarction. *Am J Cardiol* 1988; **62**: 670–74.

34. Twidale N, Taylor S, Heddle WF, Ayres BF, Tonkin AM. Morning increase in the time of onset of sustained ventricular tachycardia. *Am J Cardiol* 1988; **62**: 1204–6.

35. D'Avila A, Gebara O, Brugada P. Circadian variation in recurrent sudden death aborted by discharges from the implantable defibrillator (abstract). *Circulation* 1993; **88**(Suppl 1): I-155.

36. Muller JE, Stone PH, Turi ZG, *et al*. Circadian variation in the frequency of onset of acute myocardial infarction. *New Eng J Med* 1985; **313**: 1315–22.

37. Willich SN, Linderer T, Wegscheider K, Leizorovicz A, Alamercery I, Schroder R. Increased morning incidence of myocardial infarction in the ISAM study: absence with prior beta–adrenergic blockade. *Circulation* 1989; **80**: 853–8.

38. Muller JE, Ludmer PL, Willich SN, *et al*. Circadian variation in the frequency of sudden cardiac death. *Circulation* 1987; **75**: 131–8.

39. Frishman WH, Teicher M. Antianginal drug therapy for silent myocardial ischemia. *Am Heart J* 1987; **114**: 140–47.

40. Quyyumi AA, Crake T, Wright C, Mockus L, Fox KM. Medical treatment of patients with severe exertional and rest angina: double blind comparison of beta–blocker, calcium antagonist, and nitrate. *Br Heart J* 1987; **57**: 505–11.

41. Stone PH, Gibson RS, Glasser SP, *et al.* Comparison of propranolol, diltiazem and nifedipine in the treatment of ambulatory ischemia in patients with stable angina: differential effects on ambulatory ischemia, exercise perform-ance and anginal symptoms. *Circulation* 1990; **82**: 1962–72.

42. Rezakovic DE, Alpert JS (eds), *Nitrate Therapy and Nitrate Tolerance: Current Concepts and Controversies.* Basel: S. Karger, 1993.

43. Quyyumi AA. Circadian rhythms in cardiovascular disease. *Am Heart J* 1990; **120**: 726–33.

44. Robertson RM, Wood AJJ, Vaughn WK, Robertson D. Exacerbation of vasotonic angina pectoris by propranolol. *Circulation* 1982; **65**: 281–5.

45. Peters RW, Muller JE, Goldstein S, Byington R, Friedman LM. Propranolol and the morning increase in the frequency of sudden cardiac death (BHAT study). *Am J Cardiol* 1989; **63**: 1518–20.

Epilogue

Future Considerations

Arthur Moss

As one looks back on the past 30 years of noninvasive electrocardiologic monitoring, one can appreciate the changing emphasis from the detection of arrhythmia and ischemia to analysis of heart rate variability and repolarization phenomena. Concomitantly, there has been technical improvement in recorders and analytical systems from the tape-based devices requiring expensive decoding systems with time-consuming user interaction to digital recorders with sufficient hard disk memory to permit output directly into personal computers for sophisticated semiautomatic data analysis. New developments in signal processing of digital data permit more precise analysis of the acquired electrocardiologic data. This progress opens up new opportunities to better understand the electrocardiologic aberrations that complicate various cardiologic disorders.

At the present time, noninvasive electrophysiology is in its infancy. Many of the analytical techniques highlighted in this book assume stationarity of the recorded signal. It is quite clear that the electrophysiologic processes are dynamic with many transients, and future work will require the application of chaos and fractal theory to better appreciate the regulation and control that the central and autonomic nervous system exerts on the heart. As we better understand the control mechanisms, we should be able to appreciate the way in which various genetic and acquired diseases perturb the system.

The recorded electrocardiologic signals have their origin in cellular membrane phenomena involving the function or dysfunction of specific ionic channels. The electrocardiologic signal recorded from skin electrodes reflects the integration of electrophysiologic phenomena from millions of myocytes. Thus, genetic disorders of myocellular ionic channels should be manifest in altered static and/or dynamic electrocardiologic phenomena recorded noninvasively. In this regard, there are several promising leads to suggest that genetic cardiac disorders such as hypertrophic obstructive cardiomyopathy with altered depolarizations and the familial long QT syndrome with disordered repolarization have unique phenotypic electrocardiographic patterns that are determined, in part, by mutations of specific genes. This is an exciting area of research.

Presently, we are only scratching the surface of the clinical and basic electrophysiologic information than can be garnered from noninvasive electrocardiologic recordings. The joint combination of several simultaneously recorded and analyzed electrophysiologic signals (e.g. heart rate variability, covert T-wave alternans, and high-resolution signal averaging) with standard arrhythmia and ischemia parameters may well enhance risk stratification and help identify patients with an increased likelihood for malignant ventricular arrhythmias. The trigger mechanism that initiates life-threatening ventricular arrhythmias is poorly understood, but surely, covert transients in the autonomic influences on the heart must be playing an important role. How to decipher and dissect out these subtle neurogenic factors is an important consideration for the future. Animal studies will not suffice. Rather, noninvasive electrocardiologic recordings of individuals in their usual environment with exposure to the vicissitudes of everyday life will be required to better understand the complex interplay of environment, genes, nerves, and myocardial substrate.

Where does one start when trying to decipher and decode such complex phenomena? First, we have to establish normal standards for all these new and expanding electrocardiologic parameters, standards that require age and sex adjustment in overtly healthy individuals. We would be in a position to better understand normal electrophysiologic development of the heart if a series of recordings could be obtained on infants at periodic intervals throughout the first year of life – a time when the Purkinje and autonomic nervous systems are maturing. Cross-sectional studies with electrocardiologic recordings of healthy, overtly normal subjects in each decade of life would be an invaluable resource. With the current availability of high-frequency, digital recorders, the stored digital data could easily serve as a normal database for interested investigators, much as the MIT Holter-recorded arrhythmia database functioned in the past. In a similar manner, a centralized registry of digital recordings from patients with well-defined cardiac and noncardiac disease would reduce reduplication and expense and would accelerate progress in this field.

A fertile area of research is the use of electrocardiologic techniques to explore the role of autonomic nervous system alterations in disease mechanisms, especially those conditions in which sympathovagal factors are thought to play an important role. The role of the autonomic nervous system in essential hypertension is an important area of investigation. The question regarding the primary or secondary role of enhanced sympathetic activity in essential hypertension might be answered by longitudinal studies of subjects who are initially normotensive. Several primary neurological disorders, including Parkinson's disease, multiple sclerosis, Guillain–Barre syndrome, and orthostatic hypotension of the Shy–Drager type, are associated with altered autonomic function. In some of these disorders, changes in the autonomic nervous system may be an early manifestation of the condition and may be useful in quantifying the rate of disease progression and/or the efficacy of therapeutic interventions. This same approach may be useful in the evaluation of secondary autonomic neurologic disorders that accompany diabetes mellitus, alcoholism, and spinal cord injuries.

Although a considerable amount of emphasis in the clinical application of noninvasive electrocardiologic recordings has focused on diagnosis and disease mechanisms, the recorded signal is also useful in monitoring the safety and efficacy of various therapeutic interventions. Why is it that some patients develop torsade de pointes and other complex ventricular tachyarrhythmias with quinidine and sotalol, while other patients given the same dose of the medication do not? Can we identify patients who are risk for such arrhythmic complications by better analysis of the electrocardiologic data during, or even prior to, the initiation of the drug therapy? I suspect we will be able to develop an electrocardiologic risk profile and possibly a risk probability based on the effects of such medications on repolarization dynamics.

One promising area of investigation and clinical study that has not been included in this book, but holds much promise for the future, involves the application of chaos theory and fractal concepts to the analysis of electrocardiologic signals. As clinicians, we have been taught that stress, disease, and aging provoke erratic responses in the heart's orderly and machine-like system, thus upsetting its normal stable rhythm. Organs such as the heart are thought to function better when stable homeostasis is maintained. However, the available data indicate that this is probably not the case, at least with regard to the heart beat and its regulation by the autonomic nervous system. Rather, the heart seems to have a more irregular and unpredictable rhythm when it is young and healthy, and the rhythm becomes more regular and predictable with aging and disease. As has been pointed out in several chapters of this book, decreased heart rate variability is a strong indicator of disease.

Chaos and fractals are subjects associated with the discipline of nonlinear dynamics. Chaos associated with nonlinear dynamics is not the same as chaos in the dictionary sense where the word brings to mind complete disorganization and randomness. Chaos in the bioengineering sense refers to a constrained kind of randomness. Application of chaos theory to the fluctuations in the heart beat is interesting. If one plots the beat-to-beat variations in the heart rate over time (time-series plot), the overall plot appears ragged, irregular, and, at first glance, completely random. In fact, it is chaos with constrained randomness. As one breaks down the plot from hours into smaller and smaller intervals (minutes), the beat-to-beat fluctuations in the shorter time intervals are more rapid, but the sequence and pattern of fluctuation look somewhat like the original longer time-series plot. It is this lookalike pattern at finer and finer resolution (smaller and smaller time intervals) that is at the core of fractal theory. Thus, the beat-to-beat fluctuations in the heart can be analyzed in terms of modeling using chaos and fractal concepts. The future direction in noninvasive electrocardiology will surely involve greater participation of bioengineers with expertise in the application of time-variant algorithms, wavelet (fractal) analysis, and deterministic chaos. These nonlinear techniques are already being applied to the analysis of the frequency content of the QRS complex, heart rate variability, and repolarization dynamics. The application of chaos and fractal theory to the progressive loss of the heart's electrophysiologic complexity in the transition from health to disease and from youth to old age should greatly expand the scientific foundation and the clinical utility of noninvasive electrocardiology in the future.

Index

(Italic page numbers refer to figures and tables)